PLEASE RETURN TO:

TUMORS AND TUMORLIKE LESIONS OF THE UTERINE CORPUS AND CERVIX

CONTEMPORARY ISSUES
IN SURGICAL PATHOLOGY
VOLUME 19

SERIES EDITOR
Lawrence M. Roth, M.D.

Professor of Pathology
Director, Division of Surgical Pathology
Indiana University School of Medicine
Indianapolis, Indiana

Previously published

TUMORS AND TUMORLIKE LESIONS OF THE UTERINE CORPUS AND CERVIX

Edited by

Philip B. Clement, M.D.

Clinical Professor
Department of Pathology
University of British Columbia Faculty of Medicine
Consultant Pathologist
Department of Pathology
Vancouver General Hospital
Vancouver, British Columbia, Canada

Robert H. Young, M.D., M.R.C.Path.

Associate Professor
Department of Pathology
Harvard Medical School
Associate Pathologist
Director, Surgical Pathology
Department of Pathology
Massachusetts General Hospital
Boston, Massachusetts

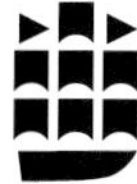

Churchill Livingstone
New York, Edinburgh, London, Madrid, Melbourne, Tokyo

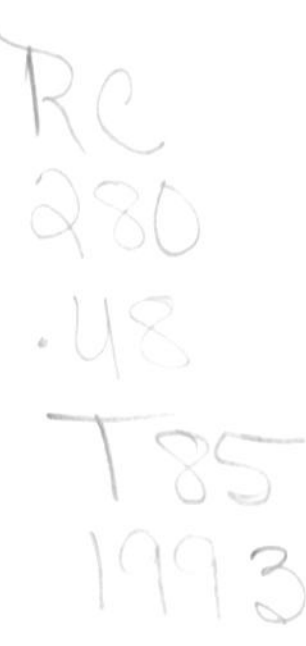

Library of Congress Cataloging-in-Publication Data

Tumors and tumorlike lesions of the uterine corpus and cervix / edited
  by Philip B. Clement, Robert H. Young.
      p. cm. – (Contemporary issues in surgical pathology ; v. 19)
    Includes bibliographical references and index.
    ISBN 0-443-08801-2
    1. Uterus–Tumors. 2. Cervix uteri–Tumors. I. Clement, Philip
  B. II. Young, Robert H. (Robert Henry), Date.   III. Series.
    [DNLM: 1. Cervix Neoplasms. 2. Uterine Neoplasms. W1 CO769MS
  v. 19 / WP 458 T925]
  RC280.U8T85 1993
  616.99'266–dc20
  DNLM/DLC
  for Library of Congress   92-48253
                                    CIP

© **Churchill Livingstone Inc. 1993**

All rights reserved. No part of this publication may be reproduced, stored in a retrieval system, or transmitted in any form or by any means, electronic, mechanical, photocopying, recording, or otherwise, without prior permission of the publisher (Churchill Livingstone Inc., 650 Avenue of the Americas, New York, NY 10011).

Distributed in the United Kingdom by Churchill Livingstone, Robert Stevenson House, 1–3 Baxter's Place, Leith Walk, Edinburgh EH1 3AF, and by associated companies, branches, and representatives throughout the world.

Accurate indications, adverse reactions, and dosage schedules for drugs are provided in this book, but it is possible that they may change. The reader is urged to review the package information data of the manufacturers of the medications mentioned.

The Publishers have made every effort to trace the copyright holders for borrowed material. If they have inadvertently overlooked any, they will be pleased to make the necessary arrangements at the first opportunity.

Acquisitions Editor: *Robert A. Hurley*
Copy Editor: *Paul Bernstein*
Production Designer: *Patricia McFadden*
Production Supervisor: *Jeanine Furino*

Printed in the United States of America

First published in 1993   7 6 5 4 3 2 1

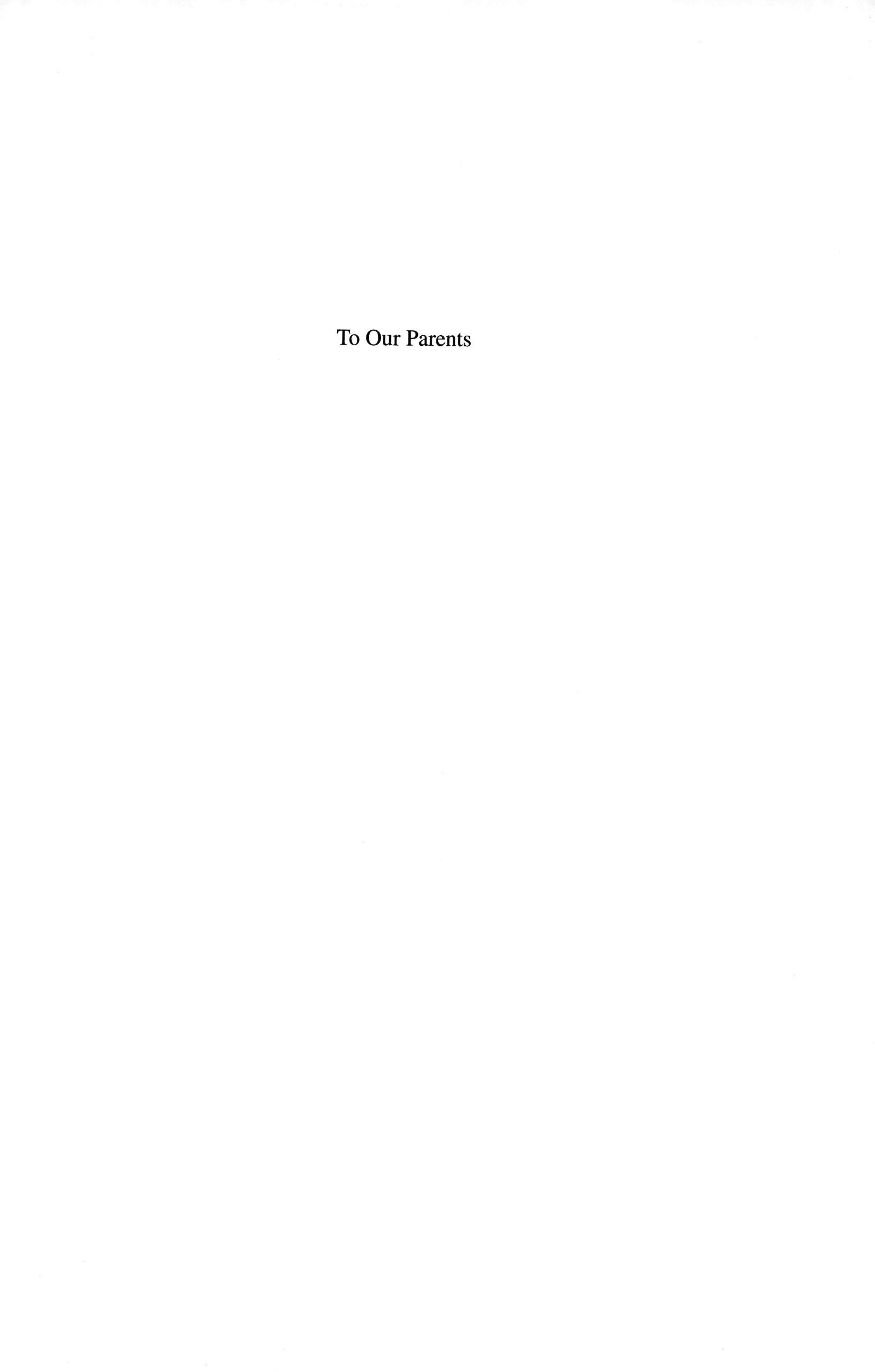

To Our Parents

Contributors

Philip B. Clement, M.D.

Clinical Professor, Department of Pathology, University of British Columbia Faculty of Medicine; Consultant Pathologist, Department of Pathology, Vancouver General Hospital, Vancouver, British Columbia, Canada

Christopher P. Crum, M.D.

Associate Professor, Department of Pathology, Harvard Medical School; Director, Women's and Perinatal Pathology Division, Department of Pathology, Brigham and Women's Hospital, Boston, Massachusetts

Janice M. Lage, M.D.

Associate Professor, Departments of Pathology, Obstetrics and Gynecology, and Pediatrics, Georgetown University School of Medicine, Washington, D.C.; Director, Surgical Pathology, Department of Pathology, Georgetown University Medical Center Hospital, Washington, D.C.; Consultant, Department of Pathology, Brigham and Women's Hospital, Boston, Massachusetts

Robert E. Scully, M.D.

Professor, Department of Pathology, Harvard Medical School; Pathologist, Department of Pathology, Massachusetts General Hospital, Boston, Massachusetts

Robert H. Young, M.D., M.R.C.Path.

Associate Professor, Department of Pathology, Harvard Medical School; Associate Pathologist and Director, Surgical Pathology, Department of Pathology, Massachusetts General Hospital, Boston, Massachusetts

Preface

This volume of *Contemporary Issues in Surgical Pathology* focuses on the wide variety of neoplasms and pseudoneoplastic lesions that involve the uterus, thereby serving as a companion to *Tumors and Tumorlike Conditions of the Ovary* (Volume 6) and *Pathology of the Vulva and Vagina* (Volume 9), previously published in this series. The surgical pathologist is confronted daily with biopsy and curettage specimens from the cervix and endometrium. When hysterectomy specimens are added, the combined material accounts for a significant proportion of the cases in almost every pathology laboratory and certainly accounts for the majority of gynecologic specimens.

As the volumes of this series are not intended to replace standard textbooks, in this monograph we concentrate on recent advances in uterine pathology, with an emphasis on newly described entities or those for which there has been significant new information. More discussion and illustrative material are devoted to uncommon or rare lesions (or variants of more common lesions) than is possible in standard textbooks of surgical or gynecologic pathology. Although the new techniques that are available may contribute helpful information in some instances and are covered where appropriate in this volume, the optimal interpretation of uterine specimens depends in most cases on careful examination of routinely stained sections, along with an appreciation of relevant clinical data. Accordingly, most of the chapters emphasize the appearances and problems encountered in hematoxylin- and eosin-stained sections. The chapters are thoroughly referenced, with an emphasis on articles published during the past two decades; we hope that most of the current pertinent papers published as of July 1992, when this book went into production, have been cited.

In the first chapter, the great array of tumorlike lesions that occur in the uterine cervix are reviewed. These lesions have diverse microscopic appearances and several of them have been recognized only recently. In the next chapter, Dr. Crum summarizes the important recent advances in the pathology of premalignant and malignant squamous lesions of the cervix, including his extensive experience with lesions associated with cervical infection by the human papillomavirus. In Chapter 3, the spectrum of precancerous glandular lesions of the cervix and the variety of invasive adenocarcinomas in this site are reviewed. In the next chapter, pseudoneoplastic lesions that involve the endometrium and myometrium are considered; this review serves as a backround for the next three chapters. Chapter 5 covers recent advances in our knowledge of the endometrial hyperplasias and their often difficult distinction from endometrial carcinomas. The same chapter summarizes current knowledge of the variety of histologic subtypes of endometrial carcinomas, as well as important prognostic parameters of these tumors, many of which are determined by the pathologist. Chapters 6 and 7 deal with pure mesenchymal and mixed epithelial-mesenchymal tumors of the uterus, respectively. Our knowledge of these two related groups has expanded considerably during the last two decades, justifying their separate coverage. In Chapter 8, a variety of primary uterine tumors not conveniently covered in the preceding chapters, as well as metastatic tumors involving the uterus, are reviewed. In the final chapter, recent developments in the pathology of trophoblastic lesions of the usual type and recently described lesions derived from intermediate trophoblast are reviewed.

We wish to thank Dr. Lawrence Roth, the Series Editor for *Contemporary Issues in Surgical Pathology*, for inviting us to edit this volume and for his words of advice. We are especially grateful to Dr. Crum and Dr. Lage for their superb and authoritative contributions, which were delivered promptly despite their very busy schedules. We are both deeply indebted to Dr. Scully, who made his customary invaluable contributions as co-author of three of the chapters. He also generously allowed us to use many gross photographs from his collection and also to take photomicrographs of many of his consultation cases, which provided illustrations in the chapters authored or co-authored by one or both of us. A number of pathologists contributed tissue slides that were essential in illustrating some unusual lesions, and these individuals are acknowledged at the appropriate point. Finally, we would like to thank Mr. Robert Hurley and the staff at Churchill Livingstone, including Mr. Paul Bernstein, Senior Copy Editor, who have all been most helpful to us. We hope that the reader will find the reviews in this monograph to be of practical help in the differential diagnosis of relatively common uterine lesions, and a reliable source of information and references when a rare lesion in this site is encountered.

Philip B. Clement, M.D.
Robert H. Young, M.D., M.R.C.Path.

Contents

1

Tumorlike Lesions of the Uterine Cervix

Robert H. Young and Philip B. Clement

A wide variety of non-neoplastic lesions occur in the uterine cervix and are prone, to varying extents, to misinterpretation. The most common error is to mistake one of these benign, but sometimes exuberant, processes as neoplastic with potentially major adverse consequences for the patient in the form of inappropriate treatment. In this chapter these lesions are reviewed with emphasis on the features that enable them to be correctly interpreted. They are considered in two major categories: glandular and nonglandular. The lesions in the former category are discussed first because they are a more homogeneous group than the latter and account for most of the diagnostic problems encountered.[1]

GLANDULAR LESIONS

The propensity for non-neoplastic glandular lesions to cause diagnostic difficulty was highlighted by one report in which 13 cases previously diagnosed as cervical "adenocarcinomas" were reviewed and five were reinterpreted as benign.[2] One reason for the problems engendered by these abnormalities is that many pathologists are not familiar with the great range of lesions and histologic spectrum in this category. These various abnormalities (Table 1-1) are considered in turn.

PAPILLARY ENDOCERVICITIS

Perhaps the commonest pseudoneoplastic glandular lesion is the florid micropapillary pattern occasionally encountered in chronic endocervicitis.[3] Stromal papillae that are usually relatively regular and that contain chronic inflammatory cells are covered with a single layer of benign endocervical columnar epithelium (Fig. 1-1). This appearance may be confused with that of endocervical adenocarcinomas with a villoglandular pattern,[4] but these tumors (see Ch. 3) usually exhibit focal cellular stratification; they always have more cytologic atypia than seen in papillary endocervicitis.

TUNNEL CLUSTERS

Fluhmann[5, 6] introduced the designation *tunnel cluster* for this common lesion (Figs. 1-2 to 1-6), which is usually an incidental microscopic finding. He demonstrated tunnel clusters in the transformation zone of 8 percent of adult women, but with the figure rising to 40 percent for women during the first trimester of pregnancy. The lesions were only found in women over 30 years of age. He described two types of tunnel clusters, types A and B, the former noncystic (Fig. 1-5) and lined by columnar epithelium, the latter cystic and lined by cuboidal or

Table 1-1. Pseudoneoplastic Glandular Lesions of the Uterine Cervix

Papillary endocervicitis
Tunnel clusters
Deep glands and cysts
Microglandular hyperplasia
Mesonephric hyperplasia
Diffuse laminar endocervical glandular hyperplasia
Endocervicosis
Glandular hyperplasia, not otherwise specified
Metaplasias (tubal, endometrioid, intestinal)
Endometriosis
Arias-Stella reaction
Changes secondary to extravasation of mucin
Infectious and reactive atypias

flattened epithelium (Figs. 1-2 to 1-4). As small cysts are seen in some type A lesions and as the two groups merge imperceptibly, in our opinion their separation is unnecessary for diagnostic purposes. Fluhmann, however, found type A tunnel clusters more frequently in older women.

In our experience, type B tunnel clusters are much more common than are type A tunnel clusters, and the only recent study of tunnel clusters, by Segal and Hart,[7] was restricted to the former, which they identified in 6 percent of hysterectomy specimens and in 10 percent of cone biopsy specimens. Almost 80 percent of the patients had at least three previous pregnancies, and all but one were multigravida. In this series, tunnel clusters were more common in the posterior lip of the cervix. Cystic lesions were observed grossly in approximately 40 percent of the cases; significant distortion of the cervical wall was encountered in one-third of this group. Rare cases have been responsible for myxometra.[8] Tunnel clusters are typically discrete, usually 0.5 to 5 mm (mean 2.4 mm) in diameter (but occasionally up to 20 mm), rounded foci composed of 20 to 50 oval, round, or irregular, closely packed tubules of varying size (Fig. 1-2). Multiple foci are present in about 80 percent of cases[7]; occasionally, the tunnel clusters are confluent. The tubules, which typically contain inspissated mucin, are separated by scanty connective tissue, and

the tunnel cluster is surrounded by normal endocervical stroma. In occasional cases of tunnel clusters, mild nuclear atypia and occasional mitotic figures (Fig. 1-6) have prompted an erroneous diagnosis of adenoma malignum ("minimal deviation adenocarcinoma")[3, 9]; this misdiagnosis was made initially in 2 of 29 cases in one study.[7] The lobulated appearance of tunnel clusters (Figs. 1-2 and 1-3) is a helpful diagnostic feature not observed in adenoma malignum. Even in cases in which this is less apparent (Fig. 1-4), tunnel clusters lack the clearly infiltrative pattern and frequent desmoplasia of adenoma malignum[9] (see Ch. 3). Like other benign disorders of the endocervical glands, tunnel clusters occasionally extend deep into the cervical wall, and the distinction of deep cystic tunnel clusters from deep nabothian cysts (see below) is sometimes arbitrary.

Tunnel clusters are presumed to represent an involutionary stage of the normal endocervical glands (clefts)[5, 6] and have no clinical significance. There is no evidence that they are hyperplastic or premalignant and, accordingly, an alternate designation that has been proposed, *adenomatous hyperplasia*,[10] should be avoided. Two unusual endocervical glandular lesions occurring in patients with Peutz-Jeghers syndrome, reported by Fetissof et al.,[11] may bear some relationship to tunnel clusters. However, the lesions were interpreted as possibly representing an in situ form of adenoma malignum.

DEEP GLANDS AND CYSTS

Endocervical glands occasionally lie as deep as 9 mm in the cervical stroma.[12, 13] This feature (Fig. 1-7), and their occasional irregular distribution, may suggest adenoma malignum. However, these glands are usually beneath normal superficial endocervical glands, are normal in size and shape, and are unassociated with any stro-

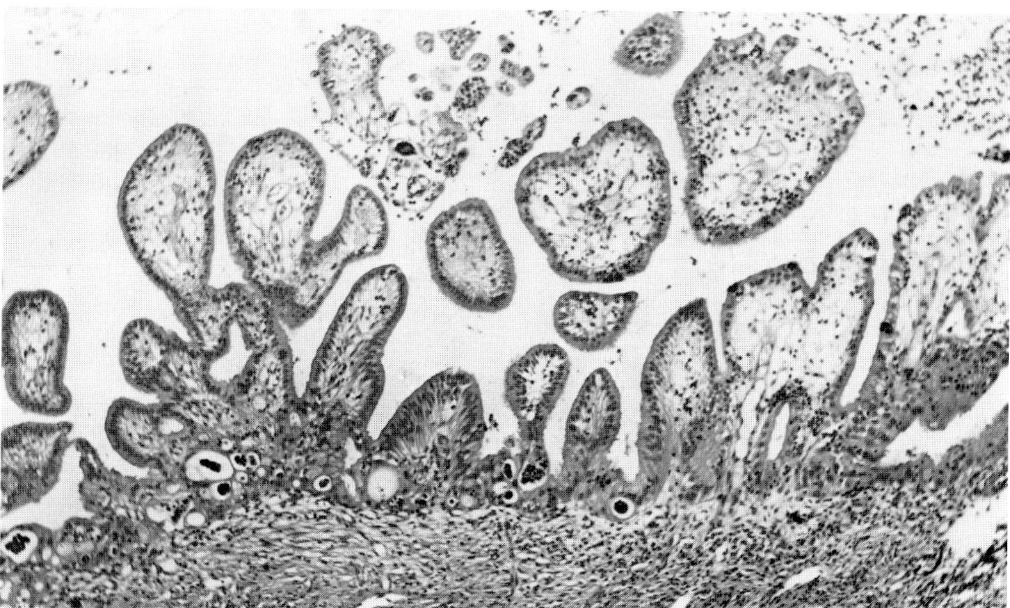

Fig. 1-1. Papillary endocervicitis. Numerous papillae protrude from the endocervical epithelium.

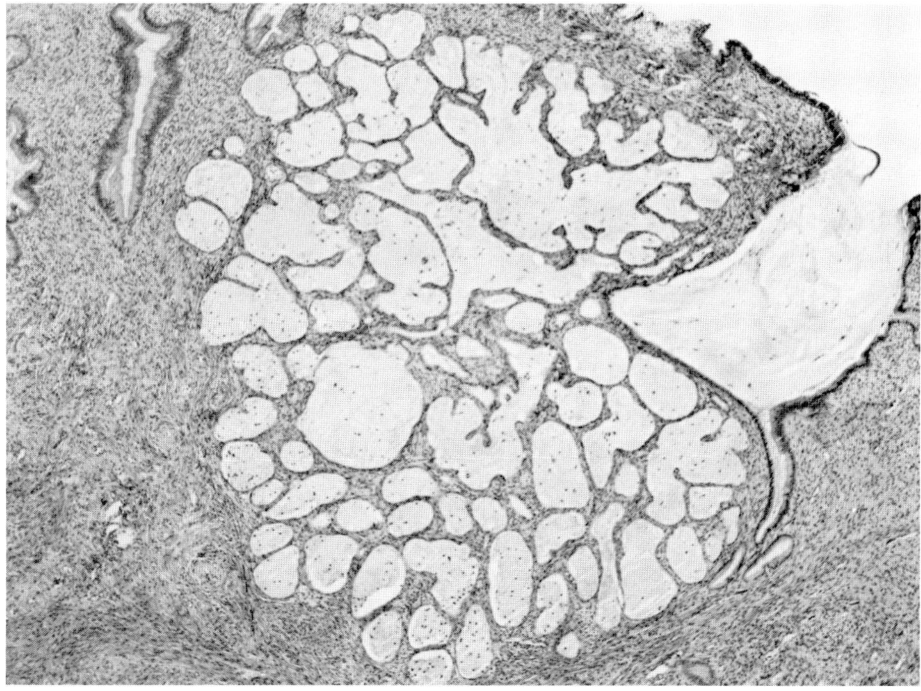

Fig. 1-2. Tunnel cluster. The lesion is well circumscribed, and composed predominantly of cystically dilated glands.

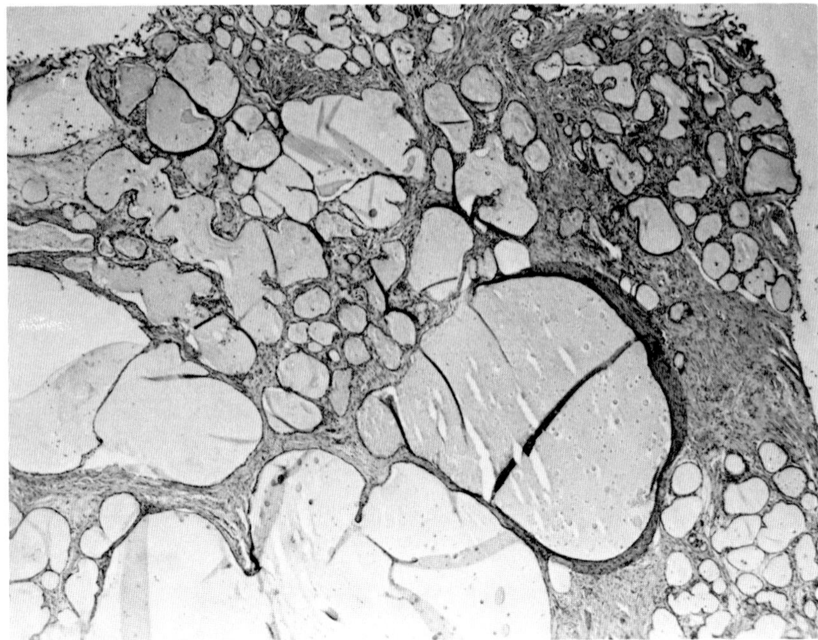

Fig. 1-3. Tunnel clusters. One large tunnel cluster with prominent dilation of its glands occupies most of the illustration, but two smaller tunnel clusters are present at the upper and bottom right.

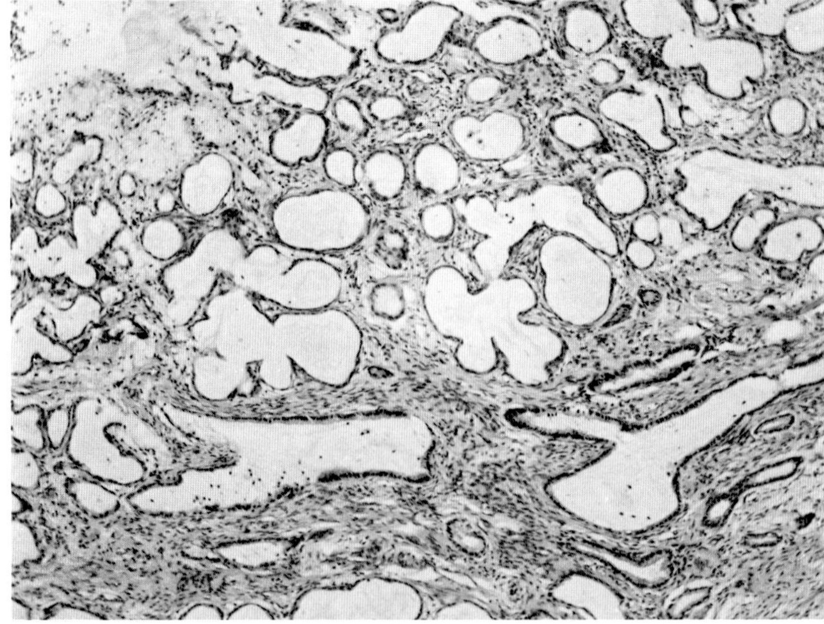

Fig. 1-4. Tunnel cluster. The well-circumscribed contour of the lesion is not evident and there is a "pseudoinfiltrative" appearance.

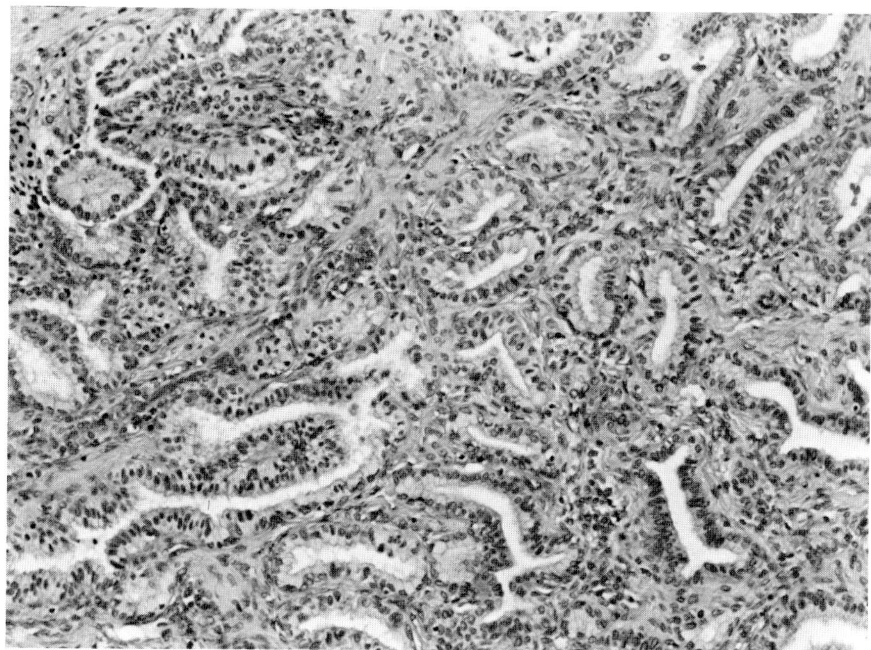

Fig. 1-5. Tunnel cluster. The glands are noncystic, closely packed, and irregular. (From Young and Clement,[1] with permission.)

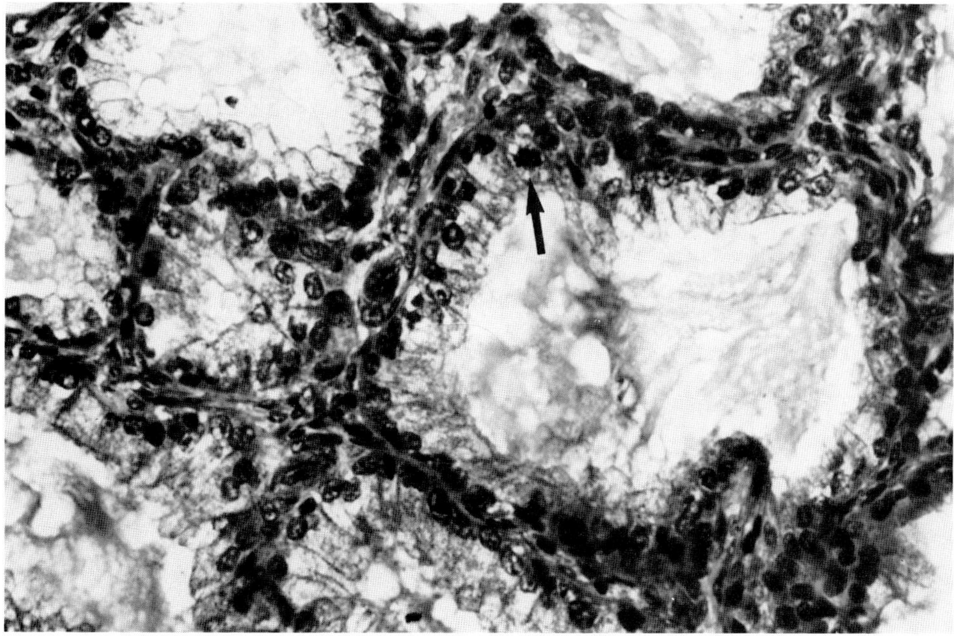

Fig. 1-6. Tunnel cluster. The cells lining the glands exhibit mild atypia and a mitotic figure (arrow). (From Young and Clement,[3] with permission.)

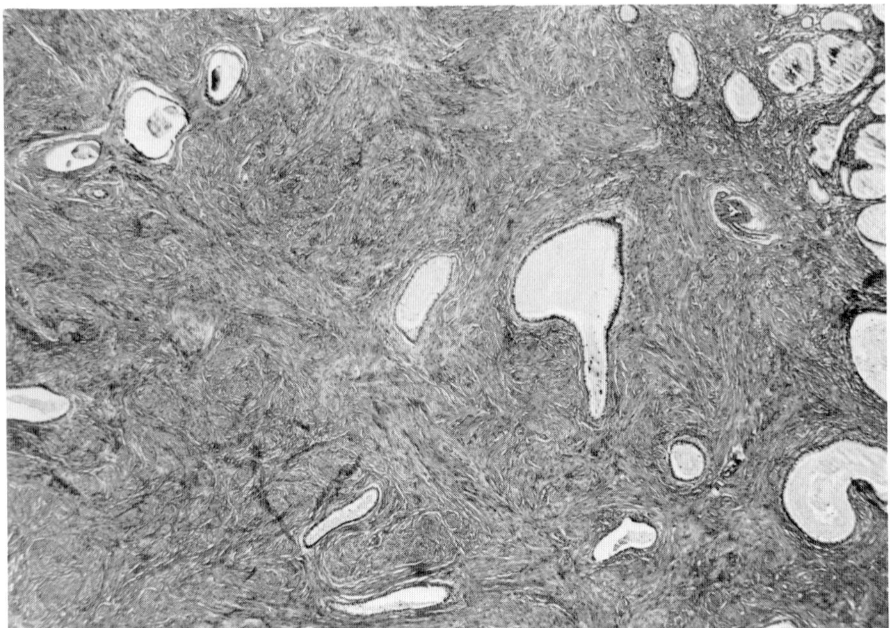

Fig. 1-7. Deep endocervical glands. Scattered endocervical glands are irregularly distributed deep to the overlying mucosa (extreme right). (From Young and Clement,[1] with permission.)

mal alteration, indicating their benign nature. Similar observations indicate the benign nature of the endometrioid glands that may be encountered deep in the cervical wall.[14]

It was recently recognized that nabothian cysts may extend through most of the cervical wall; as a result, the process may be considered neoplastic.[15] In these cases, gross examination of the cervix shows numerous mucin-filled cysts, measuring up to 1 cm in diameter, replacing the endocervical wall (Fig. 1-8). Histologic examination shows cysts lined by benign columnar, cuboidal to flattened endocervical epithelium devoid of mitotic activity (Fig. 1-9). In some cases, as alluded to earlier, tunnel clusters are present in the more superficial stroma. The differential diagnosis is with adenoma malignum, but the glands of this tumor are only occasionally cystically dilated, exhibit focal atypia, and often have an associated stromal reaction.

Rarely, other types of benign cyst may be encountered in the wall of the cervix. We have encountered one such case in which a 2.5-cm cyst was lined with a single layer of tubal-type ciliated epithelium, although in our experience cyst formation is relatively uncommon in cases of tubal metaplasia (see below). Mesonephric remnants (see p. 17) are also occasionally cystic.

MICROGLANDULAR HYPERPLASIA

Microglandular hyperplasia (MGH) is usually related to progesterone stimulation, most commonly with oral contraceptives (67 percent of the cases) and less commonly with pregnancy (7 percent of the cases).[16–23] Occasionally, however, it is seen in a patient receiving only estrogen or a patient in whom none of these associations is present. The lesion typically occurs in young

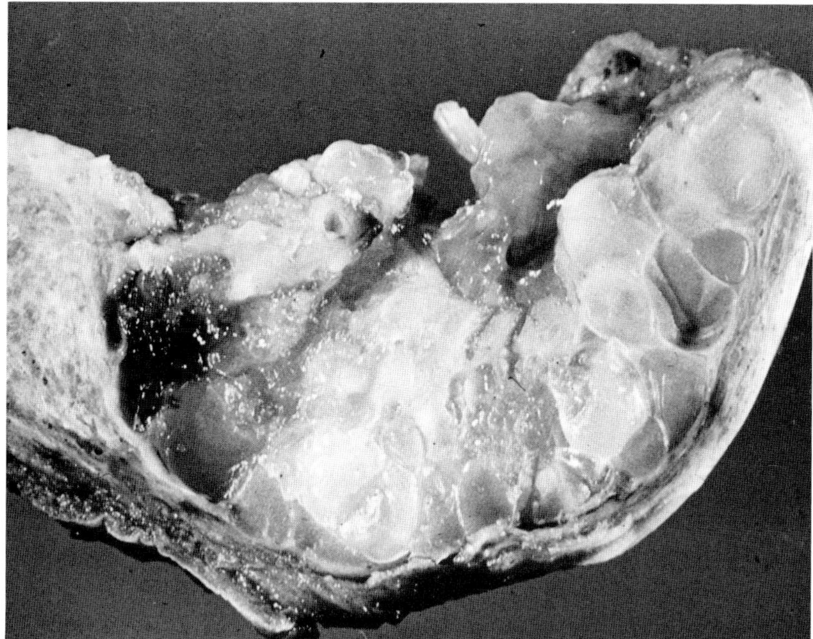

Fig. 1-8. Deep nabothian cysts. The cysts extend almost through the cervical wall. (From Young and Clement,[1] with permission; courtesy of D. Ross McLean, M.D., Edmonton, Alberta, Canada.)

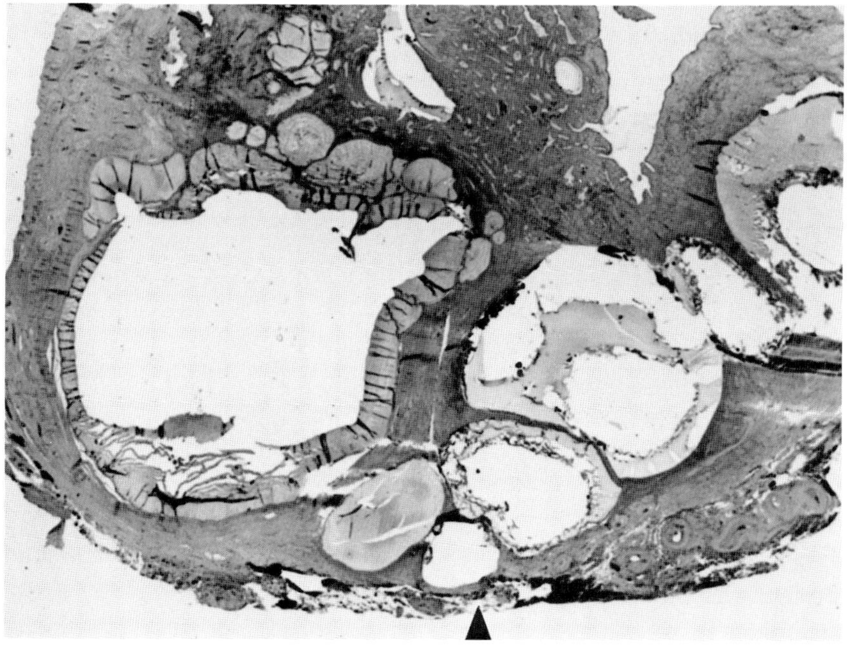

Fig. 1-9. Deep nabothian cysts. The cervical wall is largely replaced by nabothian cysts. An arrow points to paracervical connective tissue. (From Young and Clement,[1] with permission.)

women (mean, 33.5 years), but approximately 6 percent of reported cases have occurred in postmenopausal women.[16–23] The patients are usually asymptomatic but may complain of abnormal vaginal bleeding or vaginal discharge. MGH is typically an incidental microscopic finding, having been encountered in as many as 24 percent and 27 percent of the cases in two series of cone biopsies,[20] or in cone biopsy and hysterectomy specimens,[24] with this figure rising to 44 percent in those with a history of oral contraceptive use in the first study.[20] Occasionally, however, the lesion may be visible as an erosion, as a lesion that is indistinguishable from a typical cervical polyp grossly, or as a polypoid mass (Fig. 1-10) that is sometimes friable and that is rarely grossly suspicious for carcinoma.[21]

On microscopic examination, MGH may be seen as one or more polypoid fragments on the surface of the cervical mucosa, may be nonpolypoid, or alternatively may involve a portion of an endocervical polyp (Fig. 1-11). The lesion characteristically consists of closely packed glands that vary from small and round to large, irregular, and cystically dilated (Figs. 1-12 and 1-13).

They usually contain a basophilic or eosinophilic mucinous secretion, often containing many acute inflammatory cells (Fig. 1-13). There are typically many acute and chronic inflammatory cells in the intervening stroma, which is occasionally extensively hyalinized (Fig. 1-12). In some cases, small nests and large aggregates of epithelial cells are irregularly distributed in a myxoid stroma, imparting a pseudoinfiltrative pattern (Fig. 1-14). Other patterns of MGH include reticular, in which the cells, some of which may be spindle shaped, are loosely dispersed in an edematous stroma (Fig. 1-15) and solid, in which sheets of cells without gland formation are seen[25] (Figs. 1-16 to 1-18). In occasional cases, the appearance may be complicated by the presence of another non-neoplastic glandular lesion, such as papillary endocervicitis (Fig. 1-19). Exceptionally, the cells are arranged in trabeculae (Fig. 1-20) or small cords. The cells lining the glands and cysts are usually low columnar, cuboidal, or flat, with faintly basophilic or granular cytoplasm. Occasionally, the cells have abundant eosinophilic cytoplasm; in rare cases, they resemble hobnail cells (Fig. 1-21). Sub-

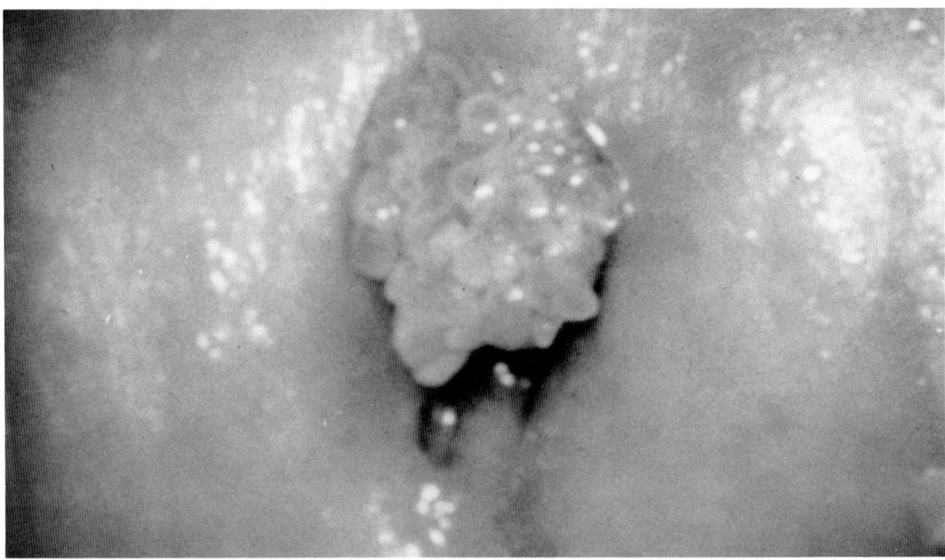

Fig. 1-10. Microglandular hyperplasia. A glistening polypoid mass protrudes from the cervical os.

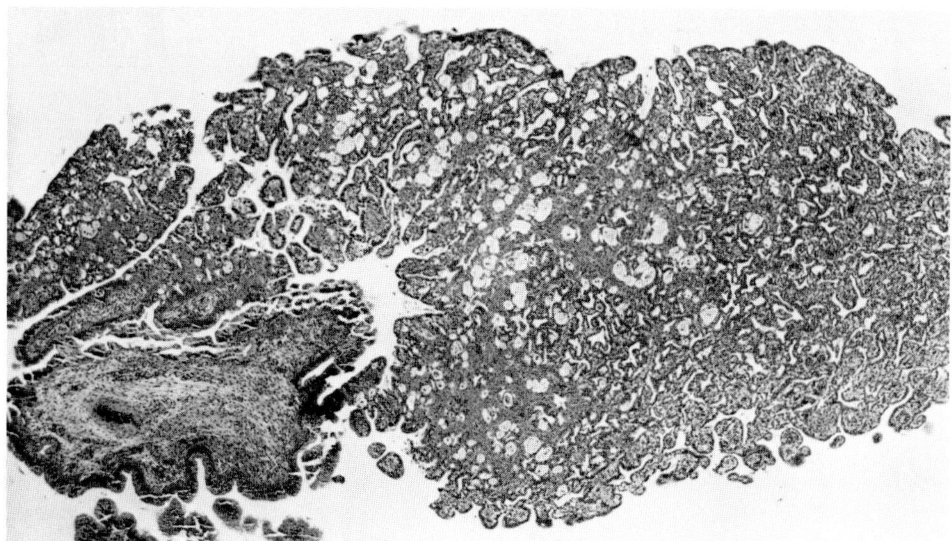

Fig. 1-11. Microglandular hyperplasia. Most of a cervical polyp has been replaced by a closely packed proliferation of small glands.

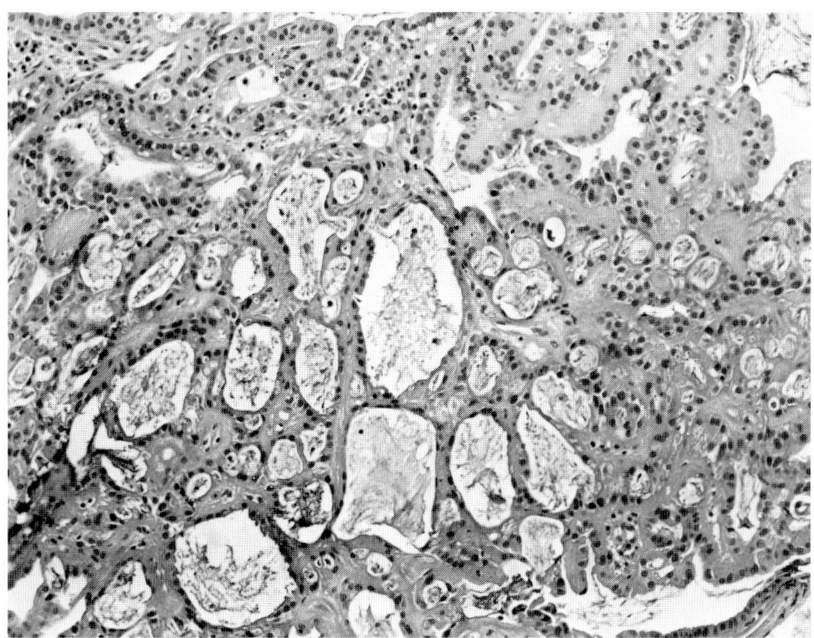

Fig. 1-12. Microglandular hyperplasia. The glands vary from small to large and cystically dilated. The stroma exhibits prominent hyalinization.

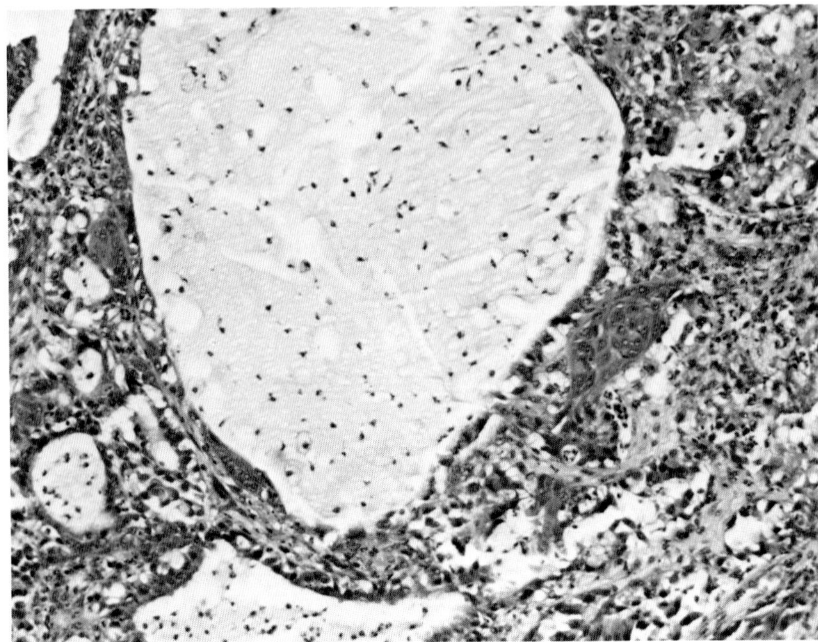

Fig. 1-13. Microglandular hyperplasia. The glands and cysts contain a mucinous secretion containing scattered inflammatory cells. Inflammatory cells are present in the stroma.

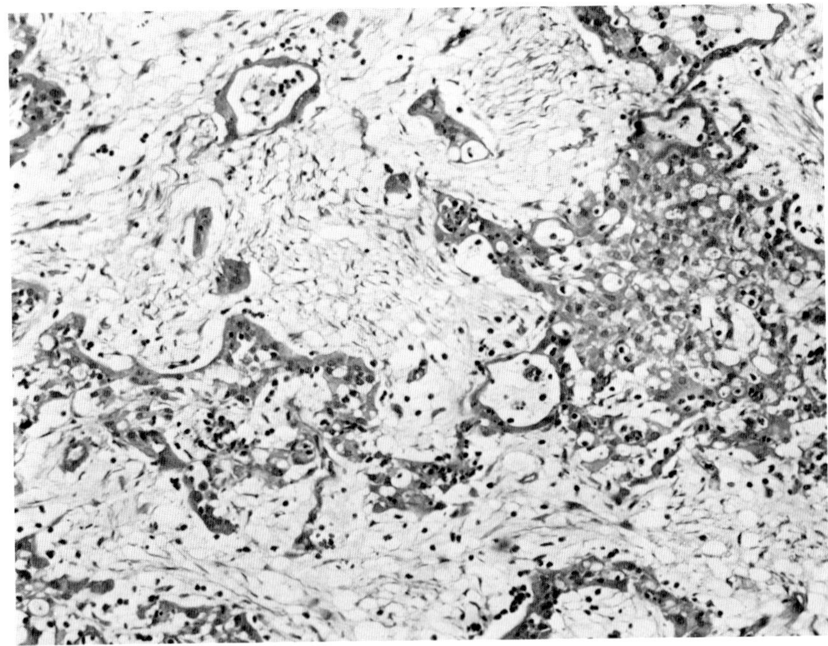

Fig. 1-14. Microglandular hyperplasia. Irregularly shaped nests of cells in a myxoid stroma simulate the infiltration of a carcinoma. (From Young and Scully,[25] with permission.)

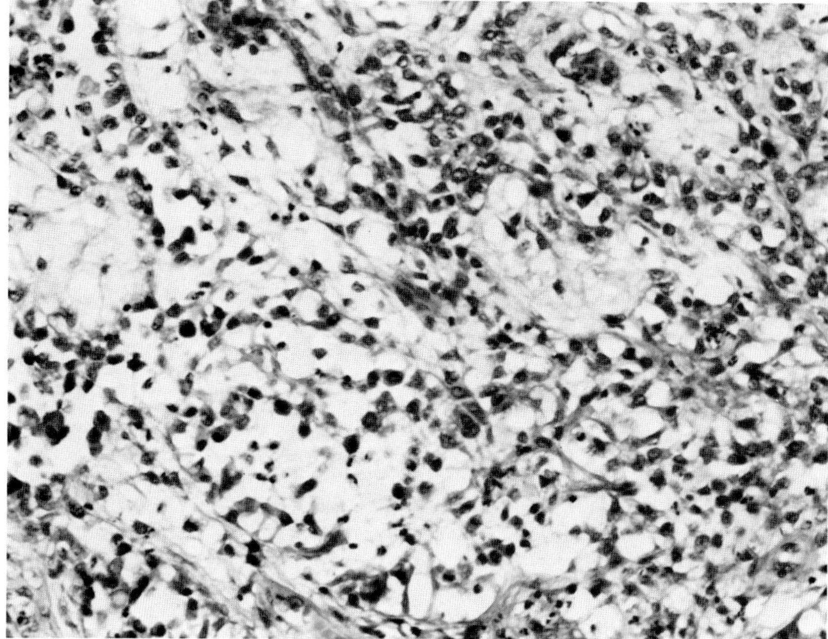

Fig. 1-15. Microglandular hyperplasia. There is a reticular pattern with loosely dispersed cells.

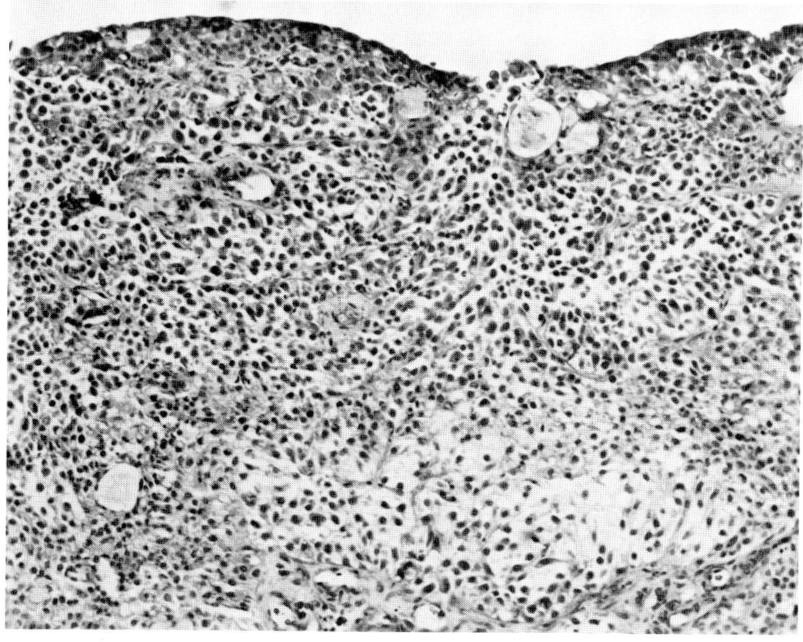

Fig. 1-16. Microglandular hyperplasia. There is a predominantly solid pattern.

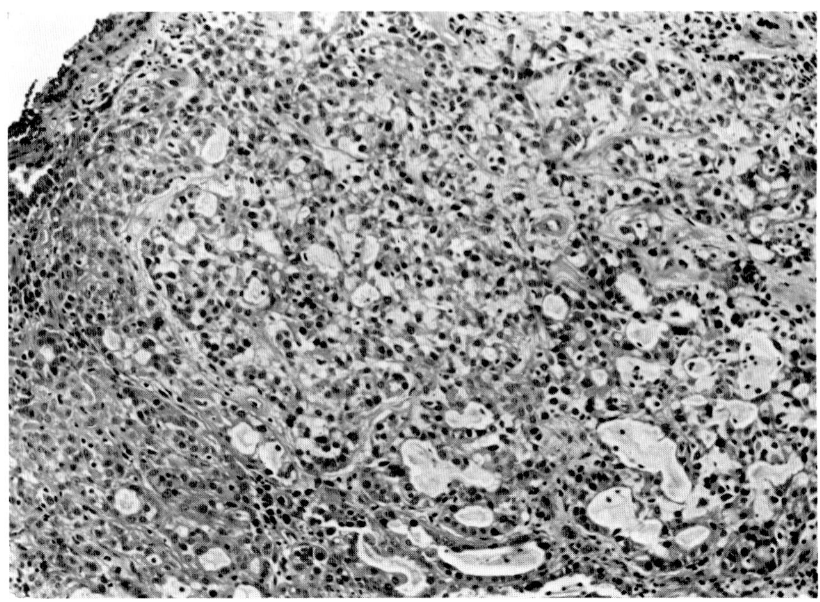

Fig. 1-17. Microglandular hyperplasia. A solid cellular proliferation is shown merging with the characteristic pattern of microglandular hyperplasia, seen best at the bottom right. (From Young and Clement,[1] with permission.)

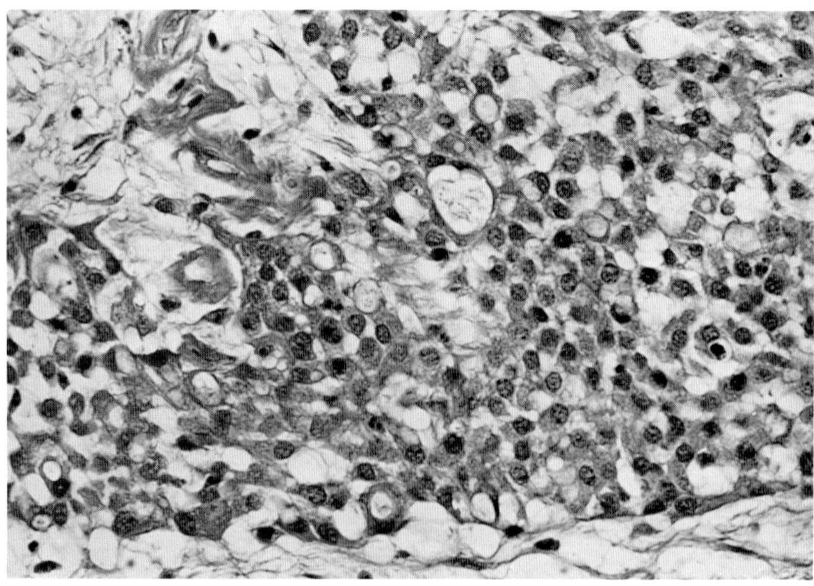

Fig. 1-18. Microglandular hyperplasia. There is a predominantly solid pattern with occasional signet-ring-like cells. (From Young and Clement,[3] with permission.)

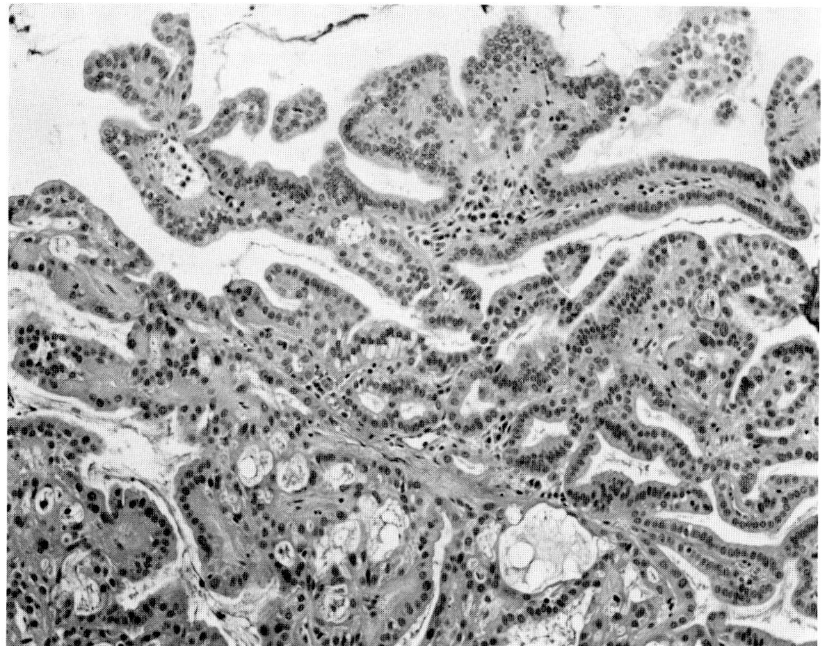

Fig. 1-19. Microglandular hyperplasia (bottom center) associated with papillary endocervicitis.

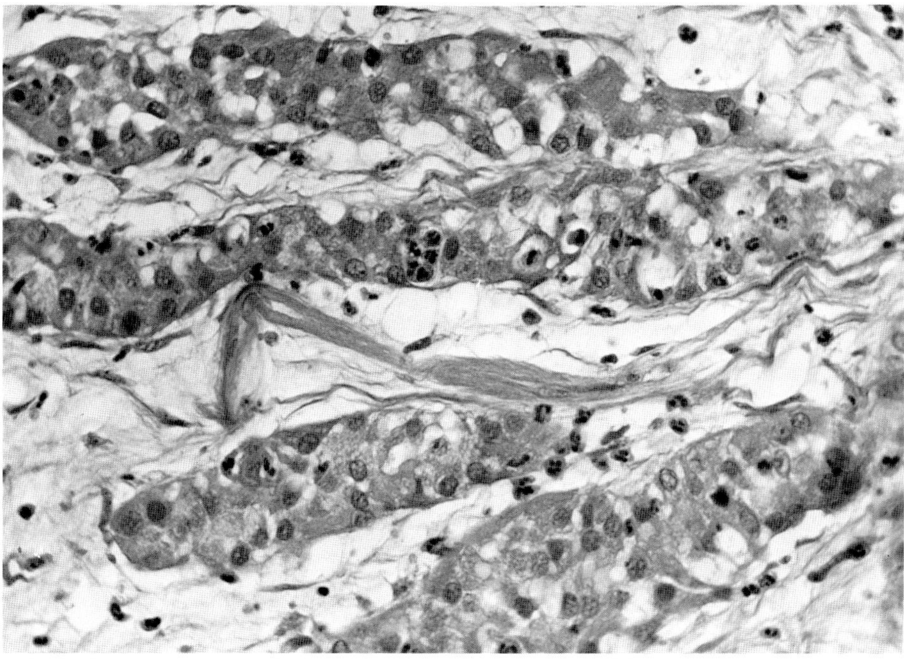

Fig. 1-20. Microglandular hyperplasia. The cells are growing in trabeculae. (From Young and Clement,[1] with permission.)

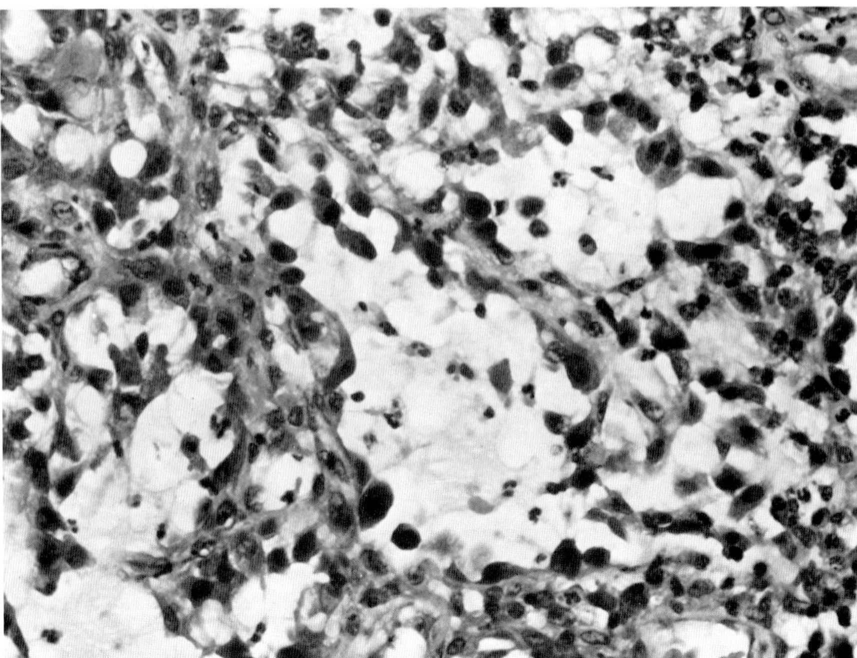

Fig. 1-21. Microglandular hyperplasia. Dilated glands are lined by cells, some of which have hyperchromatic apically located nuclei (hobnail cells). (From Young and Scully,[25] with permission.)

nuclear vacuoles, which stain positively for mucin but are negative for glycogen, are often present and may be conspicuous (Fig. 1-22). Rarely, some cells within the solid foci have pale cytoplasm and eccentric nuclei (Fig. 1-18), simulating the signet ring cells of an adenocarcinoma.[25] The nuclei of the cells are almost always small and regular, but rarely they may be mildly or even moderately atypical. Nucleoli may be visible, and hyperchromatic nuclei with a degenerative appearance are sometimes seen. Mitotic figures are generally rare, but up to one mitotic figure per 10 high-power fields (MPF) may be seen.[25]

MGH was often confused with adenocarcinoma in the past, but typical forms are usually now correctly interpreted. The adenocarcinoma most likely to be confused with MGH is clear cell carcinoma because both lesions may have tubular, cystic, and solid patterns and a hyalinized stroma. The solid foci of clear cell carcinoma usually consist of cells with abundant, clear, glycogen-rich cytoplasm, whereas those in solid foci of MGH only rarely have conspicuous clear cytoplasm and lack glycogen. Although some clear cell carcinomas may have relatively bland cytologic features and low mitotic rates, and some cases of MGH may have some degree of atypia and rare mitotic figures, the atypia and mitotic rates in clear cell carcinoma almost always exceed those of MGH. Distinguishing MGH from some well-differentiated endocervical adenocarcinomas of the usual type and endometrial adenocarcinomas of endometrioid or mucinous types may be difficult. Some of these carcinomas may have focal microglandular patterns, extensive acute inflammation, and glands filled with mucin, creating a superficial resemblance to MGH.[26] As fragments of an endometrial tumor of this type may be present in a specimen thought to be endocervical in origin, the diagnosis of MGH should be made with caution in a postmenopausal patient, particularly if its features are not characteristic.

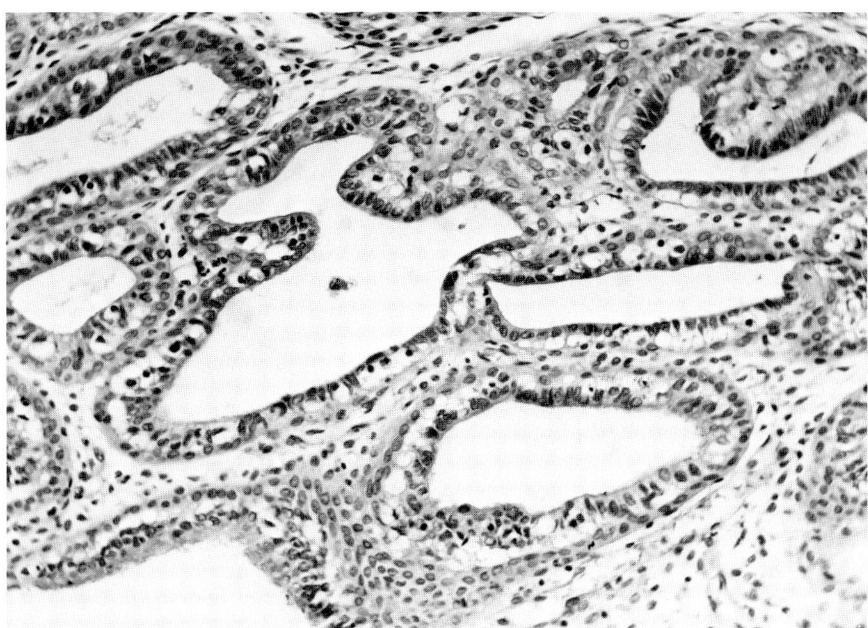

Fig. 1-22. Microglandular hyperplasia. Most of the cells lining the glands have subnuclear vacuoles. This field is unusual because of the lack of luminal mucin and paucity of inflammatory cells.

The only cervical adenocarcinoma we have seen that closely simulated MGH in areas occurred in a patient who was on oral contraceptives.[26]

Negative immunohistochemical staining for carcinoembryonic antigen (CEA) supports a diagnosis of MGH.[27] Speers et al.[28] obtained a negative result in 20 of 21 cases of MGH, the other case being focally positive. Nine of 14 adenocarcinomas were strongly positive, 4 were focally positive, and only 1 was negative. The latter result illustrates that adenocarcinomas are occasionally negative or only focally positive for CEA, a finding in agreement with other studies. In a recent study of adenoma malignum, for example, 1 of 6 tumors studied was negative, and 2 of the other 5 were only focally positive[9]; in another series, 2 of 15 typical endocervical adenocarcinomas were negative.[29] Similarly, other studies have shown that clear cell carcinoma and mesonephric adenocarcinoma are frequently CEA negative.[30, 31] Finally, in one recent series, only 55 percent of cervical adenocarcinomas were immunoreactive for CEA, although most of the nonreactive tumors were poorly differentiated and not likely to be confused with a benign lesion.[32] The above studies indicate that a negative stain for CEA should be cautiously interpreted. By contrast, intense positive staining throughout the cytoplasm is unlikely in a benign lesion and strongly suggests carcinoma.[3] Parenthetically, it can be noted that negative CEA staining also supports a benign interpretation in most of the other pseudoneoplastic glandular lesions considered here but experience with CEA staining of many of them is limited, and a diagnosis should not be rendered solely on the basis of immunohistochemical staining results. It should also be noted that normal endocervical glands and those in pseudoneoplastic lesions may exhibit a glycocalyceal pattern of CEA staining; this contrasts, however, with the diffuse cytoplasmic staining typically seen in cervical adenocarcinomas.

MESONEPHRIC HYPERPLASIA

Mesonephric remnants in the cervix are not rare, being found in approximately 10 percent of cervices.[24] Uncommonly, mesonephric remnants are so numerous that the diagnosis of adenocarcinoma is suggested, especially in those cases accompanied by cytologic atypia and mitotic activity. A recent detailed study of 41 cases of mesonephric hyperplasia has been published in which their features were compared with those of nonhyperplastic remnants and mesonephric carcinoma.[33] The cases of hyperplasia were divided into three categories: lobular mesonephric hyperplasia (31 cases) (Figs. 1-23 to 1-25), diffuse mesonephric hyperplasia (8 cases), and pure mesonephric ductal hyperplasia (2 cases) (Figs. 1-26 and 1-27).

In cases of lobular hyperplasia, round to oval, occasionally dilated, tubules are arranged in at least vaguely lobular aggregates. The tubules characteristically contain bright pink, periodic acid-Schiff (PAS)-positive hyaline material in their lumens (Fig. 1-23). In diffuse hyperplasia, no lobular grouping is apparent; in some of them, the irregular distribution of the tubules and their presence deep in the cervical wall can create a very worrisome appearance. In about one-third of both types of hyperplasia, tubules extend to within 1 mm of the endocervical surface; three-quarters have an additional component of ductal hyperplasia (Fig. 1-25).

Ductal hyperplasia is characterized by one or more large ducts that may be round or elongated, depending on the plane of section (Fig. 1-26), lined by pseudostratified epithelium that often forms small papillae. Although the tubular form of mesonephric hyperplasia is most likely to be misinterpreted as invasive adenocarcinoma, ductal hyperplasia, particularly when occurring in pure form, is usually misdiagnosed as a premalignant lesion such as endocervical glandular dysplasia or adenocarcinoma in situ. The frequently elongated form of the ducts and a usual lack of

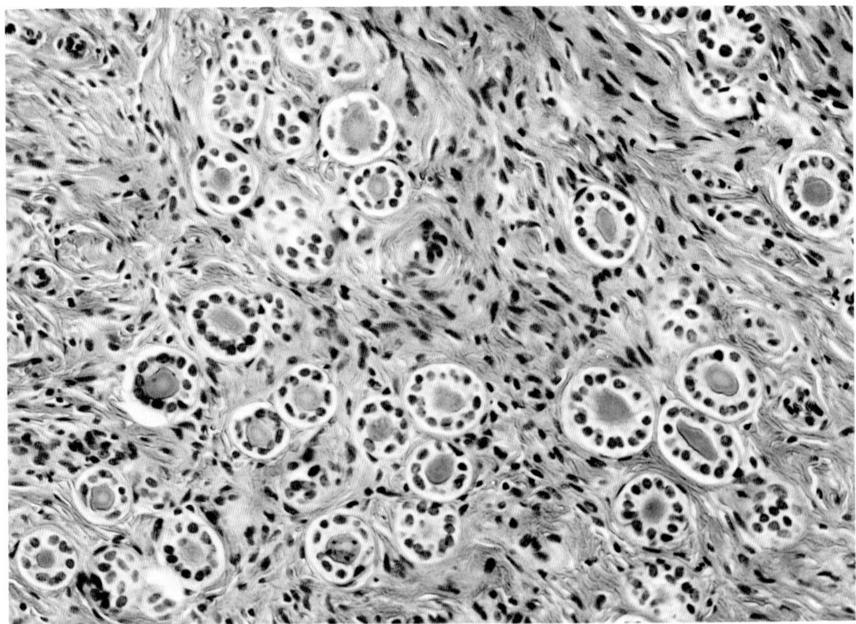

Fig. 1-23. Mesonephric hyperplasia. Small tubules contain dense material that was eosinophilic. (From Young and Clement,[1] with permission.)

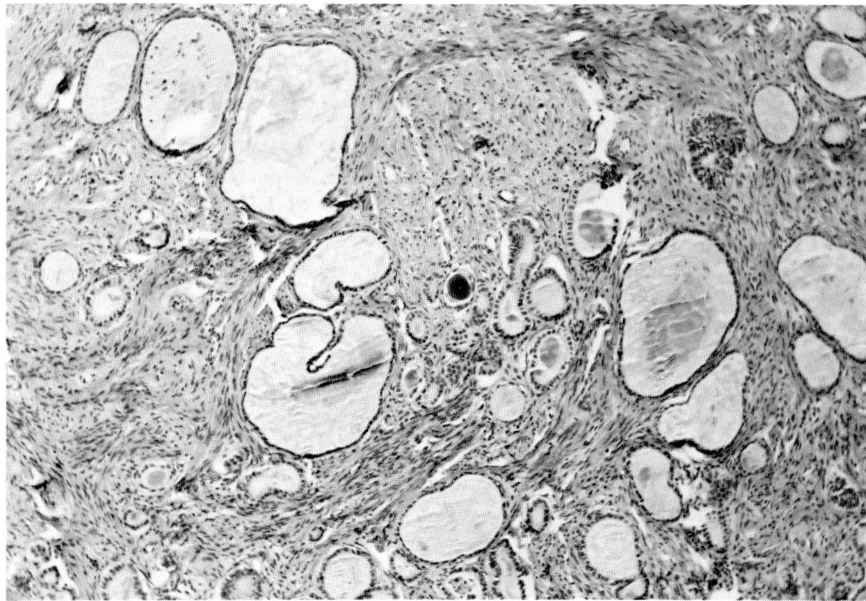

Fig. 1-24. Mesonephric hyperplasia. Many of the tubules are cystically dilated. (From Young and Clement,[1] with permission.)

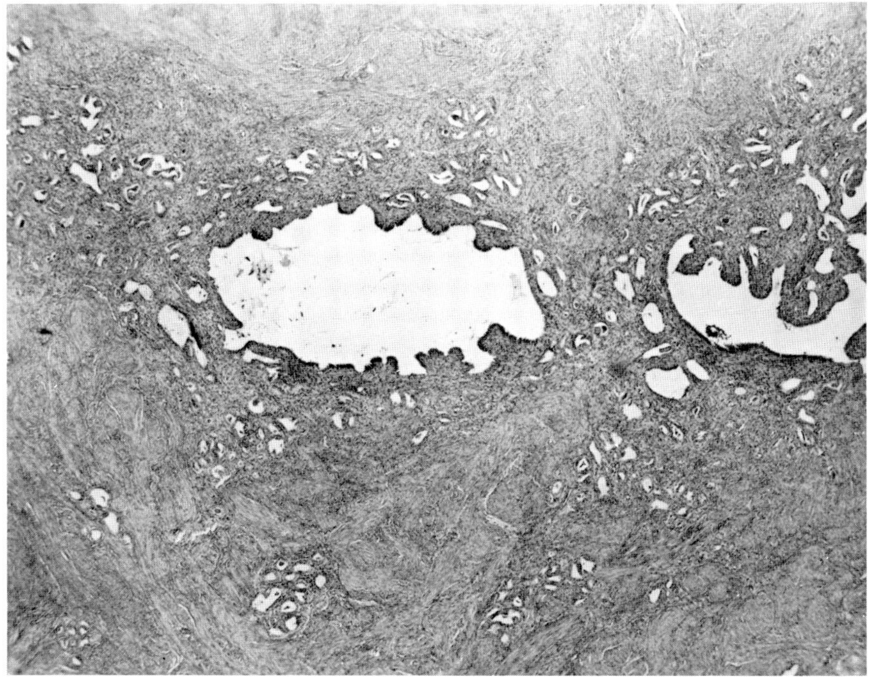

Fig. 1-25. Mesonephric hyperplasia. Lobulated aggregates of mesonephric tubules surround the main mesonephric duct. (From Young and Clement,[1] with permission.)

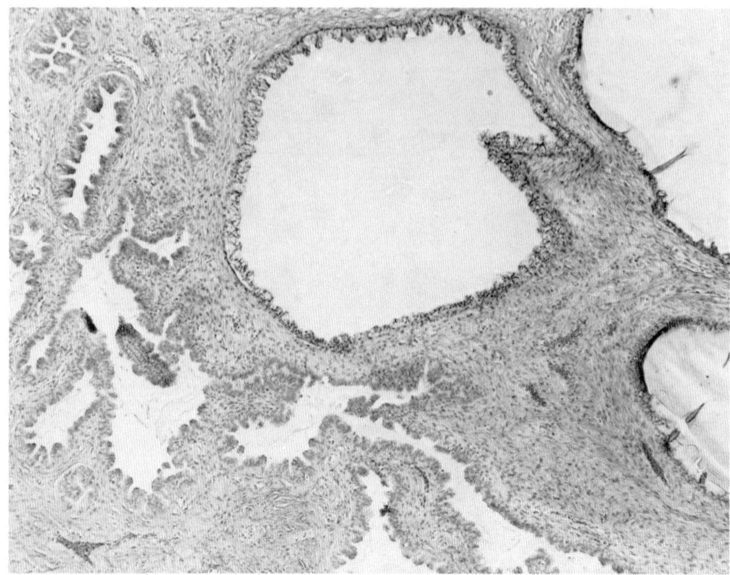

Fig. 1-26. Mesonephric ductal hyperplasia. Some of the ducts are rounded, whereas others are elongated. Pseudostratification of the lining cells is present in some of the ducts.

an association with endocervical glands are initial clues to their nature, and high power scrutiny reveals no significant cytologic atypia. Finally, the micropapillae seen in pure ductal hyperplasia are distinctive and are not a feature of premalignant glandular lesions.

Mesonephric hyperplasia must obviously be distinguished from mesonephric adeno-carcinoma (see Ch. 3), a very rare lesion that should be diagnosed only after florid mesonephric hyperplasia has been excluded. It should be noted, however, that most cases of mesonephric carcinoma have been associated with mesonephric hyperplasia.[33] In contrast to mesonephric hyperplasia, which is almost always an incidental microscopic finding, a mesonephric carci-

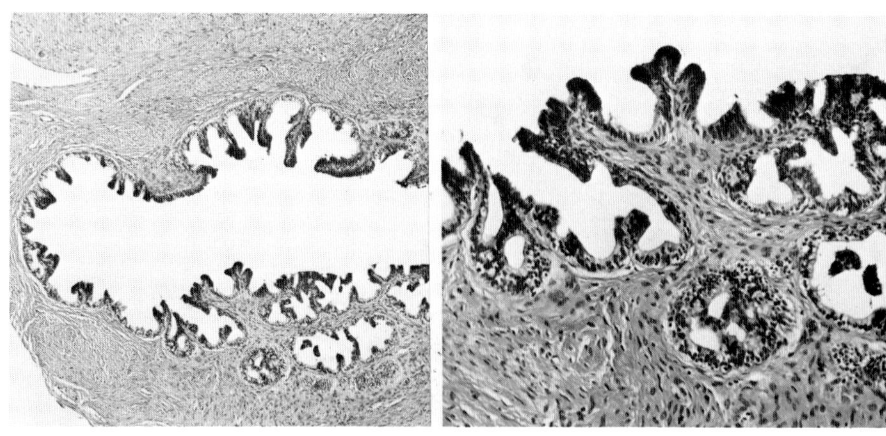

AB

Fig. 1-27. Mesonephric ductal hyperplasia. The mesonephric duct **(A)** is lined by pseudostratified cells forming small papillae **(B)**. (From Young and Clement,[1] with permission.)

noma is likely to produce a grossly visible lesion. On microscopic examination, mesonephric carcinomas are typically associated with irregular destructive invasion by the glandular elements, which are more crowded than in hyperplasia and often have an associated stromal reaction. High degrees of nuclear atypicality and prominent mitotic activity obviously favor a malignant lesion, although these features have not been present in all the carcinomas.

Mesonephric hyperplasia may be confused with other adenocarcinomas, including adenoma malignum, clear cell adenocarcinoma and, rarely, metastatic adenocarcinoma. The glands in adenoma malignum[9] are much more irregular in size and shape than are the tubules of mesonephric hyperplasia. In addition, they are lined by tall columnar mucinous cells, in contrast to the cuboidal nonmucinous epithelial cells of mesonephric tubules, and are often surrounded by an edematous or desmoplastic stromal reaction that is absent in mesonephric hyperplasia. The tubules in mesonephric hyperplasia might be confused with the tubular glands present in many clear cell adenocarcinomas of the cervix; the tubules in mesonephric hyperplasia may undergo cystic dilation, imparting a low-power appearance that may mimic that of the tubulocystic pattern of clear cell carcinoma. In contrast to mesonephric hyperplasia, however, at least some of the cells lining the glands and cysts of clear cell carcinoma have conspicuous clear, glycogen-rich cytoplasm or are of hobnail type. In addition, clear cell carcinomas with a pure tubular pattern are uncommon; solid and papillary patterns, which are not compatible with a diagnosis of mesonephric hyperplasia, are also usually present. Occasional metastatic adenocarcinomas, for example, from the breast, may consist of small tubular glands; their appearance is somewhat reminiscent of mesonephric hyperplasia (see Fig. 8-37). The carcinomas will usually focally contain cords of cells and single cells, as well as cytologic features of carcinoma inconsistent with mesonephric hyperplasia.

DIFFUSE LAMINAR ENDOCERVICAL GLANDULAR HYPERPLASIA

Diffuse laminar endocervical glandular hyperplasia refers to cases of endocervical glandular hyperplasia characterized by a diffuse distribution of closely packed endocervical glands, typically appearing as a discrete layer sharply demarcated from the underlying cervical stroma[34] (Fig. 1-28). The seven examples described occurred in patients who ranged from 22 to 48 (mean 37) years of age; only one had a history of hormone intake. All the lesions were incidental findings. Microscopic examination revealed a proliferation of moderately sized, evenly spaced, endocervical glands within the inner third of the cervical wall (Fig. 1-28). Reactive cytologic atypia was seen in some cases, but significant atypia was absent. A marked inflammatory response was present in five of the seven cases. Focal stromal edema was present in six of the cases, but a desmoplastic stromal reaction of the type often seen in cases of adenoma malignum was absent. The latter feature, along with a lack of an irregular and deep stromal infiltration and an absence of focal malignant cytologic features, aid in the distinction of diffuse laminar endocervical gland hyperplasia from adenoma malignum.

ENDOCERVICOSIS

Although in our experience this process[35] usually provides a problem in diagnosis in bladder pathology, for the sake of completeness it is worth mentioning that we have recently seen one case that did involve the bladder but that also extensively involved the outer wall of the cervix and

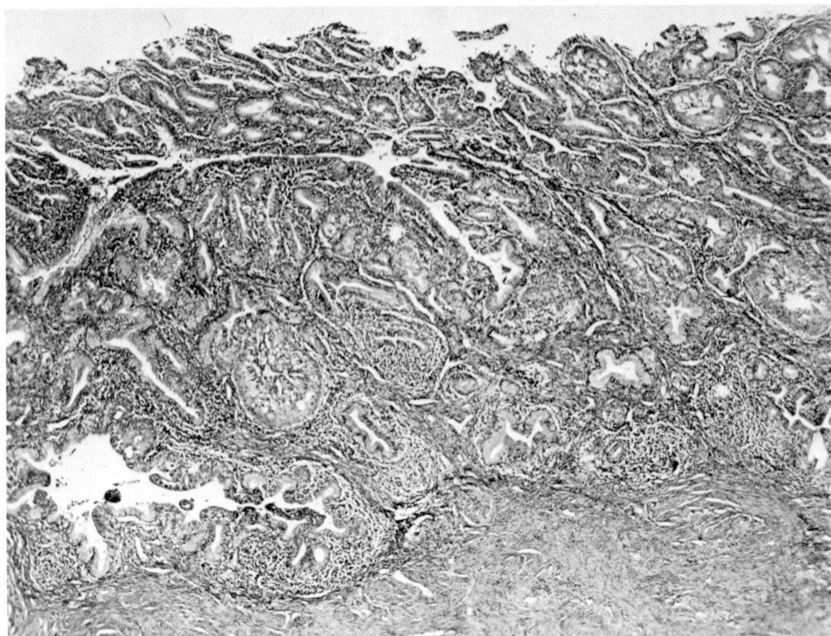

Fig. 1-28. Diffuse laminar endocervical glandular hyperplasia. Hyperplastic endocervical glands form a discrete layer that is well demarcated from the underlying stroma. (From Young and Clement,[1] with permission.)

was initially sent in for consultation with concern as to whether it represented adenoma malignum. It was helpful in diagnosis that the dilated mucinous glands of this lesion (Fig. 1-29) involved the outer wall of the cervix and were separated from the endocervical glands; in addition, the process exhibited typical features in the urinary bladder.

GLANDULAR HYPERPLASIA, NOT OTHERWISE SPECIFIED

The endocervical epithelium may be hyperplastic, sometimes floridly so, without exhibiting any of the specific aforementioned histologic patterns (Fig. 1-30). Lack of deep invasion, an orderly, sometimes lobulated, arrangement of the glands, a well-demarcated margin with the adjacent cervical stroma, the usual lack of a stromal reaction, and bland nuclear features are all features seen to varying extents in individual cases that indicate that these lesions are non-neoplastic. Other miscellaneous changes may be seen in the endocervical epithelium that may cause diagnostic difficulty. Indeed, four of the five non-neoplastic glandular lesions initially misinterpreted as adenocarcinoma in one series[2] referred to at the beginning of this chapter, appear to fall into this group rather than in any of the better defined entities already discussed. In two of these cases, the diagnostic problems resulted from the presence of irregularly shaped glands, an appearance exaggerated by poor orientation and artifactual distortion, emphasizing that, although markedly irregular gland contours are quite characteristic of adenoma malignum, they are not pathognomonic of it. In the other two cases, the worrisome appearance was largely due to the presence of "reserve cell hyperplasia" and a cribriform

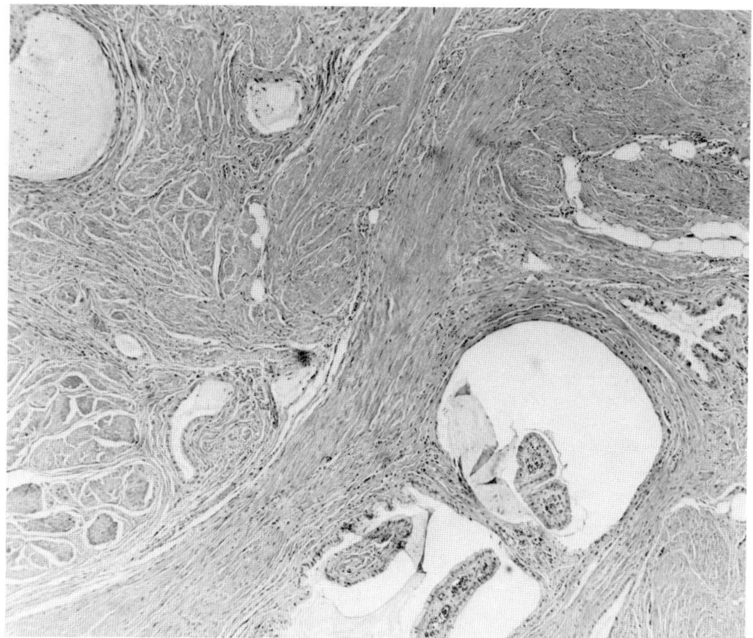

Fig. 1-29. Endocervicosis. Glands that are cystically dilated and lined by a single layer of mucinous cells are present in the outer portion of the cervix.

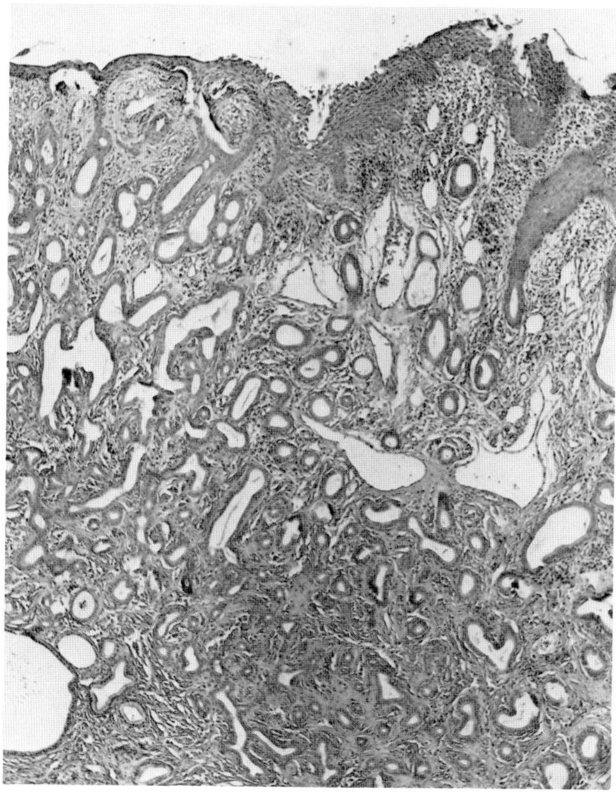

Fig. 1-30. Glandular hyperplasia, not otherwise specified. There is an irregular proliferation of benign endocervical glands.

glandular pattern. We have seen cases in which intraglandular bridging has been striking.

METAPLASIAS

Tubal Metaplasia

Tubal metaplasia of the endocervix (Figs. 1-31 and 1-32) may be misinterpreted as endocervical glandular dysplasia or adenocarcinoma in situ in histologic[36] or cytologic material.[37, 38] In one study of cervical smears from 50 women in whom the diagnosis of endocervical glandular dysplasia had been rendered, correlation with subsequent histologic material and review indicated that tubal metaplasia had been present in 76 percent of the cases.[38] In one recent series of histopathologic specimens, 2 of 11 cases were referred in consultation with such diagnoses made or entertained.[36] Tubal metaplasia is a common finding, having been found in 31 percent of the cases in a recent series of 108 cone biopsy and hysterectomy specimens.[39] As expected, its frequency was related to the number of sections examined. There was no relationship to the age of the patients. Tubal metaplasia was most common in the deeper glands of the upper endocervix but involved the surface epithelium in approximately one-third of the cases. "Tuboendometrioid metaplasia" has been related to a recent cone biopsy, being found in one-fourth of cases with such a history in a recent study.[40] In tubal metaplasia, endocervical epithelium is replaced by a single layer of ciliated cells, nonciliated cells, and peg cells, as seen in the normal tubal mucosa (Figs. 1-31 and 1-32). The admixture of cell types, absence of invasive characteristics, lack of atypia and mitotic activity, and absence of immunoreactivity for CEA are clues to the correct diagnosis. Occasionally tubal metaplasia occurs in one of the other non-neoplastic glandular lesions of the cervix discussed in this review, such as tunnel clusters or endometriosis.

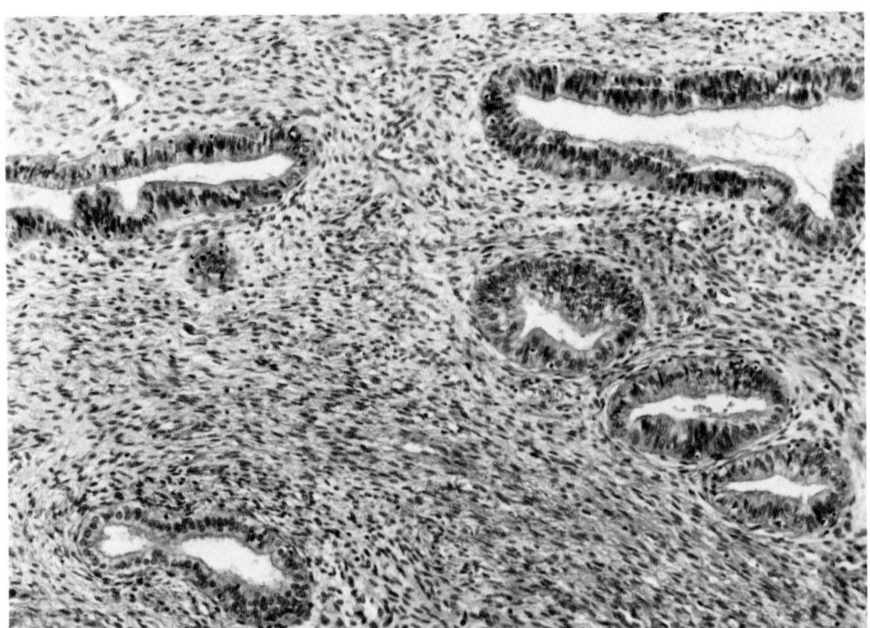

Fig. 1-31. Tubal metaplasia. Cilia are not clearly seen at this magnification.

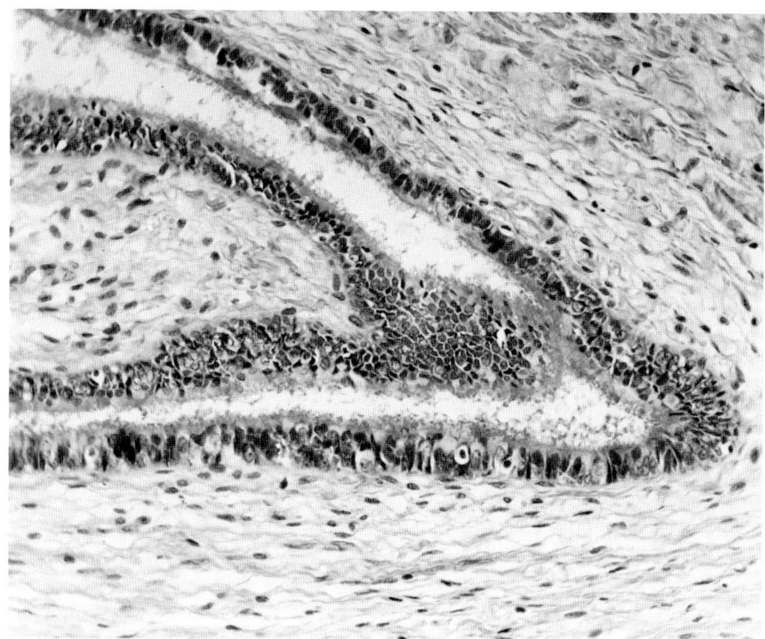

Fig. 1-32. Tubal metaplasia. The epithelium resembles that of the fallopian tube and many cilia are visible.

Endometrioid Metaplasia

Benign endometrioid glands, interpreted as ectopic endometrial glands, were found deep in the wall in 1 percent of cervices examined in one series.[14] Endometrioid glands arising by a process of metaplasia of the mucinous endocervical epithelium may also be seen. In our experience, pure endometrioid metaplasia is rare, as there is usually an additional component of tubal metaplasia; therefore, the term "*tuboendometrioid*" *metaplasia* is more appropriate.[40]

Intestinal Metaplasia

Intestinal metaplasia is the rarest form of benign glandular metaplasia seen in the uterine cervix, and is characterized by the focal presence of goblet and argentaffin cells within the endocervical glands.[41] Intestinal metaplasia in the cervix is seen more commonly in cases of adenocarcinoma in situ,[42] occasionally in benign neoplasms,[43] and in adenocarcinomas[44, 45] (see Ch. 3). As intestinal metaplasia unassociated with any degree of dysplasia is very rare, the diagnosis should only be made after careful evaluation has ruled out any cellular atypicality.

ENDOMETRIOSIS

Cervical endometriosis may be superficial (also referred to as primary) (Fig. 1-33) or deep (also referred to as secondary).[46, 47] Cervical endometriosis was found in 4 percent of patients in one recent series of hysterectomy and cone biopsy specimens[24] and in 2.4 percent of patients attending a colposcopy clinic in another series.[48] Superficial endometriosis is found in approximately 1 to 2 percent of patients in the

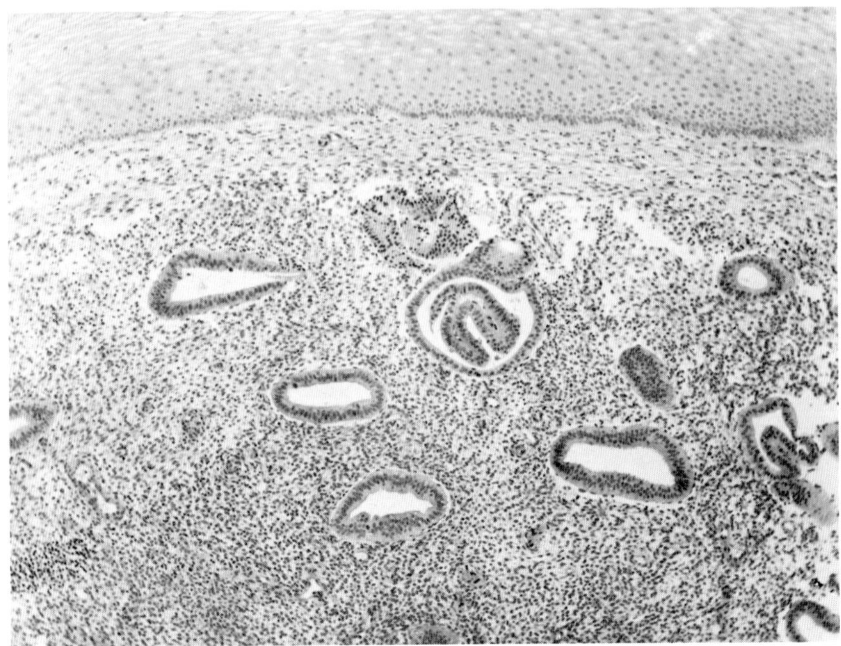

Fig. 1-33. Superficial endometriosis of cervix.

reproductive age group and, unlike deep endometriosis, is usually unassociated with generalized pelvic endometriosis. Superficial endometriosis is usually found in a patient with a history of a prior procedure, such as a cone biopsy, which has involved the cervix.[40, 48] Patients are usually in their fourth or fifth decade of life, and the lesion is an incidental finding in about one-half of these cases. Superficial endometriosis may be misinterpreted as endocervical glandular dysplasia or adenocarcinoma in situ on cytology smears. On histologic examination, the correct diagnosis is usually straightforward but may be overlooked, particularly when ulceration and edema obscures the features of the stromal component.

ARIAS-STELLA REACTION

The Arias-Stella reaction was documented within endocervical glands in 9 percent of gravid hysterectomy specimens in one study.[49] The alteration is typically fo-

cal, involving only one or two glands in each case[50] (Fig. 1-34). Glands in any part of the endocervical canal may be involved, but involvement of superficial glands is more common than that of deep glands.[49] Glands within endocervical polyps may also be affected.[51] The cytologic features are similar to those of the Arias-Stella reaction within endometrial glands (see Ch. 4) and include stratified cells with abundant vacuolated cytoplasm and enlarged pleomorphic and hyperchromatic nuclei, imparting a hobnail appearance to some of the cells (Fig. 1-34). Optically clear nuclei may also be seen. Mitoses are usually rare or absent. These atypical changes may be mistaken for adenocarcinoma in situ or clear cell carcinoma, particularly in a biopsy or cytology specimen; such diagnoses should therefore be made with caution in a pregnant patient. Clear cell carcinoma, however, will often be associated with a mass, and histologic examination will reveal features inconsistent with the Arias-Stella reaction, including the presence of invasion

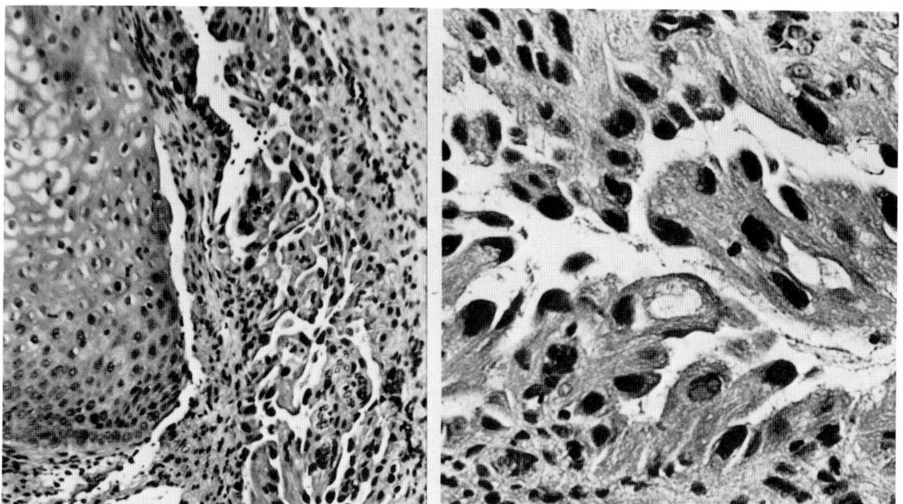

Fig. 1-34. Arias-Stella reaction. A gland adjacent to metaplastic squamous epithelium **(A)** shows the characteristic features of the Arias-Stella reaction with hobnail-like nuclei **(B)**. (From Young and Clement,[1] with permission.)

and tubular and solid patterns. Adenocarcinoma in situ, in contrast to the Arias-Stella reaction, usually exhibits uniformly atypical nuclei and relatively frequent mitotic figures, and usually lacks marked cytoplasmic vacuolation, hobnail cells, and optically clear nuclei.[52]

CHANGES SECONDARY TO EXTRAVASATION OF MUCIN

Although the lack of a stromal response often supports the benign nature of an endocervical glandular lesion, the stroma adjacent to benign glands may exhibit reactive changes, usually, but not always (Fig. 1-35), in response to mucin extravasated from a ruptured gland (Fig. 1-36). A foreign-body giant cell reaction is sometimes seen in these cases and, in some of these cases, foamy histiocytes are conspicuous. In one apparently unique case, gland rupture was associated with the dissection of mucin into the stroma and vascular lumens, the appearance raising initial concern about a primary or metastatic adenocarcinoma[1]

(Fig. 1-37). Michael and colleagues[2] described another case of a pseudoneoplastic glandular lesion with an unusual appearance interpreted by them as being due, at least in part, to the extravasation of mucin.

INFECTIOUS AND REACTIVE ATYPIAS

Cytomegalovirus (CMV) infection, usually an incidental histologic finding within the endocervix, is associated with large basophilic intranuclear inclusions within the affected endocervical epithelial cells (Fig. 1-38) and, in some cases, endothelial cells. Immunohistochemical staining for CMV antigen may be confirmatory.[53] The intranuclear inclusions, as well as associated granular cytoplasmic inclusions, are sufficiently characteristic that confusion with adenocarcinoma in situ is unlikely. In additional contrast to the latter, the cells showing the CMV-related changes are singly disposed within normal endocervical columnar cells. Brown and Wells[24] briefly described five examples of bizarre multinucleated giant cells within endocervical glands (their Fig. 1-1).

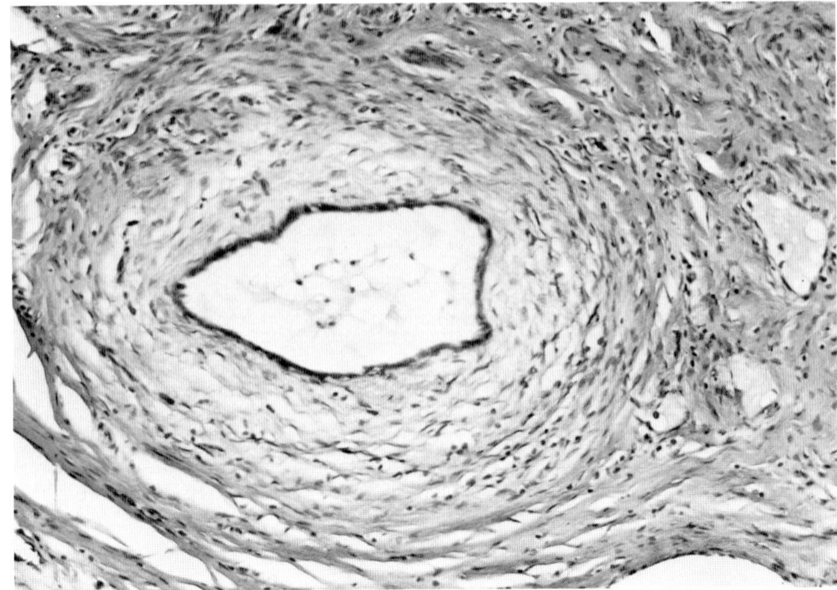

Fig. 1-35. Loose edematous stromal alteration around benign endocervical gland.

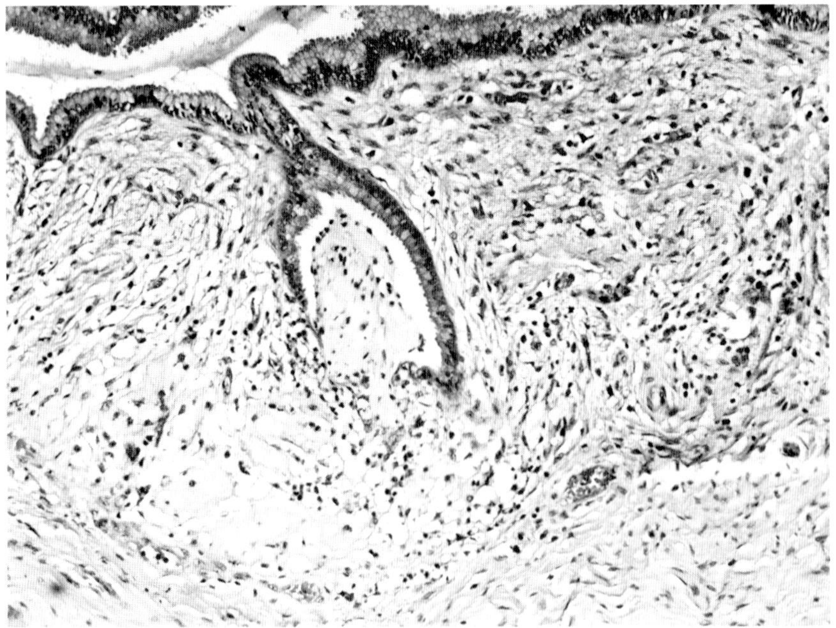

Fig. 1-36. Rupture of endocervical gland with extravasation of mucin into stroma. There is a prominent stromal reaction to the extravasated mucin.

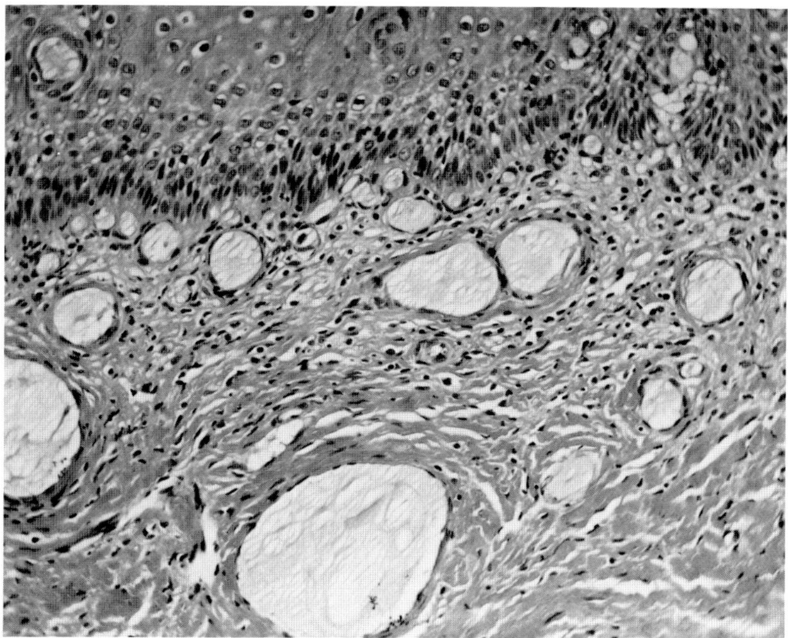

Fig. 1-37. Mucin extravasation within endocervical stroma. Some of the mucin may be within vessels.

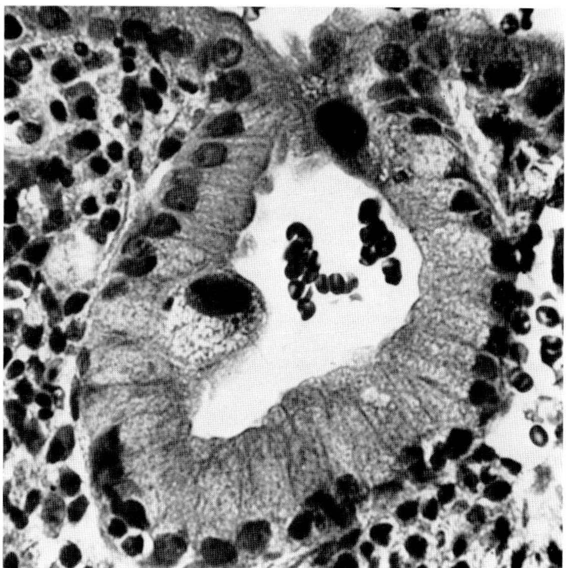

Fig. 1-38. Cytomegalic infection. Two cells lining an endocervical gland have characteristic intranuclear inclusion bodies. (From Young and Clement,[1] with permission.)

In each case, there was evidence of HPV infection elsewhere in the cervix; it was concluded that the changes were secondary to viral infection.

Herpes virus infection of the uterine cervix is quite common.[54] In typical cases, the clinician will often suspect the diagnosis, but it is not rare for the lesion to be overlooked clinically.[54] On microscopic examination, the characteristic ground glass intranuclear inclusions should establish the diagnosis with relative ease in most cases, although occasionally a misdiagnosis of a dysplastic process is made. A variety of other specific infectious diseases, whose frequency varies greatly from one part of the world to another, may involve the cervix but, with occasional exceptions, a combination of distinctive clinical, and/or pathologic features should prevent serious problems in diagnosis for the surgical pathologist.[55, 56]

Radiation to the cervix can cause markedly atypical nuclear changes (Fig. 1-40) that can be mistaken for a preneoplastic or neoplastic glandular process, particularly if the pathologist is unaware of the history.[57] In contrast to those in a neoplasm, however, the nuclear features that follow radiation are more variable from one cell to another, with bizarre forms and an absence of mitotic activity. Radiation-induced vascular and stromal changes, including post-radiation fibroblasts, may also be present.[57]

As elsewhere in the body, reactive atypia in association with marked inflammation is occasionally seen within endocervical glandular cells (Fig. 1-41). This may occur in the epithelium of any of the specific glandular lesions discussed here, for example, that of tunnel clusters (Figs. 1-42 and 1-43). In some cases, the atypical nuclei are large, hyperchromatic, and "smudgy" and are present in cells with abundant eosinophilic cytoplasm (Fig. 1-44).

NONGLANDULAR LESIONS

A wide variety of nonglandular non-neoplastic lesions within the cervix can be con-

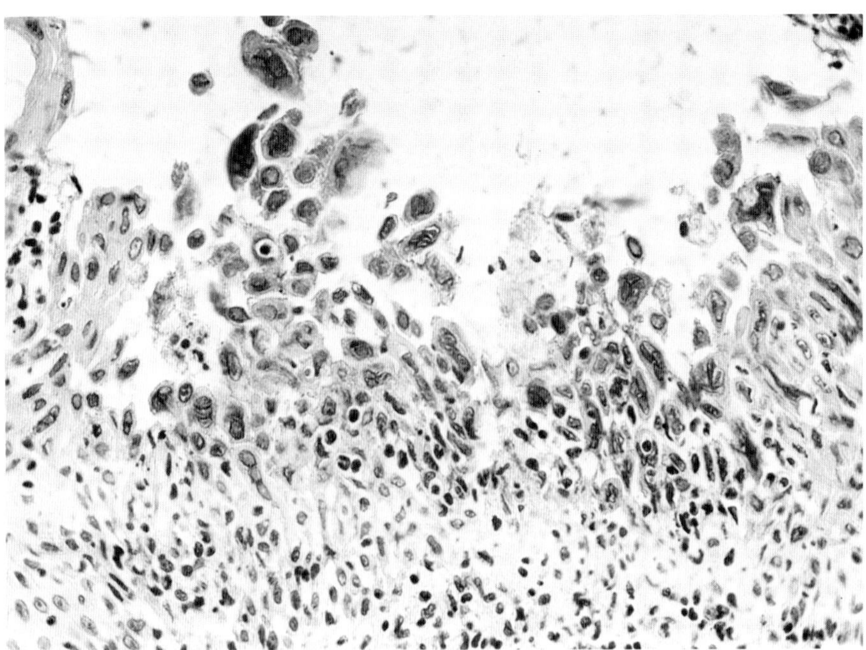

Fig. 1-39. Herpetic cervicitis. Note ground-glass intranuclear inclusions.

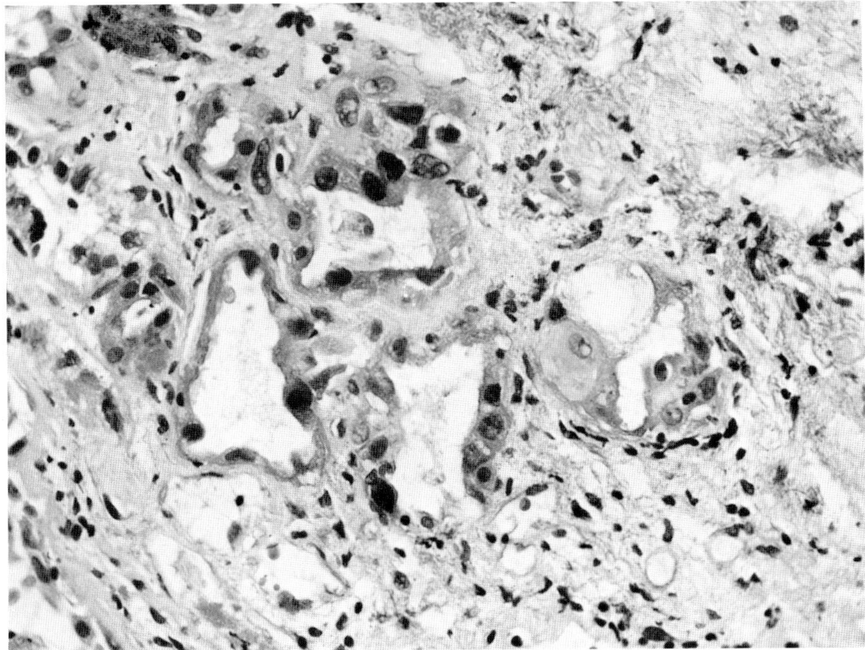

Fig. 1-40. Radiation atypia. Several endocervical glands are lined by cells with bizarre hyperchromatic nuclei. Note the fibrotic changes in the stroma.

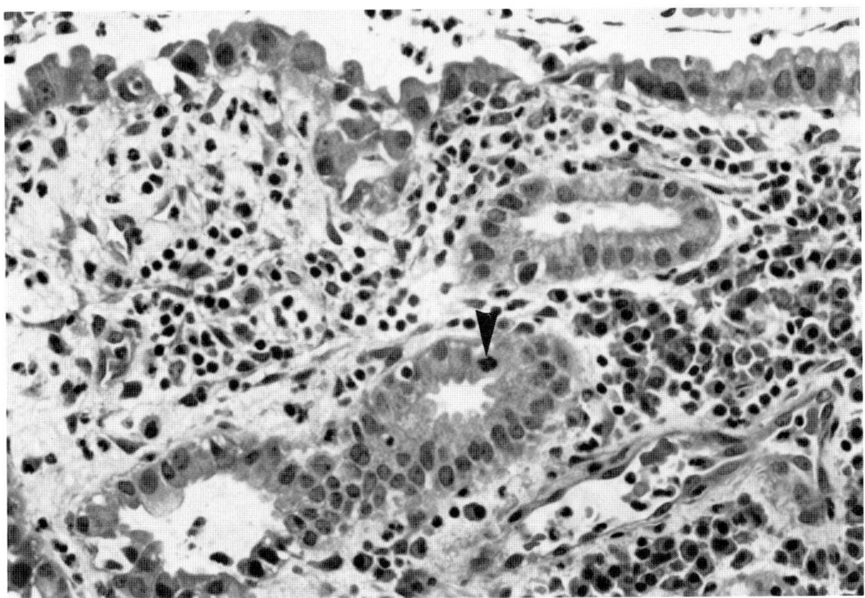

Fig. 1-41. Reactive atypia of endocervical epithelium. The glands in a case of nonspecific chronic cervicitis are lined by cells showing mild reactive nuclear atypia. Note a mitotic figure (arrow). (From Young and Clement,[1] with permission.)

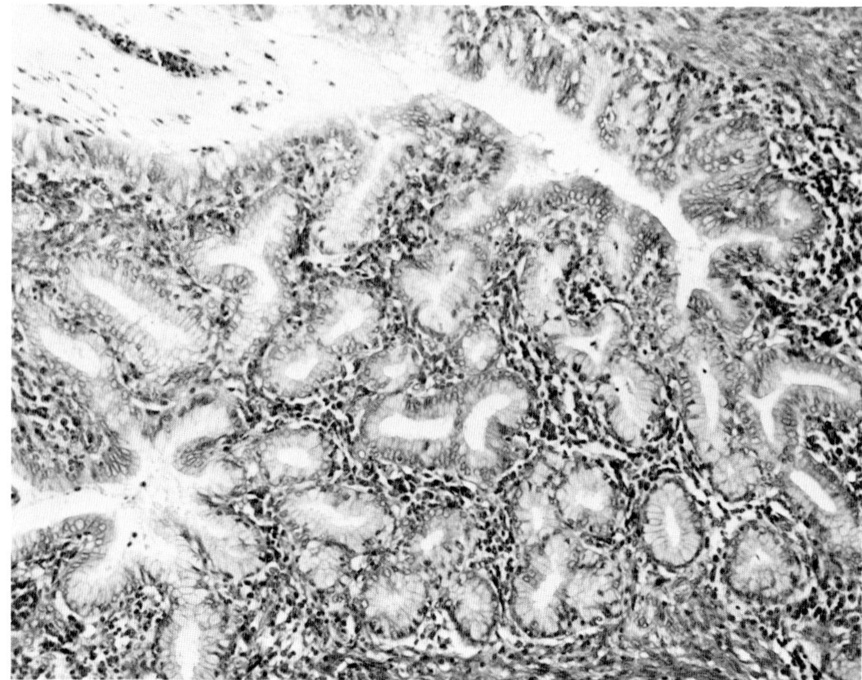

Fig. 1-42. Tunnel cluster with reactive atypia.

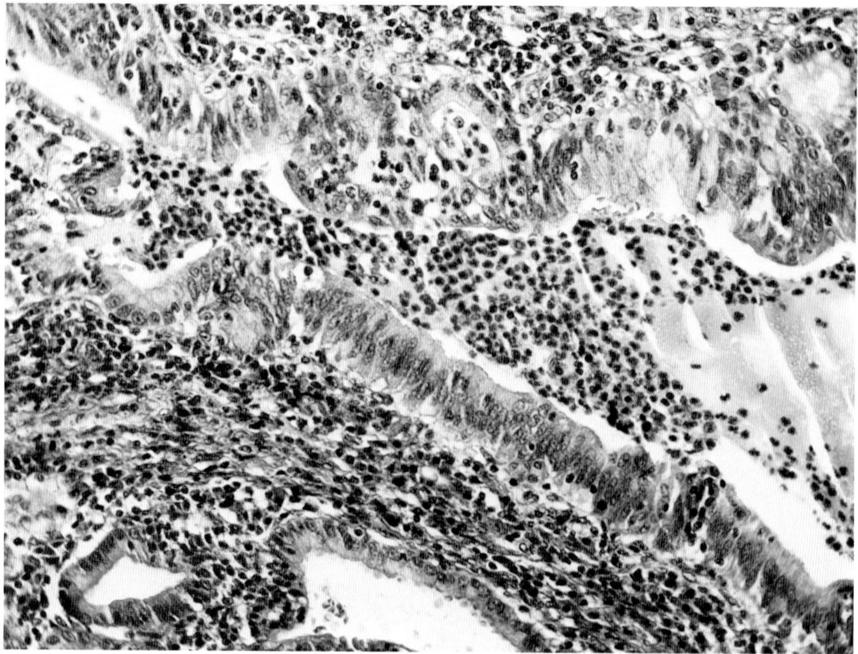

Fig. 1-43. Tunnel cluster with reactive atypia. Higher-power view of previous illustration showing cellular stratification and mild atypia.

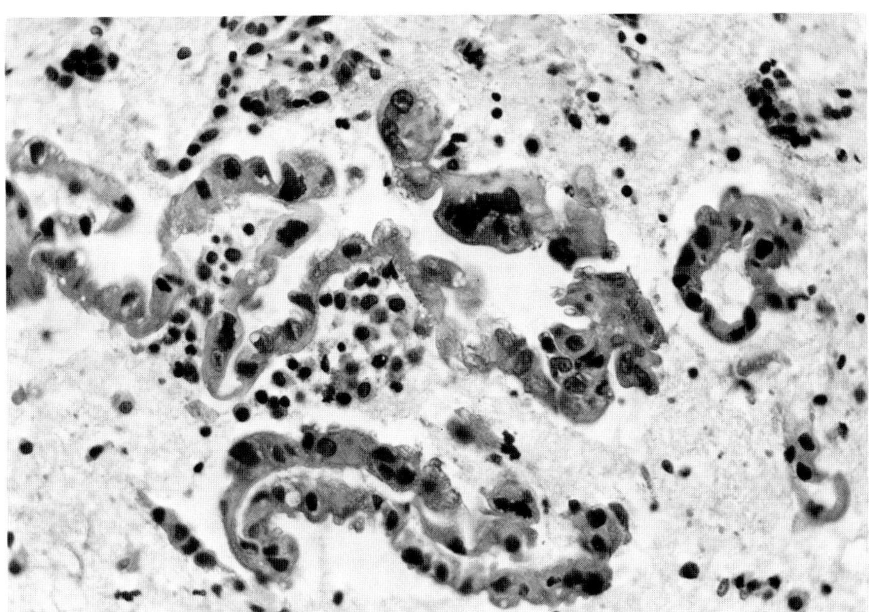

Fig. 1-44. Benign endocervical cells with abundant eosinophilic cytoplasm, that contain hyperchromatic enlarged nuclei with a degenerative appearance.

fused with neoplasms on clinical, gross, or microscopic examination (Table 1-2).

FLORID SQUAMOUS METAPLASIA

Although the appearance of squamous metaplasia does not cause any diagnostic difficulty in the great majority of cases, oc-

Table 1-2. Nonglandular Pseudoneoplastic Lesions of the Uterine Cervix

Florid squamous metaplasia
Postbiopsy pseudoinvasion of squamous epithelium
Transitional cell metaplasia
Lymphoma-like lesions
Plasma cell cervicitis
Malakoplakia and histiocytic cervicitis
Eosinophilic cervicitis
Ligneous cervicitis
Stromal endometriosis
Postoperative spindle cell nodule
Polyp with stromal atypia and atypical stromal cells
Ectopic decidua
Melanotic lesions
Miscellaneous rare lesions

casional examples of florid squamous metaplasia within many endocervical glands and clefts (Fig. 1-45) may be misinterpreted by an inexperienced observer and may even cause experienced pathologists some difficulty. Willis[58] illustrates a case of "early epidermoid carcinoma" arising in a cervical polyp that is very suspicious for florid squamous metaplasia. The low-power architectural features are often reassuring in these cases because they show that the process is occurring in foci consistent with replaced endocervical glands. In addition, the smooth contours of the metaplastic foci is in contrast to the irregular shapes seen in invasive carcinoma. In some cases, the lack of associated normal glands may cause slightly more difficulty; however, in these and other cases, high-power examination shows that the cytologic features are bland. Sometimes the focal identification of mucinous epithelial cells in the midst of the metaplastic squamous cells reinforces the diagnosis of squamous metaplasia.

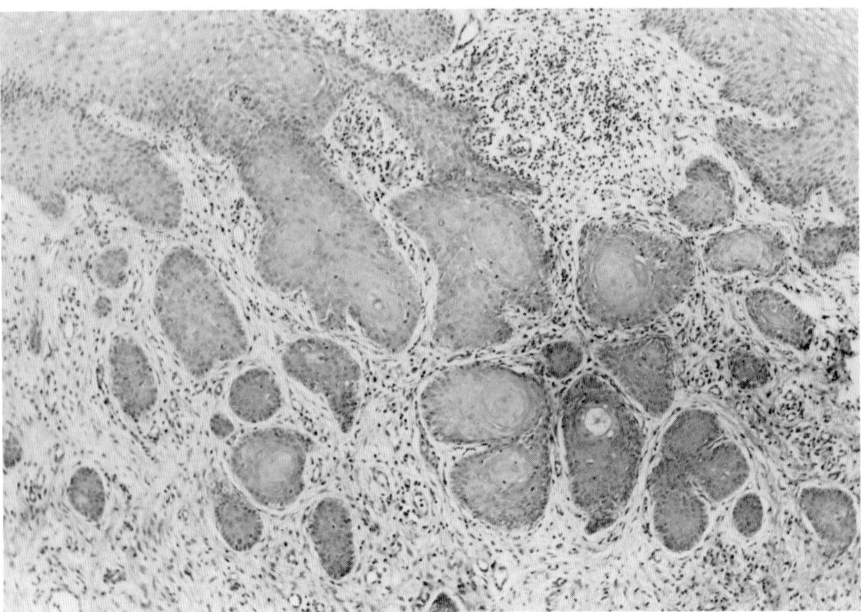

Fig. 1-45. Squamous metaplasia. Scattered nests of benign squamous epithelium are present within the superficial cervical stroma.

Postbiopsy "Pseudoinvasion" of Squamous Epithelium

Postbiopsy pseudoinvasion of squamous epithelium is a relatively rare phenomenon that may be much more problematic than florid squamous metaplasia. In these cases (Fig. 1-46), nests of squamous epithelium are present in the stroma, having been implanted there during a prior biopsy. Their occasional presence deep in the wall and the lack of an association with endocervical glands may suggest the diagnosis of squamous carcinoma; as the biopsy has often been performed for some preneoplastic abnormality of squamous epithelium, the possible diagnosis of invasive carcinoma may be considered. In addition, the squamous nests are often somewhat irregular in shape and may be associated with a fibrotic stroma secondary to postbiopsy scarring. The correct diagnosis is often suggested in these cases because the nests of epithelium are few in number—sometimes only one—

and there are no other foci of abnormal epithelium between them and the overlying mucosa, a finding that would be unusual for an invasive squamous cell carcinoma. Although of different nature, it is most convenient to mention at this juncture that traumatic neuroma of the cervix following cone biopsy has been described.[59] The lesion was noted grossly as a 20 × 15 × 5-mm firm area.

Transitional Cell Metaplasia

That the epithelium of the cervix may undergo transitional (urothelial) metaplasia is not widely recognized and is not mentioned in many standard texts but is relatively common, particularly in postmenopausal women. It is an important entity to be aware of because, on low-power examination, the lack of maturation may impart an appearance that initially suggests dysplasia. This change is usually seen in the epithe-

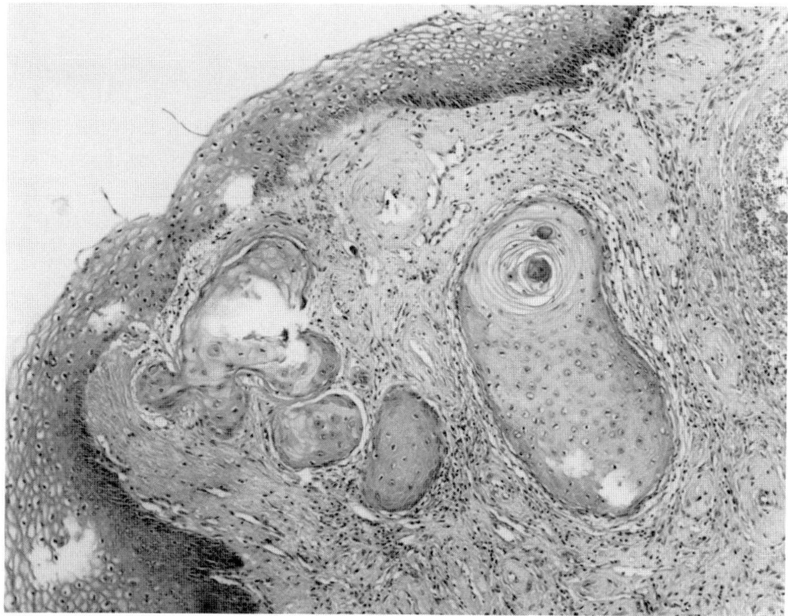

Fig. 1-46. Squamous epithelium in superficial cervical stroma postbiopsy. The abnormal arrangement of the nests suggests the possibility of microinvasion. Note the benign cytologic features of the squamous nests and the lack of atypia of the overlying epithelium.

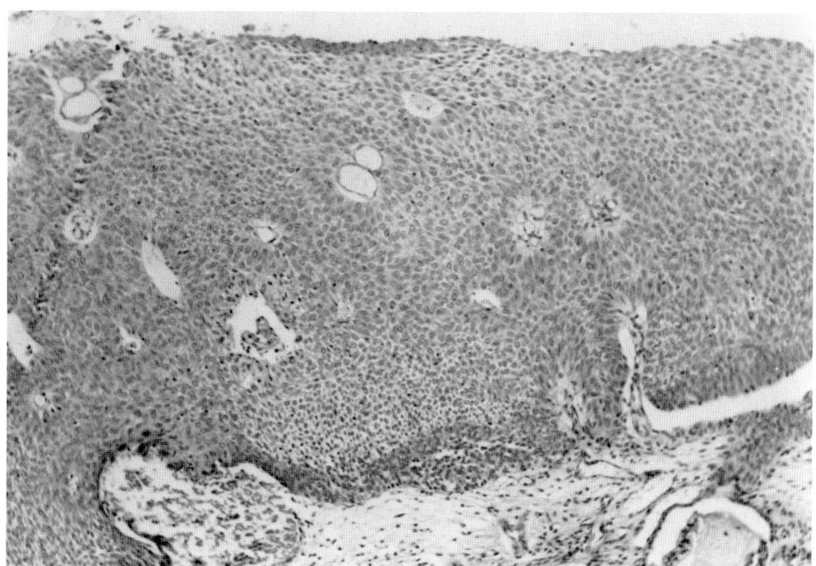

Fig. 1-47. Transitional cell metaplasia. The lack of normal maturation suggests the possibility of dysplasia on low-power examination.

lium lining the cervix, but nests of transitional cells are rarely present in the stroma, having an appearance resembling that of Walthard's nests, and indeed have been reported as such.[60] Most of the recent writing on this topic has been by Fetissof and associates, whose studies have showed that these cells frequently are argyrophilic.[61–63] In one paper,[64] changes that appear to be similar to those of transitional cell metaplasia were found in a series of transsexual women who had been treated with large doses of androgens. On microscopic examination, transitional cell metaplasia is distinguished from a dysplasia by the uniformity of the cells, lack of significant mitotic activity, and characteristic nuclear grooves within many of the nuclei (Fig. 1-47 and 1-48). In our experience, most cases of transitional cell metaplasia have entirely benign features, but we have seen cases in which the transitional cells have exhibited dysplasia and rare transitional cell carcinomas of the cervix occur (see Ch. 8).

LYMPHOMA-LIKE LESIONS

Reactive lymphoid lesions in the lower female genital tract may be florid, simulating a lymphoma. In a study of 16 of these lymphoma-like lesions, typically encountered in women of reproductive age, there were 10 cases in the cervix.[65] One patient with a cervical lesion had infectious mononucleosis that was not recognized until 10 days after a cervical biopsy disclosed an atypical lymphoid infiltrate, an observation consistent with the known association between atypical lymphoid proliferations and infectious mononucleosis seen elsewhere. In addition, we have recently seen a case of a lymphoma-like lesion in the cervix associated with, and possibly related to, CMV cervicitis.

Several gross and microscopic features help distinguish these lesions from malignant lymphoma (Table 1-3). Although the cervix appeared abnormal on pelvic examination in 70 percent of patients with lym-

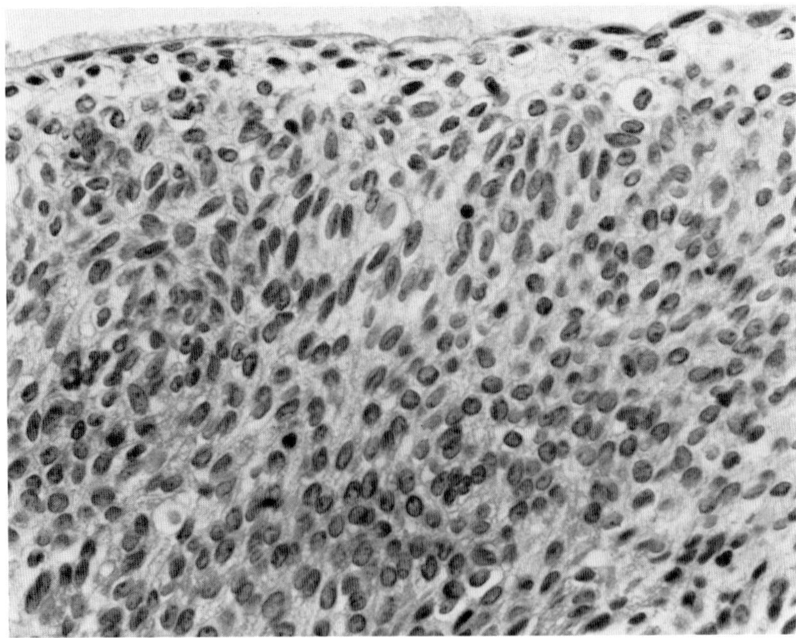

Fig. 1-48. Transitional cell metaplasia. The cells have uniform pale nuclei, many of which have longitudinal nuclear grooves.

Table 1-3. Comparison of Features of Lymphomas and Lymphoma-like Lesions

Feature	Lymphoma	Lymphoma-like
Gross mass	Usual	Seldom
Ulceration	Seldom	Usual
Surface involvement	Seldom	Frequent
Deep invasion	Usual	Seldom
Perivascular infiltrate	Frequent	Seldom
Sclerosis	Frequent	Seldom
Large cells	Monomorphic	Polymorphic
Mitoses	Frequent	Frequent
Neutrophils, lymphocytes, plasma cells in lesion	Seldom	Frequent

phoma-like lesions, and a neoplasm was suspected in three of them, cervical enlargement was not a conspicuous feature in most cases and diffuse enlargement was not encountered. In several cases, the abnormal appearance was the result of ulceration; the abnormality did not extend beyond the cervix in any case. Cervical lymphomas, in contrast, are only rarely associated with mucosal ulceration, often result in a barrel-shaped cervix, and frequently extend into the paracervical tissue or vagina.[66] The diagnosis of lymphoma of the cervix should accordingly be made with great caution if it is based solely on microscopic findings. Conversely, it should be remembered that gross abnormalities such as ulceration are compatible with a benign process.

Microscopic examination of cervical lymphoma-like lesions often shows a bandlike infiltrate in the superficial cervical

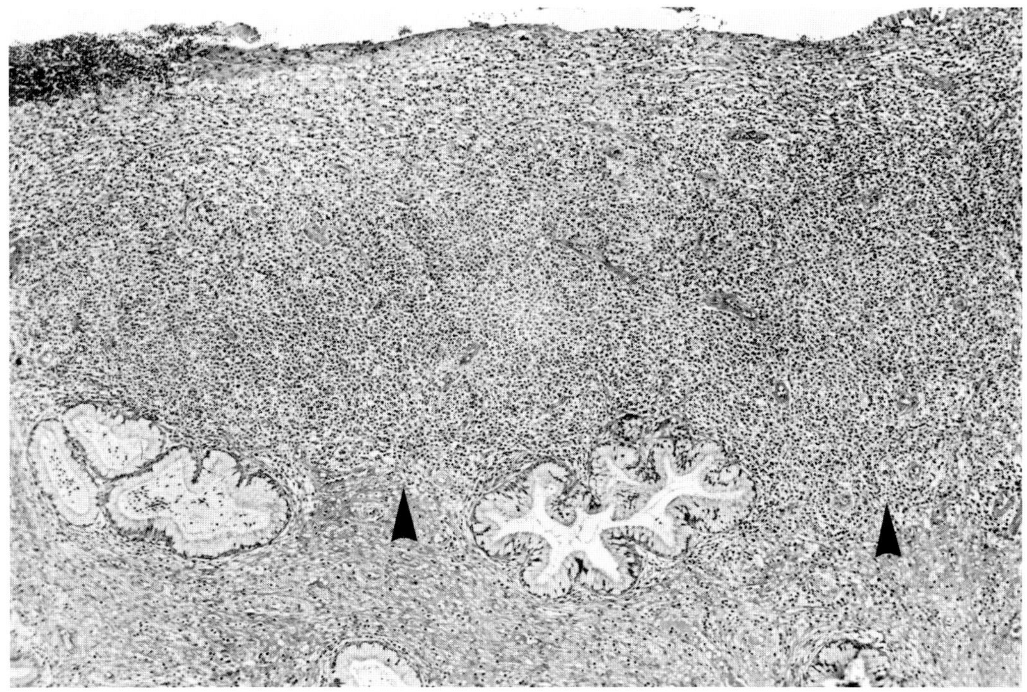

Fig. 1-49. Lymphoma-like lesion. There is a bandlike infiltrate of inflammatory cells in the superficial cervical stroma. Arrows point to the deep margin of the infiltrate. (From Young et al.,[65] with permission.)

stroma (Fig. 1-49). High-power examination reveals an infiltrate that is typically composed of large lymphoid cells with prominent mitotic activity, including cleaved and noncleaved follicular center cells and immunoblasts (Figs. 1-50 and 1-51); a starry-sky pattern may be present. Plasma cells, polymorphonuclear leukocytes, and small lymphocytes are characteristically present within the infiltrate, typically extending to the endocervical epithelium, which may be ulcerated. In contrast to lymphoma-like lesions, lymphomas typically exhibit cellular monomorphism, a perivascular distribution of the lymphoid cells, deep invasion, and prominent sclerosis. Also in contrast, surface ulceration and intralesional acute inflammatory cells and plasma cells are rarely seen in lymphomas, and there is often a spared zone of unremarkable stroma between the overlying intact epithelium and the underlying lymphomatous infiltrate. Immunohistochemical stains on paraffin-embedded material were not a diagnostic aid in the reported cases.[65]

With the exception of the above, chronic cervicitis, even when severe, rarely mimics a neoplasm on histologic examination. Striking examples of follicular cervicitis, in some cases secondary to infection by *Chlamydia trachomatis*, for example, can readily be distinguished from cases of follicular lymphoma because of the presence of germinal centers, as well as marked intraluminal, intraepithelial, and stromal inflammation, including neutrophils, transformed lymphocytes, plasma cells, and histiocytes.[67–69] Chronic plasma cell cervicitis has caused occasional problems, particularly in cytologic material. Qizilbash[70] reported a case diagnosed as either positive or suspicious for a malignant tumor but that on review and correlation with histologic findings in a cone biopsy was interpreted as being florid cervicitis with a prominent plasma cell component.

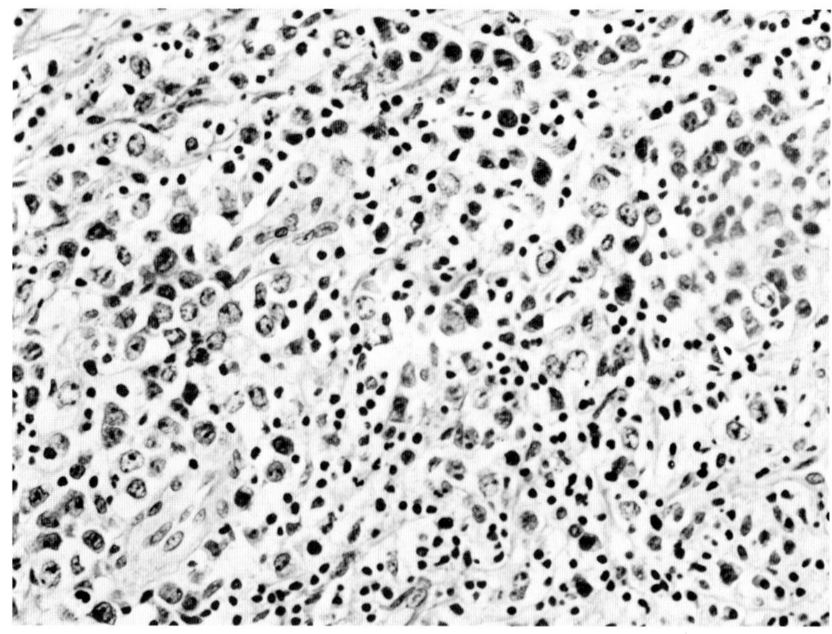

Fig. 1-50. Lymphoma-like lesion. Area from a cervical cone biopsy specimen showing centroblasts and immunoblasts with numerous small lymphocytes and occasional neutrophils. (From Young et al.,[65] with permission.)

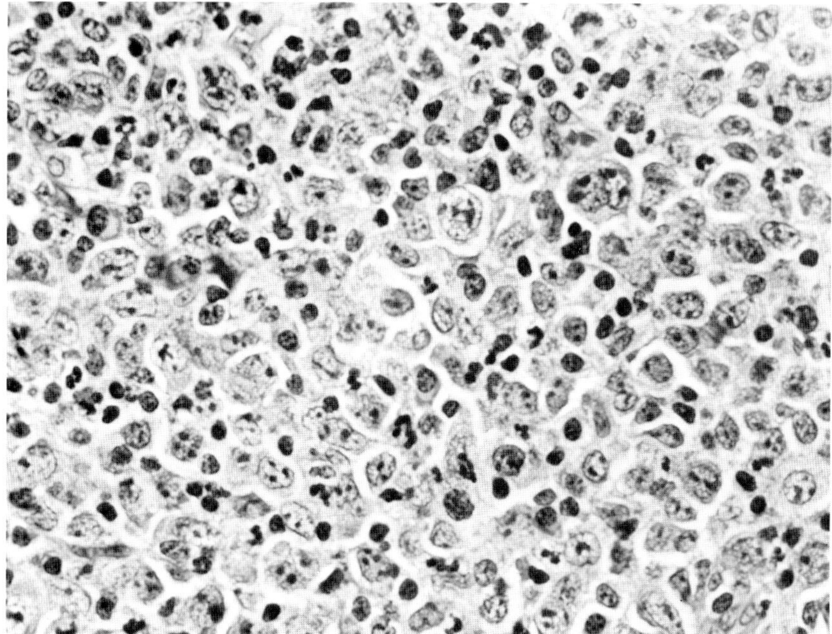

Fig. 1-51. Lymphoma-like lesion. Cervical biopsy showing sheet of large lymphoid cells with scattered plasma cells, small lymphocytes, and neutrophils. (From Young et al.,[65] with permission.)

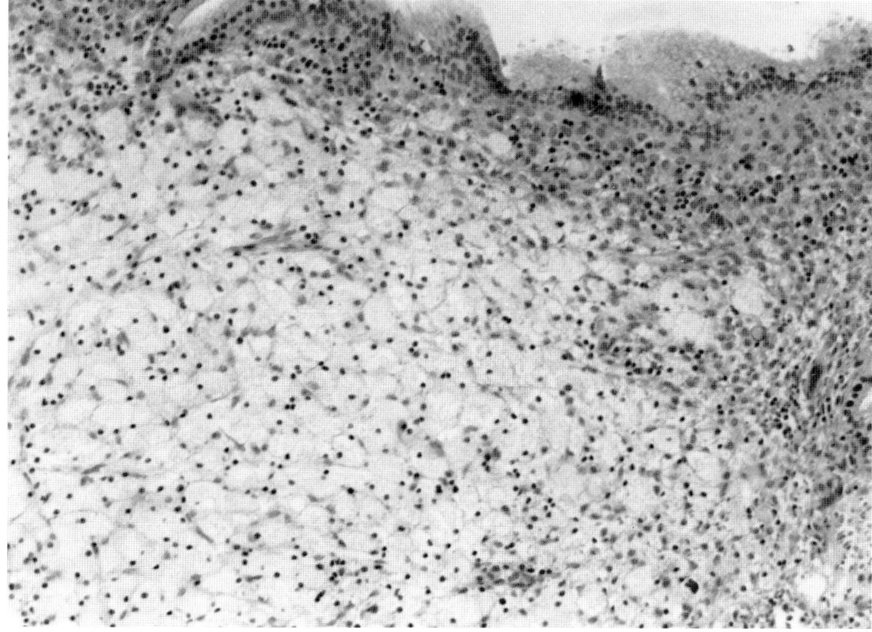

Fig. 1-52. Xanthogranulomatous endocervicitis. Numerous foamy histiocytes and scattered lymphocytes are present in the cervical stroma.

MALAKOPLAKIA AND HISTIOCYTIC CERVICITIS

Malakoplakia rarely involves the female reproductive system. Affected patients are typically but not exclusively postmenopausal. Rare examples of cervical involvement have been described, including some that have involved other sites and some that have recurred.[71–76] The gross and histologic appearances of the lesion, including the presence of diagnostic Michaelis-Guttman bodies, are similar to those seen elsewhere. We have also seen rare cases of florid cervicitis characterized by prominent numbers of foamy histiocytes (Fig. 1-52), analogous to xanthogranulomatous or histiocytic endometritis.

EOSINOPHILIC CERVICITIS

Although prominent numbers of eosinophils within the cervix most commonly represent a local inflammatory response to an invasive squamous cell carcinoma (see Ch. 2) or a glassy cell carcinoma (see Ch. 3), eosinophilic cervicitis may also occur as a tissue reaction to biopsy or curettage, or rarely, idiopathically. Of the 15 cases of uterine eosinophilia studied by Bjersing and Borglin,[77] 13 involved the cervix. All patients had had a cervical biopsy or curettage preceding the hysterectomy by 2 to 13 days (mean 4.7). The eosinophils were most frequently seen in the perivascular connective tissue within the cervical stroma. No clinical manifestations could be attributed to the eosinophilic infiltration. In another study, Divack and Janovski[78] found approximately 1 percent of unselected gynecologic specimens to contain striking tissue eosinophilia. Of 25 such cases, approximately one-third involved the cervix. Although the cases were not reported in detail, at least some of the patients had had prior biopsies performed within the previous 6 months. One of the patients, who had a history of asthma, also had a significant blood eosinophilia. Finally, d'Ablaing and Beck[79] reported a unique case of neonatal eosinophilic cervicitis. The 1,790-g infant died at 1 hour postpartum. Autopsy revealed, in addition to dysplastic kidneys and hypoplastic lungs, a well-demarcated reddish pink, 1-mm zone at the squamocolumnar junction of the cervix. Microscopic examination of this area revealed striking numbers of eosinophils within the cervical stroma associated with vascular congestion. No obvious cause for the eosinophilic infiltrate was found.

LIGNEOUS CERVICITIS

Ligneous cervicitis is a rare extraocular complication of ligneous conjunctivitis, an uncommon idiopathic form of membranous conjunctivitis that occurs predominantly, but not solely, in childhood and that is more common in females than in males.[80] Histologically, the lesions are characterized by the presence of subepithelial deposits of eosinophilic structureless material, often with overlying surface ulceration. There is characteristically little or no inflammatory infiltrate or reaction. The eosinophilic material often, but not invariably, stains positively for albumin, fibrin, and immunoglobulins but negatively for amyloid. Electron microscopic examination of the eosinophilic material shows electron-dense homogeneous and fibrillar material.[81] Blood vessels in the immediate vicinity of the lesion may show ultrastructural evidence of wide gaps between degenerate endothelial cells and an unusually thick multilaminar vascular basement membrane. The disease runs a chronic course with frequent recurrences, but spontaneous resolution sometimes occurs. The frequency of cervicovaginal involvement in cases of ligneous conjunctivitis is unknown, but in one review cervicovaginal lesions were present in almost 20 percent of female cases[80]; other rare examples have been described.[82, 83] The histologic appearances (Fig. 1-53) are identical to those seen in the conjunctiva.

STROMAL ENDOMETRIOSIS

Rarely, endometriosis is characterized by the exclusive, or almost exclusive, presence of endometriotic stroma; in our experience this process, so-called stromal endometriosis,[47] is seen disproportionately often in the uterine cervix. Six examples of this lesion in the cervix were recently reported in women aged 29 to 64 years. None of them had a history of pelvic endometriosis. Red lesions were noted on the ectocervical mucosa in three of the cases. Histologic examination in these cases shows well-circumscribed foci of closely packed cells resembling endometrial stromal cells, admixed with small blood vessels and extravasated erythrocytes within the superficial stroma of the cervix (Figs. 1-54 and 1-55). Apart from the absence or paucity of endometrial glands, the clinical and pathologic features of these lesions are similar to those of cases of typical superficial endometriosis of the cervix, as described earlier. However, in these cases of stromal endometriosis, the pure population of stromal cells may lead to confusion with malignant mesenchymal tumors, particularly low-grade endometrial stromal sarcomas, and because of the presence of many red blood cells, Kaposi's sarcoma. Awareness of this lesion, the absence of the characteristic growth pattern of an endometrial stromal sarcoma, and the presence of red blood cells between the stromal cells, rather than in preformed spaces, will facilitate the diagnosis.

POSTOPERATIVE SPINDLE CELL NODULE

In 1984, Proppe et al.[84] reported the clinical and pathologic features of 10 cases of a proliferative spindle cell lesion that devel-

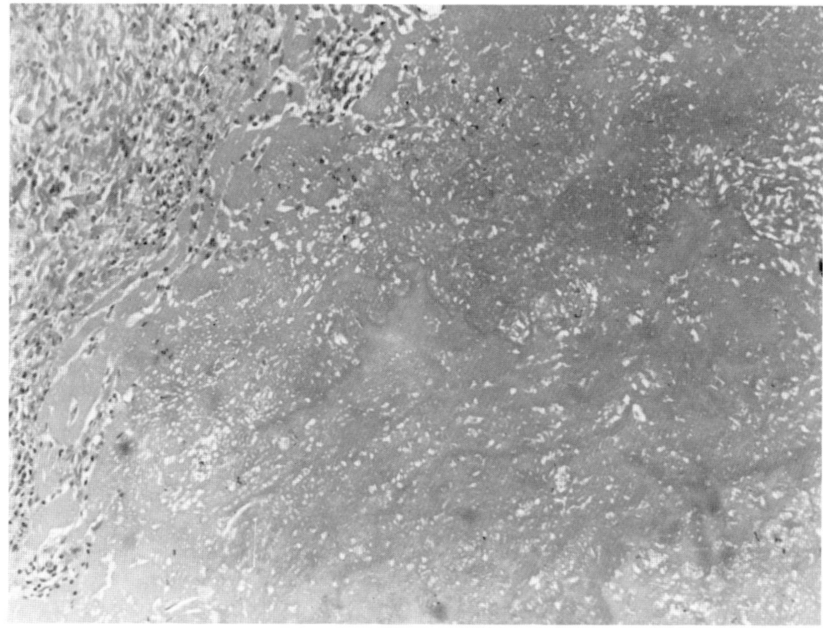

Fig. 1-53. Ligneous cervicitis. Amorphous material that was eosinophilic replaces the normal endocervical stroma. (Courtesy of Professor Harold Fox, Manchester, England.)

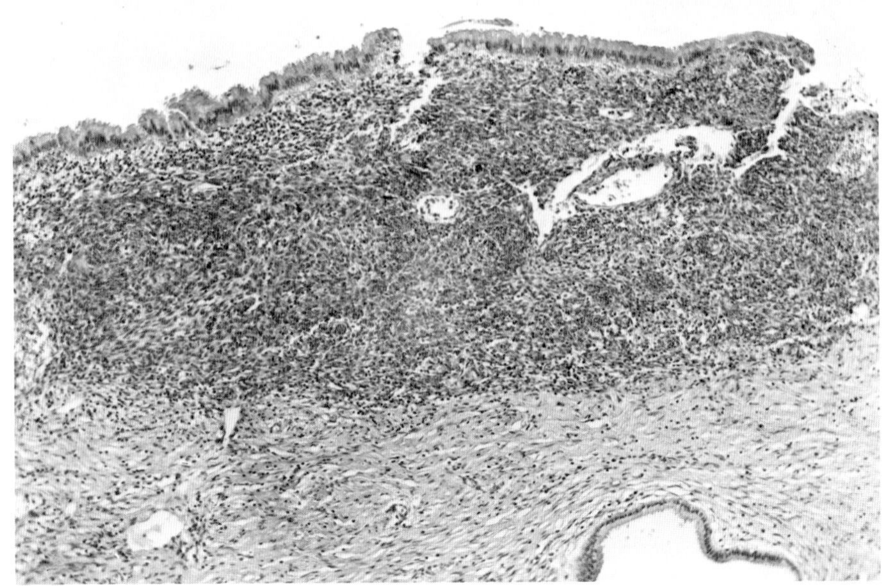

Fig. 1-54. Stromal endometriosis. A cellular bandlike proliferation is present in the superficial stroma.

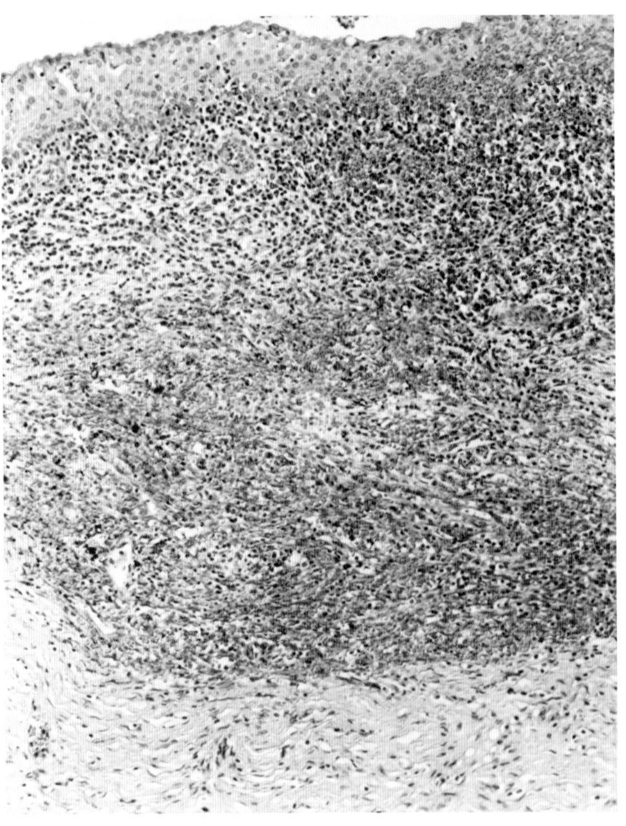

Fig. 1-55. Stromal endometriosis. Note the lack of endometrial glands.

oped shortly after an operation on the lower genitourinary tract, to which they applied the designation postoperative spindle cell nodule. The lesions resembled sarcomas (usually leiomyosarcomas) on microscopic examination and were initially often misdiagnosed as such. Subsequently, one example of this lesion has been described in the uterine cervix.[85] It occurred in a 74-year-old woman 2 weeks after an endometrial curettage had been performed.

FIBROEPITHELIAL POLYPS WITH STROMAL ATYPIA AND ATYPICAL STROMAL CELLS

In 1966 Norris and Taylor[86] drew attention to the occasional presence of atypical stromal cells within fibroepithelial polyps of the lower female genital tract, which on occasion caused the polyps to be misdiagnosed as sarcoma botryoides. Most of the polyps occur in the vagina, but occasionally they arise in the cervix.[87–89] They typically occur in women of reproductive age, who may be pregnant, but rarely they occur in children. The polyps, which may be asymptomatic or associated with postcoital bleeding, are usually 4 cm or less in greatest dimension but have occasionally been larger. Microscopic examination shows intact squamous epithelium overlying an edematous or myxoid stroma containing scattered mesenchymal cells, some of which have irregular, enlarged, hyperchromatic, and occasionally multiple or multilobed, nuclei, resembling reactive fibroblasts (Fig. 1-56). The cells have granular eosinophilic cytoplasm and delicately branched, sharply tapered cytoplasmic processes; cross-striations and longitudinal fibrils are absent. Although mitoses may be present, and even abnormal, they are usually few in number.

The major differential diagnosis in these cases is sarcoma botryoides (see Ch. 6), cervical examples of which occur in a similar age group as fibroepithelial polyps. The absence of a cambium layer is an important point of distinction from sarcoma botryoides, although a cambium layer in the latter may be only focal. Other important fea-

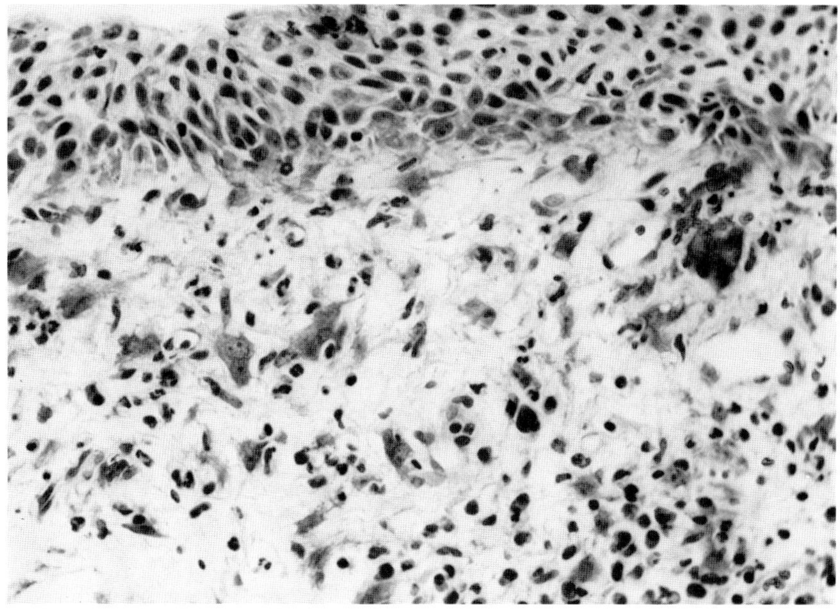

Fig. 1-56. Endocervical polyp with atypical stromal cells.

tures of sarcoma botryoides that are lacking in these polyps include the presence, at least focally, of closely packed mitotically active small cells with hyperchromatic nuclei, other cells with eosinophilic cytoplasm containing cross-striations, and invasion of the overlying squamous epithelium.

Occasionally, atypical cells similar to those seen in some fibroepithelial polyps are an incidental finding in the superficial stroma of the cervix.[90-92] In an autopsy study, these cells were found in the cervix alone in three and cervix and vagina in four of 205 cases.[92] In the cervix, the cells were confined to the ectocervix, something previously noted by one of us.[91] These cells have generally been considered of fibroblastic or myofibroblastic type, but evidence for a Schwann cell origin has been presented in one recent case.[93]

ECTOPIC DECIDUA

A cervical decidual reaction was detected on histologic examination of 36 percent of antepartum cervical biopsies in one study[94] and in 31 percent of gravid hysterectomy specimens in another.[95] The decidual cells resemble eutopic decidua and are usually confined to microscopic foci within the loose subepithelial cervical stroma (Fig. 1-57) or within the stroma of endocervical polyps.[94-102] Attenuation, erosion, or ulceration of the overlying epithelium is common. The decidual cells typically disappear by the eighth postpartum week.[94]

Rare cases of a florid decidual reaction within the cervix have taken the form of grossly visible masses during any trimester of pregnancy; some cases have been associated with antepartum bleeding.[101] Pelvic examination has revealed a polypoid, nodular, or ulcerating mass, up to 6 cm, that may mimic a malignant tumor. Histologic examination of a biopsy specimen has generally provided the correct diagnosis, but in occa-

sional cases, focal atypia of the decidual cells has resulted in diagnoses of carcinoma[100] or malignant lymphoma.[102] The mitotic inactivity and bland nuclear features of most of the decidual cells, however, should facilitate distinction from a neoplasm.

MELANOTIC LESIONS

The endocervix is the most common noncutaneous site for the blue nevus (Fig. 1-58). Until recently only approximately 50 cases had been described[103, 104] but a study from Japan in which step sections of the cervix were obtained documented what those authors preferred to call "stromal melanocytic foci" in 54 of 189 cases (28.6 percent).[105] Endocervical blue nevi are almost always an incidental gross or microscopic finding within hysterectomy or cervical biopsy specimens of adults. If seen grossly (none was in the large series from Japan), one or occasionally several, flat, blue to black, ill-defined lesions involve the endocervical mucosa. In the study from Japan noted above, 53.7 percent of the lesions involved the anterior wall, 11.1 percent the posterior wall, and 35.2 percent both walls.[105] The lesions usually do not exceed 4 mm in diameter, but two examples measured 1.5 and 2.0 cm, respectively.[103] The histologic appearance resembles that of cutaneous blue nevi, consisting of melanin-laden polygonal and spindle cells with dendritic processes, arranged in irregular clusters within the superficial endocervical stroma. The cells are argyrophilic, argentaffinic, and immunoreactive for S-100 protein.[103] Little difficulty should be encountered in distinguishing blue nevi from malignant melanoma, as the former lacks the epithelial pigmentation, junctional activity, and malignant cytologic features of the latter. One unique case with the histologic features of a cellular blue nevus has

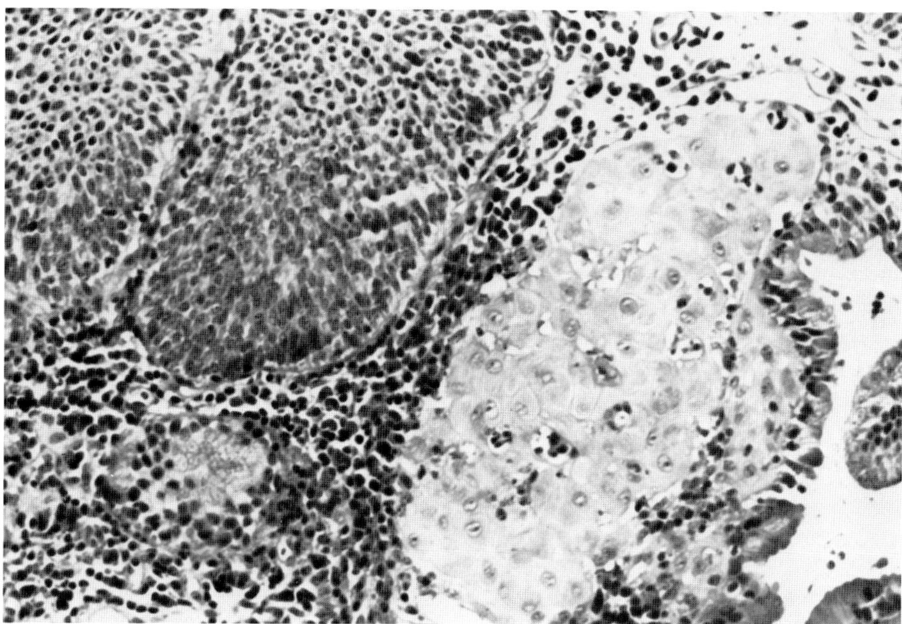

Fig. 1-57. Ectopic decidua. A nest of typical decidual cells lies in the superficial cervical stroma of a patient with severe squamous dysplasia.

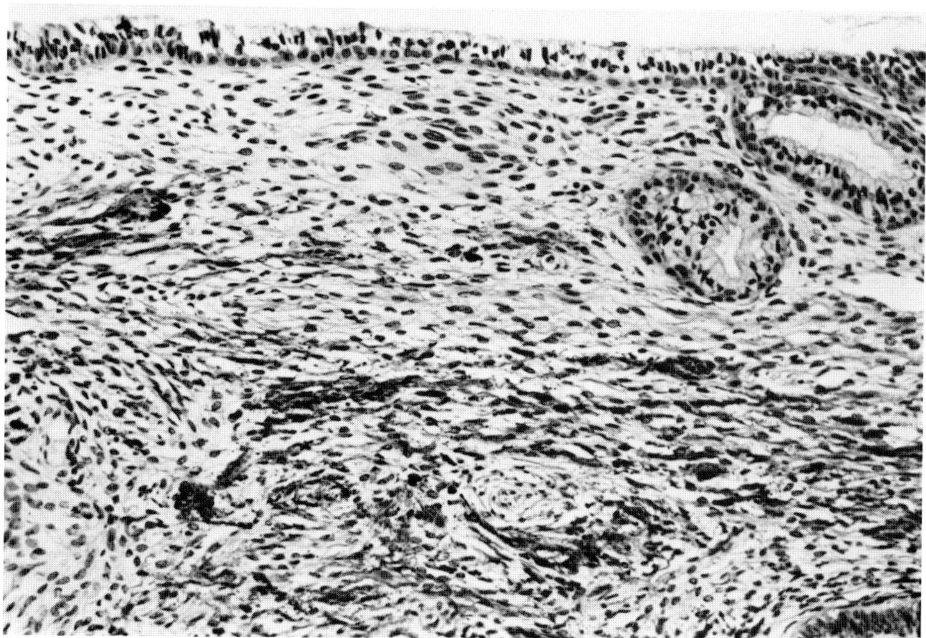

Fig. 1-58. Blue nevus of endocervix. (From Young and Clement,[3] with permission.)

been described that involved the cervix, vagina, and hymenal ring in a 19-year-old black woman.[106]

Five examples of benign melanotic pigmentation ("melanosis") of the squamous epithelium of the cervix (four cases),[107–110] or cervix and vagina (one case),[111] have been described. Irregular areas of mucosal pigmentation are typically seen on clinical examination, although some examples have been recognized only histologically. Microscopic examination typically demonstrates a proliferation of benign melanocytes within the basal layer, as well as melanin pigmentation of the basal cells. In one cervical case,[107] the melanocytic proliferation was associated with elongated rete pegs, the lesion resembling benign cutaneous lentigo.

MISCELLANEOUS RARE LESIONS

Noninfectious granulomas of the iatrogenic type, histologically resembling rheumatoid nodules, have been described in the cervix as a postoperative reaction.[112, 113] They are similar microscopically to the lesions described in other sites, for example, within the uterine corpus (see Ch. 4) and the prostate gland. Sarcoidosis rarely involves the uterine cervix.[114] Cases of ectopic tissue involving the cervix are rare, but occasional examples of sebaceous glands[115–116a] (Fig. 1-59) and hair follicles[97, 116a] have been described at this site. We have recently seen a unique case in which a cervical mass was composed of tissue that on routine microscopy resembled prostate gland tissue and stained immunohistochemically for prostate-specific antigen and prostate-specific acid phosphatase.

In addition to the Arias-Stella reaction and ectopic decidua, changes related to pregnancy may be seen in the uterine cervix. For example, occasional examples of placental site nodule (see Ch. 9) have been encountered at this location, usually in the endocervix, and rarely a cervical pregnancy may mimic a tumor on gross inspec-

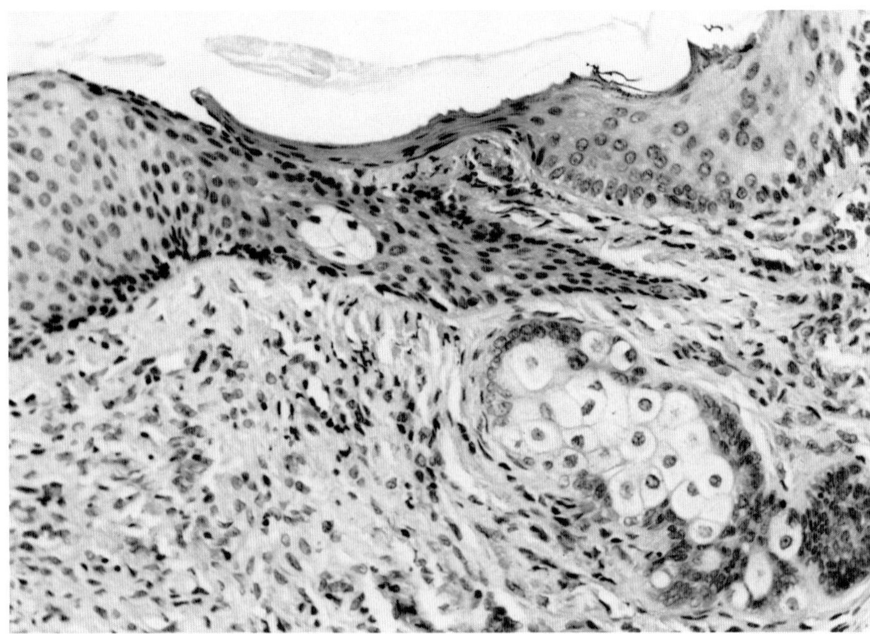

Fig. 1-59. Nests of sebaceous cells in superficial cervical stroma with smaller nest in epithelium.

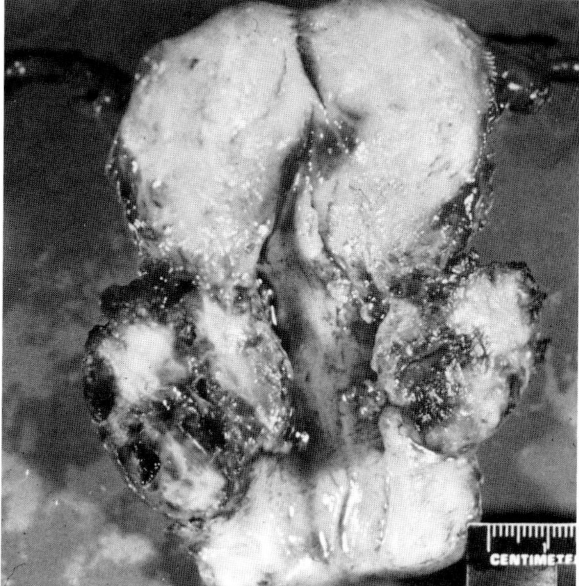

Fig. 1-60. Ectopic pregnancy in cervix, forming a tumorlike mass.

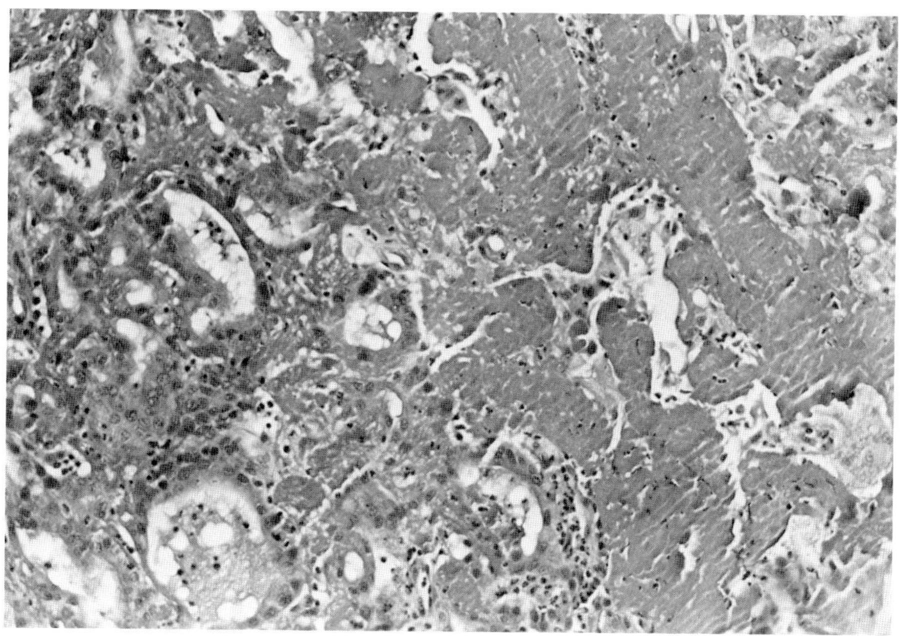

Fig. 1-61. Amyloidosis of cervix. Dense material that was eosinophilic is present in the stroma admixed with glands of microglandular hyperplasia (left).

tion as in the striking example illustrated in Figure 1-60.

Histologic changes in the cervix can be induced by the topical application of Lugol's and Monsel's solutions. Benda et al.[117] have described artifactual changes in cervical squamous epithelium associated with the use of strong iodine (Lugol's) solution in cone biopsy specimens. The changes are most pronounced in dysplastic cells and include cellular shrinkage, cytoplasmic eosinophilia and vacuolization, the development of visible intercellular spaces, and nuclear pyknosis with loss of chromatin detail. Monsel's solution (ferric subsulfate), a topical hemostatic agent, can cause tissue necrosis in the cervix that can persist for 2 weeks and impede re-epithelialization.[118] Granulation tissue in the healing phase contains iron pigment, residue from the agent that can encrust on collagen and be present in macrophages for as long as 3 months. A foreign-body giant cell can occasionally be encountered. In addition, a case of ceroid granuloma of the cervix has recently been described.[119] Finally, although it appears to be rare, based on the literature, we have recently seen a case of a patient with widespread amyloidosis, which included prominent involvement of a cervical biopsy[120] (Fig. 1-61).

REFERENCES

1. Young RH, Clement PB: Pseudoneoplastic glandular lesions of the uterine cervix. Semin Diagn Pathol 8:234, 1991
2. Michael H, Grawe L, Kraus FT: Minimal deviation endocervical adenocarcinoma: clinical and histologic features, immunohistochemical staining for carcinoembryonic antigen, and differentiation from confusing benign lesions. Int J Gynecol Pathol 3:261, 1984
3. Young RH, Clement PB: Pseudoneoplastic lesions of the lower female genital tract. Pathol Annu 24(2):189, 1989
4. Young RH, Scully RE: Cervical papillary adenocarcinoma of villoglandular type: A clinicopathological analysis of 13 cases. Cancer 63:1773, 1989
5. Fluhmann CF: Focal hyperplasia (tunnel clusters) of the cervix uteri. Obstet Gynecol 17:206, 1961
6. Fluhmann CF: The Cervix Uteri and Its Diseases. WB Saunders, Philadelphia, 1961, pp. 95–100
7. Segal GH, Hart WR: Cystic endocervical tunnel clusters. A clinicopathologic study of 29 cases of so-called adenomatous hyperplasia. Am J Surg Pathol 14:895, 1990
8. Avery DM, Alexander CB, Gore H: Adenomatous endocervical hyperplasia resulting in myxometra. Am J Obstet Gynecol 148:827, 1984
9. Gilks CB, Young RH, Aguirre P et al: Adenoma malignum (minimal deviation adenocarcinoma) of the uterine cervix: a clinicopathological and immunohistochemical analysis of 26 cases. Am J Surg Pathol 13:717, 1989
10. Sherrer CW, Parmley T, Woodruff JD: Adenomatous hyperplasia of the endocervix. Obstet Gynecol 49:65, 1977
11. Fetissof F, Berger G, Dubois MP et al: Female genital tract and Peutz-Jeghers syndrome: an immunohistochemical study. Int J Gynecol Pathol 4:219, 1985
12. Anderson MC, Hartley RB: Cervical crypt involvement by intraepithelial neoplasia. Obstet Gynecol 55:546, 1980
13. Teshima S, Shimosato Y, Kishi K et al: Early stage adenocarcinoma of the uterine cervix. Histopathologic analysis with consideration of histogenesis. Cancer 56:167, 1985
14. Noda K, Kimura K, Ikeda M, Teshima K: Studies on the histogenesis of cervical adenocarcinoma. Int J Gynecol Pathol 1:336, 1983
15. Clement PB, Young RH: Deep Nabothian cysts of the endocervix. A possible source of confusion with minimal-deviation adenocarcinoma (adenoma malignum). Int J Gynecol Pathol 8:340, 1989
16. Taylor HB, Ivey NS, Norris HJ: Atypical endocervical hyperplasia in women taking oral contraceptives. JAMA 202:185, 1967
17. Kyriakos M, Kempson RL, Konikov NF: A clinical and pathologic study of endocer-

vical lesions associated with oral contraceptives. Cancer 22:99, 1968

18. Candy MD, Abell MR: Progestogen-induced adenomatous hyperplasia of the uterine cervix. JAMA 203:323, 1968

19. Govan ADT, Black WP, Sharp JL: Aberrant glandular polypi of the uterine cervix associated with contraceptive pills: pathology and pathogenesis. J Clin Pathol 22:84, 1969

20. Nichols TM, Fidler HK: Microglandular hyperplasia in cervical cone biopsies taken for suspicious and positive cytology. Am J Clin Pathol 56:424, 1971

21. Wilkinson E, Dufour DR: Pathogenesis of microglandular hyperplasia of the cervix uteri. Obstet Gynecol 47:189, 1976

22. Leslie KO, Silverberg SG: Microglandular hyperplasia of the cervix: unusual clinical and pathological presentations and their differential diagnosis. Prog Surg Pathol 5:95, 1984

23. Chumas JC, Nelson B, Mann WJ et al: Microglandular hyperplasia of the uterine cervix. Obstet Gynecol 66:406, 1985

24. Brown LJR, Wells M: Cervical glandular atypia associated with squamous intraepithelial neoplasia: a premalignant lesion? J Clin Pathol 39:22, 1986

25. Young RH, Scully RE: Atypical forms of microglandular hyperplasia of the cervix simulating carcinoma: a report of five cases and review of the literature. Am J Surg Pathol 13:50, 1989

26. Young RH, Scully RE: Uterine carcinomas simulating microglandular hyperplasia. A report of six cases. Am J Surg Pathol 16:1092, 1992

27. Steeper TA, Wick MR: Minimal deviation adenocarcinoma of the uterine cervix ("adenoma malignum"). An immunohistochemical comparison with microglandular endocervical hyperplasia and conventional endocervical adenocarcinoma. Cancer 58:1131, 1986

28. Speers WC, Picaso LG, Silverberg SG: Immunohistochemical localization of carcinoembryonic antigen in microglandular hyperplasia and adenocarcinoma of the endocervix. Am J Clin Pathol 79:105, 1983

29. Dabbs DJ, Geisinger KR, Norris HT: Intermediate filaments in endometrial and endocervical carcinomas. The diagnostic utility of vimentin patterns. Am J Surg Pathol 10:568, 1986

30. Wahlstrom T, Lindgren J, Korhonen M, Seppala M: Distinction between endocervical and endometrial adenocarcinoma with immuno-peroxidase staining of carcinoembryonic antigen in routine histological tissue specimens. Lancet 2:1159, 1979

31. Lang G, Dallenbach-Hellweg G: The histogenetic origin of cervical mesonephric hyperplasia and mesonephric adenocarcinoma of the uterine cervix studies with immunohistochemical methods. Int J Gynecol Pathol 9:145, 1990

32. Kudo R, Sasano H, Koizumi M et al: Immunohistochemical comparison of new monoclonal antibody 1C5 and carcinoembryonic antigen in the differential diagnosis of adenocarcinoma of the uterine cervix. Int J Gynecol Pathol 9:325, 1990

33. Ferry JA, Scully RE: Mesonephric remnants, hyperplasia and neoplasia in the uterine cervix: a study of 49 cases. Am J Surg Pathol 14:1100, 1990

34. Jones MA, Young RH, Scully RE: Diffuse laminar endocervical glandular hyperplasia: a report of seven cases. Am J Surg Pathol 15:1123, 1991

35. Clement PB, Young RH: Endocervicosis of the urinary bladder. A report of six cases of a benign müllerian lesion that may mimic adenocarcinoma. Am J Surg Pathol 16:533, 1992.

36. Suh K-S, Silverberg SG: Tubal metaplasia of the uterine cervix. Int J Gynecol Pathol 9:122, 1990

37. Pacey F, Ayer B, Greenberg M: The cytologic diagnosis of adenocarcinoma in situ of the cervix uteri and related lesions. III. Pitfalls in diagnosis. Acta Cytol 32:325, 1988

38. Novotny DB, Maygarden JJ, Johnson DE, Frable WJ: Tubal metaplasia. A frequent potential pitfall in the cytologic diagnosis of endocervical glandular dysplasia on cervical smears. Acta Cytol 36:1, 1992

39. Jonasson JG, Wang HH, Antonioli DA, Ducatman BS: Tubal metaplasia of the uterine cervix: a prevalence study in patients with gynecologic pathologic findings. Int J Gynecol Pathol 11:89, 1992

40. Ismail SM: Cone biopsy causes cervical endometriosis and tubo-endometrioid metaplasia. Histopathology 18:107, 1991
41. Trowell JE: Intestinal metaplasia with argentaffin cells in the uterine cervix. Histopathology 9:551, 1985
42. Gloor E, Hurlimann J: Cervical intraepithelial glandular neoplasia (adenocarcinoma in situ and glandular dysplasia). A correlative study of 23 cases with histologic grading, histochemical analysis of mucins, and immunohistochemical determination of the affinity for four lectins. Cancer 58:1272, 1986
43. Michael H, Sutton G, Hull MT, Roth LM: Villous adenoma of the uterine cervix associated with invasive adenocarcinoma: a histologic, ultrastructural, and immunohistochemical study. Int J Gynecol Pathol 5:163, 1986
44. Fox H, Wells M, Harris M et al: Enteric tumours of the lower female genital tract: a report of three cases. Histopathology 12:167, 1988
45. Lee KR, Trainer TD: Adenocarcinoma of the uterine cervix of small intestinal type containing numerous Paneth cells. Arch Pathol Lab Med 114:731, 1990
46. Clement PB: Pathology of endometriosis. Pathol Annu 25(1):245, 1990
47. Clement PB, Young RH, Scully RE: Stromal endometriosis of the uterine cervix: a variant of endometriosis that may simulate a sarcoma. Am J Surg Pathol 14:449, 1990
48. Veiga-Ferreira MM, Leiman G, Dunbar F, Margolius KA: Cervical endometriosis: facilitated diagnosis by fine needle aspiration cytologic testing. Am J Obstet Gynecol 157:849, 1987
49. Schneider V: Arias-Stella reaction of the endocervix. Frequency and location. Acta Cytol 25:224, 1981
50. Clement PB, Young RH, Scully RE: Nontrophoblastic pathology of the female genital tract and peritoneum associated with pregnancy. Semin Diagn Pathol 6:372, 1989
51. Cariani DJ, Guderian AM: Gestational atypia in endocervical polyps—the Arias-Stella reaction. Am J Obstet Gynecol 95:589, 1966
52. Cove H: The Arias-Stella reaction occurring in the endocervix in pregnancy. Recognition and comparison with adenocarcinoma of the endocervix. Am J Surg Pathol 3:567, 1979
53. Brown S, Senekjian EK, Montag AG: Cytomegalovirus infection of the uterine cervix in a patient with acquired immunodeficiency syndrome. Obstet Gynecol 71:489, 1988
54. Josey WE, Nahmias AJ, Naib ZM: Viral and virus-like infections of the female genital tract. Clin Obstet Gynecol 12:161, 1969
55. Packer H, Turner HB, Ducaney AD: Granuloma inguinale of the vagina and uterine cervix with bone metastases. JAMA 136:326, 1948
56. Slavin G: The pathology of cervical inflammatory disease. p. 251. In Jordan JA, Singer A (eds): The Cervix. WB Saunders, Philadelphia, 1976
57. Kraus FT: Irradiation changes in the uterus. p. 457. In Norris HJ, Hertig AT (eds): The Uterus. Williams & Wilkins, Baltimore, 1973
58. Willis RA: Pathology of Tumours. p. 526. CV Mosby, St. Louis, 1948
59. Barua R: Post-cone biopsy traumatic neuroma of the uterine cervix. Arch Pathol Lab Med 113:945, 1989
60. Munsick RA, Janovski NA: Walthard cell rest of the cervix uteri. Report of a case. Am J Obstet Gynecol 82:909, 1961
61. Fetissof F, Dubois MP, Heitz PU et al: Endocrine cells in the female genital tract. Int J Gynecol Pathol 5:75, 1986
62. Fetissof F, Arbeille B, Boivin F et al: Endocrine cells in ectocervical epithelium. An immunohistochemical and ultrastructural analysis. Virchows Arch [A] 411:293, 1987
63. Fetissof F, Serres G, Arbeille B et al: Argyrophilic cells and ectocervical epithelium. Int J Gynecol Pathol 10:177, 1991
64. Miller N, Bedard YC, Cooter NB, Shaul DL: Histologic changes in the genital tract in transsexual women following androgen therapy. Histopathology 10:661, 1986
65. Young RH, Harris NL, Scully RE: Lymphoma-like lesions of the lower female genital tract. A report of 16 cases. Int J Gynecol Pathol 4:289, 1985
66. Harris NL, Scully RE: Malignant lym-

phoma and granulocytic sarcoma of the uterus and vagina. A clinicopathologic analysis of twenty-seven cases. Cancer 53:2530, 1984

67. Hare MJ, Toone E, Taylor-Robinson D et al: Follicular cervicitis—colposcopic appearances and association with Chlamydia trachomatis. Br J Obstet Gynaecol 88:174, 1981

68. Winkler B, Crum CP: Chlamydia trachomatis infection of the female genital tract. Pathogenic and clinicopathologic correlations. Pathol Annu 22(1):193, 1987

69. Paavonen J, Vesterinen E, Meyer B, Saksela E: Colposcopic and histologic findings in cervical chlamydial infection. Obstet Gynecol 59:712, 1982

70. Qizilbash AH: Chronic plasma cell cervicitis. A rare pitfall in gynecological cytology. Acta Cytol 18:198, 1974

71. Chalvardjian A, Picard L, Shaw R et al: Malakoplakia of the female genital tract. Am J Obstet Gynecol 138:391, 1980

72. Wahl RW: Malakoplakia of the uterine cervix. Report of two cases. Acta Cytol 26:691, 1982

73. Willen R, Stendahl U, Willen H, Trope C: Malacoplakia of the cervix and corpus uteri: a light microscopic, electron microscopic, and X-Ray microprobe analysis of a case. Int J Gynecol Pathol 2:201, 1983

74. Chen KTK, Hendricks EJ: Malakoplakia of the female genital tract. Obstet Gynecol 65:84S, 1985

75. Falcon-Escobedo R, Mora-Tiscareno A, Pueblitz-Peredo S: Malacoplakia of the uterine cervix. Histologic, cytologic and ultrastructural study of a case. Acta Cytol 30:281, 1986

76. Bose S, Vijayaraghavan M, Chopra P: Malakoplakia of the female genital tract. Indian J Pathol Microbiol 33:193, 1990

77. Bjersing L, Borglin NE: Eosinophilia in the myometrium of the human uterus. Acta Pathol 54:353, 1962

78. Divack DM, Janovski NA: Eosinophilia encountered in female genital organs. Am J Obstet Gynecol 84:761, 1962

79. D'Ablaing G, Beck M: Congenital neonatal eosinophilic cervicitis. Am J Obstet Gynecol 129:345, 1977

80. Hidayat AA, Riddle PJ: Ligneous conjunctivitis: A clinicopathologic study of 17 cases. Ophthalmology 94:949, 1987

81. Kanai K, Polack FM: Histologic and electron microscope studies of ligneous conjunctivitis. Am J Ophthalmol 72:909, 1971

82. Rubin A, Buck D, Macdonald MR: Ligneous conjunctivitis involving the cervix: case report. Br J Obstet Gynaecol 96:1228, 1989

83. Lee CS, Scurry J, Fortune DN, Rode J: Ligneous (pseudomembranous) inflammation of the upper female genital tract. Pathology 24:8, 1992

84. Proppe KH, Scully RE, Rosai J: Postoperative spindle cell nodules of genitourinary tract resembling sarcomas. A report of eight cases. Am J Surg Pathol 8:101, 1984

85. Kay S, Schneider V: Reactive spindle cell nodule of the endocervix simulating uterine sarcoma. Int J Gynecol Pathol 4:255, 1985

86. Norris HJ, Taylor HB: Polyps of the vagina. A benign lesion resembling sarcoma botryoides. Cancer 19:227, 1966

87. Elliott GB, Reynolds HA, Fidler HK: Pseudo-sarcoma botryoides of cervix and vagina in pregnancy. J Obstet Gynaecol Br Commonw 74:728, 1967

88. Tobon H, McIntyre-Seltman K, Rubino M: "Polyposis vaginalis" of pregnancy. Arch Pathol Lab Med 113:1391, 1989

89. Cachaza JA, Caballero JJL, Fernandez JA, Salido E: Endocervical polyp with pseudo-sarcomatous pattern and cytoplasmic inclusions: an electron microscopic study. Am J Clin Pathol 85:633, 1986

90. Elliott GB, Elliott JDA: Superficial stromal reactions of lower genital tract. Arch Pathol 95:100, 1973

91. Clement PB: Multinucleated stromal giant cells of the uterine cervix. Arch Pathol Lab Med 109:200, 1985

92. Abdul-Karim FW, Cohen RE: Atypical stromal cells of lower female genital tract. Histopathology 17:249, 1990

93. Metze K, de Angelo Andrade LAL: Atypical stromal giant cells of cervix uteri-evidence of schwann cell origin. Pathol Res Pract 187:1031, 1991

94. Johnson LD: Dysplasia and carcinoma in situ in pregnancy. p. 382. In Norris HJ,

Hertig AT (eds): The Uterus. Williams & Wilkins, Baltimore, 1973

95. Schneider V, Barnes LA: Ectopic decidual reaction of the uterine cervix. Frequency and cytologic presentation. Acta Cytol 25:616, 1981

96. Bowles HE, Tilden IL: Decidual reactions of the cervix. West J Surg Obstet Gynecol 59:168, 1951

97. Linhartova A: Unusual lesions of the uterine cervix. Int J Gynecol Obstet 10:34, 1972

98. Hennessy JP: Unusual decidual reaction of the cervix. Am J Obstet Gynecol 46:570, 1943

99. Klein J, Domeier LH: An unusual decidual reaction in the cervix. Am J Obstet Gynecol 51:423, 1946

100. Lapan B: Deciduosis of the cervix and vagina simulating carcinoma. Am J Obstet Gynecol 58:743, 1949

101. Orr CJB, Pedlow PRB: Deciduosis of the cervix manifesting as antepartum hemorrhage and simulating carcinoma. Am J Obstet Gynecol 82:884, 1961

102. Armenia CS, Shaver DN, Modisher MW: Decidual transformation of the cervical stroma simulating reticulum cell sarcoma. Am J Obstet Gynecol 89:808, 1964

103. Patel DS, Bhagavan BS: Blue nevus of the uterine cervix. Hum Pathol 16:79, 1985

104. Casadei GP, Grigolato P, Cabibbo E: Blue nevus of the endocervix. A study of five cases. Tumori 73:75, 1987

105. Uehara T, Izumo T, Kishi K, Takayama S, Kasuga T: Stromal melanocytic foci ("blue nevus") in step sections of the uterine cervix. Acta Pathol Jpn 41:751, 1991

106. Rodriguez HA, Ackerman LV: Cellular blue nevus. Clinicopathologic study of forty-five cases. Cancer 21:393, 1968

107. Schneider V, Zimberg S, Kay S: The pigmented portio: benign lentigo of the uterine cervix. Diagn Gynecol Obstet 3:269, 1981

108. Deppisch LM: Cervical melanosis. Obstet Gynecol 62:525, 1983

109. Dundore W, Lamas C: Benign nevus (ephelis) of the uterine cervix. Am J Obstet Gynecol 152:881, 1985

110. Barter JF, Mazur M, Holloway RW, Hatch KD: Melanosis of the cervix. Gynecol Oncol 29:101, 1988

111. Tsukuda Y: Benign melanosis of the vagina and cervix. Am J Obstet Gynecol 124:211, 1976

112. Christie AJ, Krieger HA: Indolent necrotizing granulomas of the uterine cervix, possibly related to chlamydial infection. Am J Obstet Gynecol 136:958, 1980

113. Evans CS, Goldman RL, Klein HZ, Kohout ND: Necrobiotic granulomas of the uterine cervix. A probable postoperative reaction. Am J Surg Pathol 8:841, 1984

114. Tsou E, Romano MC, Kerwin DM et al: Sarcoidosis of anterior mediastinal nodes, pancreas, and uterine cervix: three unusual sites in the same patient. Am Rev Respir Dis 122:333, 1980

115. Ehrmann RL: Sebaceous metaplasia of the human cervix. Am J Obstet Gynecol 105:1284, 1969

116. Watson AA, Cochran AJ: Sebaceous glands of the cervix uteri and buccal mucosa. J Pathol 98:87, 1968

116a. Robledo MC, Vasquez JJ, Contreras-Mejuto F, Lopez-Garcia G: Subaceous glands and hair follicles in the cervix uteri. Histopathology 21:278, 1992

117. Benda JA, Lamoreaux J, Johnson SR: Artifact associated with the use of strong iodine solution (Lugol's) in cone biopsies. Am J Surg Pathol 11:367, 1987

118. David JR, Steinbronn KK, Graham AR, Dawson BV: Effects of Monsel's solution in uterine cervix. Am J Clin Pathol 82:332, 1984

119. Al-Nafussi AI, Hughes D, Rebello G: Ceroid granuloma of the uterine cervix. Histopathology 21:282, 1992

120. Copeland W, Hawley PC, Teteris NJ: Gynecological amyloidosis. Am J Obstet Gynecol 153:555, 1985

2

Papillomavirus-Related Changes and Premalignant and Malignant Squamous Lesions of the Uterine Cervix

Christopher P. Crum

This chapter addresses recent advances in two broad areas of the field of cervical neoplasia. The first is genital human papillomaviruses (HPV), their relationship to squamous neoplasia, and their role in the classification of squamous precursor lesions in the uterine cervix. The second is the diagnosis of invasive squamous neoplasia, including microinvasive squamous cell carcinoma and the recognition of a variety of subsets of cervical squamous cell carcinoma. Changes in our understanding of the former have been due in part to the evolution of molecular biology and related technologies that have rapidly altered our perception of the pathogenesis and therapeutic approach to intraepithelial squamous lesions of the lower female genital tract. This technology can be applied on several different levels, resulting in changes in knowledge of basic disease processes at one extreme to promises of tests that will alter therapy on the other. This chapter reviews existing information in this field and addresses the following issues: (1) an overview of HPV and cervical neoplasia, (2) the morphologic basis for papillomavirus-related changes and their relationship to molecular biology, (3) the practical histologic and cytologic diagnosis based upon the above, followed by (4) approaches to excluding invasion, including the interpretation of the endocervical curettage and early (microinvasive) invasive carcinoma, and (5) the differential diagnosis of invasive squamous carcinoma of the cervix.

PREMALIGNANT LESIONS

OVERVIEW AND RELATIONSHIP TO PAPILLOMAVIRUSES

Each year in the United States, approximately 3 percent of young women develop an HPV-related cervical abnormality; approximately 1 million women are treated for genital warts annually in this country.[1, 2] The major risk factor for cervical cancer is number of sexual partners, with number of partners for the male consort, age at first intercourse, parity, smoking, barrier contraception, immune status, low socioeconomic status, and, possibly, oral contraceptive use also being associated.[3–8] Nonwhites have a two- to threefold higher incidence and mortality from cervical cancer.[9]

Predictably, the above risk factors are associated with both the risk of cancer and the acquisition of cervical precancers and genital warts, although the link between parity and cervical intraepithelial neoplasia (CIN) is less clear.[10] The factors influencing the acquisition of "occult" HPV infection (in the form of HPV DNA only in the absence of cytologic or clinical evidence of disease) appear similar, based on recent

51

studies using polymerase chain reaction analysis.[11] The precise relationship between the prevalence of HPV DNA in the population and cancer risk remains to be determined.[6]

The techniques used to detect HPV include Southern blot hybridization, dot or slot-blot hybridization, in situ hybridization, and the polymerase chain reaction (PCR).[5, 12–14] The first two techniques analyze cellular DNA that has been bound to nitrocellulose membranes using radioactive HPV DNA probes. In situ hybridization involves the detection of the HPV nucleic acids in a tissue section by visualizing a reagent that marks the site of the HPV (Fig. 2-1). The PCR makes it possible to amplify the target HPV DNA about a 100,000-fold in vitro prior to binding the DNA to a membrane and performing hybridization.[14, 15] Hence, this technique is the most sensitive, albeit the most susceptible to false-positive results, because of contamination of samples. A recent adaptation of both PCR and in situ hybridization has facilitated the detection of nucleic acids in individual cells with a high degree of sensitivity.[16] Using these techniques, investigators have been able to define not only the distribution of HPV nucleic acids in cervical lesions but also profile populations harboring HPV

DNA. In population studies, the frequency of HPV DNA detection by the most sensitive technique—PCR—is approximately 30 percent.[11]

More than 60 human papillomaviruses have been identified; the types most commonly associated with genital disease are summarized in Table 2-1.[17] In-depth studies of these viruses have demonstrated a variety of mechanisms by which cancer-associated viruses may exert their influence over the host cells. Three of the most interesting mechanisms include (1) expression of critical viral oncogenes (E6 and E7) that alter the function of host tumor suppressor genes (Rb and P53)[18, 19]; (2) integration of the virus into the host chromosome, which most commonly occurs in cancers and is preferentially associated with those HPV types[18] associated with cancers[20–24]; and (3) alterations in regulation of viral expression, such as influenced by the viral transcriptional (upstream) regulatory region (URR).[25] Such alterations may be of substantial importance in view of the fact that so-called low-risk papillomaviruses may contain genomic alterations that increase their risk of association with invasive cancers.[26]

One of the unresolved issues in papillomavirus research is the significance of occult or latent HPV. Although a multitude of

Table 2-1. Genital Papillomavirus Types

Type	Isolated From	Associated Primarily With
6, 11	Condyloma Laryngeal papilloma	Condylomata (vulva, cervix)
16	Cervical carcinoma	HSIL, cervical carcinoma
18	Cervical carcinoma	Cervical squamous, adenocarcinomas, and small cell carcinomas
30	Laryngeal carcinoma	SIL
31	Cervical SIL	HSIL, cervical carcinoma
33	Cervical carcinoma	HSIL, cervical carcinoma
34	Cutaneous Bowen's disease	SIL
35	Cervical adenocarcinoma	HSIL, cervical carcinoma
39, 40	Penile SIL	SIL, cervical carcinoma
42–44	Vulvar papilloma	LSIL, normal mucosa
45, 51, 52, 56	Cervical SIL	SIL, cervical carcinoma

Abbreviations: SIL, squamous intraepithelial lesion (not otherwise specified); LSIL, low-grade squamous intraepithelial lesion; HSIL, high-grade squamous intraepithelial lesion. (From de Villiers,[17] with permission.)

Fig. 2-1. Distribution of human papillomavirus type 16 (HPV 16) mRNA and capsid proteins in a high-grade squamous intraepithelial lesion (HSIL) of the cervix. **(A)** Hematoxylin and eosin stained section; **(B)** after hybridization with an S-35-labeled HPV 16 RNA probe; note the intense signal in the superficial cells in this darkfield image; **(C)** after staining for capsid proteins with an antibody to the L1 protein; nuclear staining (arrows) parallels the distribution of MRNA, illustrating the link between epithelial maturation, DNA replication and transcription, and capsid assembly. (From Crum and Roche,[114] with permission.)

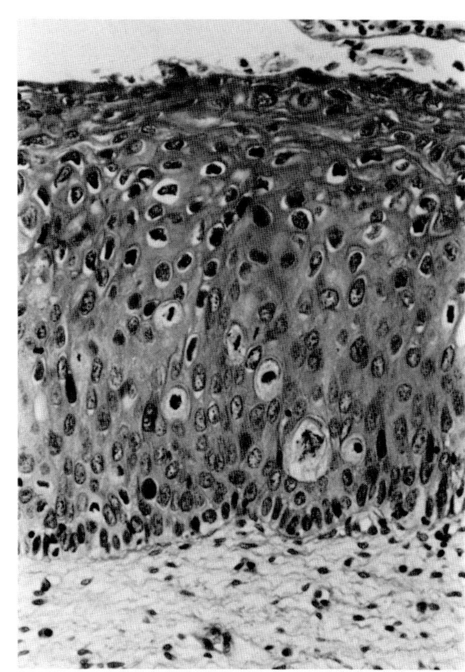

A

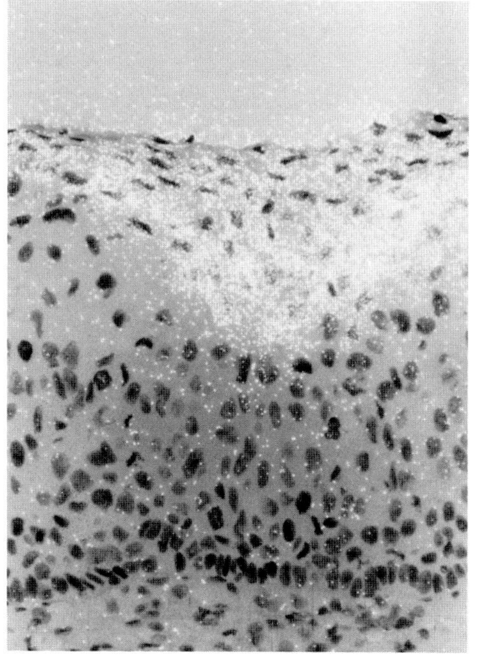

B

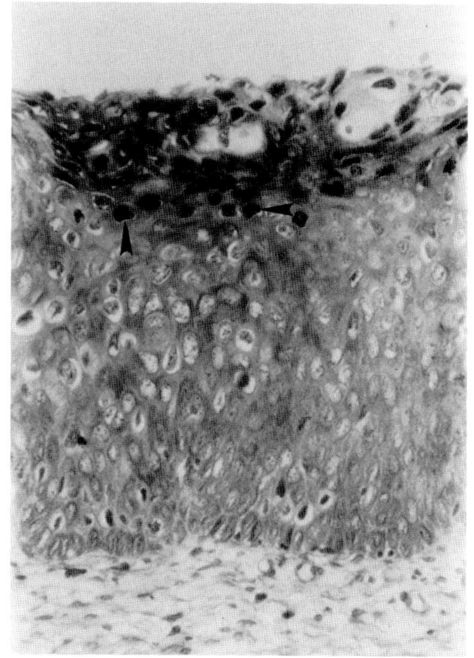

C

studies have demonstrated HPV nucleic acids in normal squamous epithelium, the precise location of these nucleic acids remains unclear. The most sensitive techniques for detecting HPV DNA in situ (including the in situ PCR technique recently described by Nuovo) have failed to demonstrate HPV nucleic acids in normal squamous epithelial cells, even those adjacent to lesional tissue. Thus, precisely what latent infection represents is unresolved. What is clear is the following:

1. Occult HPV DNA is identified in the genital mucosa in up to 30 percent of the population by the most sensitive PCR techniques.[11]
2. The presence of "occult" HPV DNA may be associated with recurrent disease in patients with a history of condylomata.[27, 28]
3. The natural history of occult infection in the absence of a clinical history of disease or abnormal smear is not defined.[28]
4. Many occult infections may be due to HPV types with minimal clinical importance.[11]
5. Recurrent cervical lesions following ablative therapy frequently are related to types other than the original, suggesting that type-specific immunity may occur. Conversely, recurrent lesions in immunosuppressed women are usually associated with the same HPV type.[29]

MOLECULAR PATHOLOGY

There is a relationship between the morphology of precursor lesions and the HPV types with which they are associated. In some instances, this association is strong, and parallels morphometric and DNA ploidy indices.[30–32] For example, conventional exophytic condylomata of the cervix, like those of the vulva, are closely associated with HPV types 6 or 11.[33] By contrast, most lesions containing HPV 16 fulfill the histologic criteria for CIN (high-grade squamous intraepithelial lesion). A variety of other HPV types associate with either condylomata (i.e., types 42 to 44) or CIN (i.e., types 31, 33, 35). HPV 18 is unique because it segregates most commonly in invasive cancers, including adenocarcinomas, squamous cell carcinomas, and small cell carcinomas.[34–36] Preliminary studies indicate that this preference of certain HPV types for groups of neoplasms parallels overall oncogenic potential. For example, HPV 6 or 11 (6/11) does not possess the capacity to immortalize cells in culture, whereas HPV 16 and 18 do; HPV 18 has a higher capacity to immortalize cells in culture than type 16.[25] Whether this explains the greater potential for HPV 18 to be associated with cancer is unclear. However, HPV 18 associated neoplasms invariably contain integrated HPV 18 sequences,[21] suggesting that these properties (transformation and integration potential) may operate in vivo to hasten the evolution of invasive neoplasia once a lesion develops.[36]

Although the concept remains untested, there is reason to hypothesize that the widespread differences in morphology among cervical precursor lesions may be related to different HPV types. If this is true, the traditional notion that the spectrum of cervical precursors is simply a biologic continuum through which all lesions progress would bear re-evaluation.

It is important to emphasize that lesion morphology may not parallel the HPV type present. This observation is most evident in the so-called "flat condyloma" of the cervix, which has a relatively bland morphology, but which occasionally contains HPV 16 or viral DNAs of similar oncogenic capacity.[33, 37] Moreover, lesions containing potentially "high-risk" viral DNAs may exhibit a morphologic spectrum that includes both bland-appearing condylomata as well as CIN.[38] The location of an individual lesion will likely influence its appearance, with portio lesions tending to be well differentiated in contrast to endocervical lesions, which appear less well differentiated.[39, 40] These observations must be taken into consideration when pondering the potential spectrum of lesions encountered in the cervix. An additional variable which must be superimposed upon the above is the manner in which the observer decides whether a lesion is a high-grade or low-grade precursor lesion, in that one pathologist's flat condyloma may be another's moderate dysplasia or vice versa. Without clear agreement on criteria for diagnosis, diagnostic concordance between examiners, and correlation with HPV DNA type, will vary.

DIAGNOSIS OF PRECURSOR LESIONS

This section applies the above information to the management of patients with cervical precursor lesions. The criteria for the cytologic and histologic diagnosis of

squamous intraepithelial lesions are discussed in detail (Table 2-2).

Nonspecific Changes Mimicking Koilocytosis: Defining the Threshold for Diagnosis

A by-product of the latency concept has been the increased focus on the use of molecular biologic techniques to define the lower limits of morphologically detectable HPV infection. Currently, management protocols of women with abnormal Papanicolaou smears dictate that any cervical lesion that is found should be removed.[39] Defining exactly what constitutes a lesion has been difficult. As expected, attention to koilocytotic atypia as a diagnostic feature of both warts and precancerous lesions may have resulted in the cytologic and histologic overuse of this term.[41] Broadening the criteria for the diagnosis of this cellular change has an immediate impact on clini-

Table 2-2. Selection of Criteria for Diagnosis of Cervical Intraepithelial Squamous Lesions

Findings	Diagnosis	Management
Negative; no transformation zone seen	Descriptive	Repeat if indicated
Acanthosis; parakeratosis; nonspecific halos; atrophy	Descriptive	Follow
Severe inflammation; reparative atypia	Descriptive	Culture; rule out *Chlamydia;* follow
Superficial cell atypia, maturation; minimal basal atypia	LSIL (CIN I, condyloma)	Remove
Koilocytosis; maturation; diffuse atypia	HSIL (CIN II)	Remove
Minimal koilocytosis or maturation; diffuse atypia	HSIL (CIN III)	Remove
Fragments of SIL/neoplastic squamous epithelium in the ECC	Strips of neoplastic squamous epithelium (specify amount, grade [if consistent with SIL], and if invasive carcinoma is suspected)	Cone biopsy if T zone is not visualized; otherwise treat conservatively or repeat examination, depending on colposcopic findings
Very scant SIL/neoplastic epithelium in the ECC	Descriptive (determine whether canal is involved clinically)	Repeat or cone

Abbreviations: CIN, cervical intraepithelial neoplasia; ECC, endocervical curettage; HSIL, high-grade intraepithelial lesion; LSIL, low-grade intraepithelial neoplasia; SIL, squamous intraepithelial lesion. (From Crum and Nuovo,[115] with permission.)

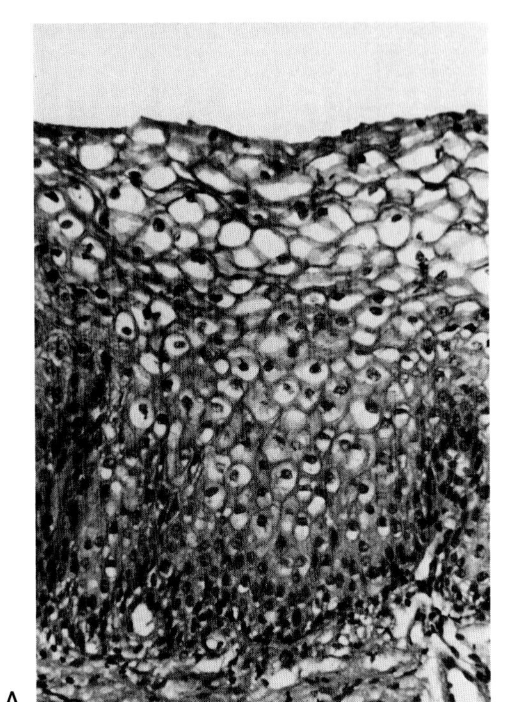

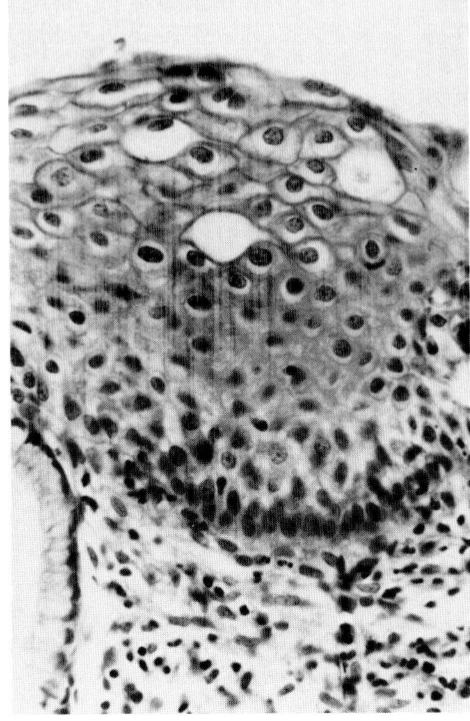

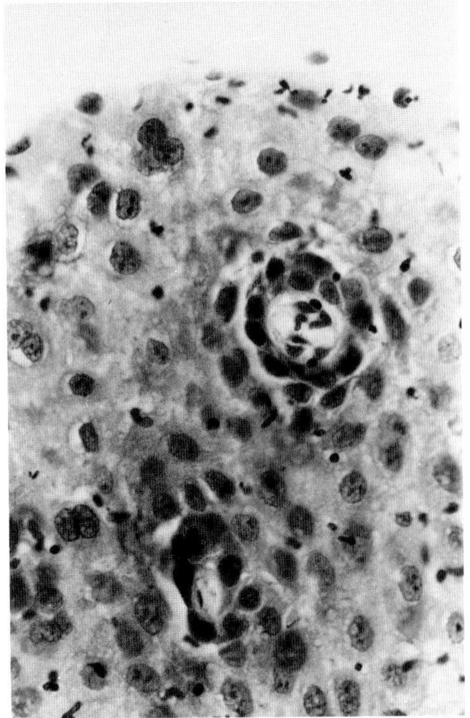

Fig. 2-2. Nonspecific and specific histologic correlates of human papillomavirus (HPV)-related intraepithelial lesions. **(A & B)** Cytoplasmic halos without nuclear abnormalities are uncommonly associated with HPV nucleic acids. **(C)** Reactive epithelial changes with mild nuclear enlargement and a few binucleate forms; note that hyperchromasia and irregular nuclear shapes or size are minimal in this HPV-negative lesion. (*Figure continues.*)

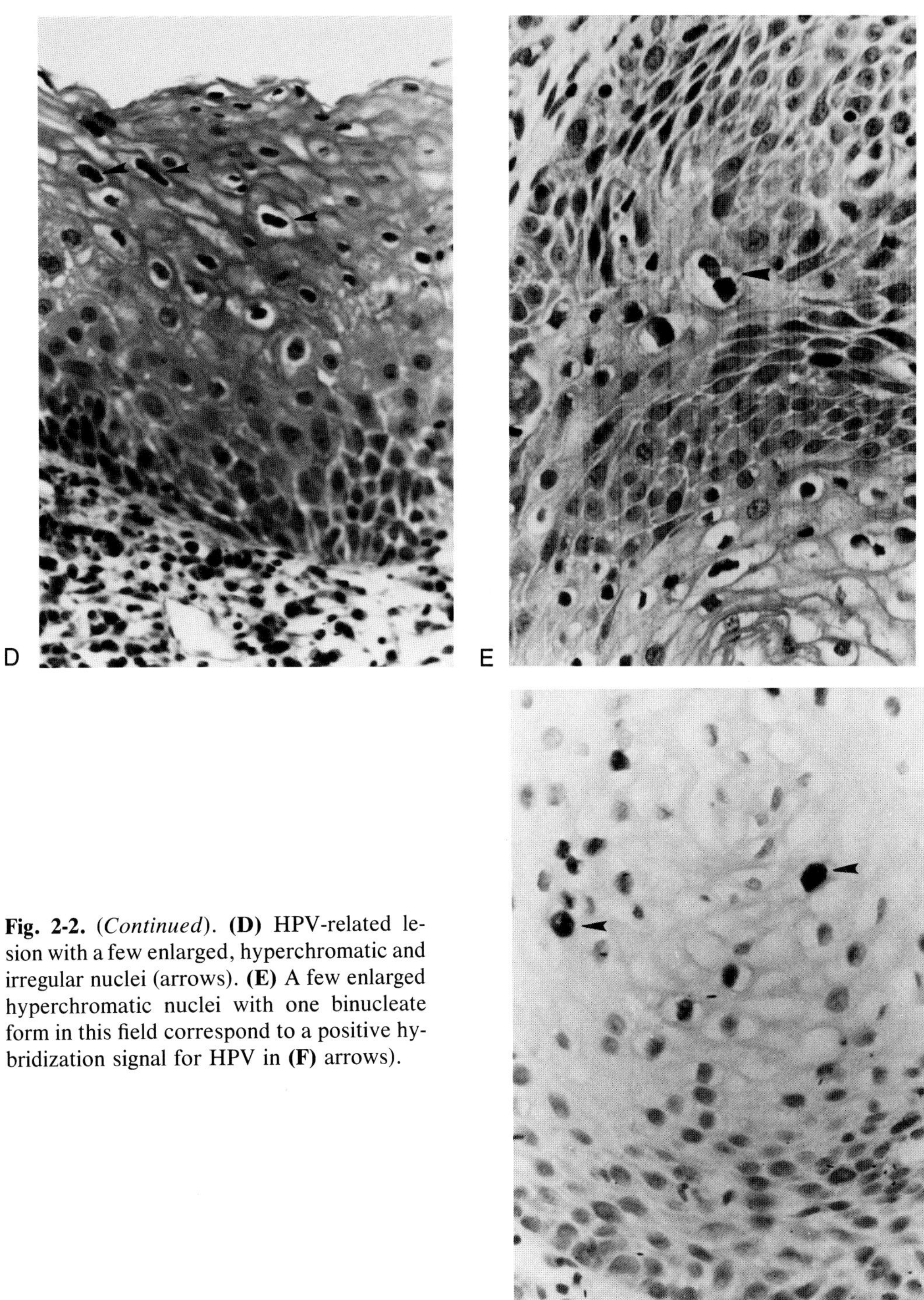

Fig. 2-2. (*Continued*). **(D)** HPV-related lesion with a few enlarged, hyperchromatic and irregular nuclei (arrows). **(E)** A few enlarged hyperchromatic nuclei with one binucleate form in this field correspond to a positive hybridization signal for HPV in **(F)** arrows).

cians and their patients, who are burdened by the information that HPV infection is widespread and is associated with neoplasia, and thus are "held hostage" to the uncertainties of cytologic and histologic interpretation.[42] Although one might assume that mild cytologic atypia in the biopsy or Papanicolaou smear indicates a low-grade or subtle condyloma, studies designed to correlate such findings with HPV infection have failed to support this concept consistently[43] (Fig. 2-2).

Because of the clinical and social ramifications of a diagnosis of HPV-related disease, it is imperative that minimal or nonspecific changes not be misinterpreted as HPV-related lesions. There is no evidence that such lesions are premalignant, and they frequently do not contain HPV nucleic acids.[43, 44] Precisely how the pathologist should go about excluding a nonspecific abnormality may vary, but the fundamental parameter that justifies a diagnosis of a low-grade intraepithelial lesion versus a reactive process is the presence of nuclear atypia. The problem is determining the degree of nuclear change that justifies this diagnosis. For some, "moderate" atypia, particularly when accompanied by perinuclear halos, justifies the diagnosis.[45] I follow a similar philosophy, with a three-step approach to ruling in or out an HPV-related lesion. In the first step, the general epithelial architecture is evaluated for features (albeit nonspecific) that associate with HPV-related lesions, including acanthosis, expansion of the lower epithelial cell layers, papillomatosis, and perinuclear halos.[43, 44] This is a useful first step, inasmuch as such changes are somewhat more likely to be associated with intraepithelial lesions than are patterns that characterize immature metaplasia or reactive/reparative changes with inflammatory cells in the epithelium. The second and most important step is to identify conspicuous anisonucleosis (i.e., 2 to 3× size differences) and variable intensity (polychromasia) in chromatin staining with differences in nuclear

texture. These parameters are usually mild, and occasionally moderate, in degree in reactive/reparative epithelia. If present in association with a squamous proliferation that, on low-power magnification, has characteristics of a lesion, the likelihood of an HPV-related lesion is stronger.[42, 45] The final step is to identify bi- or multinucleated cells. I find these cells to be present in more than 95 percent of all classic low-grade lesions, including condylomata or CIN I. They are, however, not specific, and cannot serve effectively as an initial screening parameter. If the first two categories suggest condyloma, the final parameter (bi- or multinucleation) will virtually always be present if the abnormality is HPV related (Fig. 2-2E).

The value of this exercise is that it is a systematic approach to differentiating HPV-related lesions from nonspecific reactive processes. The latter may contain multinucleation, nuclear "atypia," and variable nuclear size and staining. In particular, reactive processes in immature inflamed squamous epithelium may occasionally contain all of these features and be extremely difficult to distinguish from a high-grade squamous intraepithelial lesion (HSIL). In such cases, the pathologist may have no choice but to make a diagnosis of an HPV-related lesion or to classify the lesion as a squamous atypia of uncertain significance. In such cases, it is my practice to state a preference for either a lesion or a reactive process, if possible, while still stressing that the diagnosis is uncertain. "Borderline lesions," particularly those in which the diagnosis hinges on the identification of koilocytosis, usually turn out to be HPV negative on review (Fig. 2-2C).

Defining Squamous Intraepithelial Lesions

Squamous intraepithelial lesions (SIL) have traditionally been viewed as a continuum of change rather than representing morphologically or biologically distinct steps through which all precursors must pass.[46] However, efforts have been made to refine the spectrum by DNA analysis. For example, lower-grade lesions characterized morphometrically and by DNA microspectrophotometry are principally diploid or polyploid in DNA content and have a tendency to regress. By contrast, higher-grade lesions frequently are aneuploid, demonstrate greater degrees of cytologic atypia, and are more likely to progress.[30] Nevertheless, the consistent distinction of true precancerous lesions from cytologically and histologically similar lesions that are benign is impossible, notwithstanding the capacity of the above techniques to segregate lesions into general groups. If one reviews the number of papillomaviruses involved in squamous lesions of the cervix (Table 2-1) and embraces the hypothesis that morphologic diversity is a reflection, in part, of infection by HPV DNA types with divergent biologic effects, the futility of predicting behavior strictly from morphology alone is obvious.

Nasielle et al. observed that slightly less than two-thirds of mildly dysplastic lesions and one-third of moderate dysplastic lesions regressed during follow-up.[47, 48] Problems encountered in most studies, however, include length of follow-up, lack of illustrated or defined criteria for determining the grade of an individual lesion, and the potential alteration of the natural history of a lesion by biopsy.[46–48]

The time for a lesion to "progress" from a low-grade to a high-grade process or eventually to invasive cancer has never been determined. This may be impossible to resolve given the heterogeneity of cancer precursors in general. In an attempt to understand what might happen, mathematical models based on data from several studies in women of different ages with different epidemiologic risk factors have been developed. Barron and Richart have calculated the mean time to progression between grades of intraepithelial lesions at approximately 5 years.[49] The mean time to progression of HSIL (CIN III) to invasive disease is also uncertain and has been calculated to be 1 to 30 years, with a reasonable estimate of 10 to 13 years.[50–52]

Diagnosis begins with analysis of the Papanicolaou smear. The value of the Papanicolaou smear lies in the sampling of the cervix at regular intervals.[53] Theoretically, the mortality from cervical cancer can be reduced by at least 70 percent with screening every 3 years.[54–56] The length of the ideal interval is a subject of controversy, although it is currently reasonable to assume that if a woman has two or three consecutive negative yearly smears, she may be followed at less frequent but regular intervals. Only 5 to 7 percent of women have never had a Papanicolaou smear, but it is estimated that 37 percent of women with invasive cancer fall into this group.[56] Approximately one-third of women with invasive cancer, however, have had a negative Papanicolaou smear during the preceding 5 years.[9] It is assumed that sampling error or reader error contributes to this lack of correlation in most cases, although it is possible that a subset of invasive cancers develop rapidly in the absence of a precursor lesion of long standing.[36, 54]

The false-negative rates found in sampling have been reduced by the use of both the Ayers spatula and endocervical sampling, such as aspiration.[57] Recently, the endocervical brush has become the preferred method for obtaining endocervical material, reducing the frequency of inadequate smears to less than 2 percent.[58] Determining the laboratory "false-negative" rate depends on the parameters used in its calculation. For example, if errors are calculated on the basis of total smears processed, the false-negative rates are usually less than 1 percent. However, if false-negative rates are calculated by dividing the false negatives by the total number of positives (including false-negatives), the proportion of positive smears incorrectly diagnosed as negative in the course of processing a large volume of smears is placed at 11 to 23 percent.[59]

Classification of Papanicolaou smear abnormalities has traditionally included normal (group I), uncertain (group II), abnormal consistent with precancer (group III), high-grade CIN (group IV), and invasive cancer (group V). This has recently been replaced by the Bethesda classification, in which groups II to V are divided into nonspecific atypia and abnormal,[60] as outlined in Table 2-1. The latter includes three groups: abnormal of uncertain significance, low-grade intraepithelial lesion, and high-grade intraepithelial lesion. The value of this approach is the clear segregation of nonspecific abnormalities and reduction of the number of classifications for intraepithelial lesions. The latter terminology is designed to avoid the use of intraepithelial neoplasia, which has been increasingly difficult to define in the face of HPV-related changes and condylomata. However, such terms as CIN or dysplasia may be included to clarify the message. This classification conforms loosely to the concept that there are low-risk and high-risk intraepithelial lesions as defined above, although it must be stressed that it is impossible to make these distinctions consistently on the basis of cytology alone.[60]

Because the distinction of precursors with low versus high risk may not be possible, the goal of the pathologist is to identify lesions which should be removed rather than be concerned with nuances of grading (Table 2-2). In fact, with the simplification in Papanicolaou smear interpretation to include only low-grade and high-grade squamous intraepithelial lesions (LSIL and HSIL), concurrent changes in the classification of biopsy material is timely.

It is my practice to grade intraepithelial lesions on the basis of the distribution and severity of nuclear atypia. Low-grade squamous intraepithelial lesions, which include flat and exophytic condylomata and some immature variants, exhibit nuclear atypia principally in the surface epithelium, with milder variations in nuclear morphology and staining in the lower epithelial layers. By contrast, HSIL will encompass those in the category of CIN as classically described, wherein nuclear atypia will be present in both the lower and upper epithelial layers and variations in nuclear morphology and staining intensity will be greater in the parabasal cells. Although the classification will not be biologically precise, for reasons outlined above, it carries some advantages. First, it eliminates the use of two terms that are becoming increasingly confusing: *condyloma* and *CIN*. Some lesions in the former group fail to behave like benign warts, and some in the latter are not true precancers. The term "lesion" protects the pathologist (and clinician) from the potentially confusing image produced by the diagnosis of "condyloma" or "CIN." For similar reasons, the term *koilocytotic atypia* should probably not be used as a diagnostic term, but as a criterion for lesion recognition.

Low-Grade Squamous Intraepithelial Lesions

LSIL include exophytic and flat condylomata and variants (Fig. 2-3). The typical cervical condyloma may vary in appearance from flat to slightly raised to that resembling condyloma acuminata of the vulva. Accordingly, the degree of papillomatosis observed histologically will vary. The distinguishing features are thickening of the epithelium (acanthosis) and koilocytotic atypia in the mid and upper portions of the epithelium. Koilocytotic atypia is defined as the presence of nuclear atypia with variation in nuclear size and shape, wrinkling of nuclei, polychromasia and binucleate forms, and perinuclear halos. The perinuclear halos tend to vary in appearance, in shape and conformation, with a distinct zone of clearing between the nu-

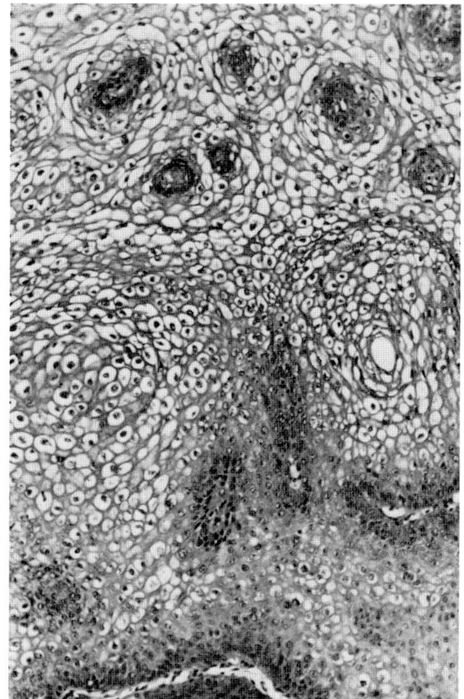 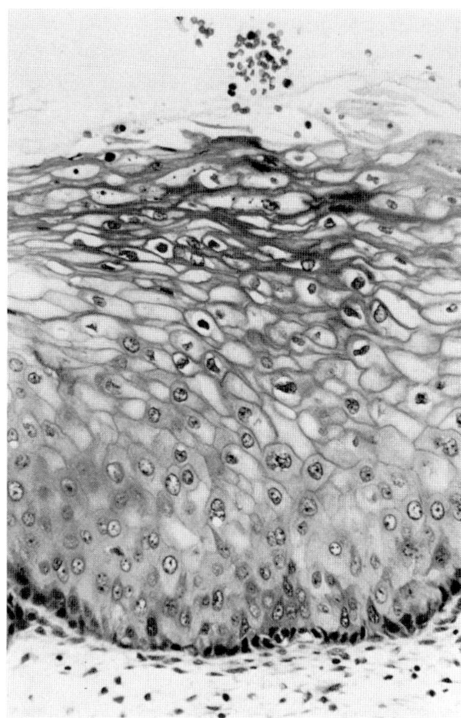

A   B

Fig. 2-3. The spectrum of low-grade squamous intraepithelial lesions (LSIL). **(A)** Exophytic condyloma; **(B)** flat condyloma.

cleus and cytoplasmic membrane. Important features of exophytic condyloma are the presence of minimal nuclear atypia in the lower half of the epithelium, a low mitotic index, and absence of abnormal mitoses. Flat condylomata have a similar appearance, although the parabasal epithelium may be slightly more atypical in appearance. Accordingly, this group of lesions may be associated with HPV 16 nucleic acids or other "high-risk" HPV types, as described previously.[30, 33, 61]

A major problem in the two-tiered system is the proper placement of lesions that demonstrate indeterminate degrees of cytologic atypia in the lower epithelial layers, an example of which is illustrated in Figure 2-4. These lesions, variably classified as flat condyloma, CIN I, and very mild or mild dysplasia, can be classified in either low-grade or high-grade categories. However, they are probably best classified as LSIL, inasmuch as cytologic/histologic correlation will be arduous if lesions are classified as high grade on the basis of relatively minor degrees of atypia in the lower cell layers. However, if conspicuous nuclear atypia is present in the parabasal cells, the lesion should be classified as an HSIL (Fig. 2-5).

High-Grade Squamous Intraepithelial Lesions

HSIL include two variants: CIN with koilocytotic atypia (i.e., CIN II, moderate dysplasia) and CIN without koilocytotic atypia (i.e., CIN III, severe dysplasia, carcinoma-in-situ). Lesions in the former category exhibit features of both condyloma and CIN. Cell maturation is present in the

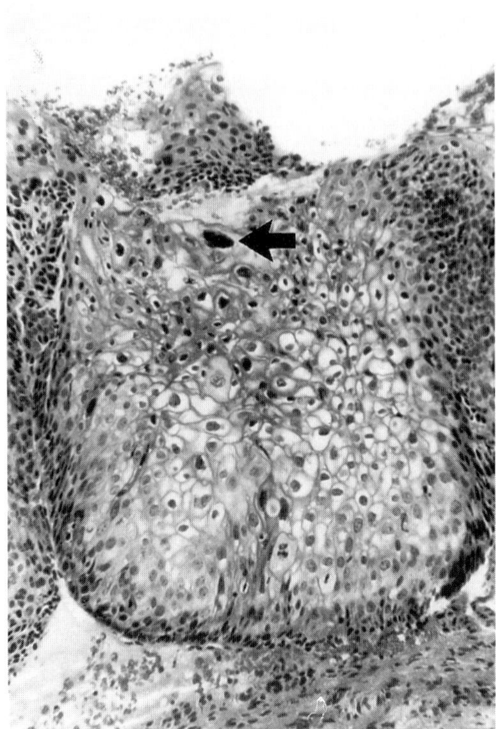

Fig. 2-4. HSIL resembling LSIL. This HPV 16 associated lesion resembles a flat condyloma but exhibits greater cellularity and nuclear crowding in the parabasal cells (compare to Fig. 2-3). Note in addition the greatly enlarged and coarsely chromatic superficial cell nucleus (arrow).

upper half of the epithelium, usually with koilocytotic atypia. The koilocytes may be identical to those in flat condyloma, but commonly differ by the presence of smaller, more concentric halos, and dense, hyperchromatic and pleomorphic nuclei. The epithelial surfaces of CIN II and CIN III lesions frequently contain horizontally arranged parakeratotic cells with abnormal nuclei. In addition, nuclear atypia is present in the lower half of the epithelium in at least a portion of the lesion (Fig. 2-5A,B). The picture may be of a mixed lesion, with a combination of flat condyloma and CIN.[46, 62, 63]

In CIN without koilocytotic atypia (CIN III, severe dysplasia-CIS), there is minimal maturation or koilocytotic atypia, although they may be combined with areas resembling CIN I or II. Cells with a high nuclear-to-cytoplasmic ratio are present throughout the epithelium (Fig. 2-5C,D). Paradoxically, high-grade CIN lesions often exhibit a more homogeneous population of neoplastic cells, with less variation in nuclear size and staining than do lower-grade CIN lesions. However, the nuclei are crowded, enlarged, hyperchromatic and contain a higher mitotic index than conventional basal cells or immature metaplasias.

Pitfalls in Classification

It is important to stress that when classifying lesions on the basis of the distribution and degree of nuclear atypia, maturation of the epithelium in the lesion plays a minor role, notwithstanding the fact that high-grade lesions tend to be less well differentiated. A small subset of low-grade lesions (condylomata) may appear immature when they involve the more proximal (endocervical) regions of the transformation zone. These so-called atypical metaplasias have been previously discussed.[40, 64] A portion of these lesions, specifically those associated with or resembling exophytic condylomata, are associated with HPV 6 nucleic acids and display a population of metaplastic appearing cells with mild nuclear atypia and a very low mitotic index (Fig. 2-6). It is acceptable to term these and similar immature lesions as low grade if they demonstrate sufficient nuclear atypia to be termed a lesion but contain no other features (other than immaturity) of an HSIL. The potential pitfalls in assuming all these lesions are benign (ref. 40 and Ward BE, Crum CP: unpublished observations) will be discussed subsequently. A second and potentially more serious pitfall is the assumption that features of condyloma denote a benign process. Figure 2-7 illustrates a common finding of koilocytotic atypia or superficial mat-

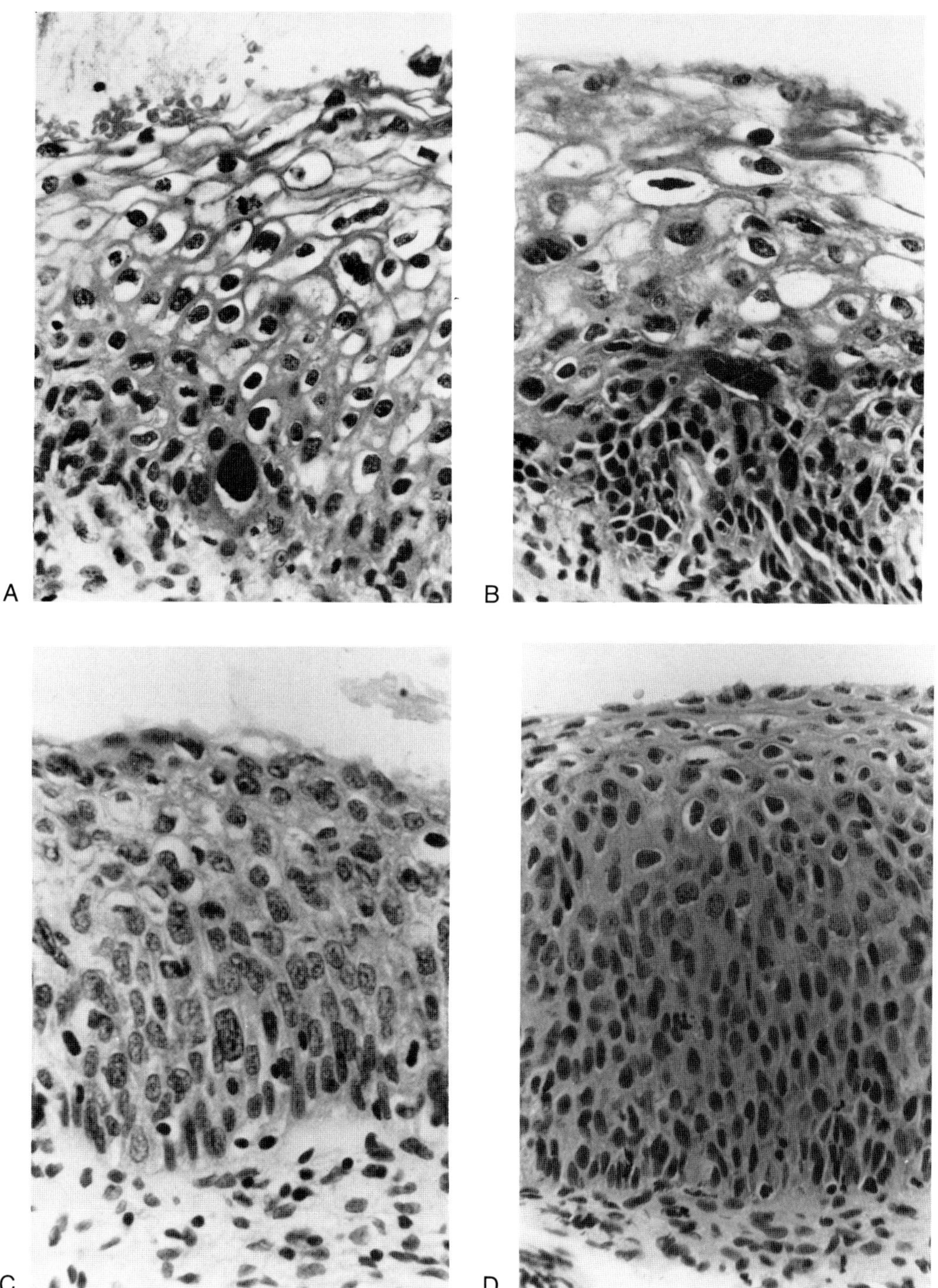

Fig. 2-5. The spectrum of high-grade squamous intraepithelial lesions (HSIL). **(A & B)** Well-differentiated HSILs with conspicuous nuclear enlargement and atypia in the parabasal cells. **(C & D)** Less well-differentiated HSILs with a similar distribution of nuclear atypia.

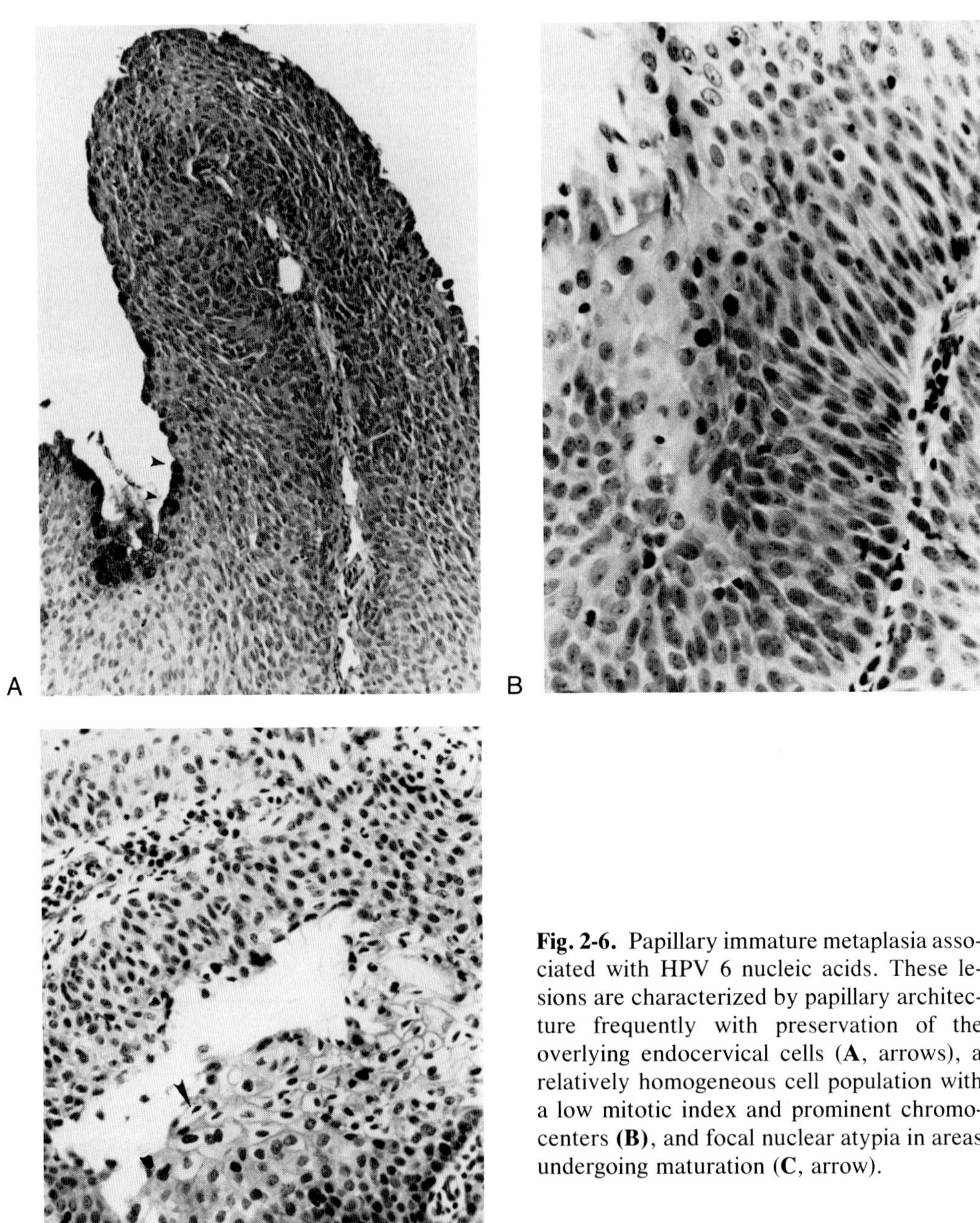

Fig. 2-6. Papillary immature metaplasia associated with HPV 6 nucleic acids. These lesions are characterized by papillary architecture frequently with preservation of the overlying endocervical cells (**A**, arrows), a relatively homogeneous cell population with a low mitotic index and prominent chromocenters (**B**), and focal nuclear atypia in areas undergoing maturation (**C**, arrow).

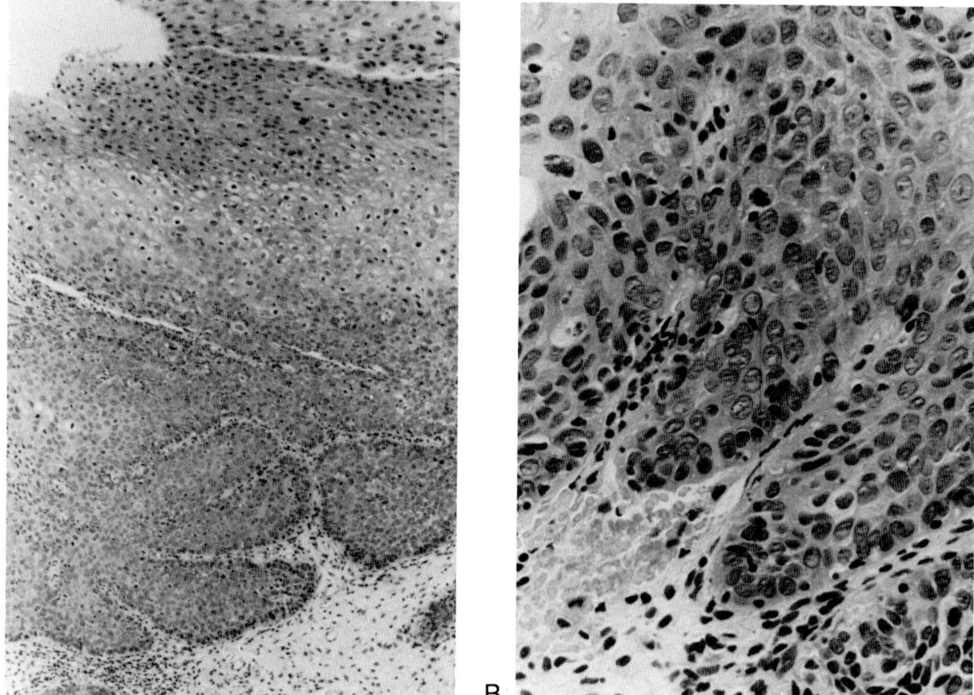

Fig. 2-7. Well-differentiated SIL with superficial maturation. **(A)** On low power the lesion appears to be low grade; **(B)** at higher power, there is parabasal cell atypia. (From Tabbara et al.,[65] with permission.)

uration with underlying parabasal cell atypia associated with a high-risk HPV type. This is relatively common in HSIL lesions associated with high-risk HPV types, emphasizing the importance of evaluating all layers of the epithelium.

Pitfalls in Cytologic/Histologic Correlation

Clearly, depending on the criteria used for diagnosis, the success in achieving reproducibility of histologic classification and correlating Papanicolaou smear and histology will vary. At the root of the problem is establishing what histologic (hence cytologic) changes deserve to be classified as low and high grade, respectively, and what this means to the clinician. If a three- or four-tiered classification system stressing maturation is used, concordance between observers will be poor (because of the many nuances of grade) but will likely occur within one grade in most cases. A two-tiered system will produce better concordance overall (by focusing on relatively fewer parameters combined with the inherent limitation of choices) but will carry the disadvantage that lack of concordance will not be between, say, mild and moderate or moderate and severe dysplasia but between high and low grade. Predictably, if the clinician makes major therapeutic decisions over whether the lesion is classified as "low" or "high" grade, a two-tiered system will not ultimately serve the patient. On the other hand, if the clinician is aware of the limitations in predicting lesion behavior and is concerned primarily with lesion distribution and excluding carcinoma, this will not be a problem.[65]

In summary, the problems of a two-tiered system are several and can be divided into biologic and practical categories. In the biologic category, (1) a portion of LSIL by anyone's classification system will contain potentially oncogenic HPV types; and (2) a lesion may be undersampled, appear as an LSIL, yet be associated with an adjacent HSIL. As a corollary, the Papanicolaou smear of a potentially progressive lesion may be read as LSIL because of either of the above. Undersampling may occur in the vertical plane, wherein superficial sampling of a HSIL reveals only mature atypical cells (Fig. 2-7), or on a horizontal plane, wherein a lesion exhibiting two components (low and high grade) is not uniformly sampled.

Are these major problems? Within the context of correlative conferences between clinicians and cytopathologists, the problems in grading discrepancy between cytology and histology can be resolved easily in the vast majority of cases in which a lesion is found in both specimens. The greatest problems in Papanicolaou smear/histology correlation occur when (1) the smear is *overcalled* as LSIL and resolved when nothing is present histologically; and (2) the smear is clearly abnormal, but nothing is present histologically. In the latter case, repeat colposcopy is usually performed in 4 to 6 months.[42, 65] In the author's experience, up to one-third of LSIL Papanicolaou smear diagnoses will not be corroborated on biopsy, even when review of the smear confirms an abnormality. Conversely, up to 20 percent will be confirmed as HSIL on biopsy. This argues for both realistic expectations when triaging patients with LSIL diagnoses on Papanicolaou smear, as well as caution in following up these patients, if colposcopy is not immediately performed or is initially negative.

Molecular Diagnosis: Pros and Cons

With the development of technologies for detecting and classifying HPV DNA in the genital tract, there is considerable interest in the feasibility of HPV testing as an adjunctive technique for diagnosing HPV-related diseases of the cervix. This can be approached on at least four levels: (1) the use of HPV DNA testing to reduce the "false-negative" rate of screening Papanicolaou smears; (2) To evaluate screening smears with squamous atypia of uncertain significance; (3) To detect occult or latent HPV infection; and (4) to modify therapy of patients with morphologically distinct HPV-related lesions.

Reducing False-Negative Papanicolaou Smears. The Papanicolaou smear clearly carries a significant false-negative rate, and the component of false-negative rates that is most preventable is the misreading of Papanicolaou smears. The addition of HPV DNA testing to reduce this would employ rescreening of negative smears which were HPV DNA positive. Studies indicate that approximately 20 percent of such smears will be found to contain abnormal cells that were missed on the first analysis.[28, 41] However, it is not clear (1) how efficiently routine viral testing would reduce false-negative rates for Papanicolaou smear interpretation, (2) what the impact of such a program would be on morbidity and mortality related to cervical cancer, and (3) what the cost would be of achieving an incremental improvement in morbidity and mortality. On one hand, approximately one-third of the nearly 7,500 women who die of cervical cancer-related causes each year had a negative Papanicolaou smear in the 5 years before diagnosis, and conceivably may have benefitted from more intensive screening.[66] On the other hand, the cumulative cost of delivering this test indiscriminately would be extremely high and its value to women who already receive regular examinations is questionable.

HPV DNA Testing to Evaluate Borderline Papanicolaou Smears. In this scenario, HPV DNA testing would be used to fine-tune the management of women with Papanicolaou smear abnormalities of uncertain significance. In a recent study of "nondiagnostic" squamous atypia, it was found that those associated with HPV DNA were more likely to remain abnormal on follow-up and correlate with the presence of a distinct cervical lesion (Nuovo G: personal communication). The principal objections to using HPV DNA testing to resolve these borderline abnormalities, however, are the inherent false-negative rate of HPV DNA sampling and the requirement that any persistent cytologic abnormality be evaluated by colposcopy under any circumstances.

Detecting Occult or Latent HPV Infection. By definition, programs aimed at detecting occult infection would require sampling large populations. Unlike the first approach, HPV-positive patients would be notified that they carried the infection and be counseled to return for routine cytologic follow-up. However, the significance of HPV DNA in the absence of cytologic or histologic abnormalities is unknown. Furthermore, the rate of conversion of subclinical infection to clinical disease and the factors influencing this conversion are unknown. There is also the risk of considerable emotional morbidity in the knowledge that one carries occult HPV infection with no alternative but to adhere to the currently accepted practice of a regular Papanicolaou smear.

HPV DNA Testing to Modify Therapy. Because the accepted approach to cervical intraepithelial lesions is to remove them, HPV DNA testing has little value in the management of women prior to ablative therapy. In cases in which lesions are extensive or the patient has concomitant immunosuppression, HPV DNA testing may be useful for identifying extensive infections with "low-risk" HPV types, possibly providing for an approach centering on a period of follow-up rather than proceeding directly to extensive ablation. However, there is no evidence that making such decisions requires more than careful histologic interpretation. Moreover, most commercially available techniques for HPV DNA detection categorize HPV DNA positives using groups of more than one probe (i.e., 6/11, 16/18, 31/33/35). Depending on the hybridization conditions specified by the detection technique, specifying precisely what HPV DNA is present may be impossible. Because there is no evidence that the probe types in some groups identify infections with the same natural history, the "prognostic" value of categorizing lesions as positive for "6/11," "16/18," and "31/33/35" is questionable.

In summary, HPV DNA testing remains an experimental technique that has provided insights into the distribution of papillomaviruses in the population and their association with neoplasia. As such it has been a useful tool for gathering information about epidemiology, the significance of certain morphological changes, and follow-up studies. This technology may be producing as many questions as it answers concerning the relationship between HPV and the risk of disease. It is reasonable to assume that widespread testing under optimal conditions would reduce the false-negative Papanicolaou smear rate and would possibly increase the rate of early detection. Whether such a program would alter the death rate from cervical cancer is unknown.

Excluding Invasive Carcinoma: Positive Endocervical Curettage

Positive endocervical curettage (ECC) is an established component of the colposcopic triage process.[67] Its value increases inversely with the adequacy of the colposcopic evaluation. Hatch et al. found that ECC provided information in addition to, or in lieu of, the biopsy in 1.2, 16, and 31 percent of satisfactory, unsatisfactory, and negative colposcopic examinations, respectively.[68] Drescher and co-workers reported that 49 versus 18 percent of inadequate and adequate colposcopies, respectively, were associated with a positive ECC.[69] The precise role of ECC as a guide to therapy after a satisfactory colposcopic exam is controversial. Soissan et al. and Krebs and Wheelock found that 0.8 and 1.5 percent of adequately evaluated patients with positive ECC had associated invasive cancer.[70, 71] Dinh et al. found the figure to be slightly higher (nearly 4 percent) for women 45 years and older.[72] This contrasts with from 4 to 9 percent of cases with inadequate colposcopy and a positive endocervical curettage, and as high as 18 percent for women aged 45 or older.[72–73]

Despite the presence of some, albeit small, risk of invasive cancer in patients with adequate colposcopy and a positive ECC, most colposcopists adopt a conservative approach in such cases, deferring cone biopsy if the colposcopic examination was adequate, the canal clearly visualized, the lesion small, and the amount of neoplastic epithelium in the ECC minimal.[71, 73, 74] El-Dabh et al. suggested a conservative approach to all cases of LSIL with adequate colposcopy and a positive ECC, citing no examples of more severe disease in association with this finding.[75] Spirtos demonstrated a strong correlation between a positive ECC and disruption of the ectocervical lesion, presumably indicating contamination.[76] However, these investigators stressed that not all cancers could be ruled out by colposcopy, biopsy, and ECC. There is little momentum to eliminate the ECC. It is considered a standard,

albeit uncertain, part of the colposcopic triage.[77]

A final question concerns the value of the ECC at the time of conization, including the importance of cone margins in predicting residual disease. Husseinzadeh et al. found that 36 percent of cases with positive endocervical margins on cone biopsy but a negative post-cone ECC had residual disease at hysterectomy.[78] This figure rose to 80 percent in cases in which both the endocervical margins and post-cone ECC were positive.[78] For this reason, the combination of margin evaluation and post-cone ECC may provide information concerning risk of residual disease. Others, however, have stressed that negative endocervical curettage does not rule out residual disease above the cone excision line.[79]

For the pathologist, interpretation of the ECC requires (1) assuring adequacy, (2) identifying high-grade or low-grade lesional epithelium, and (3) excluding endocervical glandular neoplasia. As detailed in Table 2-2, the term *strips of neoplastic epithelium* is synonymous with the presence of HSIL (usually without stroma) in the ECC. If strips of condylomatous epithelium (LSIL) are present, the pathologist should take care to qualify the diagnosis, particularly if the colposcopist does not visualize a lesion deep in the canal. Moreover, if the amount of neoplastic epithelium is scant (in an otherwise adequate ECC), this should be commented on, since it may not correlate with the clinical impression of canal involvement. In the latter two instances, the decision concerning conization will depend on the cytology and colposcopic findings as well as other clinical factors.[77]

MICROINVASIVE SQUAMOUS CELL CARCINOMA

Depending on the age of the patient and the adequacy of the colposcopic evaluation, up to 7 percent of HSIL of the cervix are associated with superficial invasion.[80, 81] Accordingly, a subset of invasive squamous cell carcinoma of the cervix is termed "microinvasive carcinoma," on the assumption that a portion of early invasive cancers can be treated conservatively by cone biopsy or simple hysterectomy. Tumors exceeding the criteria for microinvasion are managed with radical hysterectomy or radiation therapy. In recent years, the proportion of invasive cervical carcinoma that have invaded less than 5 mm in depth at diagnosis has increased more than 10-fold and currently is approximately 21 percent.[82, 83]

For the pathologist, several concerns must be met when determining whether a cervical squamous cell carcinoma is microinvasive. They include (1) identifying invasion, (2) distinguishing it from noninvasive mimics, (3) and applying correctly the criteria for microinvasion. It should be emphasized that the diagnosis of microinvasion is histologic and can only be made on a cone specimen. The specimen must have uninvolved margins and the pathologist must examine a sufficient number of sections, usually one for every 2 mm of cone thickness.

Diagnosis of Invasion

The criteria for invasion include an inflammatory desmoplastic response in the adjacent stroma, focal conspicuous maturation of the neoplastic epithelium with prominent nucleoli, blurring of the epithelial stromal interface, and loss of palisading nuclei at the epithelial-stromal border (Fig. 2-8A–D). The additional cytoplasm observed in the maturing foci will often stand out by its pink appearance due to keratinization (Fig. 2-8A). Two additional and related features include scalloping of the margins at the epithelial-stromal interface, and the apparent "folding or duplication" of the neoplastic epithelium. These features are helpful when faced with an intense inflammatory response, which may obscure desmoplasia on one hand and blur the epithelial-stromal inferface on the other.[84]

Differential Diagnosis of Invasion

A previous review of 265 cases of presumed microinvasion sent to the Gynecologic Oncology Group determined that approximately one-third were overdiagnosed intraepithelial lesions,[85] underscoring the potential problems in interpretation. The most important mimics of microinvasion are tangentially sectioned glands involved by CIN, cautery or crush artifact, and previous biopsy sites. Intraepithelial lesions associated with underlying inflammation, from either secondary infection or previous biopsy, must be evaluated carefully to avoid the overdiagnosis of invasion when the epithelial-stromal interface is disrupted by the inflammatory process.

Confirming "Microinvasion"

Cone biopsy is necessary if the lesion (1) does not appear grossly invasive clinically or colposcopically, and (2) is not clearly deeper than 3 mm in the original biopsy or (depending on the clinician) does not exhibit capillary-lymphatic space invasion. Once the cone biopsy is performed, the measurement of depth of invasion should be made from the most superficial epithelial-stromal interface of the adjacent intraepithelial process. This is best accomplished using an ocular micrometer.

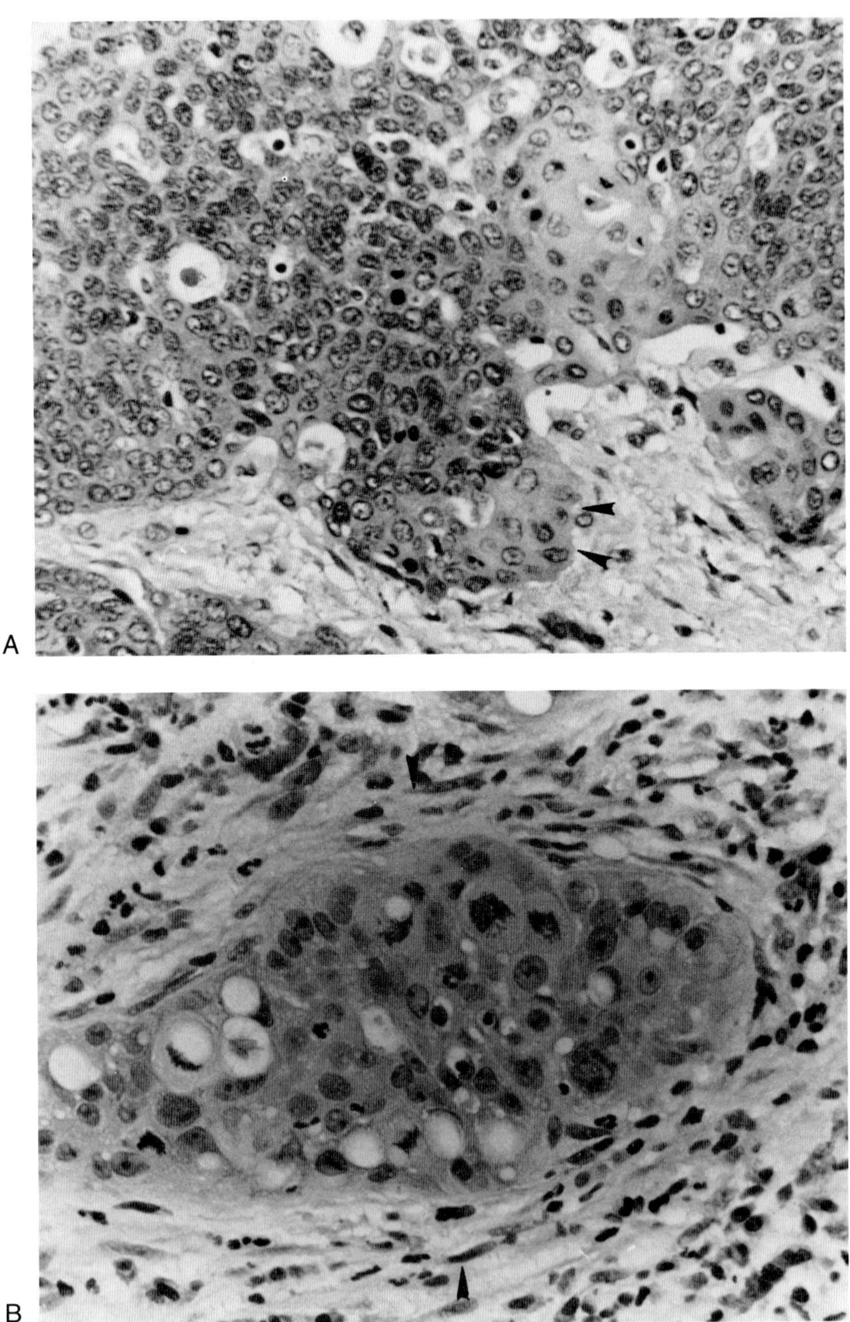

Fig. 2-8. Diagnosis of stromal invasion. **(A)** Scalloping of epithelial stromal border with loss of cellular polarity with maturation (arrows). **(B)** Desmoplastic stromal response (arrows). (*Figure continues.*)

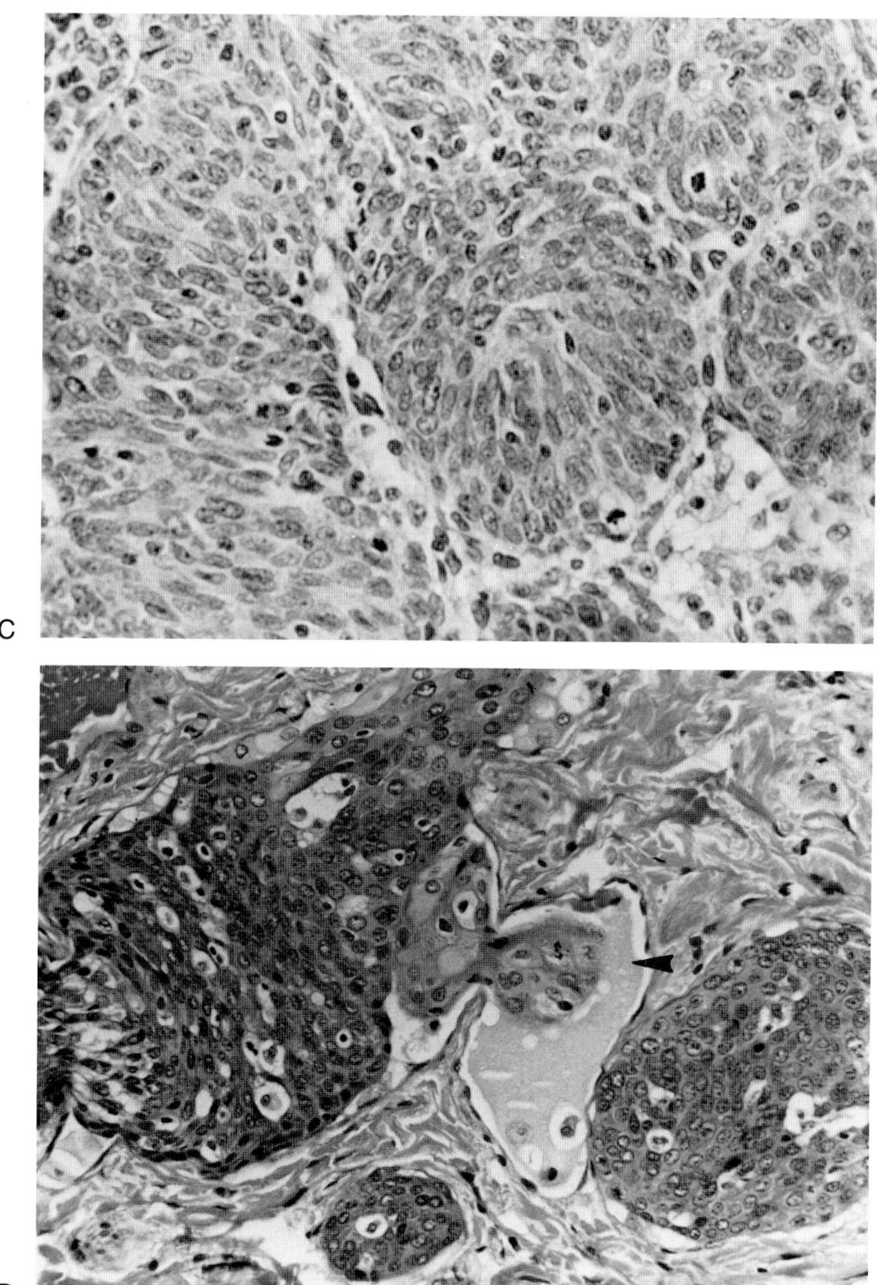

Fig. 2-8. (*Continued*). **(C)** Folding or reduplication of the epithelium. **(D)** Capillary lymphatic space invasion (arrows). (From Crum and Nuovo,[115] with permission.)

Three issues of potential concern when considering microinvasion are tumor depth, confuence of growth pattern, and capillary-lymphatic space invasion. Although microinvasion was originally defined as any lesion less than 5 mm in depth, the risk of lymph node metastases increases with depths over 3.0 mm.[86, 87] Hence, a diagnosis of microinvasion (as defined by the therapeutic alternative of simple hysterectomy) requires that the lesion extend not beyond 3.0 mm into the stroma.

Both confluent growth patterns and capillary lymphatic space invasion correlate with depth of invasion,[88, 89] but their independent value is less clear. Confluence has been defined as anastomosing tongues of epithelium with pushing borders or a lesion front of greater than 1 mm.[83] Despite a report emphasizing the prognostic importance of confluent patterns of invasion, some investigators have not found confluence to be an independent factor, once depth of invasion is controlled for.[86, 87, 90] However, lesion width may be important, as discussed below.[85, 91]

Capillary-lymphatic (CL) space invasion occurs in up to 57 percent of cases of early invasion, and its significance remains controversial.[87] CL space invasion increases in frequency as a function of lesion depth that increases the risk of lymph node metastases.[85–90] However, no studies have established that CL space invasion is a critical factor in lesions of 3.0-mm depth or less.[86–88] Van Nagell et al. found that none of 17 patients with CL space invasion and lesions invading less than 3.0 mm had metastases in their lymph node specimens. Despite this, the nomenclature committee of the SGO has not accepted the diagnosis of microinvasion if CL space invasion is present. In standard practice, most oncologists will request that the presence of CL space invasion be reported; they will probably proceed with a radical hysterectomy if it is seen in a lesion less than 3.0 mm in depth. For this reason, overinterpretation of CL space invasion must be avoided. This requires a careful distinction of CL space invasion from artifacts due to inflammation or retraction[88] (Fig. 2-8D).

Depth of invasion remains the most intensively studied parameter. Several studies have shown that the risk of pelvic lymph node metastases is less than 0.9 percent for lesions invading up to 3 mm, but the risk has ranged from 4.3 to 13.9 percent for lesions invading 3.1 to 5.0 mm.[83, 86, 87] Thus, the cutoff point for simple hysterectomy is placed at 3.0 mm. The importance of width is less clear. Burghardt and Holzer proposed that tumor volume be taken into account as a more precise predictor of recurrence and metastases. They reported that lesions of less than 420 mm[3] rarely recur.[91] Unfortunately, determining tumor volume is tedious and is not universally accepted. In lieu of this approach, the greatest width of the lesion can be determined and reported by examining the histologic sections. There is an association among width, recurrence, and metastases, although the precise limits are unclear. A width of 10 mm is proposed by some investigators as a limit for conservative therapy with lesions less than 3.0 mm in depth.[92]

In summary, a diagnosis of microinvasive carcinoma requires an invasive lesion extending to or less than 3.0 mm in depth with no evidence of CL space invasion and free margins on the cone biopsy. Determination of greatest width is also advisable, although the precise width which should serve as a cutoff is unclear.

INVASIVE SQUAMOUS CELL CARCINOMAS

VIRAL ETIOLOGY

There is a strong association between HPV nucleic acids and invasive squamous cell carcinoma of the cervix[93] (Table 2-1), with up to 92 percent of cancers containing a high-risk HPV type.[93] These findings are in accordance with the concept that most carcinomas develop from HPV-related precursors. However, two caveats are in order. One is that some squamous carcinomas are not associated with HPV nucleic acids; preliminary studies indicate that such tumors may have a poorer prognosis.[94] The second caveat is that certain HPV types, such as HPV 18, are not typically associated with precursors, in contrast to invasive neoplasms.[21, 36] Thus, it may be possible to identify subsets of squamous carcinoma with more aggressive biology on the basis of these parameters.

With regard to the above, HPV 18 has been preferentially associated with small cell carcinomas and adenocarcinomas of the cervix, further linking this virus with neoplasms with different cell types and greater aggressive potential. With respect to small cell carcinomas, most have HPV 18, but this subset cannot consistently be distinguished morphologically from those with HPV 16.[95] The proportion of adenocarcinomas containing HPV-nucleic acids has varied, with recent studies indicating that a very high proportion of these neoplasms contain HPV nucleic acids as well.[96, 97] The relationship between other variants of squamous cell carcinoma—basaloid, papillary, and verrucous variants—and HPV remains to be determined.

CONVENTIONAL SQUAMOUS CELL CARCINOMA

Most squamous cell carcinomas evolve from a precancerous lesion. Up to two-thirds of CIN III lesions will progress to cancer if untreated; the time course for this evolution has been estimated at 3 to 20 years.[50, 98] Squamous cell carcinoma developing rapidly, without a defined precursor, has also been reported rarely.[99] The mean age for patients with invasive cancer is approximately 51 years, in contrast to approx-

imately 28 years for CIN III. A subset of invasive cancers, termed *occult carcinomas,* are clinically inapparent Stage Ib lesions of greater than 3.0 mm in depth. The mean age for occult carcinoma is estimated at 43 years, and the 5-year survival of 96 percent distinguishes this group from clinical stage IB invasive carcinoma (86 percent 5-year survival).[80]

Survival correlates with the stage of disease when diagnosed. Spread to regional nodes (stage III) occurs principally through the superficial and deep lymphatics draining to the iliac and obturator, hypogastric and common iliac, and sacral lymph nodes.[100] Approximately two-thirds of invasive squamous carcinomas are stage I or II when diagnosed. The actuarial 5-year survival drops abruptly from more than 70 percent for stage II to 30 percent to 35 percent for stage III neoplasms.[92]

Squamous cell carcinomas have been classified according to either degree of squamous differentiation (grades I to III) or cell type. Reagan et al. subdivided squamous cancer of the cervix into (1) large cell keratinizing carcinoma, (2) large cell nonkeratinizing carcinoma, and (3) small cell carcinoma,[101] in part on the presumption that large cell keratinizing carcinomas are radioresistant relative to nonkeratinizing carcinomas (Fig. 2-9). Moreover, small cell carcinomas were observed to have the worst overall prognosis.[88] In a review of five large series by Reagan and Fu, the average 5-year survival for stage I tumors treated by radiation therapy was 54 percent, 84 percent, and 42 percent for keratinizing, nonkeratinizing, and small cell carcinomas, respectively.[102]

With the exception of small cell undifferentiated carcinoma (see Ch. 8), classification according to cell type is not universally accepted. Not all investigators have observed differences in survival between keratinizing and nonkeratinizing tumors. Randall et al. found that keratinizing tumors had a greater tendency to recur locally after

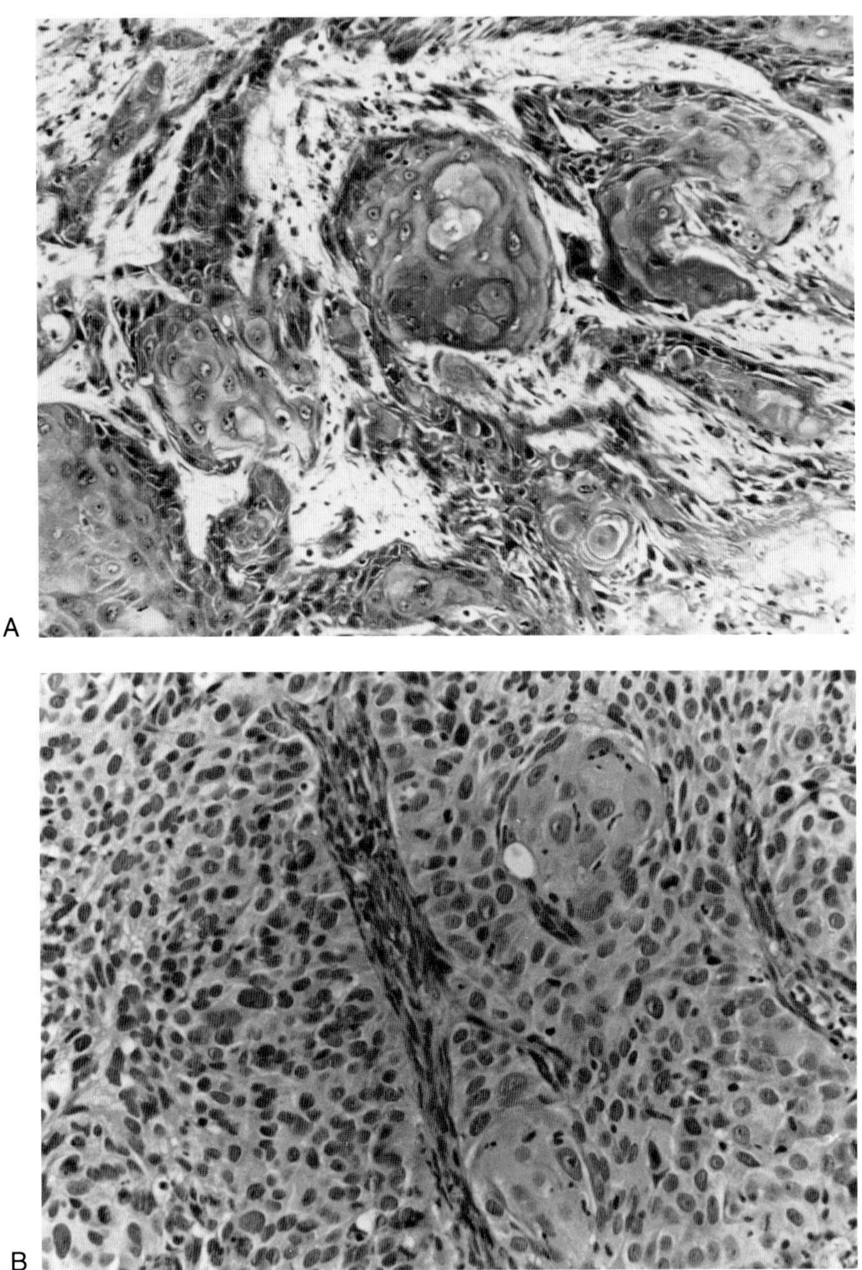

Fig. 2-9. Invasive squamous cell carcinoma. **(A)** Well differentiated (keratinizing). **(B)** moderately differentiated (large cell nonkeratinizing). (*Figure continues.*)

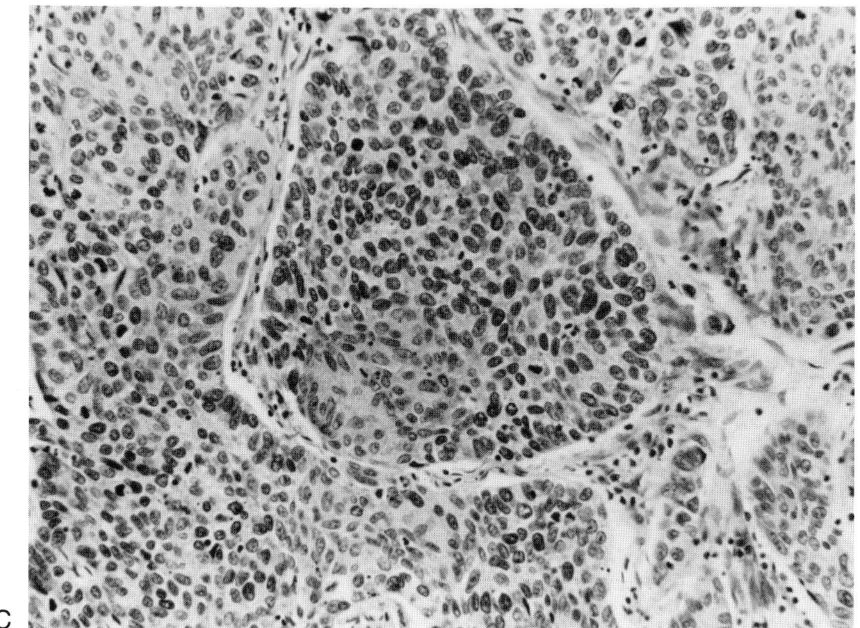

Fig. 2-9. (*Continued*). (**C**) poorly differentiated (large or small cell nonkeratinizing).

radiotherapy but that the frequency of distant metastases was the same for both cell types.[103] An alternative and currently accepted approach to grading is to classify squamous cell carcinomas as well, moderately, or poorly differentiated.

The distinction between well-differentiated (large cell keratinizing) squamous cell carcinoma and moderately differentiated (large cell nonkeratinizing) squamous cell carcinoma is based primarily on the presence of intercellular bridges and keratin pearls in the former, although focal individual cell keratinization may be present in the latter.[102] The small cell group as originally defined by Reagan et al. was reserved for nonkeratinizing squamous cell carcinomas composed of small cells. In retrospect, this group overlapped somewhat with other nonkeratinizing lesions, and recently it has become apparent that most of these neoplasms are morphologically and functionally identical to small cell undifferentiated

carcinoma (oat cell carcinoma, argyrophilic carcinoma, neuroendocrine carcinoma)[88] (see Ch. 8). Nevertheless, there exists a subset of small cell squamous carcinomas that lack the characteristic argyrophylia and immunohistochemical features of neuroendocrine carcinomas, and histologically, exhibit sharply demarcated nests of tumor cells similar in appearance to high-grade precursor lesions (Fig. 2-9C). The differential diagnosis and the potential differences in biologic behavior of this group with small cell undifferentiated carcinomas of the cervix, are discussed in Chapter 8.

Rare Variants of Squamous Cell Carcinoma

Lymphoepithelioma-like Carcinoma

Lymphoepithelioma-like carcinoma, also referred to in the literature as "medullary carcinoma with marked lymphoid infiltration[104]" (Hamazaki) and "circumscribed carcinoma of the uterine cervix with marked lymphocytic infiltration,[105]" resembles its morphologic counterpart in the nasopharynx. The tumor is composed of uniform round cells with clear to eosinophilic cytoplasm, vesicular nuclei, and prominent nucleoli, disposed singly or in small noncohesive groups within a dense inflammatory infiltrate[106] (Fig. 2-10A). In occasional foci, the neoplastic cells form cohesive syncytial nests with more obvious epithelial features. Areas of obvious keratinization or glandular differentiation are absent. The inflammatory infiltrate may be predominantly lymphoplasmacytic or occasionally may consist of large numbers of eosinophils. Immunohistochemistry has confirmed the epithelial nature of the larger cells and the T-cell nature of the lymphoid infiltrate. Thus far, cervical lymphoepithelioma-like carcinomas have been negative for Epstein-Barr virus DNA. The biologic behavior and therapeutic sensitivity of these tumors in the cervix remains to be completely defined, although current knowledge suggests that they do not differ significantly in their behavior from conventional nonkeratinizing squamous cell carcinomas of the cervix.

Sarcomatoid Squamous Cell Carcinoma

Rare squamous cell carcinomas of the cervix are characterized by a prominent component of malignant spindle cells, potentially mimicking a sarcoma.[107] A minor component of otherwise typical, well to moderately differentiated squamous cell carcinoma, which tends to occur within the superficial parts of the tumor, is also usually present, merging imperceptibly with the spindle cell component. The cells of the latter are typically highly pleomorphic, with large nuclei that have coarse chromatin and often prominent nucleoli. Mitotic figures are numerous and often atypical. Intracytoplasmic periodic acid-Schiff (PAS)-positive hyaline droplets have been observed in occasional cases. The spindle cells may be associated with a pronounced desmoplastic reaction, especially in the deeper parts of the tumor. Cytokeratin immunoreactivity and ultrastructural findings have confirmed the squamous nature of the spindle cells.[107] Although only a small number of cases have been reported, follow-up evaluation of these tumors suggests that they are highly aggressive.

Verrucous Carcinoma

Verrucous carcinomas are extremely rare in the cervix.[108] I have seen a single nonreferred case during the past 13 years. Verrucous carcinomas characteristically occur in older women, usually present as a large sessile lesion resembling a condyloma, and may be underdiagnosed cytologically and histologically as either normal or a variant of condyloma. On histologic examination, these lesions exhibit both an exophytic and endophytic growth pattern, the latter composed of bulbous pegs of well-differentiated epithelium that have a well-circumscribed pushing margin with the underlying stroma (Fig. 2-10B). This border is maintained even in deeply invasive tumors. There is minimal to absent nuclear atypia, and mitotic figures if present, are usually confined to the basal cells. An intense inflammatory infiltrate has been associated with verrucous carcinoma of the cervix but is, in itself, nonspecific. The differential diagnosis includes large exophytic condylomata with crypt involvement, in situ or invasive papillary squamous carcinoma (marked nuclear atypia), and well-differentiated squamous cell carcinoma (some nuclear atypia and irregular nests of invasive tumor). Given the extreme rarity of this lesion, the diagnosis of verrucous carcinoma must be made with caution, and the diagno-

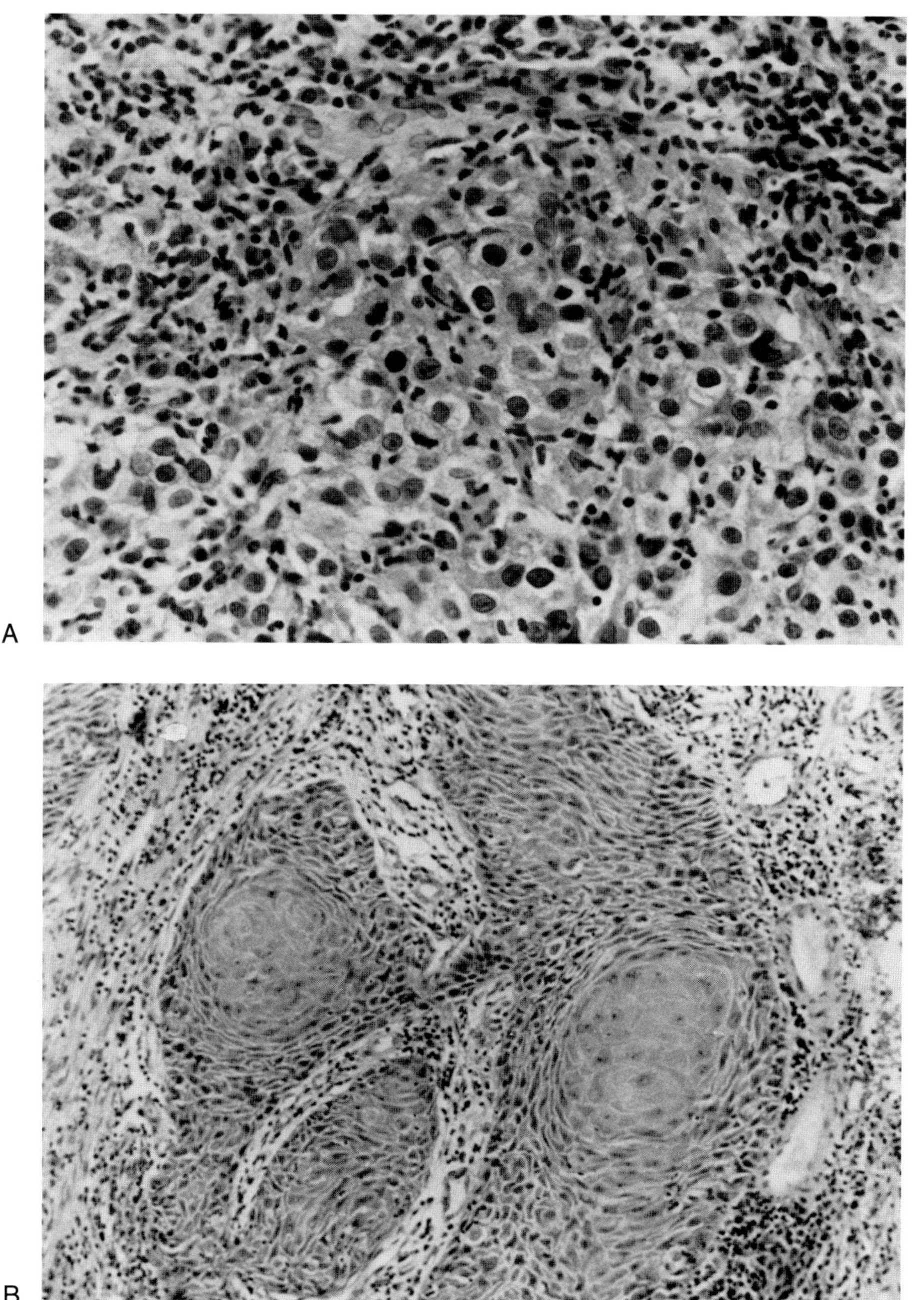

Fig. 2-10. (A) Lymphoepithelioma-like carcinoma. The cells are arranged in noncohesive arrangements with an intense inflammatory infiltrate. **(B)** Verrucous carcinoma. Note the bland cytologic features. (*Figure continues.*)

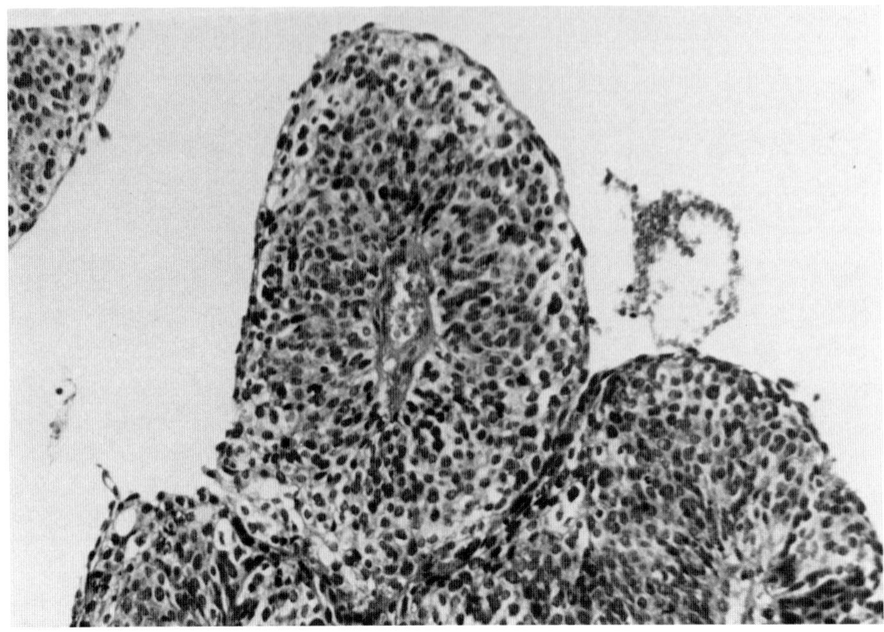

Fig. 2-10. (*Continued*). **(C)** Papillary squamous cell carcinoma. This lesion exhibits a conspicuous papillary architecture lined by neoplastic squamous cells, similar to high-grade SIL (carcinoma in situ) or transitional cell carcinoma of the bladder. Such lesions can usually be distinguished from variants of condylomata or other papillary lesions by the degree of nuclear atypia, and are presumed to be invasive carcinoma until proven otherwise. (Fig. C from Crum and Nuovo,[115] with permission.)

sis may be difficult without multiple biopsies or hysterectomy. Local excision is not usually possible, and direct extension into the endometrium[108] or invasion of adjacent pelvic tissues may occur. No verrucuous carcinomas of the cervix have metastasized to lymph nodes, although the recurrence rates have been as high as 50 percent.[83, 109] It should be noted that occasional otherwise typical verrucuous carcinomas may have an associated component of conventional squamous cell carcinoma.[108] In such cases, the conventional component should be recognized and reported accordingly.

Papillary Squamous Cell Carcinomas

Papillary neoplasms of the cervix encompass a broad spectrum of benign, potentially malignant, and clearly malignant lesions of the cervix; papillomas are summarized in Chapter 8. Papillary lesions have been described in the cervix, ranging from those resembling transitional cell papillomas to those diagnosed as papillary carcinoma in situ.[110–112] Papillary lesions with marked squamous atypia (carcinoma in situ) may be associated with invasion and probably should be considered invasive until proven otherwise[113] (Fig. 2-10C).

REFERENCES

1. Meisels A, Morin C: Human papillomavirus and cancer of the uterine cervix. Gynecol Oncol 12:S111, 1981
2. U.S. Centers for Disease Control, National Institutes of Health. MMWR 23:306, 1983
3. Vessey M, Grice D. Carcinoma of the cer-

vix and oral contraceptives: epidemiological studies. Biomed Pharmacother 43:157, 1989

4. Layde PM, Broste SK: Carcinoma of the cervix and smoking. Biomed Pharmacother 43:161, 1989

5. Koutsky LA, Galloway DA, Holmes KK: Epidemiology of genital human papillomavirus infection. Epidemiol Rev 10:122, 1988

6. Kjaer SK, Teisen C, Haugaard BJ et al: Risk factors for cervical cancer in Greenland and Denmark: a population-based cross-sectional study. Int J Cancer 44:40, 1989

7. Kessler II: Perspectives on the epidemiology of cervical cancer with special reference to the herpes virus hypothesis. Cancer Res 34:1091, 1974

8. Brinton LA, Reeves WC, Brenes MM et al: The male sexual factor in the etiology of cervical cancer among sexually monogamous women. Int J Cancer 44:199, 1989

9. Dunn JE, Crocker DW, Rube IF et al: Cervical cancer occurrence in Memphis and Shelby County, Tennessee, during 25 years of its cervical cytology screening program. Am J Obstet Gynecol 150:861, 1984

10. Brinton LA, Reeves WC, Brenes MM et al: Parity as a risk factor for cervical cancer. Am J Epidemiol 130:486, 1989

11. Schiffman MH, Bauer HM, Lorincz At et al: Comparison of southern blot hybridization and polymerase chain reaction methods for the detection of human papillomavirus DNA. J Clin Microbiol 29:573, 1991

12. Southern EM: Detection of specific sequences among DNA fragments separated by gel electrophoresis. J Mol Biol 98:503, 1975

13. Beckman AM, Myerson D, Daling JR et al: Detection of HPV DNA in condylomas by in-situ hybridization with biotinylated probes. J Med Virol 16:265, 1985

14. Shibata D, Fu YS, Gupta JW, Shah KV et al: The detection of human papillomavirus in normal and dysplastic tissues by the polymerase chain reaction. Lab Invest 59:555, 1988

15. Saiki RK, Scharf S, Faloona F et al: Enzymatic amplification of beta-globin genomic sequences and restriction site analysis for diagnosis of sickle cell anemia. Science 230:1350, 1985

16. Nuovo GJ, MacConnell P, Forde A, Delvenne P: Detection of human papillomavirus DNA in formalin-fixed tissues by in situ hybridization after amplification by polymerase chain reaction. Am J Pathol 139:847, 1991

17. De Villiers E-M: Heterogeneity of human papillomavirus group. J Virol 63:4898, 1989

18. Dyson N, Howley PM, Munger K, Harlow E: The human papillomavirus-16 E7 oncoprotein is able to bind to the retinoblastoma gene product. Science 243:934, 1989

19. Werness BA, Levine AJ, Howley PM: Association of human papillomavirus types 16 and 18 E6 proteins with p53. Science 248:79, 1990

20. Crum CP, Mitao M, Levine RU, Silverstein S: Cervical papillomaviruses segregate within morphologically distinct precancerous lesions. J Virol 54:675, 1985

21. Cullen AP, Reid R, Campion M, Lorincz AT: Analysis of the physical state of different human papillomavirus DNAs in intraepithelial and invasive cervical neoplasm. J Virol 65:606, 1991

22. Lehn H, Villa LL, Marziona F et al: Physical state and biological activity of human papillomavirus genomes in precancerous lesions of the female genital tract. J Gen Virol 69:187, 1988

23. Schwartz E, Freese UK, Gissman L et al: Structure and transcription of human papillomavirus sequences in cervical carcinoma cells. Nature 314:111, 1985

24. Gissman L, Wolnick L, Ikenberg H et al: Human papillomavirus type 6 and 11 DNA sequences in genital and laryngeal papillomas and in some cervical cancers. Proc Natl Acad Sci USA 80:560, 1983

25. Romanczuk H, Villa LL, Schlegel R, Howley PM: The viral transcriptional regulatory region upstream of the E6 and E7 genes is a major determinant of the differential immortalization activities of human papillomavirus types 16 and 17. J Virol 65:2739, 1991

26. Rando RF, Groff DE, Chirikjian JG, Lancaster WD: Isolation and characterization

of a novel human papillomavirus type 6 DNA from an invasive vulvar carcinoma. J Virol 57:353, 1986

27. Ferenczy A, Mitao M, Nagai N, Silverstein SJ, Crum CP: Latent papillomavirus and recurring genital warts. N Engl J Med 313:784, 1985

28. Lorincz AT, Shiffman MH, Jaffurs WJ et al: Temporal associations of human papillomavirus infection with cervical cytologic abnormalities. Am J Obstet Gynecol 162:645, 1990

29. Nuovo GJ, Pedemonte BA: Human papillomavirus types and recurrent genital warts. JAMA 263:1223, 1990

30. Fu YS, Reagan JW, Richart RM: Definition of precursors. Gynecol Oncol 12:S220, 1981

31. Fu YS, Huang I, Beaudenon S et al: Correlative study of human papillomavirus DNA, histopathology, and morphometry in cervical condyloma and intraepithelial neoplasia. Int J Gynecol Pathol 7:297, 1988

32. Crum CP, Ikenberg H, Richart RM, Gissman L: Human papillomavirus type 16 in early cervical neoplasia. N Engl J Med 310:880, 1984

33. Willett GD, Kurman RJ, Reid R et al: Correlation of the histologic appearance of intraepithelial neoplasia of the cervix with human papillomavirus types. Int J Gynecol Pathol 8:18, 1989

34. Smotkin D, Gerek JS, Fu YS et al: Human papillomavirus deoxyribonucleic acid in adenocarcinoma and adenosquamous carcinoma of the uterine cervix. Obstet Gynecol 68:241, 1986

35. Stoler MH, Walker AN, Mills SE; Small cell neuroendocrine carcinoma of the cervix: a human papillomavirus type 18 associated cervix cancer, abstracted. Lab Invest 60:92A, 1989

36. Kurman RJ, Shiffman RM, Lancaster WD et al: Analysis of individual human papillomavirus types in cervical neoplasia: a possible role for type 18 in rapid progression. Am J Obstet Gynecol 159:293, 1988

37. Franquemont D, Ward B, Andersen W, Crum CP: Prediction of ''high risk'' cervical papillomavirus infection by biopsy morphology. Am J Clin Pathol 92:577, 1989

38. Mitao M, Nagai N, Levine RU et al: Human papillomavirus type 16 infection of the uterine cervix: A morphological spectrum with evidence of late gene expression. Int J Gynecol Pathol 5:287, 1986

39. Koss LG, Stewart FW, Foote FW et al: Some histological aspects of behavior of epidermoid carcinoma in situ and related lesions of the uterine cervix. Cancer 16:1160, 1963

40. Crum CP, Egawa K, Fu YS et al: Atypical immature metaplasia (AIM): a subset of human papillomavirus infection of the cervix. Cancer 51:2214, 1983

41. Ward BA, Burkett BJ, Peterson C et al: Cytological correlates of cervical papillomavirus infection. Int J Gynecol Pathod 9:297, 1990

42. Crum CP: The Bethesda System: a perspective. Am J Clin Pathol 96:S2, 1991

43. Nuovo GJ, Blanco JS, Silverstein SJ, Crum CP: Histologic correlates of papillomavirus infection of the vagina. Obstet Gynecol 72:770, 1988

44. Nuovo GJ, Nuovo MA, Cottral S et al: Histological correlates of clinically occult human papillomavirus infection of the uterine cervix. Am J Surg Pathol 12:198, 1988

45. Mittal KR, Chan W, Demopoulos RI: Sensitivity and specificity of various morphological features of cervical condylomas. An in situ hybridization study. Arch Pathol Lab Med 114:1038, 1990.

46. Richart RM: Cervical intraepithelial neoplasia. p. 301. In Sommers SC (ed): Pathology Annual. Appleton & Lange, E. Norwalk, CT, 1973

47. Nasielle K, Nasielle M, Vaclavinkova V: Behavior of moderate cervical dysplasia during long term follow-up. Obstet Gynecol 61:609, 1983

48. Nasielle K, Roger V, Nasielle M: Behavior of mild cervical dysplasia during long term follow-up. Obstet Gynecol 67:665, 1986

49. Barron BA, Richart RM: A statistical model of the natural history of cervical carcinoma based on a prospective study of 557 cases. JNCI 40:343, 1968

50. Barron BA, Cahill MC, Richart RM: A statistical model of the natural history of cervical neoplastic disease: the duration of

cervical carcinoma-in-situ. Gynecol Oncol 6:196, 1978

51. Coppelson LW, Brown B: Observations on a model of the biology of carcinoma of the cervix. Am J Obstet Gynecol 122:127, 1975

52. Gustafsson L, Adami H-O: Natural history of cervical neoplasia; consistent results obtained by an identification technique. Br J Cancer 60:132, 1989

53. Guzick DS: Efficacy of screening for cervical cancer: a review. Am J Public Health 68:125, 1978

54. U.S. Center for Disease Control, National Institutes of Health. MMWR 38:650, 1989

55. U.S. Center for Disease Control, National Institutes of Health. MMWR 38:659, 1989

56. National Cancer Institute: Cancer Control Objectives for the Nation: 1985-2000. In NIH Publ No. 86-2880. NCI Mono No. 2. NCI, Bethesda, MD, 1986

57. Richart RM: An evaluation of the "true" false-negative rate in cytology. Am J Obstet Gynecol 89:723, 1964

58. Taylor PT, Andersen WA, Barber SR et al: The screening Papanicolaou smear: contribution of the endocervical brush. Obstet Gynecol 70:734, 1987

59. American Medical Association Council on Scientific Affairs: Quality assurance in cervical cytology: the Papanicolaou smear. JAMA 262:1672, 1989

60. National Cancer Institute Workshop: The 1988 Bethesda system for reporting cervical/vaginal cytologic diagnoses. JAMA 262:931, 1988

61. Durst M, Gissman L, Ikenberg H, zur Hausen H: A papillomavirus DNA from a cervical carcinoma and its prevalence in cancer biopsy samples from different geographic regions. Proc Natl Acad Sci USA 80:3812, 1983

62. Winkler BW, Crum CP: Chlamydia trachomatis infection of the female genital tract: pathogenetic and clinico-pathologic correlations. p. 193. In Rosen PP, Fechner R (eds): Pathology Annual. Appleton & Lange, E. Norwalk, CT, 1985

63. Crum CP, Mitao M, Winkler B et al: Localizing chlamydial infection in cervical biopsies with the immunoperoxidase technique. Int J Gynecol Pathol 3:191, 1984

64. Ward BE, Saleh AM, Williams J, Crum CP: Papillary "immature metaplasia" of the cervix: a distinct subset of exophytic cervical condyloma associated with HPV nucleic acids. A reevaluation. Mod Pathol 5:391, 1992

65. Tabbara S, Saleh AM, Barber S et al: The Bethesda classification: histologic, cytologic and viral correlates. Obstet Gynecol 79:338, 1992

66. Dunn JE, Schweitzer V: The relationship of cervical cytology to the incidence of invasive cervical cancer and mortality in Alameda County, California, 1960 to 1974. Am J Obstet Gynecol 139:868, 1981

67. Shingleton HM, Gore H, Austin JM: Outpatient evaluation of patients with atypical Papanicolaou smears: contribution of endocervical curettage. Am J Obstet Gynecol 126:122, 1976

68. Hatch KD, Shingleton HM, Orr JW, Jr, et al: Role of endocervical curettage in colposcopy. Obstet Gynecol 65:403, 1985

69. Drescher CW, Peters WA, Roberts JA: Contribution of the endocervical curettage in evaluating abnormal cervical cytology Obstet Gynecol 62:343, 1983

70. Soisson AP, Molina CV, Benson WL: Endocervical curettage in the evaluation of cervical disease in patients with adequate colposcopy. Obstet Gynecol 71:109, 1988

71. Krebs HB, Wheelock JB: Endocervical curettage after cryotherapy for cervical intraepithelial neoplasia. J Reprod Med 30:379, 1985

72. Dinh TA, Dinh TV, Hannigan EV et al: Necessity for endocervical curettage in elderly women undergoing colposcopy. J Reprod Med 34:621, 1989

73. Oyer R, Hanjani P: Endocervical curettage: does it contribute to the management of patients with abnormal cervical cytology? Gynecol Oncol 25:204, 1986

74. Swan RW: Evaluation of colposcopic accurcy without endocervical curettage. Obstet Gynecol 53:680, 1979

75. El-Dabh A, Rogers RE. Davis TE, Sutton GP: The role of endocervical curettage in satisfactory colposcopy. Obstet Gynecol 74:159, 1989

76. Spirtos NM, Schlaerth JB, d'Ablaing G III, Morrow CP: A critical evaluation of the endocervical curettage. Obstet Gynecol 70:729, 1987

77. Crum CP, Taylor PT: Intraepithelial squamous lesions of the cervix. p. 179. In Knapp RC, Berkowitz RS (eds): Gynecologic Oncology. Macmillan, New York, 1992

78. Husseinzadeh N, Carter V, Wesseler T: Significance of positive endocervical curettage in predicting endocervical involvement in patients with cervical intraepithelial neoplasia. Gynecol Oncol 35:358, 1989

79. Presley JJ, Hernandez E, Mudfort E, Miyazawa K: Endometrial and endocervical curettage findings at the time of cervical conization. J Reprod Med 32:99, 1987

80. Boyes DA, Worth AJ, Fidler HK: The results of treatment of 4389 cases of preclinical squamous cell carcinoma. J Obstet Gynaecol Br Commonw 77:769, 1973

81. Savage EW: Microinvasive carcinoma of the cervix. Am J Obstet Gynecol 113:708, 1972

82. Ng ABP, Reagan JW: Microinvasive carcinoma of the uterine cervix. Am J Clin Pathol 52:511, 1969

83. Robert ME, Fu YS: Squamous cell carcinoma of the uterine cervix—a review with emphasis on prognostic factors and unusual variants. Semin Diagn Pathol 7:173, 1990

84. Wilkinson EJ, Komorowski RA: Borderline microinvasive carcinoma of the cervix. Obstet Gynecol 51:472, 1977

85. Sedlis A, Sall S, Tsukada Y et al: Microinvasive carcinoma of the uterine cervix: a clinicopathologic study. Am J Obstet Gynecol 133:64, 1979

86. Benson WL, Norris HJ: A critical review of the frequency of lymph node metastasis and death from microinvasive carcinoma of the cervix. Obstet Gynecol 49:632, 1977

87. Roche WD, Norris HJ: Microinvasive carcinoma of the cervix. The significance of lymphatic invasion and confluent patterns of growth. Cancer 36:180, 1975

88. Van Nagell JR, Greenwell N, Powell DF: Microinvasive carcinoma of the cervix. Am J Obstet Gynecol 145:981, 1983

89. Creasman WT, Fetter BF, Clarke-Pearson DL et al: Management of stage IA carcinoma of the cervix. Am J Obstet Gynecol 153:164, 1985

90. Hasumi K, Sakamoto A, Sugano H: Microinvasive carcinoma of the uterine cervix. Cancer 45:928, 1980

91. Burghardt E, Holzer E: Diagnosis and treatment of microinvasive carcinoma of the uterine cervix. Obstet Gynecol 49:641, 1977

92. Ferenczy A: Anatomy and histology of the cervix. p. 119. In Blaustein A (ed): Pathology of the Female Genital Tract. Springer-Verlag, New York, 1982

93. zur Hausen H: Papillomaviruses as carcinomaviruses. p. 1. In Klein G (ed): Advances in Viral Oncology. Raven Press, New York, 1989

94. Riou G, Favre M, Jennel D et al: Associations between poor prognosis in early stage invasive cervical cancers and nondetection of HPV DNA. Lancet 335:1171, 1990

95. Ambros RA, Park J-S, Shah KV et al: Evaluation of the histologic, morphometric, and immunohistochemical criteria for the differential diagnosis of small cell carcinomas of the cervix with particular reference to human papillomavirus types 16 and 18. Mod Pathol 4:586, 1992

96. Stoler M, Greer C, Shick E et al: The association and type distribution of HPVs in adenocarcinoma of the uterine cervix, abstracted. Mod Pathol 5:69A, 1992

97. Crum CP, Nuovo GJ: Genital Papillomaviruses and Related Neoplasms. Raven Press, New York, 1991; p 167

98. Fidler HK, Boyes DA, Worth AJ: Cervical cancer detection in British Columbia. J Obstet Gynaecol Br Commonw 75:392, 1968

99. Schiller W, Daro AF, Gollin HA et al: Small pre-ulcerative invasive carcinoma of the cervix—the spray carcinoma. Am Obstet Gynecol 65:1088, 1953

100. Krantz KE: The anatomy of the human cervix, gross and microscopic. p. 57. In Bandau RJ, Moghiss K (eds): The Biology of the Cervix. University of Chicago Press, Chicago, 1973

101. Reagan KW, Mamanic MS, Wentz WB: Analytical study of the cells in cervical

squamous cell cancer. Lab Invest 6:241, 1957

102. Reagan KW, Fu YS: Histologic types and prognosis of cancers of the uterine cervix. Int J Radiol Oncol Biol Phys 5:1015, 1979

103. Randall ME, Constable WC, Hahn SS et al: Results of the radiotherapeutic management of carcinomas of the cervix with emphasis on the influence of histologic classification. Cancer 62:48, 1988

104. Hamazuki M, Fujita H, Ara T et al: Medullary carcinoma with marked lymphoid infiltration of the uterine cervix. Jpn J Cancer Clin 14:787, 1968

105. Hasumi K, Sugano H, Sakamoto G et al: Circumscribed carcinoma of the uterine cervix with marked lymphocytic infiltration. Cancer 39:2503, 1977

106. Mills SE, Austin MB, Randall ME: Lymphoepithelioma-like carcinoma of the uterine cervix. Am J Surg Pathol 9:883, 1985

107. Steeper TA, Piscioli F, Rosai J: Squamous cell carcinoma with sarcoma-like stroma of the female genital tract. Clinicopathologic study of four cases. Cancer 52:890, 1983

108. Spratt DW, Lee SC: Verrucous carcinoma of the cervix. Am J Obstet Gynecol 129:699, 1977

109. Benedet JL, Clement PB: Verrucous carcinoma of the cervix and endometrium. Diagn Gynecol Obstet 2:197, 1987

110. Tiltman AJ, Atad J: Verrucous carcinoma of the cervix with endometrial involvement. Int J Gynecol Pathol 1:221, 1982

111. Kistner RW, Hertig AT: Papillomas of the uterine cervix—the malignant potentiality. Obstet Gynecol 6:147, 1955

112. Qizilbash A: Papillary squamous tumors of the uterine cervix. A clinical and pathological study of 21 cases. Am J Clin Pathol 61:508, 1974

113. Randall ME, Andersen WA, Mills SE et al: Papillary squamous cell carcinoma of the uterine cervix. A clinicopathologic study of nine cases. Int J Gynecol Pathol 5:1, 1986

114. Crum CP, Roche JK: Molecular pathology of the lower female genital tract: the papillomavirus model. Am J Surg Pathol 14:S1, 1990

115. Crum CP, Nuovo G: The cervix. p. 1557. In Sternberg S (ed): Diagnostic Surgical Pathology. Raven Press, New York, 1989

3

Premalignant and Malignant Glandular Lesions of the Uterine Cervix

Robert H. Young, Philip B. Clement, and Robert E. Scully

PREINVASIVE GLANDULAR LESIONS AND MICROINVASIVE ADENOCARCINOMAS

The first section of this chapter deals with the spectrum of endocervical glandular dysplasia (EGD), adenocarcinoma in situ (AIS), and microinvasive (early invasive) adenocarcinoma (MIA).[1] Compared with their squamous counterparts, these lesions are relatively uncommon; only recently have they received significant attention in the literature. However, they are almost certainly more prevalent than generally appreciated because they tend to be underdiagnosed cytologically and histologically. With the exception of AIS, the lesions considered here are not yet fully defined histologically, and knowledge of their behavior is incomplete. Although it is believed that a proportion of clinically invasive adenocarcinomas are preceded by AIS, and probably by EGD, the number is unknown. In contrast to adenocarcinomas with obvious invasion, these lesions are typically unassociated with clinical signs and symptoms but are detectable by cervicovaginal cytologic smears in most cases. As their cytologic features have been well reviewed elsewhere, they are not considered here.[2-10] The many pseudoneoplastic glandular lesions of the endocervix that may be confused with AIS on histologic examination are discussed in detail in Chapter 1. The discussion of EGD will follow that of AIS because it is less well defined.

ADENOCARCINOMA IN SITU

Clinical Features

Since the report of Friedell and McKay in 1953,[11] a large number of studies on AIS of the cervix have appeared[12-57] and have provided evidence that it is a precursor of invasive adenocarcinoma. In contrast to most precursor lesions, however, AIS is less frequently diagnosed than its invasive counterpart, having accounted for only about 10 percent of endocervical adenocarcinomas diagnosed at three institutions.[20, 26, 28] This low figure is at least partially attributable to the underdiagnosis of AIS.

The age range of patients with AIS is 20 to 85 years, but the median and mean ages, which in most series are in the fourth decade, are 10 to 15 years lower than those of patients with invasive adenocarcinoma.[2, 23, 26, 27, 29, 39] Almost 20 percent of the patients in one series had a history of treated squamous cervical intraepithelial neoplasia (CIN).[33] Women with AIS are usually asymptomatic but occasionally complain of abnormal bleeding or discharge,[4, 20, 23, 26, 29] which in some cases are secondary to other uterine lesions. A visi-

85

ble lesion is rare.[39] The colposcopic findings are frequently abnormal, in many cases secondary to synchronous CIN, but no findings are specific for AIS.[23, 29]

In almost all cases, the patient has an abnormal cytologic smear at presentation; dysplastic columnar cells, dysplastic squamous cells, atypical reserve cells, or combinations thereof may be seen.[15, 29, 33, 39] Atypical glandular cells have been present in the smears of 50 to 93 percent of the patients in several recent series.[3, 15, 20, 25, 29] A review of smears after a histologic diagnosis of AIS usually increases the frequency of positive diagnoses, in one series of cases from 50 to 67 percent.[29] In the same series, the detection rate of AIS by both cytology and biopsy was proportional to the extent of the lesion.[29] By contrast, in a recent study of 72 cases of AIS by Jaworski et al.,[27] "virtually all" the cases of AIS were diagnosed prospectively by cytological examination; this high detection rate was independent of the presence or absence of atypical squamous cells.

Microscopic Features

AIS typically occurs in the transformation zone and appears to begin at or near the squamocolumnar junction.[21, 27] As a result, glands involved by AIS may be covered by normal, metaplastic, or dysplastic squamous epithelium (see below). AIS typically involves both the surface columnar and underlying glandular epithelium; less commonly it is confined to the glands, typically admixed with normal glands. Very rarely, only the surface columnar epithelium is affected.[13, 23, 27] AIS almost always involves the necks of the glands and, in some cases, deeper portions of the glands as well.[27] Deep gland involvement in the absence of superficial gland involvement was not seen in any of the 72 cases studied by Jaworski et al.[27] but was reported in two cases by Betsill and Clark.[4] Noda et al.[18]

found that deep involvement is more common in the endometrioid form of cervical AIS. AIS is most commonly unicentric, but multifocality has been documented in approximately 15 percent of cases.[20, 23, 29]

AIS may assume a variety of patterns. Most commonly, the involved glands have a normal distribution (Fig. 3-1), a relatively normal configuration and are lined, usually entirely, but sometimes only in part (Fig. 3-2), by stratified cells with moderate to severe nuclear atypia (Fig. 3-3). Glands that are somewhat abnormal in contour or that are cystically dilated (Fig. 3-4), as well as some of the glandular processes discussed in Chapter 1, may also be involved by AIS. The lesional cells may replace the epithelium lining the endocervical lumen or that lining endocervical glands. They may line papillae with fibrous cores that project into involved glands or that replace the surface epithelium. A cribriform pattern may be present and, in some cases, solid sheets of cells obliterate gland lumens. Rare cases of AIS have been confined to endocervical polyps.[4]

AIS is characterized by pseudostratified or stratified columnar cells with malignant nuclear features. The involved epithelium is usually recognizable as abnormal on low-power examination because the cellular stratification and nuclear atypia makes it appear darker than the normal glandular epithelium (Fig. 3-1). When AIS involves only a portion of an endocervical gland, it is usually sharply demarcated from the normal epithelium (Fig. 3-2). The lesional cells have enlarged fusiform nuclei oriented perpendicular to the lumen, are variably hyperchromatic, and contain fine to coarse chromatin and nucleoli that are typically small; macronucleoli are seen in a minority of cases.[27] Occasionally, the glands are lined by more pleomorphic large polygonal cells (AIS-type 2 of Gloor and Ruzicka[17]). Mitotic figures are typically frequent and juxtaluminal and may be abnormal. Individual cell necrosis with intraepithelial nuclear

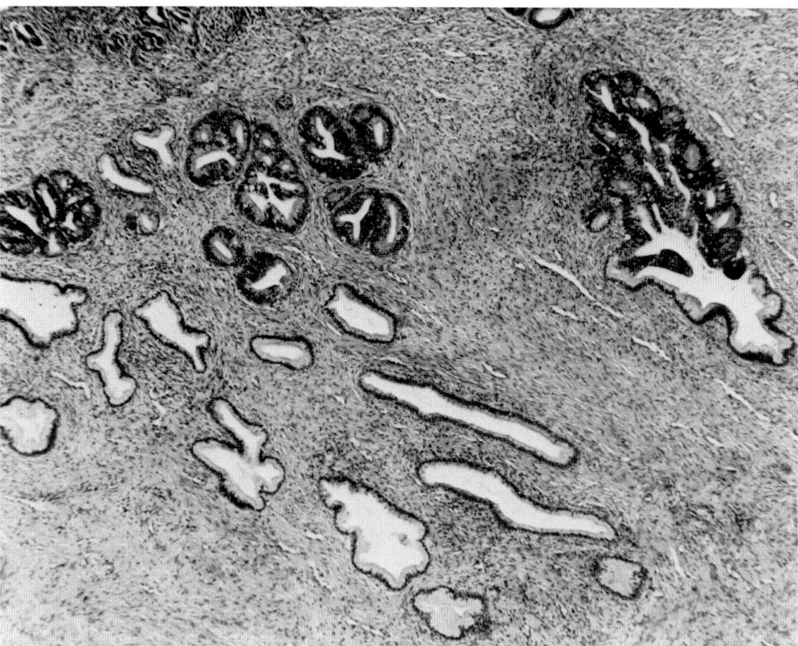

Fig. 3-1. Adenocarcinoma in situ. The abnormal epithelium differs greatly in appearance from the normal epithelium. Note the partial involvement of a large gland toward the upper right.

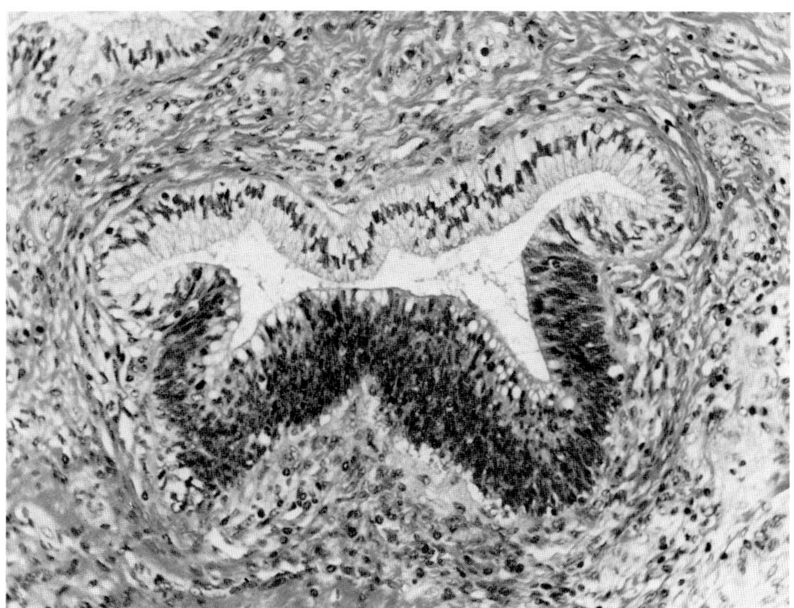

Fig. 3-2. Adenocarcinoma in situ. Only a portion of an endocervical gland is involved.

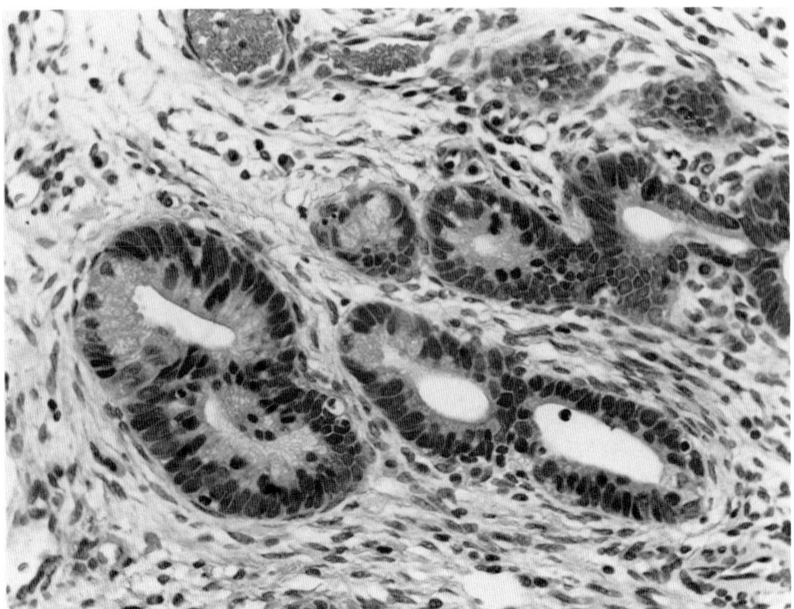

Fig. 3-3. Adenocarcinoma in situ. Several endocervical glands are lined by stratified cells with atypical nuclei and occasional mitotic figures.

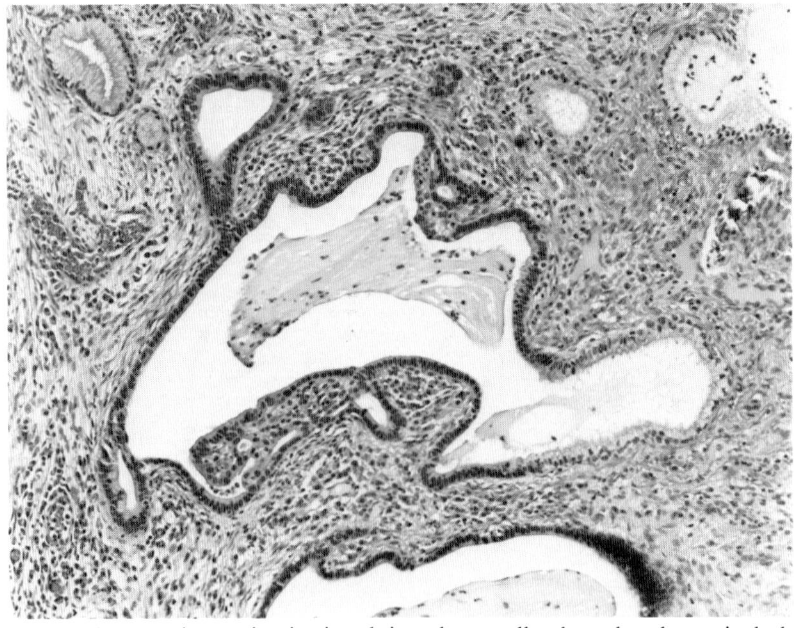

Fig. 3-4. Adenocarcinoma in situ involving abnormally shaped endocervical gland.

debris (apoptosis) is relatively frequent.[1, 27] The malignant cells occasionally exfoliate into the gland lumens.[19]

In the typical or "endocervical" form of AIS, the lesional cells have moderate amounts of predominantly juxtaluminal cytoplasm that stains variably positive for mucin, although the latter is diminished in amount compared to the mucin content of normal endocervical cells.[27] The presence of mucin-rich goblet cells (and, less commonly, argentaffin cells and Paneth cells) are characteristic of the "intestinal" form of AIS.[20, 22, 27] Histochemical stains reveal a predominance of sialomucins over sulfomucins, in contrast to their distribution in normal endocervical glands and the endocervical type of AIS.[22] The "endometrioid" variant of AIS is characterized by an absence of stainable mucin.[21, 27] The frequency of the endocervical, intestinal, and endometrioid subtypes in one recent large series of AIS was 95.8 percent, 29 percent, and 16 percent, respectively; the two less common subtypes were almost invariably admixed with the endocervical subtype.[27]

A number of less common variants of AIS have been described. Adenosquamous carcinoma in situ[17] usually resembles high-grade squamous CIN, with the additional finding of intracellular mucin in some of the neoplastic cells.[34] Rarer variants include serous papillary carcinoma in situ,[35] glassy cell carcinoma in situ,[36] clear cell adenocarcinoma in situ, which may contain hobnail as well as clear cells,[37] and AIS with a prominent signet-ring cell component.[13] Rare examples of AIS have been characterized by cells with abundant, foamy cytoplasm, presumably due to lipid accumulation.[17]

A number of studies have addressed the longitudinal and lateral extent and depth of AIS. In a study of 21 cases, Ostor et al.[20] found a mean longitudinal extent of 7 mm (range, 0.5 to 30 mm). In the study by Bertrand et al.,[23] 18 of their 19 cases extended less than 25 mm up the canal; and

one lesion extended 29.9 mm. In the same study, AIS involved one quadrant in 15 percent of cases, two quadrants in 30 percent, three quadrants in 35 percent, and four quadrants in 20 percent. In the study by Ostor et al., lateral involvement of AIS in cone biopsy specimens ranged from 0.5 mm to 25 mm (mean, 12 mm). Andersen and Arffmann[29] found the area of involvement by AIS to be less than 20 mm^2 in 36 percent, 20 to 100 mm^2 in 26 percent, 101 to 299 mm^2 in 19 percent, and more than 300 mm^2 in 19 percent of 31 cases. In the same study, the depth was 2 mm or less in 81 percent of cases, 3 mm in 9.5 percent, and 3.5 to 5 mm in 9.5 percent.[29]

Associated Lesions. There is a strong association between AIS and squamous CIN. The percentage of cases of AIS with synchronous CIN has varied from 48 to 90.[1, 4, 13, 14, 17, 21, 23, 25, 27, 29, 33, 39, 51] A coexistent microinvasive or invasive squamous cell or adenosquamous carcinoma is present in occasional cases.[13, 17, 20, 26, 27, 29, 33, 51] Colgan and Lickrish[32] have shown that the age of the patient, the topography of the AIS, and the presence or absence of invasive adenocarcinoma are unaffected by the coexistence of squamous CIN.

An association between AIS and endocervical glandular dysplasia (EGD) (see below) has been noted in only a few studies. Jaworski et al.[27] noted areas of EGD in "some" of their cases of AIS, and observed a transition between the two lesions. Similarly, Gloor and Hurlimann[22] found EGD (their cervical intraepithelial glandular neoplasia [CIGN] grades I and II) in 22 of 23 cases of AIS (their CIGN grade III). Early invasive adenocarcinoma (see below) should obviously be carefully searched for in specimens with AIS, and has been found in 10 percent,[22] 13 percent,[33] 22 percent,[29] and 43 percent[23] of cases. There appears to be no correlation between the extent of AIS and the presence of early invasive adenocarcinoma in the same specimen. Indeed, even small foci of AIS were accompanied by early invasion in one study.[23] The association between AIS and clinically invasive adenocarcinoma is discussed below. Occasionally, AIS is an incidental finding in a hysterectomy specimen performed for endometrial hyperplasia or carcinoma.[11, 23, 28]

Immunohistochemistry and Other Special Techniques. Most studies have shown that the cytoplasm of the lesional cells of AIS is typically immunoreactive for carcinoembryonic antigen (CEA)[38, 39, 40, 41, 42]; in one study, however, less than 10 percent of the cases were CEA positive.[28] These findings are in contrast to the typical CEA nonreactivity of benign glandular lesions that may be confused with AIS (see Ch. 1). Variable immunoreactivity for other antigens has been reported, including low- and high-molecular-weight cytokeratins, epithelial membrane antigen, B72.3, secretory component, amylase, 3-fucosyl-N-acetyllactosamine (AGF 4:48), CA 125, CA 19-9, IC5, and chromogranin, as well as loss of appropriate blood group antigens, although the diagnostic utility of these techniques has not yet been established.[10, 38, 41–44]

A number of other special techniques have been applied to the study of AIS. Using video image analysis, Jaworski and Jones[46] studied Feulgen-stained cell suspensions of AIS in three cases and found that two of the lesions were tetraploid and one was diploid.[46] Two groups of investigators have found increased nucleolar organizer regions (AgNORs) in AIS.[47, 48] Darne et al.[48] found mean counts of 200.7 in AIS, compared to 79.8 and 299 for normal endocervical glands and invasive adenocarcinomas, respectively. There was, however, significant overlap in the counts between cases of AIS and invasive adenocarcinoma, limiting the discriminatory value of this technique. Darne et al.[48] found elevated AgNOR counts in adjacent morphologically normal endocervical glands compared to remote normal endocervical glands, in contrast to a lack of such a finding in a similar study by Cullimore et al.[47] Morphometry of AIS performed on cytologic smears[4] and

tissue sections[19] indicates that this technique may have a role in distinguishing AIS from EGD.

Evidence Supporting Precancerous Potential. A number of observations, some of which have been noted above, support the precancerous nature of AIS:

1. As expected with a precursor lesion, AIS typically occurs in women 10 to 15 years younger than those with invasive adenocarcinoma of the cervix.
2. AIS is commonly associated with microinvasive adenocarcinoma or invasive adenocarcinoma in the same cone biopsy or hysterectomy specimen. In one series of invasive adenocarcinomas of the cervix, AIS was found adjacent to the invasive tumor in 46 of 52 cases.[15]
3. AIS may precede invasive adenocarcinoma in the same patient. Boon et al.[15] found that 18 of 52 patients with invasive cervical adenocarcinomas had had "negative" endocervical biopsies performed 3 to 7 years prior to the diagnosis of the invasive adenocarcinoma. Review of these biopsies revealed that foci of AIS had been overlooked on initial examination in five cases. More recently, Kashimura et al.[49] reported the case of an invasive cervical adenocarcinoma that developed 5 years after a biopsy had revealed AIS, and found a similar case in the German literature, in which the interval was 11 years.[49]
4. A high frequency of HPV-related antigens (especially types 16 and 18) has been reported in EGD, AIS, and invasive adenocarcinoma.
5. There is histologic similarity between AIS and invasive adenocarcinomas.

Treatment

If a diagnosis of AIS is suspected or established by a cytologic smear, punch biopsy, or curettage, most patients undergo a cone biopsy, permitting histologic confirmation of the diagnosis and determination of the presence or absence of stromal invasion. In a patient in whom preservation of fertility is not a consideration, hysterectomy has been recommended after the conization.[26] In young patients in whom preservation of fertility is a consideration, or in patients who are poor operative candidates, the cone biopsy may be curative. In the study cited above, Bertrand et al.[23] recommended that a therapeutic conization encompass the transformation zone and be at least 5 mm deep to include the deep portions of the endocervical glands and at least 25 mm long.

In patients treated by conization, involvement of the resection margins of the cone biopsy specimen is predictive of residual AIS in the subsequent hysterectomy specimen. Combining the results of seven studies in the literature[12–14, 20, 23, 26, 33] reveals that residual AIS was found in 64 percent of hysterectomy specimens when the cone biopsy margins were involved, in contrast to only 8.5 percent when the margins were negative. Additional treatment in the form of another cone biopsy, or hysterectomy is clearly needed when the margins contain tumor. Even patients with negative cone margins, however, are at risk for residual disease. Any patient treated conservatively should have careful follow-up that includes frequent cervicovaginal smears.

MICROINVASIVE ADENOCARCINOMA

Microinvasive (early invasive) adenocarcinoma (MIA) of the cervix has received little attention in the literature, in contrast to its squamous cell counterpart, and at present, there is no concensus regarding criteria for its diagnosis. Indeed, Yeh et al.[50] recently concluded that the variety of proposed diagnostic criteria "are too ambiguous to be applied uniformly" and have suggested abandoning the term. This lack of concensus will likely persist for the foreseeable future because of the small number of cases available for study and the problems inherent in the histological recognition of early stromal invasion in cases of AIS.

The mean age of the patients with MIA (44 years) in one study was between that of patients with AIS (39 years) and those with clinically invasive adenocarcinoma (49 years).[2] In another study, the mean age of patients with MIA was 40.2 years compared to 35.8 years for patients with AIS.[13] Although the clinical manifestations usually do not differ from those of AIS, five of seven patients in one series presented with postcoital bleeding,[23] and 6 of 22 patients in another series had colposcopic changes suggestive of early invasion.[21] Cytologic smears in patients with MIA have shown changes similar to those in patients with AIS.[15, 21]

MORPHOLOGY AND DEFINITIONS OF MICROINVASIVE ADENOCARCINOMA

Early lesions, the counterpart of microinvasive squamous cell carcinoma FIGO stage IA1, may appear as irregular budlike projections, small glands, or uncommonly, solid nests of cells that arise from foci of AIS. The invasive foci may be associated with a stromal reaction that consists of a fibroblastic response with a chronic inflammatory cell infiltration.[13, 51] The invasive cells typically resemble those of AIS. Occasionally they are squamoid with abundant eosinophilic cytoplasm and enlarged, rounded nuclei with chromatin clearing and prominent nucleoli.[31, 51] The presence of these squamoid cells within the glands of AIS should suggest the possibility of early stromal invasion in another plane of section, and deeper sections should be obtained.[1] Yavner et al.[52] have found that the study of sections stained immunohistochemically for laminin or type IV collagen may be useful in finding foci of early invasion, which are usually associated with gaps in the basement membrane.

In later stages of MIA, the invasive focus is measurable in two or three dimensions, corresponding to FIGO stage IA2 microinvasive squamous cell carcinoma. Low-power examination reveals an aggregate of malignant glands that lack the orderly arrangement of normal endocervical glands or those involved by AIS. The invasive glands are typically separated by cervical stroma but may be crowded or even confluent, and are typically haphazardly disposed although the invasive focus in such cases is usually still within the zone of endocervical stroma occupied by normal glands. The finding of malignant glands deep to this zone, rarely the finding of lymphatic invasion, or both, provide confirmatory evidence of invasion. The presence of a stromal response is often helpful in indicating the probability of invasion. In occasional MIAs, the invasive glands have morphologic features closely resembling those of AIS, including an absence of a stromal response.[1] The depth of the glands, as well as their focal confluence and irregular architecture, to varying extents are helpful in individual cases (Figs. 3-5 and 3-6), although the assessment of invasion in some cases is exceptionally difficult.

Most investigators have defined MIA (of the FIGO IA2 type) as a tumor that invades the endocervical stroma to a depth of less than 5 mm[13, 14, 18, 21, 29] as measured from the mucosal surface of the endocervical canal; the corresponding figure in other studies has been only 2 mm.[4] This measurement is problematic, however, in that most MIA probably arise from the endocervical glands rather than from the surface epithelium; in such cases, the site of origin of the invasive focus may no longer be recognizable. Burghardt[51] suggested that tumor volume may be a more appropriate criterion of early invasion and defines a "microcar-

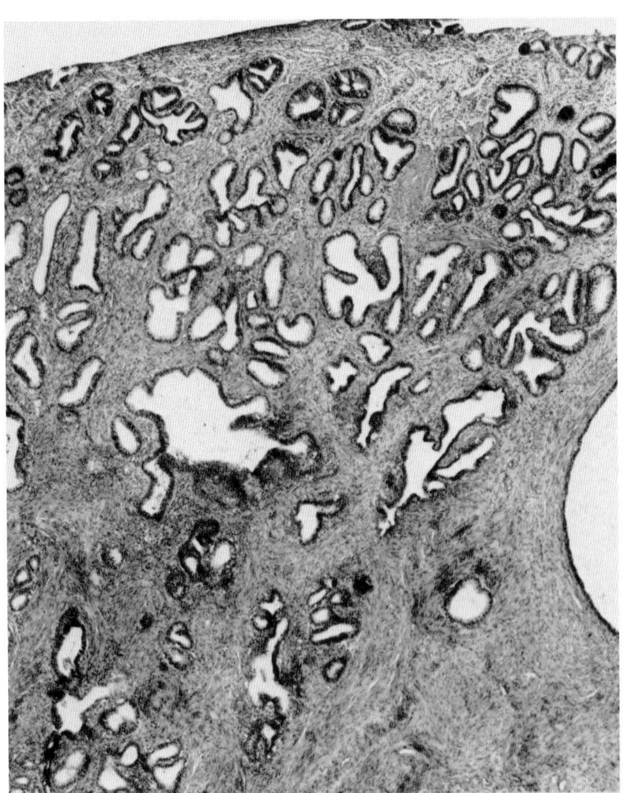

Fig. 3-5. Invasive endocervical-type adenocarcinoma. Although superficial glands have an arrangement consistent with adenocarcinoma in situ, the arrangement of the underlying glands and the depth of infiltration are diagnostic of invasive adenocarcinoma.

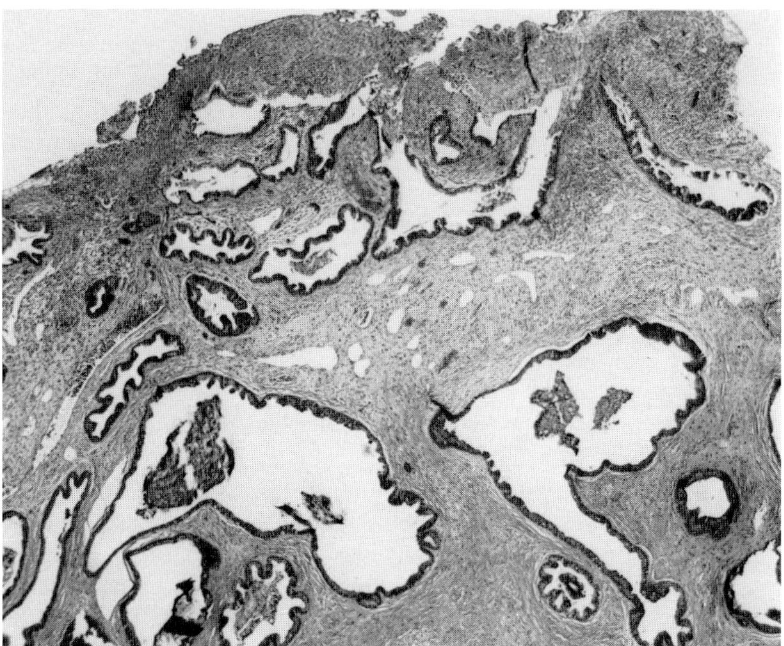

Fig. 3-6. Invasive endocervical-type adenocarcinoma. The disorderly arrangement and shapes of the atypical glands are diagnostic of invasive adenocarcinoma.

cinoma'' (which may be squamous, glandular, or adenosquamous) as one in which the invasive focus is less than 500 mm³. Three-dimensional measurement of small tumors, however, is probably not practical in routine practice. Additional studies should be performed to determine if MIA is definable using two-dimensional measurements, as with FIGO stage IA2 microinvasive squamous carcinomas (less than 50 mm²).

Follow-up Studies

In Burghardt's study, there were four patients with microcarcinomas (two microadenocarcinomas and two microadenosquamous carcinomas) and four somewhat larger tumors (with volumes between 500 and 1000 mm³.[51] Four of the eight patients were treated by radical hysterectomy and pelvic lymphadenectomy, three by radical hysterectomy without lymphadenectomy, and one by cone biopsy. Six of the patients,

including the woman treated only by cone biopsy, were followed for over 5 years with no evidence of recurrence. Other follow-up studies have been of cases defined only by depth of invasion. Teshima et al.[21] followed 22 cases of MIA (defined as less than 5 mm of stromal invasion) that included endocervical (12), endometrioid (8), and clear cell (2) subtypes. Only one patient had a recurrence (in the vagina, 2.3 years after radical hysterectomy); the primary tumor in that case was 3 mm in depth. In the series conducted by Berek et al.,[53] there were no nodal metastases in six patients who had tumors that were less than 2 mm deep, whereas positive nodes were found in 11 percent (2/18) of patients with 2 to 5 mm of invasion.[23] In addition, pulmonary metastases appeared in one patient with a tumor that invaded to a depth of 5 mm, although the tumor in that case was poorly differentiated.[23] These observations, albeit on a small number of cases, suggest that early invasive adenocarcinomas are associated with a negligible risk of nodal metastases when they invade the stroma for a distance of less than 2 mm, but that there is a low but definite risk of nodal metastases or pelvic recurrence when the lesions invade the stroma for depths of 2 to 5 mm.

Treatment

The currently recommended minimal treatment for MIA (however defined) is hysterectomy, even in cases in which the lesion appears completely excised by cone biopsy. In the study of MIAs (defined by less than 5 mm depth of invasion) by Andersen and Arffmann,[29] four of six patients with MIA in cone biopsy specimens in which the lesions appeared to be completely excised were found to have "residual disease" in the hysterectomy specimens. Many patients with lesions regarded as MIA have also had pelvic lymphadenectomy performed as part of their treatment. However, if the designation MIA is to have

clinical utility, its ultimate definition (if the lesion is definable) should be that of a lesion in which there is a negligible risk of nodal involvement. Additional studies of cervical adenocarcinomas with early stromal invasion are required. The pathologic descriptions of the lesions in such studies should include measurements of the invasive focus in at least two dimensions, so that results of various studies can be more easily compared.

ENDOCERVICAL GLANDULAR DYSPLASIA

It has been recognized only during the past 20 years that the endocervical columnar epithelium may exhibit a spectrum of precancerous changes that are less severe than those that characterize AIS (Figs. 3-7 and 3-8). Most of the earliest studies identified such changes on cytologic smears studied both routinely[2] and morphometrically,[54] with only rare cases in which dysplastic

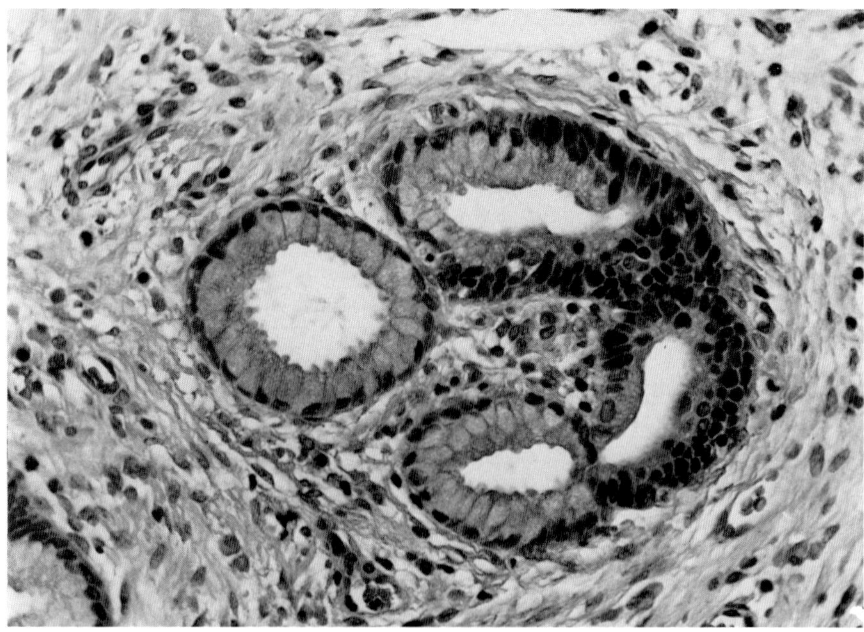

Fig. 3-7. Endocervical glandular dysplasia. The nuclei of the glandular lining cells are moderately atypical in the glands on the right side.

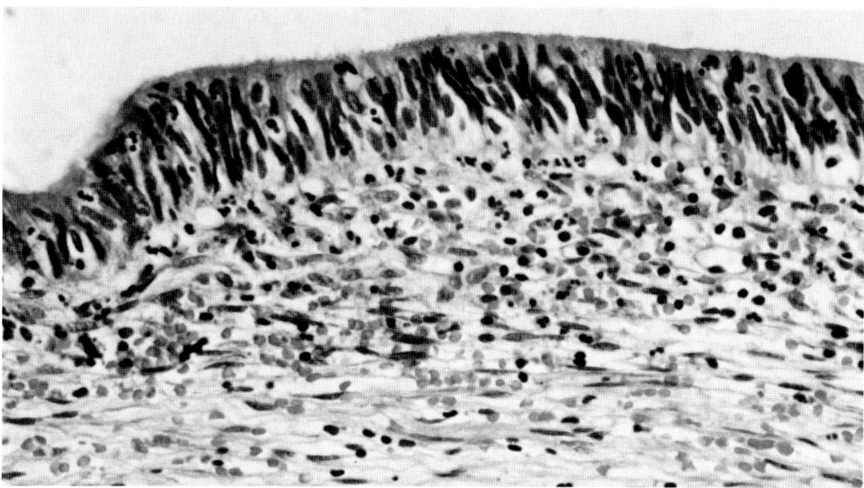

Fig. 3-8. Endocervical glandular dysplasia. The endocervical lining epithelium is stratified with moderately atypical nuclei.

changes less severe than those of AIS were documented on histologic specimens.[57] More recently, a number of histologic studies have made attempts to define these changes, which have been referred to as *endocervical glandular dysplasia* (EGD).[1, 17, 19, 22, 25, 55]

Gloor and Hurlimann[22] found foci of EGD (their cervical intraepithelial glandular neoplasia [CIGN] grades I and II) of both endocervical and intestinal types in 22 of 23 cases of AIS (their CIGN grade III). The cells of CIGN I had slightly hyperchromatic nuclei without significant stratification; occasional mitotic figures were present. CIGN II had pseudostratified crowded hyperchromatic nuclei with more frequent mitotic figures and diminished intracellular mucin. More recently, Brown and Wells[55] identified 17 cases of EGD (one of which merged with foci of AIS) in 105 cases of squamous CIN III within cone biopsy and hysterectomy specimens. The mean age of the patients was 36.9 years (range, 27 to 50), within the range of those with AIS. These investigators subclassified their cases of pure EGD into low-grade EGD (nine cases) and high-grade EGD (seven cases). The latter lesion was characterized by nuclear stratification (greater than two-thirds of the epithelial height), enlarged, elongated, hyperchromatic, occasionally vesicular nuclei, pleomorphic nuclei with densely clumped chromatin, and an increased nuclear-to-cytoplasmic ratio. Mitotic figures were rare (less than 1 per glandular profile). Most of the glands had an abnormal profile, with irregular branching and budding and intraluminal cellular tufts and low papillae lacking stromal cores. Low-grade EGD exhibited a spectrum of appearances ranging from glandular epithelium with minimal abnormalities to changes similar to but less severe than those of high-grade EGD. Nuclear enlargement, elongation, and hyperchromasia were noted, but vesicular nuclei were not as common as in the high-grade lesions, and stratification was limited to the basal two-thirds of the epithelium. Mitotic figures were not seen. Glandular profiles were abnormal and were similar to those of high-grade EGD. Both low-grade and high-grade lesions had a decrease in intracellular mucin, and subnuclear vacuoles were a common finding. The atypical glands were located ''randomly'' in the endocervix and occasionally were high in the endocervical canal. The amount of atypical epithelium varied from a small focus within an otherwise normal gland to diffuse involvement of many glands. Almost all the cases of EGD studied by Brown et al.[56] and Griffin et al.[44] had cytoplasmic immunoreactivity for both human milk fat globule 1 and amylase, a staining pattern similar to that observed in cases of AIS. As might be expected of a precursor lesion, Brown and Wells[55] estimated that EGD was 16 times more common than AIS.

Because of what appears to be a morphologic continuum (as in squamous CIN) and the subjectivity of the proposed criteria, the distinction between high-grade EGD and AIS, as Brown and Wells[55] noted, will likely prove problematic and of limited clinical utility in routine practice. Jaworski[1] suggested that all lesions regarded as less than AIS be presently categorized as EGD (without subdivision into grades). The minimal criteria used by Jaworski[1] for EGD include nuclear atypia and some evidence of cellular turnover, specifically apoptotic bodies and occasional mitotic figures (two or fewer per gland). Although there is some evidence to suggest a neoplastic progression from EGD to AIS,[55] further study of EGD is needed to determine what proportion of cases of AIS are preceded by EGD, what proportion of cases of EGD progress to AIS, and the time interval between the appearance of EGD and AIS.[1]

INVASIVE ADENOCARCINOMA

In the older literature, adenocarcinomas were generally reported to account for only 5 percent of cervical carcinomas,[58–62] but much higher figures have been recorded in more recent studies,[63–65] and these tumors now account for approximately 14 percent of cervical carcinomas.[66] To a large extent, their increased frequency among all carcinomas of the cervix is relative, due to a decrease in the incidence of invasive squamous cell carcinomas, which are more

readily identified in their preinvasive stages by cytologic examination, but some studies have suggested that an actual increase in frequency of adenocarcinomas has also occurred. Several reports have provided evidence that the human papillomavirus (particularly HPV 18) may have a significant role in the causation of these tumors and their precursors.[67, 68] Evidence was presented in one study that suggested an association with oral contraceptive use[69] and was supported by a large epidemiologic study that concluded that extended use of oral contraceptives was a risk factor for all cervical carcinomas, but particularly for adenocarcinomas.[70] However, a more recent study did not agree with the findings in prior studies.[71] In addition, in another study of the frequency of adenocarcinoma in Japanese and New Zealand women, there was no significant difference despite the much greater use of oral contraceptives in New Zealand.[72]

Adenocarcinoma of the cervix almost always occurs in adults, being very rare in the first decade and uncommon in the second. The average age in the majority of reported series is in the range of 44 to 54 years.[73–96] The patients present with abnormal uterine bleeding in approximately 80 percent of the cases. Occasional women complain of vaginal discharge or pain. In some cases, the symptoms are attributable to the presence of a mucinous ovarian tumor, either metastatic from the cervix or an independent primary tumor.[97–99] The tumor causes no symptoms in 20[61, 75] to 39 percent[77] of cases. In such cases, it is usually discovered because of an abnormal Papanicolaou smear, although cytologic examination is less sensitive in its detection than in the detection of squamous cell carcinoma. In one report, 51 percent of patients with cervical adenocarcinoma had normal cytologic findings, and only 20 percent of patients without a grossly visible lesion had a positive result.[86] The gross appearance of the tumors varies greatly. Some are de-

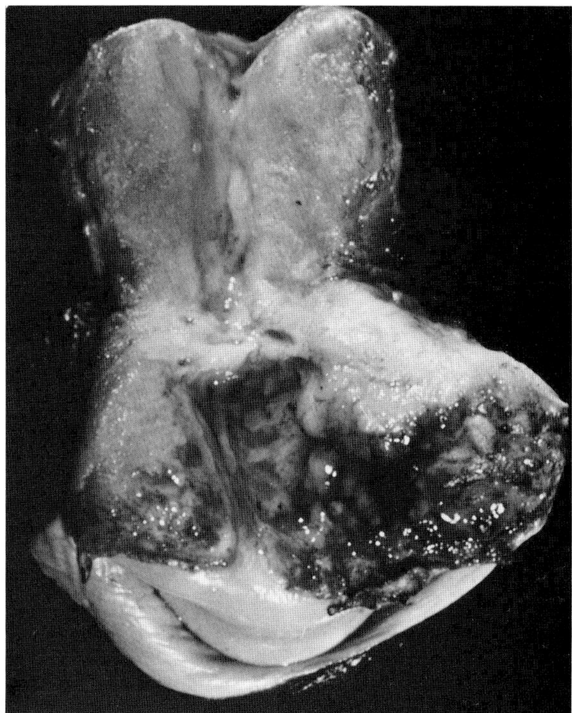

Fig. 3-9. Invasive adenocarcinoma. There is extensive destruction of the cervix by an ulcerating tumor.

structive ulcerated lesions (Fig. 3-9), others are elevated granular masses (Fig. 3-10), and still others are strikingly polypoid (Fig. 3-11). Some tumors produce little or no mucosal abnormality presenting as a barrel-shaped cervix (Fig. 3-12). In 20 to 30 per-cent of cases, the cervix appears normal or is thought to exhibit only benign changes.[88] Adenocarcinomas may cause considerable diagnostic difficulty on microscopic examination because of their relative rarity and varied patterns and because of the potential

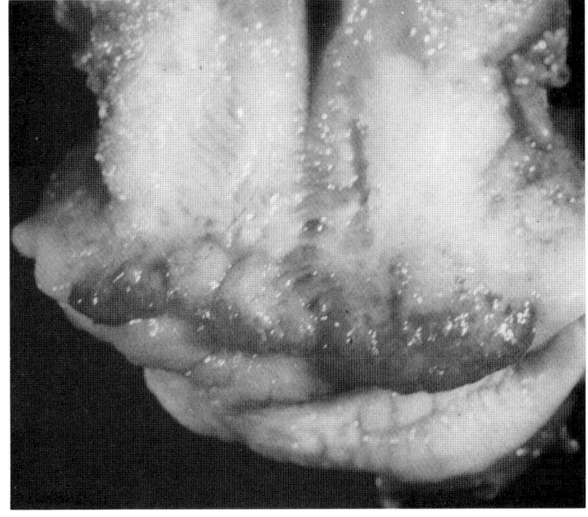

Fig. 3-10. Invasive adenocarcinoma. An elevated slightly nodular mass that was light brown in the fresh state is shown circumferentially involving the cervix.

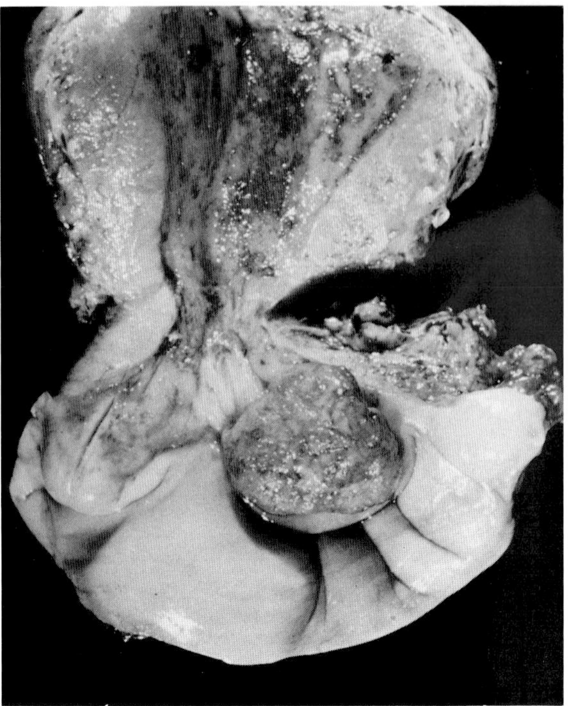

Fig. 3-11. Invasive adenocarcinoma. The tumor is polypoid.

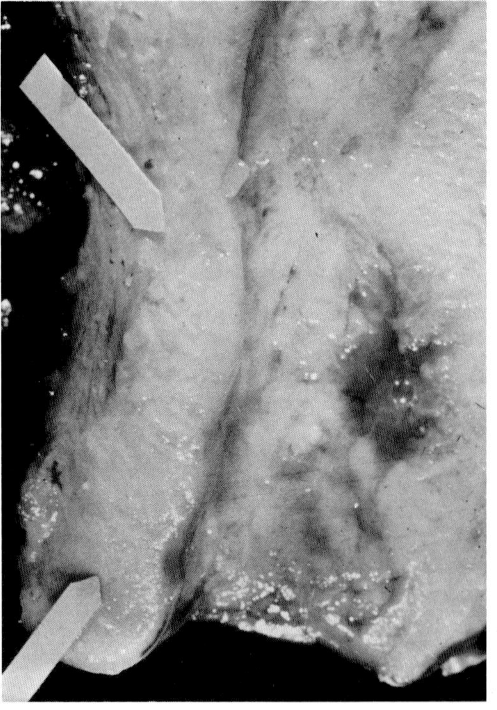

Fig. 3-12. Invasive adenocarcinoma. The cervical wall is thickened.

for confusing them with the non-neoplastic glandular lesions discussed in Chapter 1. A histologic classification of these tumors is presented in Table 3-1. The various microscopic subtypes are discussed separately. Those in the mixed group (category 5) are not discussed specifically, as the features of the individual components are similar histologically to their appearance in pure form. A tumor is placed in this group when, rarely, a neoplasm has more than one component of a specific subtype, each accounting for at least 10 percent of the neoplasm.

ENDOCERVICAL-TYPE ADENOCARCINOMA

Adenocarcinomas of typical or endocervical type account for approximately 70 percent of cervical adenocarcinomas. Most of them are moderately to well differentiated mucinous adenocarcinomas characterized by glands of medium size (Figs. 3-13, 3-14) that are lined by atypical stratified co-

Table 3-1. Classification of Cervical Adenocarcinoma and Related Tumors

1. Adenocarcinoma
   a. Endocervical type
      Variants
         (i) Adenoma malignum (minimal deviation adenocarcinoma)
         (ii) Villoglandular
   b. Endometrioid
   c. Clear cell
   d. Serous
   e. Mesonephric
   f. Intestinal type
   g. Signet ring cell

2. Adenosquamous carcinoma
      Variant
         Glassy cell carcinoma

3. Adenoid basal carcinoma

4. "Adenoid cystic" carcinoma

5. Adenocarcinoma, mixed (specify subtypes)

6. Adenocarcinoma and "carcinoid"/small cell carcinoma (see Ch. 8)

7. Metastatic adenocarcinoma (see Ch. 8)

lumnar cells some of which contain mucin. In some cases, however, the glands are very small (Fig. 3-15); at the other extreme some may be large and cystically dilated, sometimes containing abundant basophilic mucin (Fig. 3-16) or, less commonly, an eosinophilic secretion (Fig. 3-17). The arrangement of the glands is very variable; some are widely spaced, others form closely packed aggregates with a cribriform pattern (Fig. 3-18). Rarely, a microglandular pattern is present, but a close resemblance to microglandular hyperplasia has been observed by us in only one case of a patient who was on oral contraceptives (Fig. 3-19).[100] The tumors rarely contain large cysts (Fig. 3-20) and may contain solid areas (Fig. 3-21) that cannot be distinguished from poorly differentiated squamous cell carcinomas if viewed in isolation. Papillae may be present both on the surface (Fig. 3-22) and within gland lumens (Fig. 3-23) but are uncommonly conspicuous. One tumor that was associated with chorionic gonadotropin production contained anaplastic cells, including giant cells that stained immunohistochemically for hCG.[101] The tumors may elicit little or no stromal reaction, a desmoplastic stroma, or occasionally a prominent fibromatous stroma. Endocervical-type adenocarcinomas may be components of mixed tumors, for example, adenocarcinoma and small cell carcinoma,[102, 103] and, as noted for EGD and AIS, premalignant squamous lesions are found in the adjacent epithelium in as many as 43 percent of the cases.[104, 105]

The distinction of endocervical-type adenocarcinomas from endometrial adenocarcinomas may be difficult, particularly when a fractional curettage has not been performed or when tumor is present in both endocervical and endometrial curettage specimens. Although abundant intracellular mucin favors an endocervical origin, some endometrial adenocarcinomas are mucinous (see Ch. 5), and some endocervical type adenocarcinomas have little intracellu-

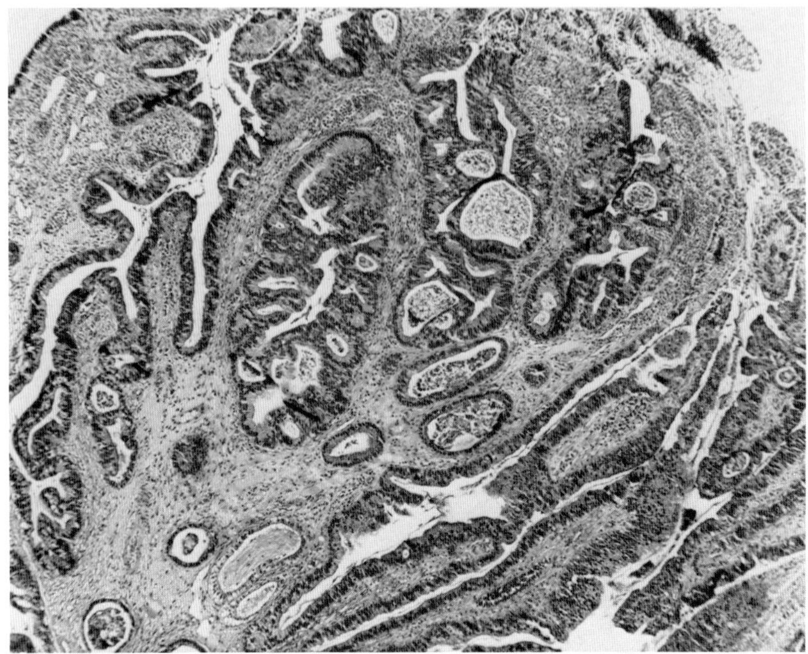

Fig. 3-13. Endocervical-type adenocarcinoma.

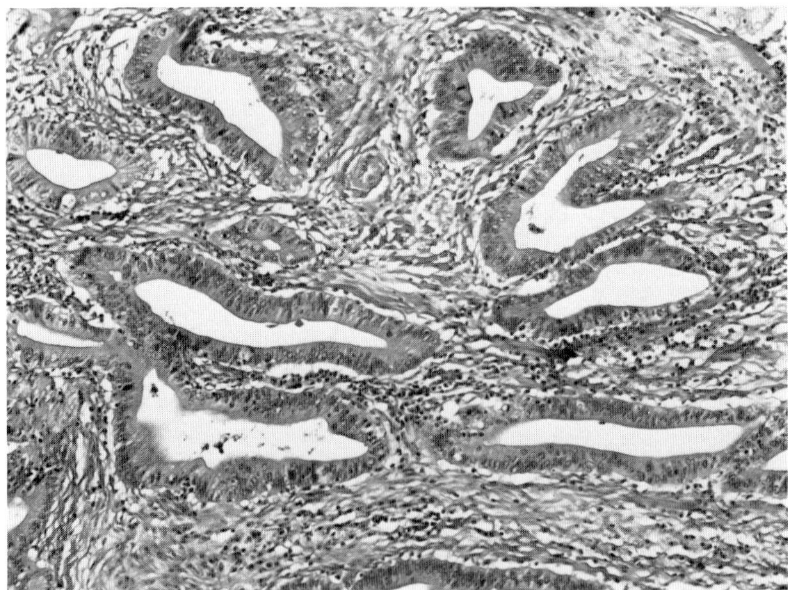

Fig. 3-14. Endocervical-type adenocarcinoma. The glands are lined by stratified columnar cells.

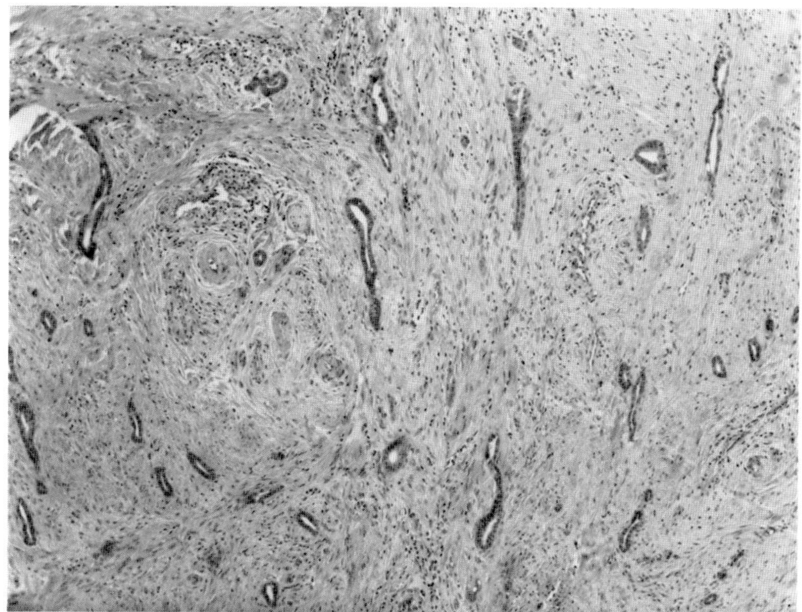

Fig. 3-15. Endocervical-type adenocarcinoma. The glands are widely spaced and many of them are very small.

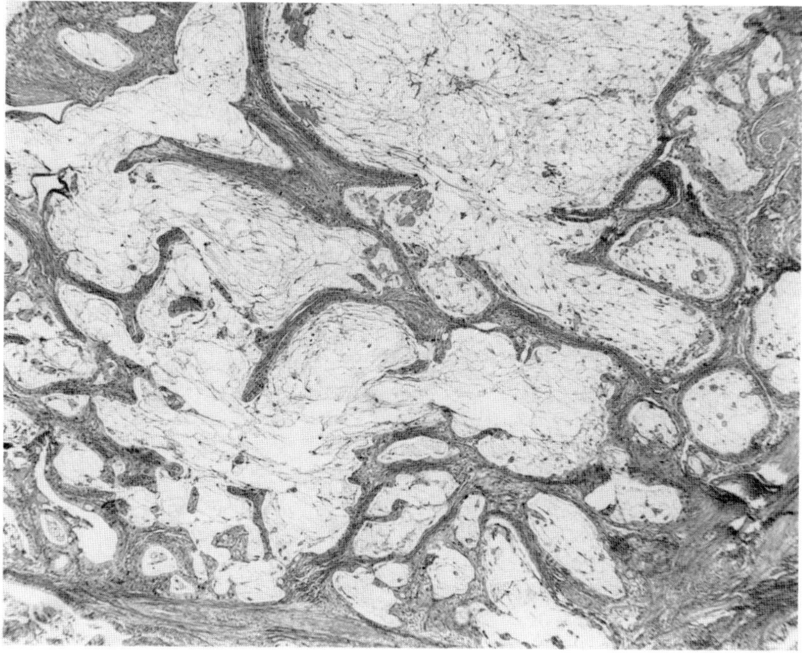

Fig. 3-16. Endocervical-type adenocarcinoma. Dilated glands contain mucin that was basophilic.

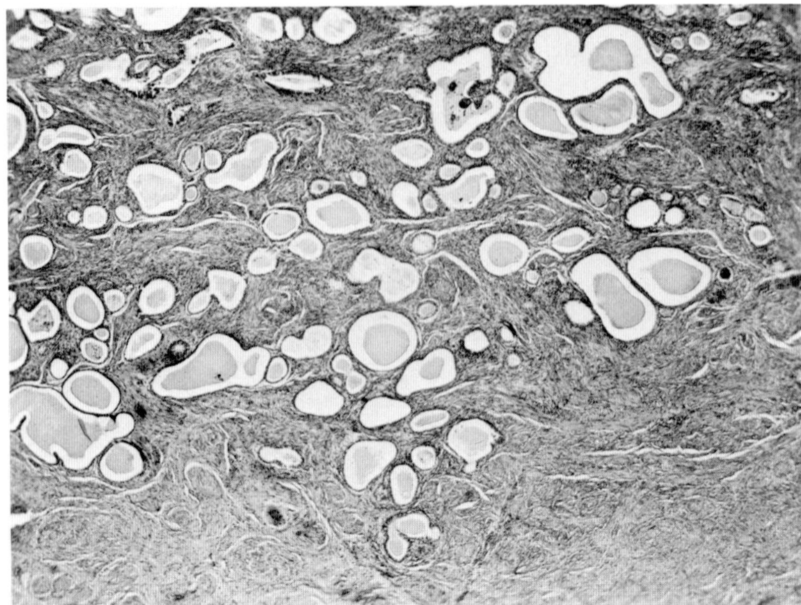

Fig. 3-17. Endocervical-type adenocarcinoma. The glands contain a secretion that was eosinophilic. The appearance simulates that of mesonephric hyperplasia.

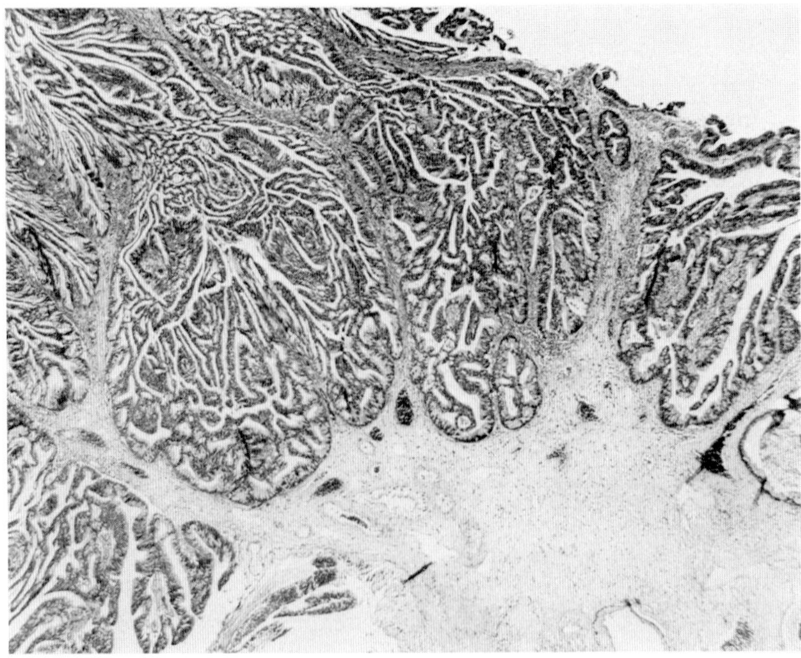

Fig. 3-18. Endocervical-type adenocarcinoma. The glands are confluent and have a focal cribriform pattern.

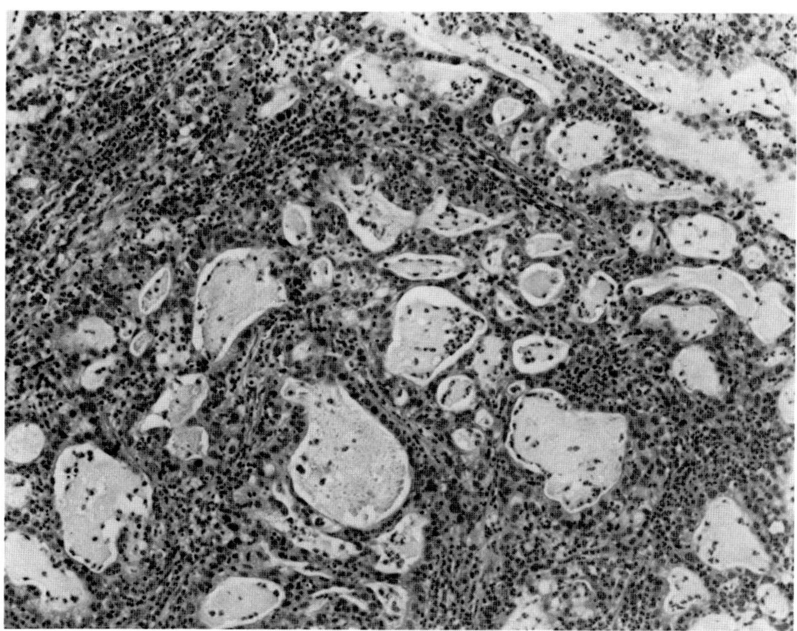

Fig. 3-19. Endocervical-type adenocarcinoma. This neoplasm, from a patient on oral contraceptives, has a pattern simulating that of microglandular hyperplasia with focal glandular dilatation, luminal mucin with inflammatory cells, and stromal inflammatory cells.

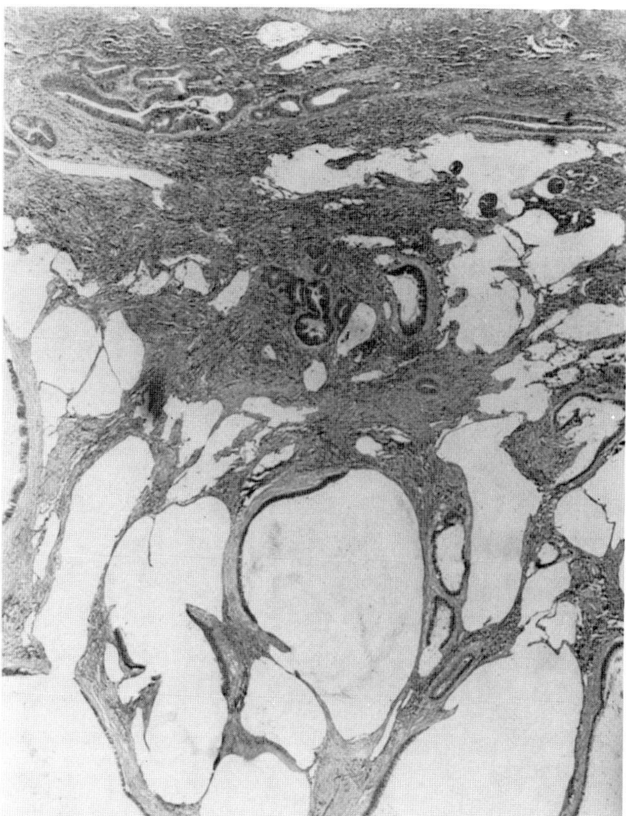

Fig. 3-20. Endocervical-type adenocarcinoma. The glands in the deep portion of the neoplasm are cystically dilated.

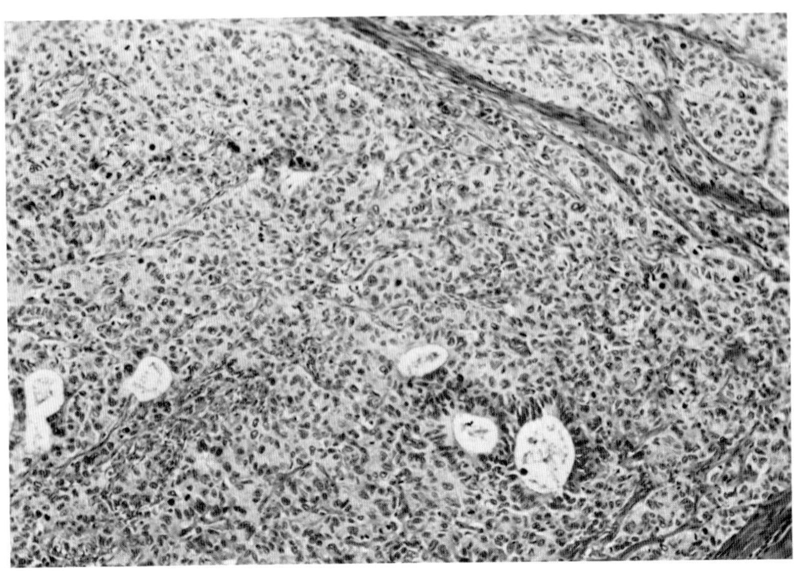

Fig. 3-21. Endocervical-type adenocarcinoma. Most of the tumor has a solid pattern but there is focal glandular differentiation.

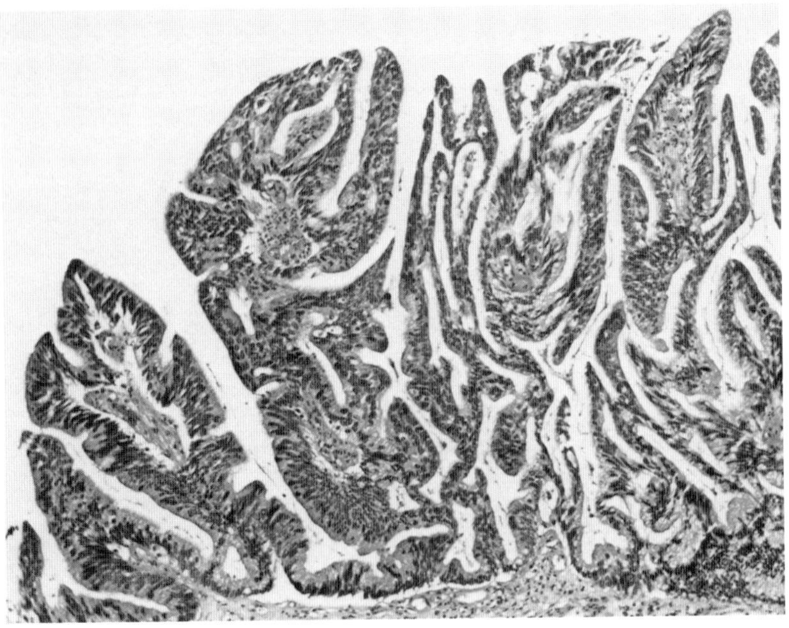

Fig. 3-22. Endocervical-type adenocarcinoma. Tumor lining the endocervical mucosa has a papillary pattern.

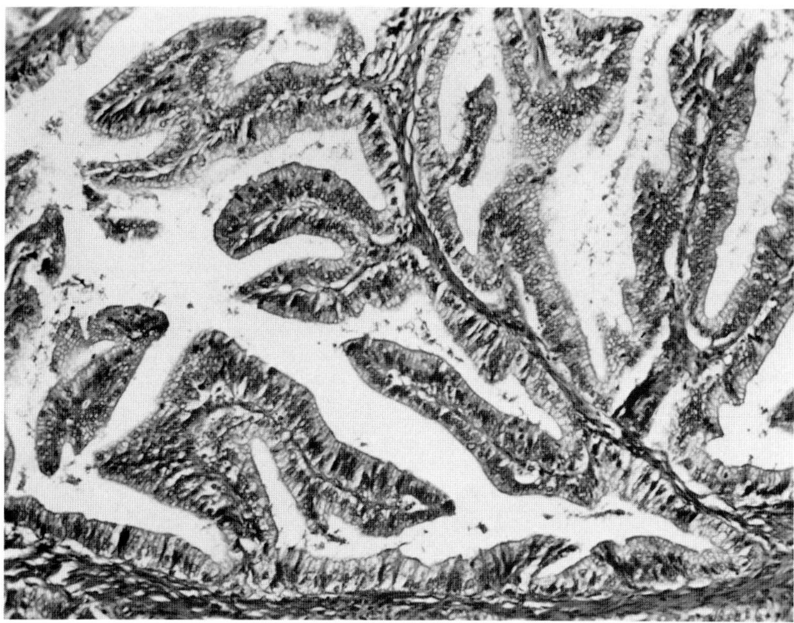

Fig. 3-23. Endocervical-type adenocarcinoma. Papillae project into glands.

lar mucin, and therefore, this criterion is not reliable. The nature of the stroma of the tumor may be helpful; in endometrial carcinomas it may resemble normal endometrial stroma and may contain lipid-laden foam cells, whereas in the cervical tumors such features are absent. Foci of acanthomatous change favor an endometrial origin but are not diagnostic. The finding of atypical endometrial hyperplasia in the specimen is strong evidence of an endometrial derivation. Although some studies[106, 107] have suggested that the more frequent staining of endocervical adenocarcinoma for carcinoembryonic antigen (CEA) may help in its distinction from endometrial adenocarcinoma, other studies have indicated that this staining is not a reliable discriminatory feature in individual cases.[108–110] Kudo et al.[45] have reported that 90 percent of cervical adenocarcinomas were immunoreactive with a new monoclonal antibody, IC5; the corresponding figure for CEA immunoreactivity was only 55 percent. None of their endometrial carcinomas showed cytoplasmic positivity with either antibody although

apical staining for both was seen in 40 percent of the cases. Hysteroscopy is often helpful in identifying the site of origin of the tumor. In some cases, a determination cannot be made until a hysterectomy specimen has been examined. Very rare endocervical-type adenocarcinomas superficially resemble mesonephric hyperplasia (Fig. 3-17) because of prominent eosinophilic secretion in gland lumens but the lining of the glands by mucinous cells excludes a mesonephric lesion. Differentiation from endometrioid carcinoma is discussed under the latter heading. The features of microglandular hyperplasia and other pseudoneoplastic glandular lesions that facilitate their distinction from adenocarcinoma are discussed in Chapter 1.

Adenoma Malignum (Minimal Deviation Adenocarcinoma)

The term *adenoma malignum* is used for cervical adenocarcinomas characterized by mucinous glands, the great majority of which have a deceptively benign histologic appearance.[111–116] An alternative designation, *minimal deviation adenocarcinoma*, is preferred by some.[112] Because of its unique pathologic features and clinical associations we restrict the term *adenoma malignum* to the mucinous tumors to which it was originally applied by McKelvey and Goodlin,[111] although others[114] have used the term to embrace several other types of deceptively benign appearing adenocarcinomas of the cervix as well.

Adenoma malignum, which accounts for approximately 10 percent of cervical adenocarcinomas, occurs over a wide age range, but as far as we are aware has not been reported in a patient under 20 years. In one large series, the average age was 42 years, and one-third of the patients were in the reproductive age group.[116] The presenting manifestations are usually menometrorrhagia and menorrhagia; some patients complain of a mucoid vaginal discharge. Ten cases of adenoma malignum have been reported in patients with the Peutz-Jeghers syndrome.[116–120]

On gross examination, the cervix is often firm or indurated and the mucosal surface may be hemorrhagic, friable or mucoid. Sectioning of the wall typically discloses yellow or tan-white tissue (Fig. 3-24); cysts up to 2 cm in diameter are occasionally prominent. Microscopic examination discloses closely to widely spaced glands that vary from small to large and are often irregular in size and shape (Fig. 3-25). They are occasionally cystically dilated and may exhibit papillary infolding. Most of the glands are lined by innocuous-appearing mucin-containing columnar epithelial cells with basal nuclei (Fig. 3-26). Thorough sampling of the tumor in a hysterectomy specimen, however, almost always shows at least occasional glands that are lined by obviously malignant epithelium and in some cases, foci of less well-differentiated adenocarcinoma are found. A desmoplastic stromal response is usually present around at least

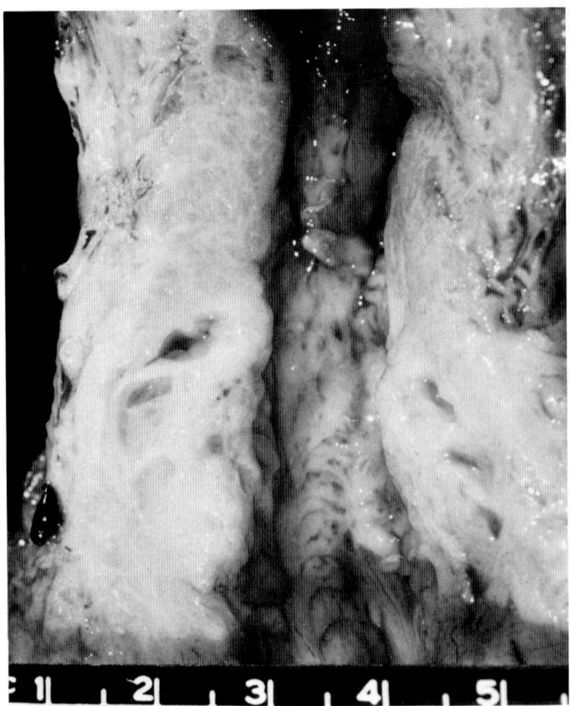

Fig. 3-24. Adenoma malignum. The endocervical wall is thickened and replaced by tumor that was tan-white. Several cysts are visible. (From Gilks et al.,[116] with permission).

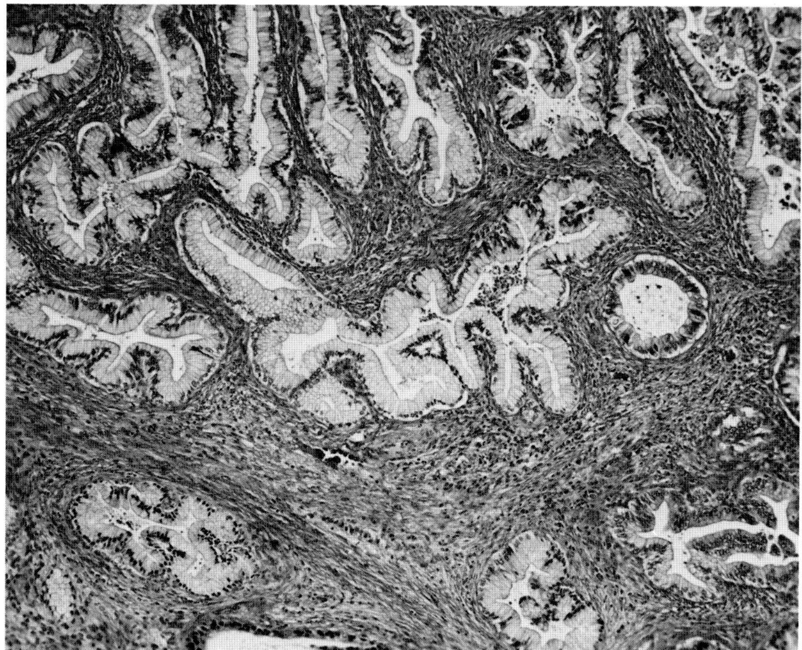

Fig. 3-25. Adenoma malignum. Most of the glands are lined by well-differentiated endocervical-type epithelium. (From McGowan et al.,[119] with permission).

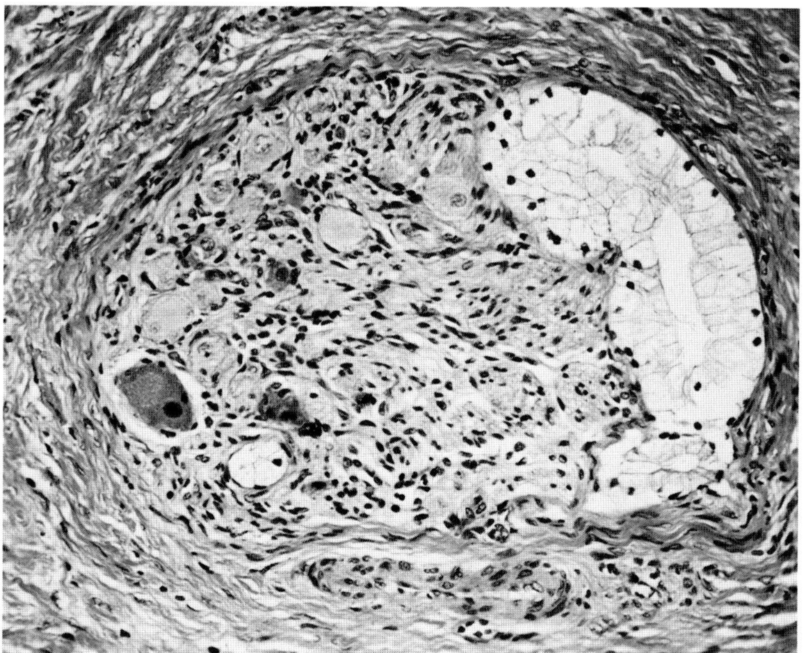

Fig. 3-26. Perineural invasion by adenoma malignum showing bland cytologic features of neoplastic cells. (From Young et al.,[120] with permission).

some of the glands in most cases and may be a prominent feature (Fig. 3-27). Vascular invasion is seen in approximately one-half of cases and perineural invasion in approximately one-sixth of them[116] (Fig. 3-26). In most cases, the tumor is deeply invasive of the cervical wall, and transmural extension or spread to the parametrium is seen in approximately 40 percent of cases, and the myometrium is involved in a similar proportion of cases.

The deceptively benign histologic appearance of adenoma malignum results in frequent diagnostic difficulties, particularly when only small biopsy specimens are available for examination and the diagnostic features recognizable in hysterectomy specimens may be absent. For example, in one series the initial biopsy specimens were misinterpreted as benign in one-third of cases, and in one case, the tumor was overlooked in a hysterectomy specimen.[116] In distinguishing the glands of adenoma malignum from abnormally shaped benign endocervical glands, the typical stromal response associated with the former may be helpful in indicating the infiltrative nature of the glands, although this change is not seen around most neoplastic glands, is often absent in small biopsy specimens, and is sometimes seen in association with benign glandular proliferations. The finding of glands lined by clearly malignant epithelium, as well as vascular or perineural invasion, establishes the diagnosis. In the absence of diagnostic features on biopsy, adenoma malignum should be considered when large, abnormally shaped glands are present. In some superficial biopsy specimens, especially if there is artifactual distortion, the abnormalities may be insufficient to warrant a diagnosis of carcinoma, but any worrisome proliferation as well as a clinical suspicion of carcinoma should lead to additional biopsies. The latter should be as deep as feasible because diagnostic features may be more apparent in deeper portions of the tumor. The features of the various non-neoplastic lesions with which adenoma malignum is apt to be confused

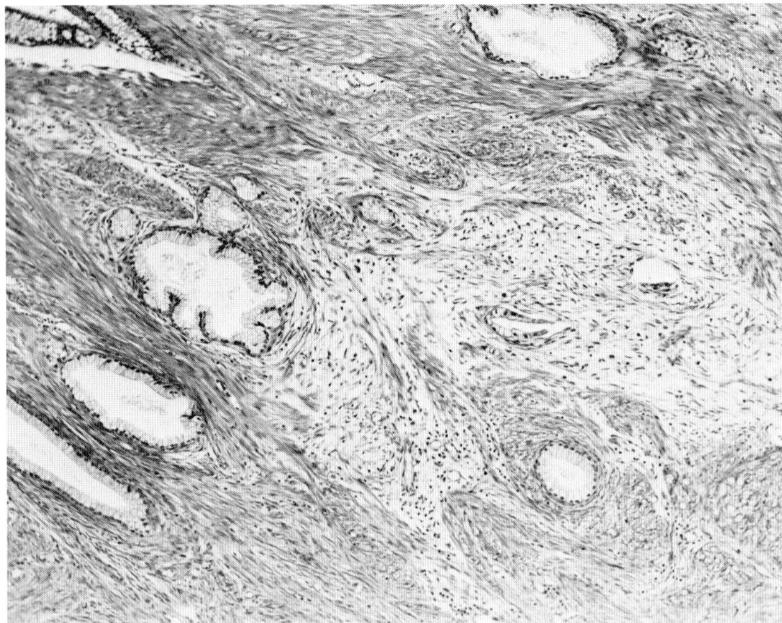

Fig. 3-27. Adenoma malignum. There is a pale-appearing stromal reaction around some of the glands.

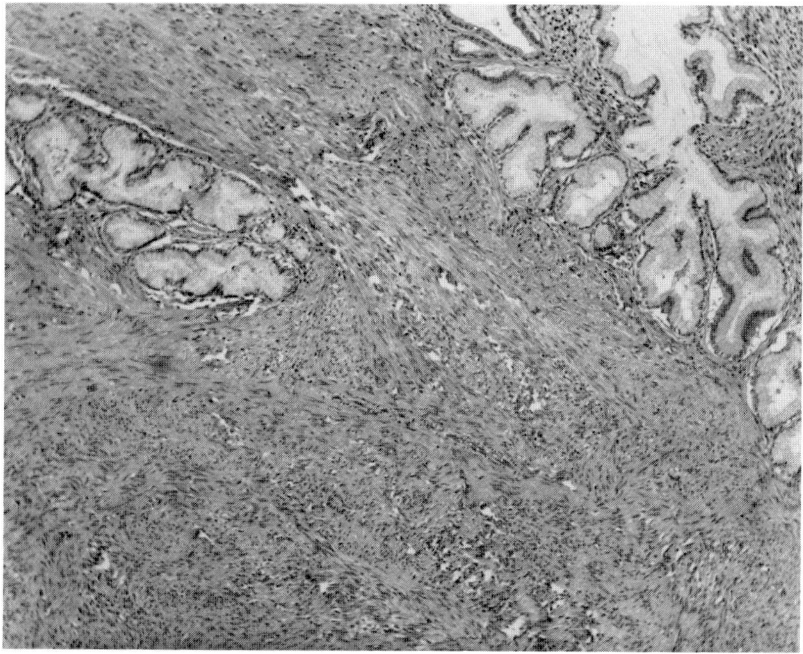

Fig. 3-28. Adenomyoma of cervix. Endocervical-type glands within the smooth muscle of this lesion may lead to a misdiagnosis of adenoma malignum if the myomatous nature of the smooth muscle is not appreciated.

are discussed in Chapter 1. A rare benign neoplasm which may enter into the differential diagnosis with adenoma malignum is a cervical adenomyoma whose glandular component is of typical endocervical type (Fig. 3-28). The glands in such a lesion may be haphazardly arranged, suggesting adenoma malignum. The major clues to the diagnosis of adenomyoma in such cases are an appreciation of the leiomyomatous nature of the muscle between the glands and the well-circumscribed margin of the lesion, although the latter is dependent on a generous biopsy. Because of the often subtle nature of the histologic features in cases of adenoma malignum, clinical information such as a gross appearance suggestive of carcinoma, a mucoid vaginal discharge, or the presence of the Peutz-Jehgers syndrome should alert the pathologist to the possibility of adenoma malignum. The cytologic features of adenoma malignum may

be subtle, as expected from its histologic appearance, and thorough sampling of the endocervical canal is important as only some of the tumor cells have diagnostic cytological features.[121]

Kaku and Enjoji[113] found argyrophil cells in five of eight cases of adenoma malignum and Fetissof et al.[122] suggested that Grimelius-positive endocrine cells might be characteristic of this lesion. Gilks et al.[116] reported argyrophil cells in six of 15 cases. The endocrine nature of the argyrophil cells in the latter study was confirmed by staining for serotonin in four cases. While these cells can be demonstrated commonly in adenoma malignum, and in its possibly preinvasive form,[122] their presence is only suggestive and not diagnostic of the tumor. Michael et al.[115] found that immunohistochemical staining for CEA was focally positive in five cases of adenoma malignum, while only areas of reserve cell hyperplasia were positive in five benign glandular lesions. Steeper and Wick[123] compared four cases of adenoma malignum, all of which were CEA positive, to seven cases of microglandular hyperplasia, all of which were negative. Gilks et al.,[116] however, found CEA staining of adenoma malignum so focal as to limit its diagnostic utility in biopsy specimens, a conclusion supported by another recent study.[124] It is important to emphasize that when adenoma malignum is immunoreactive for CEA, the staining is intracytoplasmic[124] as well as glycocalyceal. By contrast, only the latter pattern of staining is seen in normal endocervical epithelium and benign glandular lesions.

Controversy has surrounded the prognosis of adenoma malignum. Only one of the five patients in the series of McKelvey and Goodlin[111] survived for a long period. By contrast, four of five patients in the series of Silverberg and Hurt[112] were disease-free for at least 3 years, leading those authors to suggest that the poor prognosis in the earlier series was the result of inadequate ther-apy. If the series reported after 1963 are combined only 16 of 57 patients with a follow-up period of at least 2 years were alive without evidence of recurrence, 33 had died of their disease, 6 were alive with recurrences, and 2 had died of other causes. Of the patients whose tumors were staged, 6 of 12 patients with stage I tumors and 12 of 15 patients with stage II tumors died of their disease.[116] Kaku and Enjoji[113] compared the outcome of patients with adenoma malignum with that of patients with typical well-differentiated adenocarcinoma of the cervix also treated at their institution and found that the survival rate of those with adenoma malignum was significantly worse.

Villoglandular Papillary Adenocarcinoma

This recently described variant of adenocarcinoma usually occurs at a younger age (average, 35 years) than does cervical ade-

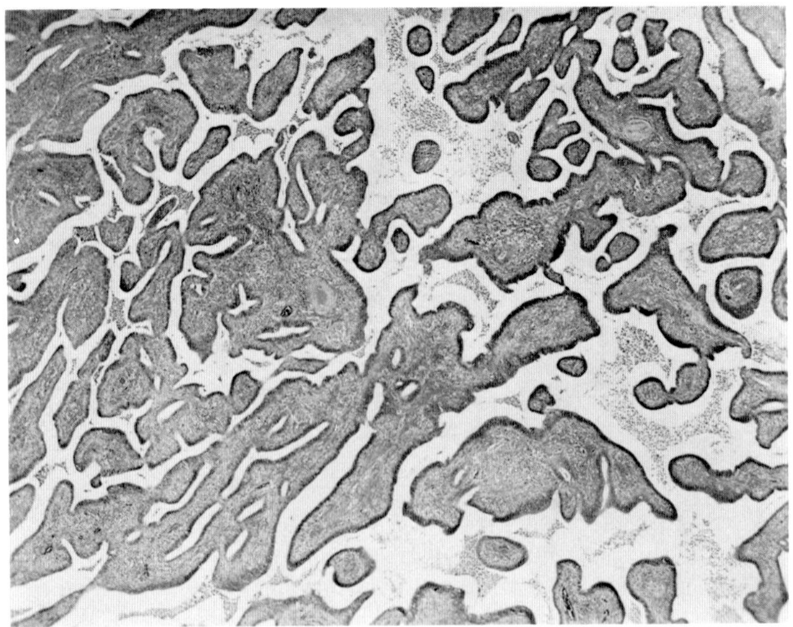

Fig. 3-29. Villoglandular papillary adenocarcinoma. Surface component of tumor showing villoglandular pattern and abundant cellular fibrous stroma.

nocarcinoma in general and is associated with a favorable prognosis.[125–127] Its cardinal feature is a surface papillary component of variable thickness with papillae that are usually tall and thin, but occasionally short and broad, and that have a fibromatous stromal core (Figs. 3-29 and 3-30). Occasional small cellular papillae may bud off the surfaces of the larger papillae, but cellular budding of the extent seen in serous papillary carcinomas is absent. The invasive portion of the tumors is typically composed of elongated branching glands separated by a fibromatous stroma similar to that present in the papillae (Fig. 3-31), but occasionally the stroma is desmoplastic or myxoid at the advancing margin of the tumor. The stroma of both the papillae and the invasive component often contains many acute and chronic inflammatory cells. The tumors are generally well circum-scribed, with only small foci of irregular invasion of the cervical stroma. The papillae and glands are usually lined by stratified nonmucinous columnar cells, but some of them are lined by a single layer of mucinous cells, a single layer of nonmucinous cells,or both. In occasional cases intracellular mucin is not demonstrable; such cases may belong in the endometrioid rather than the endocervical adenocarcinoma category. The tumor cells typically exhibit mild to moderate nuclear atypicality (Fig. 3-30) and contain scattered mitotic figures. A rare tumor has a component of villoglandular adenoma. Lymphatic or vascular invasion is rarely observed. The adjacent cervical glandular epithelium often shows adenocarcinoma-in-situ.

In the initial series of cases of this tumor, a hysterectomy was performed in 12 cases and only a cone biopsy in one case.[125] The

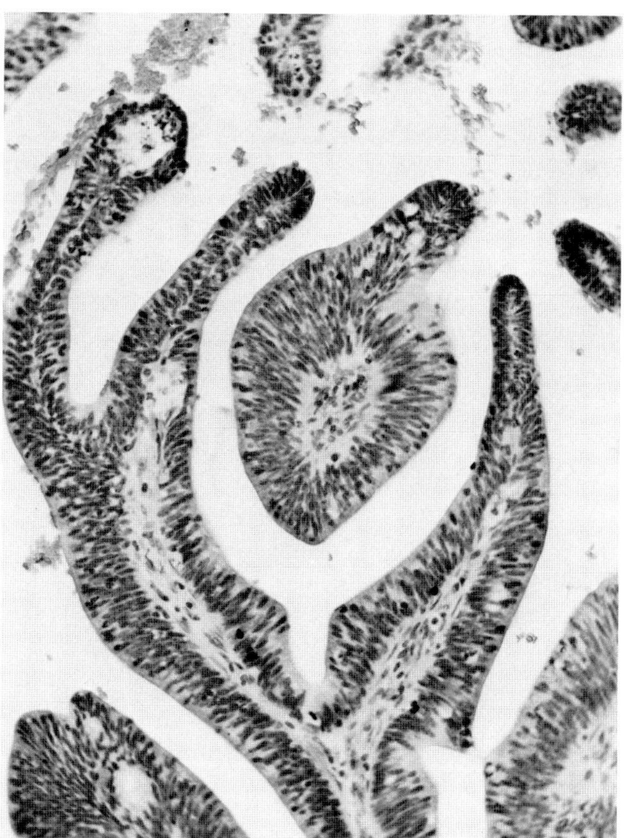

Fig. 3-30. Villoglandular papillary adenocarcinoma. Papillae are lined by stratified moderately atypical cells. (From Young and Scully,[125] with permission).

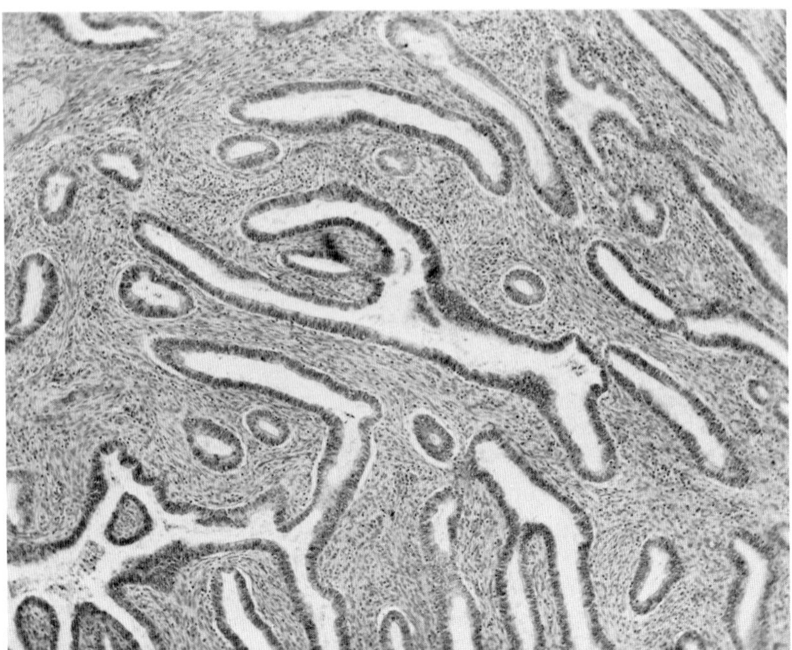

Fig. 3-31. Villoglandular papillary adenocarcinoma. Branching glands, many of which are elongated, are separated by prominent cellular fibrous stroma. (From Young and Scully,[125] with permission.)

cone biopsy specimen and four of the hysterectomy specimens contained no residual tumor. In six cases, the adenocarcinoma was confined to the inner third of the cervical wall and in two cases there was deep invasion. Follow-up evaluation of 2 to 14 years duration, including more than 5 years in 10 cases, revealed no evidence of recurrent tumor. In two subsequent studies of a total of 27 cases, no recurrences or metastases have developed.[126, 127] In five of these patients, only excisional or cone biopsy was performed. The young age of many of the patients and the excellent prognosis of this tumor suggest that it may be managed by a cone biopsy and careful follow-up, if the tumor is noninvasive or microinvasive, well differentiated, and without vascular space invasion or involvement of resection margins. We recently observed two unpublished cases of villoglandular adenocarcinoma of the cervix that were deeply invasive and metastasized to lymph nodes.

They were more cytologically atypical than the usual villoglandular tumor.

Villoglandular adenocarcinomas of the cervix must be differentiated from papillary adenocarcinomas of serous and clear cell types. The very rare serous carcinoma has irregular fine papillae with conspicuous cellular budding in contrast to villoglandular carcinomas that have minimal cellular budding. The cytologic atypia in serous carcinomas is usually more pronounced than that seen in villoglandular papillary adenocarcinomas and psammoma bodies are more common in serous than in the villoglandular papillary adenocarcinomas. The papillae of clear cell carcinoma lack a villous character and often have hyalinized cores, in contrast to those of the villoglandular tumors. The presence of other patterns of clear cell carcinoma as well as their composition of clear and hobnail cells also facilitate its diagnosis. Focal villoglandular areas can occur in otherwise nonpapillary adenocarcinomas of the cervix, but the term "*villoglandular papillary adenocarcinoma*" should be reserved for tumors having an exclusive or almost exclusive villoglandular pattern.

The differential diagnosis of villoglandular papillary adenocarcinoma also includes several benign lesions. Fingerlike papillae may be seen in chronic endocervicitis, but they are lined by a single layer of bland-appearing mucinous cells (see Ch. 1). Foci in villoglandular adenocarcinomas in which papillae are lined by a single layer of bland-appearing cells of müllerian type may resemble a müllerian papilloma[128] (Ch. 8), but the atypia in other areas of the carcinoma facilitates its diagnosis. Also, the müllerian papilloma almost always occurs in children, although we have seen rare cases in adults. In an adult patient a lesion for which the diagnosis of müllerian papilloma is being considered should be sampled extensively to exclude a villoglandular carcinoma. A lesion closely related to the müllerian papilloma is the rare cervical villoglandular papillary adenoma (see Ch. 8), which has an architecture similar to that of the papillary adenocarcinoma, but contains uniformly well differentiated cells. It must be emphasized, however, as noted above, that an occasional villoglandular tumor has both benign and malignant components. Two cases of "villous adenoma" of the cervix of intestinal type associated with underlying invasive adenocarcinoma have been reported.[129, 130] In one of the cases, the invasive adenocarcinoma was well differentiated with nuclear features similar to those of the villous portion of the tumor, whereas in the other case, the invasive portion of the tumor had more atypical nuclear features than the villous component. Both were characterized by the presence of intracellular mucin. The presence of invasive carcinoma in those two cases indicates that the finding of a villoglandular lesion of the cervix, even if it is lined by only slightly atypical cells, should warrant investigation to

exclude an underlying adenocarcinoma. The more or less sharp circumscription of villoglandular papillary adenocarcinomas and their prominent fibromatous stroma in part or all of the tumor occasionally raise the question of a müllerian adenofibroma (see Ch. 7). The atypicality of the epithelial component of the carcinomas, however, exceeds that of an adenofibroma, and the papillae are thinner and more villous in contrast to the typically broader polypoid fronds of an adenofibroma. In a superficial biopsy specimen, however, these two lesions may be difficult to distinguish.

ENDOMETRIOID ADENOCARCINOMA

These tumors are histologically similar to endometrioid adenocarcinomas of the uterine corpus (Fig. 3-32). When endocervical-type adenocarcinomas contain relatively little mucin, as they sometimes do, a superficial resemblance to endometrioid adenocarcinoma often results. Careful search in these cases, sometimes with the additional help of mucin stains, usually discloses endocervical features, warranting the diagnosis of endocervical-type adenocarcinoma. In our experience, true endometrioid carcinomas of the cervix are uncommon. Features that are helpful in the distinction of endometrioid carcinoma of the cervix from endometrioid adenocarcinoma of the corpus that has spread to the cervix are similar to those previously mentioned for distinguishing endocervical-type carcinomas from endometrial carcinomas. One endometrioid adenocarcinoma of the cervix arose from cervical endometriosis.[131] Kaminski and Norris[112] reported seven "minimal deviation adenocarcinomas of endometrioid type" that occurred in patients from 31 to 76 years of age. Three of five patients for whom follow-up information was available were free of disease 9 to 11 years postoperatively, one died of her disease at 14 years, and one died of a serous carcinoma of the

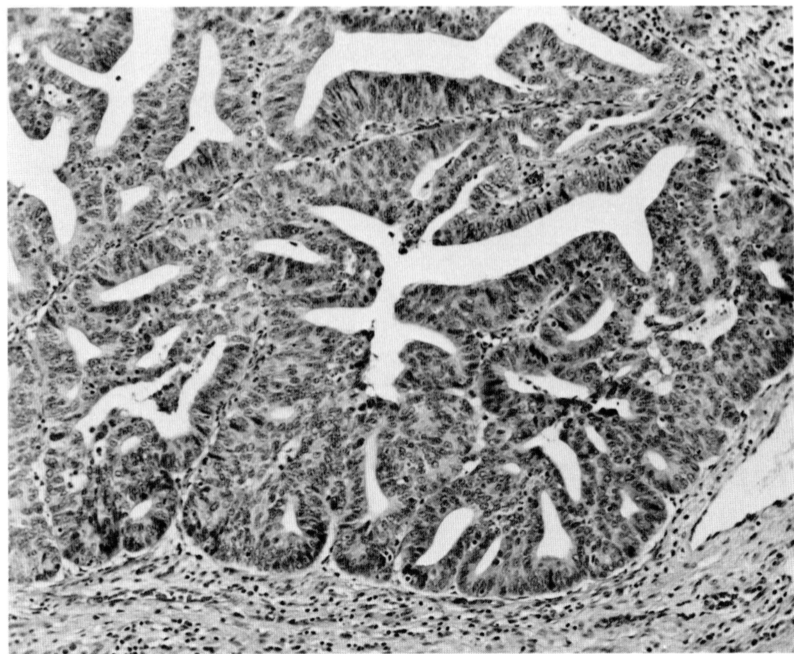

Fig. 3-32. Endometrioid adenocarcinoma. The tubular glandular pattern is indistinguishable from that of endometrioid adenocarcinoma of the uterine corpus.

ovary 9 years postoperatively. More recently, Rahilly and colleagues[132] have described two additional cases in patients who were well 1 year and 6 months after radical hysterectomy. We have seen several tumors that appear to fall in this category (Figs. 3-33 and 3-34). In one of the cases reported by Rahilly et al.,[132] the subtle nature of the abnormality caused it to be overlooked in a cone biopsy specimen.

CLEAR CELL ADENOCARCINOMA

Clear cell adenocarcinoma has been of interest over the past two decades because approximately two-thirds of young patients with this tumor have been exposed to diethylstilbestrol (DES) in utero.[133] This tumor is also encountered in the absence of DES exposure in females of all ages, reaching a peak frequency in postmenopausal women.[134–136] In most series of cervical adenocarcinomas prior to the DES era, clear cell adenocarcinoma accounted for approximately 5 percent of cases. The tumor may be located on the exocervix or in the endocervix; all the tumors that have developed in patients with DES exposure have involved the exocervix, sometimes extending into the endocervix. The tumors are typically nodular or polypoid, but are occasionally sessile with little abnormality of the overlying mucosa. Microscopic examination reveals three basic patterns: tubulocystic (Figs. 3-35 and 3-36), solid, and papillary (Fig. 3-37). In the tubulocystic pattern, tubules and cysts of varying size are lined by hobnail (Fig. 3-35), flat (Fig. 3-36), or clear cells. The cysts often contain mucin, and rarely intracytoplasmic mucin is present in occasional cells. The solid pattern is characterized by nests and sheets of cells containing abundant, clear, glycogen-rich cyto-

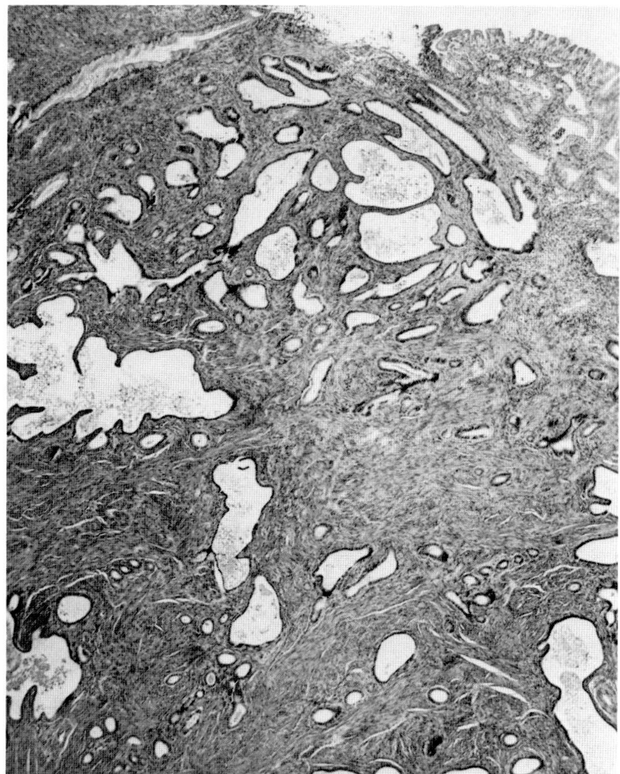

Fig. 3-33. Endometrioid adenocarcinoma, low grade. The invasive glands, many of which are cystically dilated, are not associated with a stromal reaction.

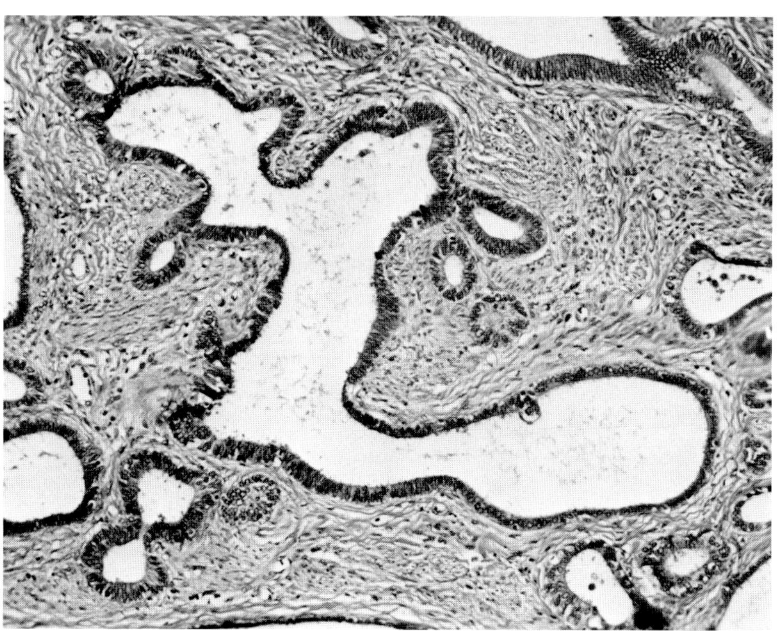

Fig. 3-34. Endometrioid adenocarcinoma, low grade. The glands are lined by stratified, minimally atypical cells that lack mucin.

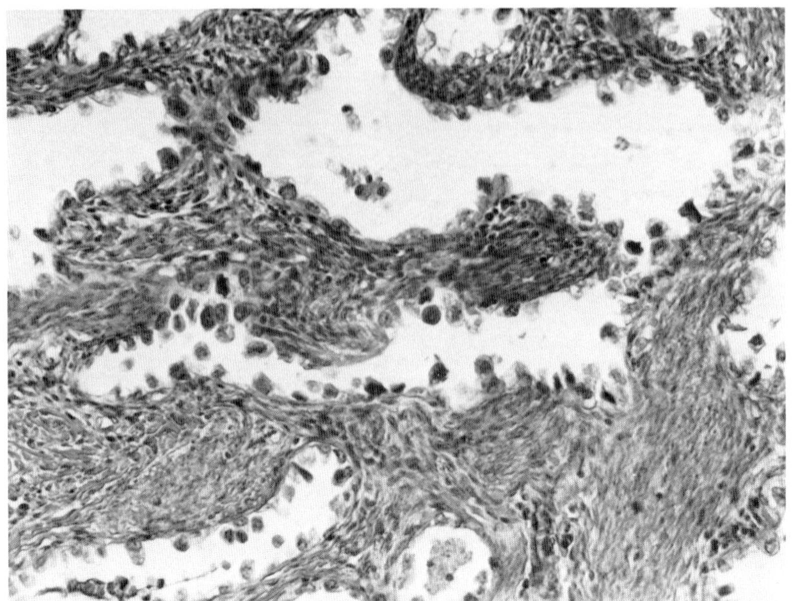

Fig. 3-35. Clear cell adenocarcinoma. Tubular glands are lined by hobnail cells.

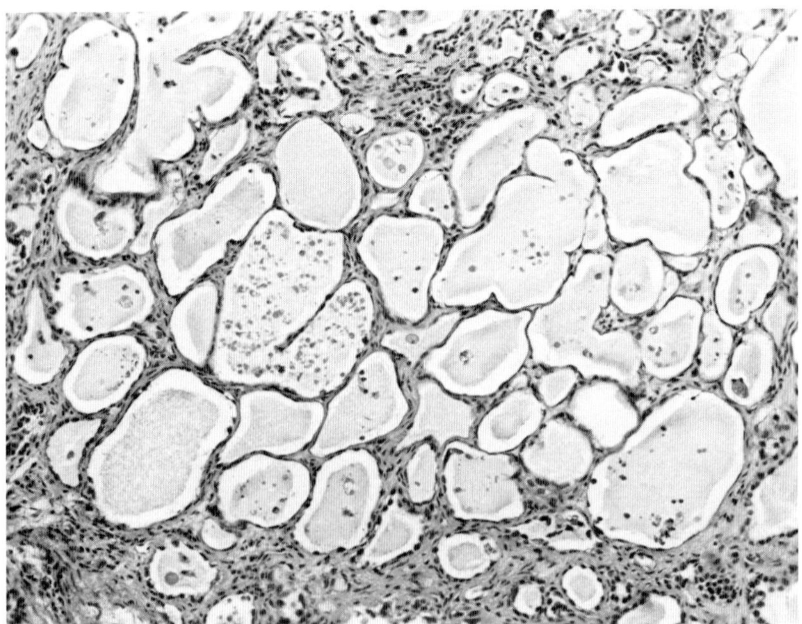

Fig. 3-36. Clear cell adenocarcinoma, tubulocystic pattern. The cysts are lined by flattened cells and appear deceptively benign.

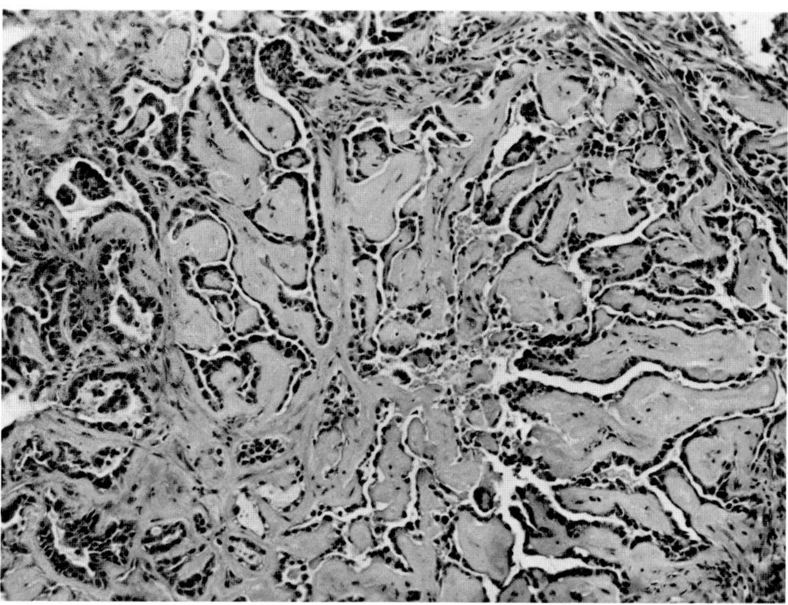

Fig. 3-37. Clear cell adenocarcinoma. The tumor has many papillae with extensive hyalinization of their cores.

plasm. The least common of the three patterns, the papillary, is characterized by numerous papillae extending into the tubules or cysts. The papillae vary from small and delicate with inconspicuous fibrovascular cores to larger with more prominent fibrovascular cores that are often extensively hyalinized (Fig. 3-37). The stroma of nonpapillary tumors is also occasionally prominently hyalinized.

Differentiation of clear cell adenocarcinomas from other types of cervical adenocarcinoma is almost always possible because of the typical microscopic features of the former tumors. In a small biopsy specimen, however, it may be difficult to distinguish clear cell adenocarcinoma from microglandular hyperplasia; even then, the cytologic atypia encountered in clear cell carcinoma, the usual lack of intracellular mucin, and the absence of the typical patterns of microglandular hyperplasia facilitate the differential diagnosis. Rarely, the Arias-Stella reaction (see Ch. 4) involves the endocervix[137] and the cells of this lesion may be confused with the hobnail cells of clear cell adenocarcinoma. In the pregnancy-associated lesion, however, the association with pregnancy is usually evident, a papillary tufting pattern, if present, is uniform instead of irregular, and the nuclei tend to be dark and homogeneous, exhibiting no mitotic activity. In young children, the very rare yolk sac tumor of the cervix, which may be composed, at least in part, of clear cells, may be confused with clear cell adenocarcinoma. The variety of distinctive patterns of this tumor, especially a reticular pattern with Schiller-Duval bodies, and the primitive appearance of its cells facilitate the diagnosis. In difficult cases, immunostaining for α-fetoprotein (AFP) may be helpful although it should not be relied on entirely to establish the diagnosis. Finally, the rare primary alveolar soft part sarcoma of the cervix (see Ch. 8) should not be confused with a clear cell carcinoma that has an organoid pattern and cells with eosinophilic cytoplasm. The distinctive architecture of the former tumor and its characteristic PAS-positive intracytoplasmic crystals help in the differential diagnosis. Metastatic renal cell carcinoma is always a consideration when the tumor is made up exclusively of clear cells and contains little or no luminal mucin.

SEROUS PAPILLARY ADENOCARCINOMA

There are only a few reviews[138] or original articles[139] in which this tumor is mentioned specifically, although cases appear to have been included under the general designation "papillary adenocarcinoma" in some reports. Abell and Gosling[58] illustrated one tumor that resembled a serous papillary adenocarcinoma, and Marcus and Marcus[82] noted a similarity between some examples of adenocarcinoma of the cervix and ovarian serous papillary carcinoma. In our experience the cervical form of the tumor is rare, and some of the cases that have been illustrated probably were clear cell papillary adenocarcinomas.[140] Only one report specifically devoted to this tumor has appeared.[141] The three patients in that series were 32, 33, and 69 years of age. The microscopic features are identical to those of serous papillary carcinomas of the ovary and uterine corpus (Fig. 3-38). In view of the paucity of reported cases, the behavior of this tumor is uncertain. One might expect it to have a prognosis similar to that of its endometrial counterpart, but two of three patients in the one report on this tumor were alive and well 5 years after treatment; follow-up was of insignificant duration in the third case. The diagnosis of primary serous carcinoma of the cervix should be made only after spread from the ovary, fallopian tube, or endometrium has been excluded.

MESONEPHRIC ADENOCARCINOMA

Mesonephric adenocarcinoma is one of the rarest subtypes of cervical adenocarcinoma.[142–148] Most of the "mesonephric carcinomas" reported in the older liter-

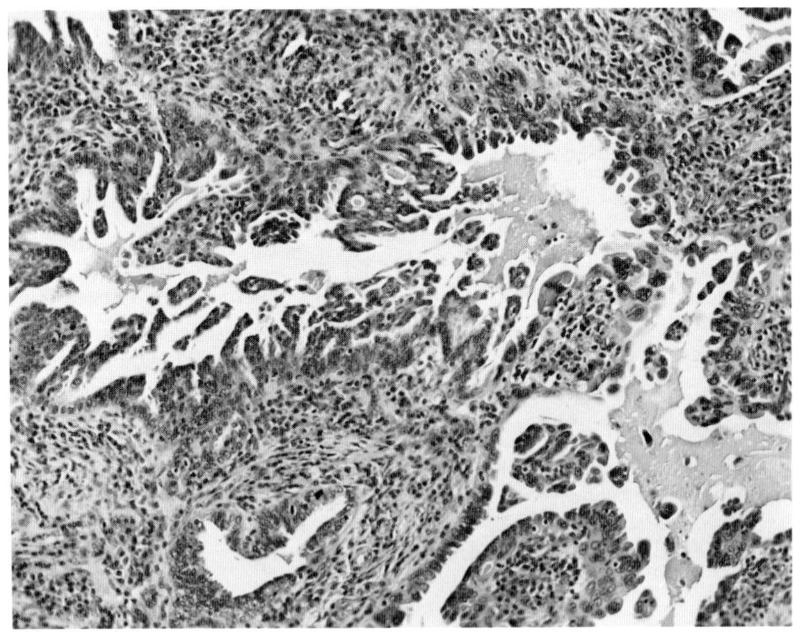

Fig. 3-38. Serous papillary adenocarcinoma. Numerous small papillae and cellular buds are evident. (From Young and Scully,[180] with permission.)

ature are examples of clear cell adenocarcinoma, although some reports have probably also included occasional additional examples of "true" mesonephric adenocarcinoma.[134, 148] The rarity of this tumor is borne out by a recent study of a consultation series in which there were only four cases of carcinoma in contrast to 41 cases of mesonephric hyperplasia.[146] The four patients with carcinoma ranged from 36 to 58 (mean, 49) years of age. Information concerning the gross appearance of the cervix was available in two of the cases; in one of them it was normal, and in the other there was slight induration of the anterior wall without a discrete mass. Microscopic examination reveals a variety of appearances, but in general a tubulo-glandular pattern predominates (Figs. 3-39 and 3-40). The tubules and glands, which may be closely apposed, or separated by stroma, are usually small and round but are occasionally larger and resemble endometrioid glands (Fig. 3-40) or are cystic. The lumens typically contain bright pink or red hyaline material, which is negative on mucin staining. Rarely, the tubulo-glandular pattern merges with a solid undifferentiated growth. Mesonephric carcinomas usually extensively invade the cervical wall and also usually extend close to the overlying endocervical mucosa, sometimes eroding it. Mesonephric hyperplasia is often present at the periphery of the tumor[146] (Fig. 3-39).

Mesonephric carcinomas appear to have a poor prognosis on the basis of the small number of reported cases. One patient in the above series had a vaginal apex recurrence at 7 years and underwent excision of the recurrent tumor, followed by radiation therapy; she was well 15 months later. A second patient died of disease within 3 years of presentation, while an extensive pelvic recurrence in a third patient developed at 6 years, and she died 1 year later; follow-up in the fourth case was of insignificant duration.[146]

The major differential diagnosis of mesonephric carcinoma is with mesonephric hyperplasia (see Ch. 1). Mesonephric carci-

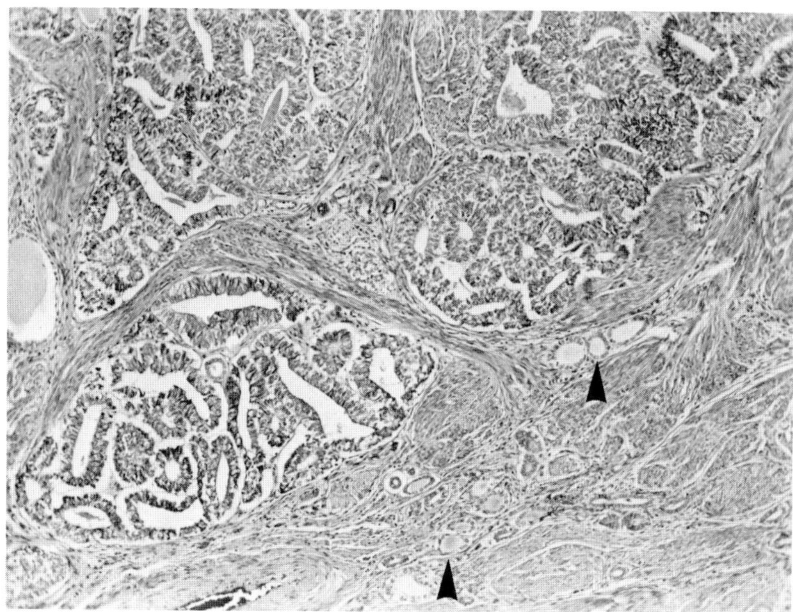

Fig. 3-39. Mesonephric adenocarcinoma. Large tubular glands of adenocarcinoma (upper left) and smaller tubules representing foci of mesonephric hyperplasia in adjacent portion of cervical wall (arrows).

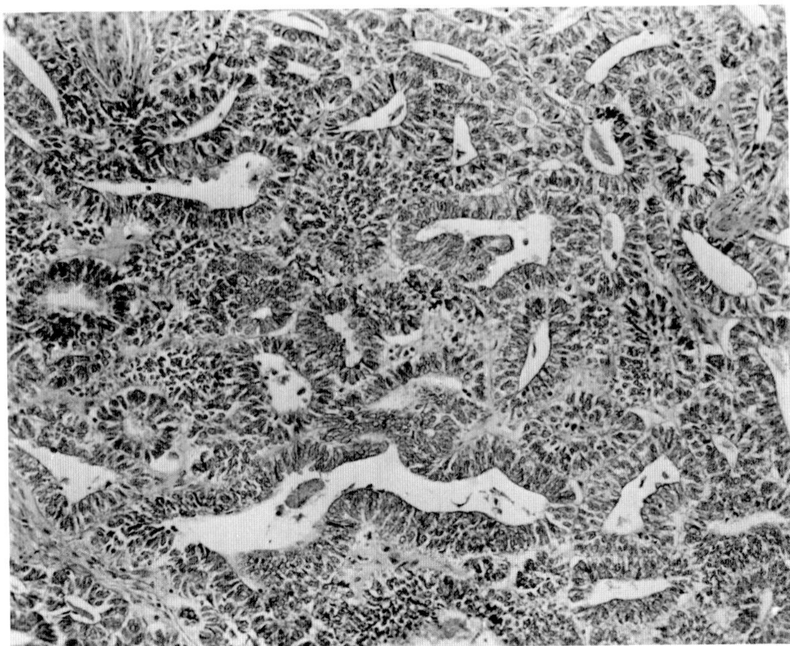

Fig. 3-40. Mesonephric adenocarcinoma. The glands are lined by stratified epithelial cells and simulate those of an endometrioid adenocarcinoma.

noma must be distinguished from other adenocarcinomas of the cervix, with the major forms in the differential diagnosis being adenoma malignum, endometrioid carcinoma, serous carcinoma, and clear cell carcinoma. The differing microscopic features of these tumors have already been described. Metastatic adenocarcinomas (see Ch. 8) also sometimes come into consideration but lack the distinctive features of mesonephric carcinoma.

INTESTINAL-TYPE ADENOCARCINOMA

The occurrence of cervical adenocarcinomas with unequivocal intestinal features was first reported by Azzopardi and Hou,[149] who described a cervical adenocarcinoma containing numerous argentaffin and Paneth cells. However, tumors that resembled intestinal adenocarcinomas microscopically had been reported previously, although the specific designation "intestinal"

was not used. Some investigations have found that 3.5 to 5.5 percent of cervical adenocarcinomas are of the colloid type, a subtype of "intestinal" adenocarcinoma.[80, 150] In the only report devoted soley to colloid carcinomas,[150] two of the three patients presented with a mucoid vaginal discharge. Three other cases of intestinal-type cervical adenocarcinoma have been described in detail.[130, 151, 152] One of them, mentioned earlier, was noteworthy because the superficial component of the tumor resembled a villous adenoma of the intestinal tract.[130] A primary intestinal-type adenocarcinoma (Fig. 3-41) obviously has to be distinguished from an intestinal adenocarcinoma that has spread to the cervix.

SIGNET-RING CELL ADENOCARCINOMA

Signet-ring cells may be seen within otherwise typical cases of cervical adenocarcinoma and within adenosquamous carcino-

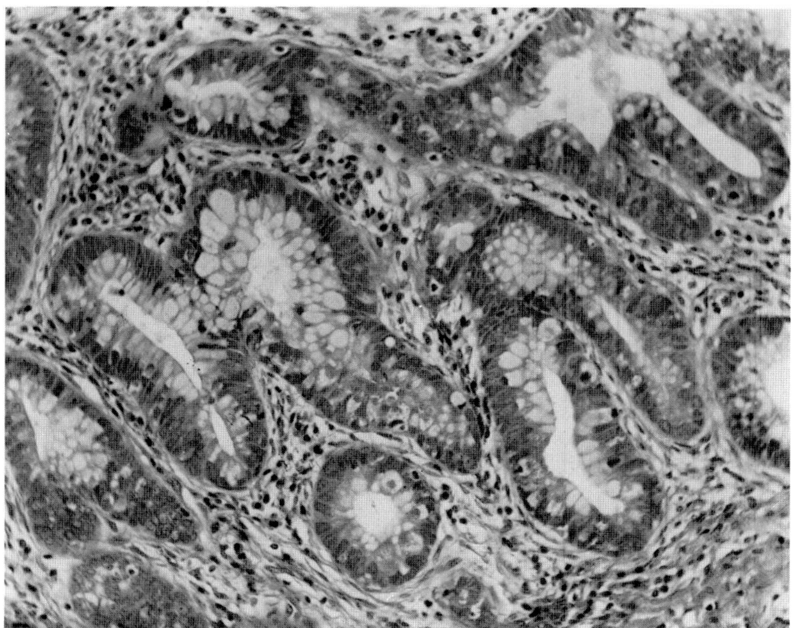

Fig. 3-41. Intestinal type adenocarcinoma. Many goblet cells are present in the lining epithelium of the glands.

mas as discussed below. In one series, 6 of 37 poorly differentiated adenocarcinomas contained some signet-ring cells.[88] Pure or almost pure signet-ring cell carcinomas are exceedingly rare[153, 154] (Fig. 3-42), and are less common than metastatic signet-ring cell carcinoma (see Ch. 8), which must be excluded before a primary cervical signet-ring cell carcinoma is diagnosed. It should be remembered that cells resembling signet-ring cells, but lacking mucin, are rarely seen in squamous cell carcinomas.[155]

Adenosquamous Carcinoma

These tumors[156–159] account for approximately one-third of all cervical carcinomas that have a glandular component.[77] A figure of approximately 50 percent was reported in one series of pregnant women,[160] but a more recent study disclosed no increase in frequency in pregnant patients.[161] The glandular component in adenosquamous carcinomas is almost always of endocervical type. If the glands are of endometrioid type, the tumor should be placed in the endometrioid category, but such tumors are rare. Occasional cervical adenosquamous carcinomas contain bland squamous morules (Fig. 3-43), but the squamous component in adenosquamous carcinomas is usually moderately to severely atypical. In poorly differentiated tumors, the coexistence of squamous and glandular elements may be appreciated only on close scrutiny, and in some cases, mucin stains may be essential to demonstrate poorly formed glands or intracellular mucin. In occasional cases, the mucinous component of the tumor takes the form of a signet-ring cell carcinoma.

Several studies have highlighted the problem of defining the histologic criteria for adenosquamous carcinoma of the cervix. Teshima et al.[162] showed with special stains that 59 percent of nonkeratinizing large cell squamous cell carcinomas, 58 percent of nonkeratinizing small cell squamous cell carcinomas and 14 percent of ke-

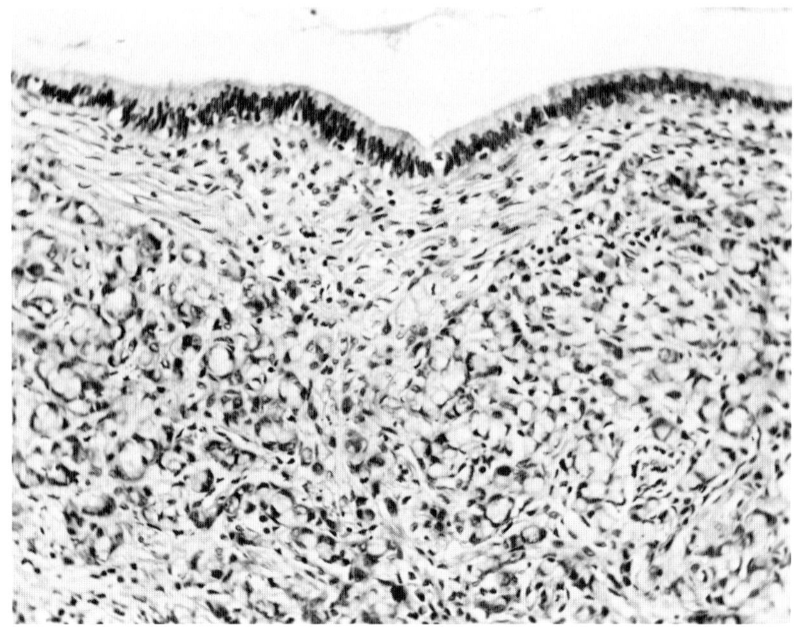

Fig. 3-42. Signet-ring cell adenocarcinoma.

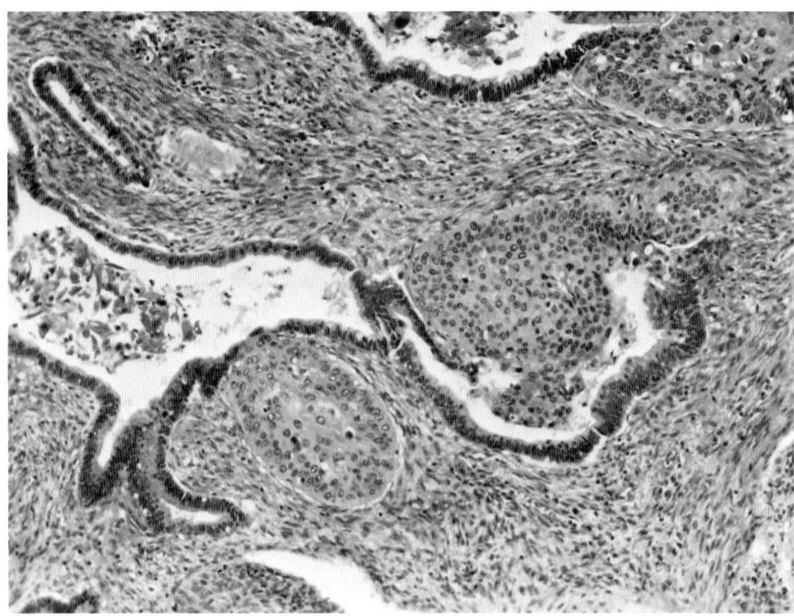

Fig. 3-43. Adenosquamous carcinoma. Nests of cytologically malignant squamous cells are present in association with malignant glandular epithelium.

ratinizing squamous cell carcinomas contained mucin. In another study of tumors thought to be squamous cell carcinomas on the basis of hematoxylin and eosin (H&E)-stained sections, special staining revealed intracellular mucin in 35 percent of the cases.[163] These findings illustrate that the definition of adenosquamous carcinoma is to some extent arbitrary but, in keeping with World Health Organization (WHO) criteria for histologic typing of tumors, it is appropriate to confine the diagnosis to tumors that contain mucin or glands in addition to squamous elements that are recognizable without the use of special stains. Adenosquamous carcinomas have been stated to have a poorer prognosis than pure adenocarcinomas of the cervix,[76] but a recent study showed a prognosis for stage I adenosquamous carcinomas similar to that of squamous cell carcinomas.[164]

Glassy Cell Carcinoma

Glucksmann and Cherry[157, 160] considered the entity that they designated glassy cell carcinoma the most undifferentiated form of adenosquamous carcinoma of the cervix. It accounted for 20 percent of the tumors they placed in the adenosquamous category and for 1.6 percent of all their cervical carcinomas. In two other series it accounted for 1.3 percent[36] and 5.3 percent[165] of cervical carcinomas. This tumor occurs in a somewhat younger age group than adenocarcinoma in general, with a median age of 31 years in one series.[166] In another series, 15 of 18 patients were 34 years or less.[167] The tumors are typically large and often polypoid. Microscopic examination reveals sheets of large cells with abundant eosinophilic or amphophilic, ground-glass or finely granular cytoplasm, prominent cell borders, large nuclei with prominent nucleoli, a high mitotic rate, and often a stromal inflammatory infiltrate composed predominantly of eosinophils and plasma cells[36, 165–172] (Fig. 3-44). Rare foci of squamous or glandular differentiation and intracellular mucin may be present. Tumors with significant components of glassy cell carcinoma and typical adenocarcinoma[169] should be regarded as mixed carcinomas. Occasionally, an associated in situ carcinoma composed of glassy cells is seen.[36] The major tumor to be differentiated from glassy cell carcinoma is the large cell nonkeratinizing squamous cell carcinoma. The latter tumor, however, lacks a ground-glass appearance of the cytoplasm of its cells, usually does not exhibit the prominent nucleoli seen in glassy cell carcinoma, and shows more than a minor degree of squamous differentiation. In a recent study, large cell nonkeratinizing squamous cell carcinomas with some features of glassy cell carcinoma were found to have a prognosis similar to that of glassy cell carcinoma.[166] The glassy cell carcinoma may also be difficult to distinguish from the rare lymphoepithelioma-like carcinoma of the cervix (see Ch. 2). The cells in the latter neoplasm tend to grow singly rather than as cohesive groups and lack the characteristic cytoplasmic features of glassy cell carcinoma. Likewise the massive lymphocytic infiltration of the former tumor is not present in the latter.

ADENOID BASAL CARCINOMA

Adenoid basal carcinoma[173–177] usually occurs in postmenopausal patients, at an average age of 64 years.[177] There is a higher frequency in black patients. The patients are usually asymptomatic, and the tumor is often discovered as a result of an abnormal cytologic smear, with subsequent cervical conization. The cervix is normal on pelvic and gross pathologic examination in most of the cases. Microscopic examination reveals widely separated or occasionally closed packed small, round, oval, or lobulated nests of uniform basaloid cells with

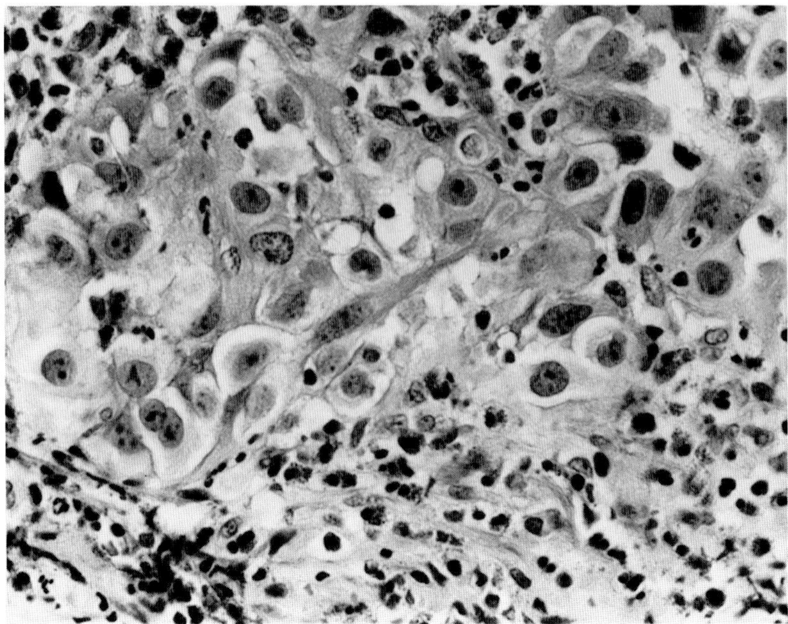

Fig. 3-44. Glassy cell carcinoma. The tumor cells have abundant ground-glass cytoplasm, well-defined cytoplasmic membranes, and prominent nucleoli. Many inflammatory cells, some of which are eosinophils, are present. (From Young and Scully,[180] with permission.)

peripheral palisading (Fig. 3-45). Lumens may form in the centers of the nests (Fig. 3-46) and may be cystically dilated (Fig. 3-47). The spaces can be lined by mucinous epithelium, cells with clear cytoplasm, basaloid cells, or flattened cells; some of the nests may show squamous (Fig. 3-48) or transitional cell differentiation. There is rarely more than an occasional mitotic figure, and there is typically no stromal response to the nests of tumor. A premalignant squamous abnormality or microinvasive squamous cell carcinoma is usually present in the adjacent cervix and is responsible for the associated abnormal cytologic smears. In some cases, adenoid basal carcinoma merges with typical squamous cell carcinoma. The cells of adenoid basal carcinoma stain immunohistochemically for cytokeratin, but do not stain for S-100 protein.[177]

This tumor has a favorable prognosis. In a recent study, 10 of 13 patients with follow-up data were alive and well 2 to 10 years after the diagnosis.[177] Two other pa-tients died of unrelated causes without evidence of recurrence. Only 1 patient died as a result of the cervical tumor, which differed from the others in that series being high grade and having an infiltrative pattern with a marked stromal response, features absent in the typical cases.

"ADENOID CYSTIC" CARCINOMA

Patients with "adenoid cystic" carcinoma are usually postmenopausal, with an average age of 72 years.[177] Like adenoid basal carcinoma, there seems to be an increased frequency in blacks. The patients usually present with abnormal uterine bleeding and typically have an obvious cervical mass, which varies greatly in size and may be exophytic or endophytic. Microscopic examination shows nests of cells often with a focal cribriform pattern (Figs. 3-49 and 3-50) resembling that seen in adenoid cystic carcinoma of the salivary glands, as well as sheets, trabeculae, and

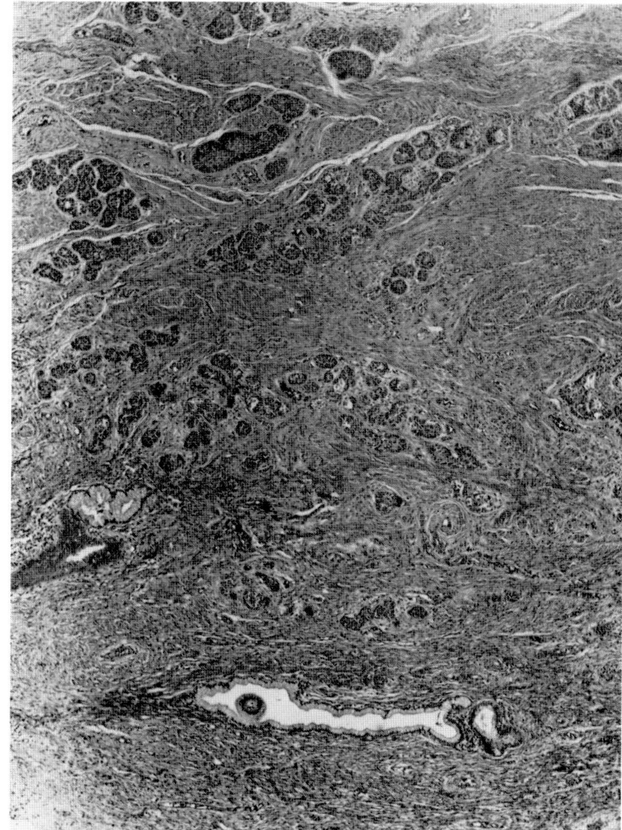

Fig. 3-45. Adenoid basal carcinoma. Small nests of basaloid cells extensively infiltrate the cervical wall. (From Young and Scully,[180] with permission.)

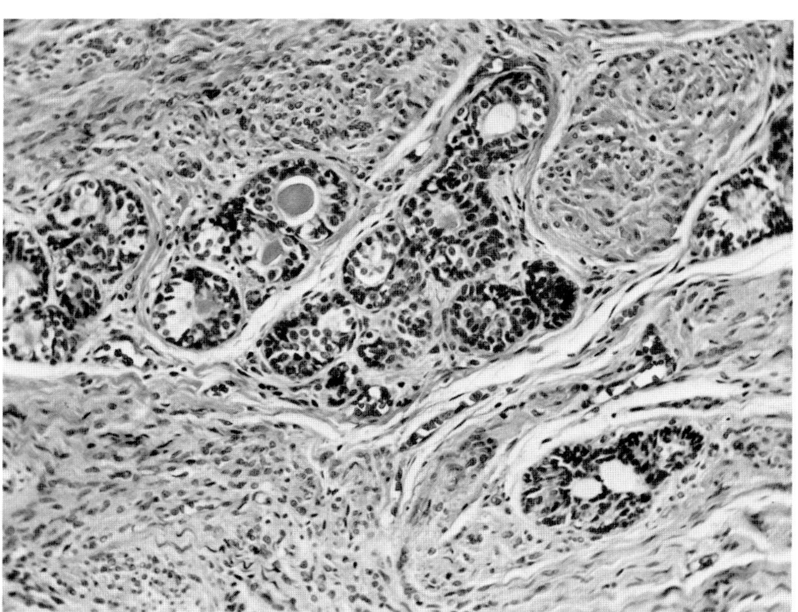

Fig. 3-46. Adenoid basal carcinoma. Small lumens are present within some of the nests of basaloid cells.

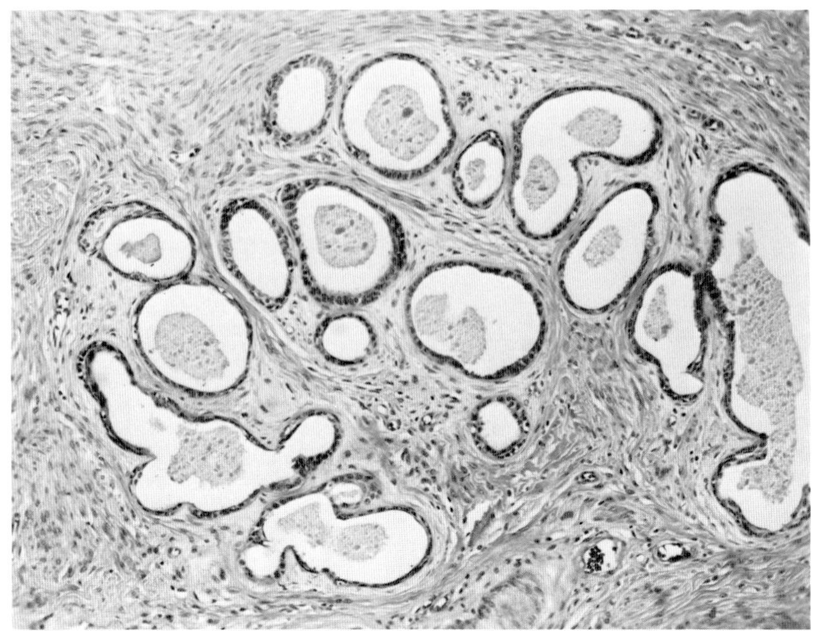

Fig. 3-47. Adenoid basal carcinoma. Small cysts are present.

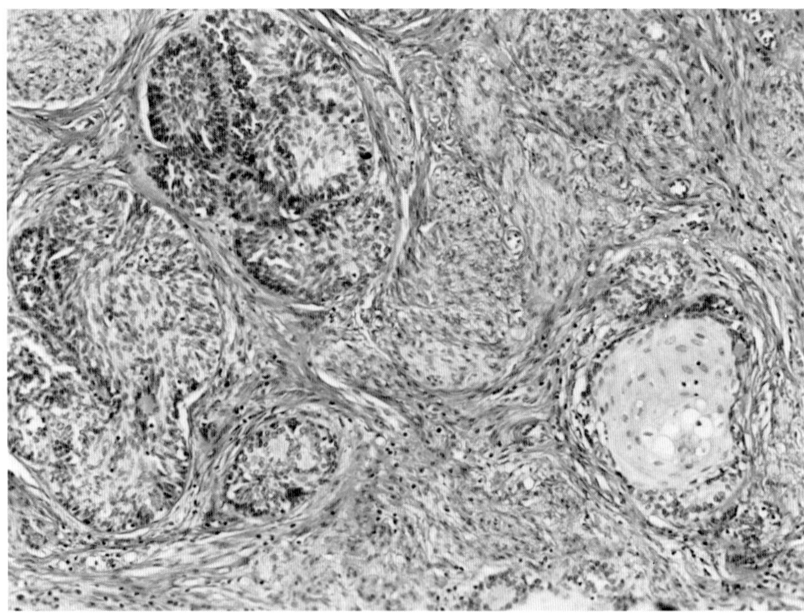

Fig. 3-48. Adenoid basal carcinoma. A focus of squamous differentiation is evident at the right.

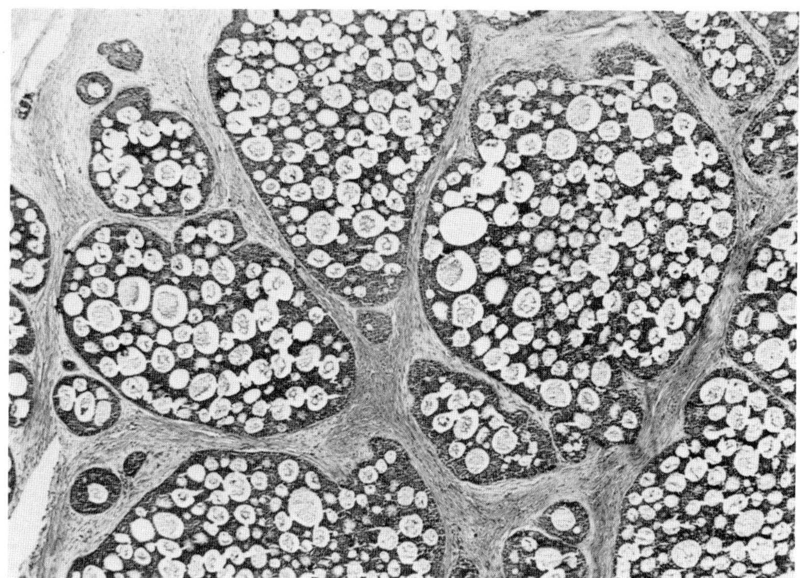

Fig. 3-49. Adenoid cystic carcinoma. The rounded nests have a cribriform pattern.

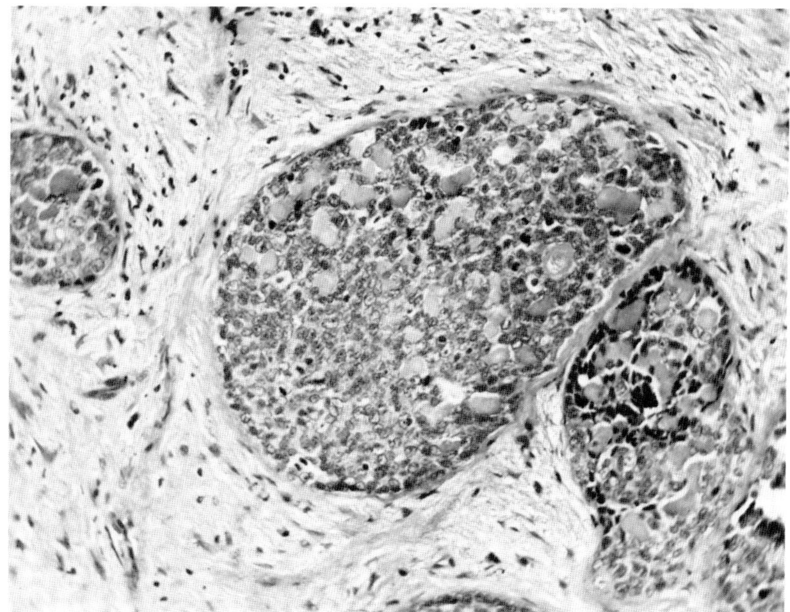

Fig. 3-50. Adenoid cystic carcinoma. The nests contain small rounded spaces containing hyalinized material that was eosinophilic.

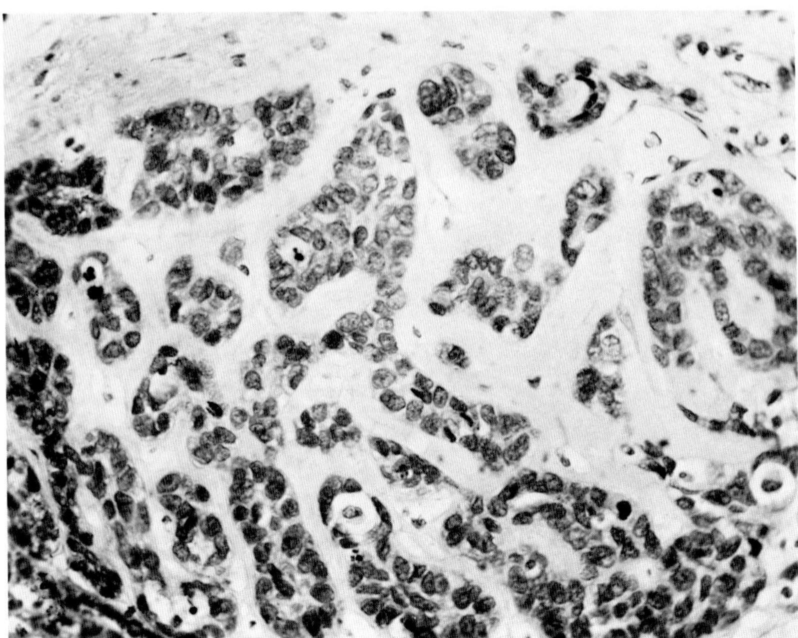

Fig. 3-51. Adenoid carcinoma. The tumor cells are forming trabeculae separated by hyalinized material.

cords (Fig. 3-51). The glandular lumens may contain hyaline or mucinous material. There is usually at least focal palisading of cells at the periphery of tumor nests. The neoplastic cells are larger than those of adenoid basal carcinoma and have more pleomorphic nuclei. The mitotic rate is generally high; necrosis is typically present and may be extensive. An additional difference from adenoid basal carcinoma is the presence of a stromal response, which may be myxoid, fibroblastic or hyaline. In approximately 20 percent of adenoid cystic carcinomas of the cervix, solid foci of undifferentiated carcinoma are present, giving rise to the use of the designation "solid variant" of adenoid cystic carcinoma by one group.[178] Small foci of squamous differentiation are seen in some cases,[177, 178] indicating that the use of the designation adenoid cystic carcinoma for these cervical tumors does not imply an identity to the salivary gland tumor of a similar name, but rather a resemblance to it. In addition, unlike adenoid cystic carcinomas of salivary gland origin, the cervical tumors rarely contain myoepithelial cells, as evidenced by the failure of staining for such cells with S-100 protein, although ultrastructural examination has shown suggestive, but not conclusive, evidence of myoepithelial differentiation.[179] For these reasons, we recommend using "adenoid cystic" in quotation marks for the cervical tumors. In most cases, cervical "adenoid cystic" carcinomas are distinctly different from adenoid basal carcinomas, but in approximately 20 percent of adenoid cystic carcinomas a minor component of small nests and cords of basaloid cells, similar to those of adenoid basal carcinoma is present. "Adenoid cystic carcinoma" has a much worse prognosis than adenoid basal carcinoma. Only 4 of 12 patients in a recent study were alive and free of disease at the time of the last follow-up evaluation[177]; the other patients had either died of their tumor or had recurrent tumor when last seen.

REFERENCES

1. Jaworski RC: Endocervical glandular dysplasia, adenocarcinoma in situ, and early invasive (microinvasive) adenocarcinoma of the uterine cervix. Semin Diagn Pathol 7:190, 1990
2. Bousfield L, Pacey F, Young Q et al: Expanded cytologic criteria for the diagnosis of adenocarcinoma in situ of the cervix and related lesions. Acta Cytol 24:283, 1980
3. Nguyen G-K, Jeannot AB: Exfoliative cytology of in situ and microinvasive adenocarcinoma of the uterine cervix. Acta Cytol 28:461, 1984
4. Betsill WL, Jr, Clark AH: Early endocervical glandular neoplasia. I. Histomorphology and cytomorphology. Acta Cytol 30:115, 1986
5. Clark AH, Betsill WL, Jr: Early endocervical glandular neoplasia. II. Morphometric analysis of the cells. Acta Cytol 30:127-134, 1986.
6. Ayer B, Pacey F, Greenberg M, Bousfield L: The cytologic diagnosis of adenocarcinoma in situ of the cervix uteri and related lesions. I. Adenocarcinoma in situ. Acta Cytol 31:397, 1987
7. Ayer B, Pacey F, Greenberg M: The cytologic diagnosis of adenocarcinoma in situ of the cervix uteri and related lesions. II. Microinvasive adenocarcinoma. Acta Cytol 32:318, 1988
8. Pacey F, Ayer B, Greenberg M: The cytologic diagnosis of adenocarcinoma in situ of the cervix uteri and related lesions. III. Pitfalls in diagnosis. Acta Cytol 32:325, 1988
9. Lee KR, Manna EA, Jones MA: Comparative cytologic features of adenocarcinoma in situ of the uterine cervix. Acta Cytol 35:117, 1991
10. Kudo R, Sagae S, Hayakawa O et al: Morphology of adenocarcinoma in situ and microinvasive adenocarcinoma of the uterine cervix. A cytologic and ultrastructural study. Acta Cytol 35:109, 1991
11. Friedell GH, McKay DG: Adenocarcinoma in situ of the endocervix. Cancer 6:887, 1953
12. Weisbrot IM, Stabinsky C, Davis AM: Adenocarcinoma in situ of the uterine cervix. Cancer 29:1179, 1972
13. Qizilbash AH: In-situ and microinvasive adenocarcinoma of the uterine cervix. A clinical, cytologic and histologic study of 14 cases. Am J Clin Pathol 64:155, 1975
14. Christopherson WM, Nealon N, Gray LA, Sr: Noninvasive precursor lesions of adenocarcinoma and mixed adenosquamous carcinoma of the cervix uteri. Cancer 44:975, 1979
15. Boon ME, Baak JPA, Kurver PJH et al: Adenocarcinoma in situ of the cervix: an underdiagnosed lesion. Cancer 48:768, 1981
16. Boon ME, Kirk RS, Rietveld-Scheffers PEM: The morphogenesis of adenocarcinoma of the cervix—a complex pathological entity. Histopathology 5:565, 1981
17. Gloor E, Ruzicka J: Morphology of adenocarcinoma in situ of the uterine cervix: a study of 14 cases. Cancer 49:294, 1982
18. Noda K, Kimura K, Ikeda M, Teshima K: Studies on the histogenesis of cervical adenocarcinoma. Int J Gynecol Pathol 1:336, 1983
19. Roon EV, Boon ME, Kurver PJH, Baak JPA: The association between precancerous-columnar and squamous lesions of the cervix: a morphometric study. Histopathology 7:887, 1983
20. Ostor AG, Pagano R, Davoren RAM et al: Adenocarcinoma in situ of the cervix. Int J Gynecol Pathol 3:179, 1984
21. Teshima S, Shimosato Y, Kishi K et al: Early stage adenocarcinoma of the uterine cervix. Histopathologic analysis with consideration of histogenesis. Cancer 56:167, 1985
22. Gloor E, Hurlimann J: Cervical intraepithelial glandular neoplasia (adenocarcinoma in situ and glandular dysplasia). A correlative study of 23 cases with histologic grading, histochemical analysis of mucins, and immunohistochemical determination of the affinity for four lectins. Cancer 58:1272, 1986
23. Bertrand M, Lickrish GM, Colgan TJ: The anatomic distribution of cervical adenocarcinoma in situ: implications for treatment. Am J Obstet Gynecol 157:21, 1987
24. Fu YS, Berek JS, Hilborne LH: Diagnostic

problems of in situ and invasive adenocarcinomas of the uterine cervix. Appl Pathol 5:47, 1987

25. Luesley DM, Jordan JA, Woodman CBJ et al: A retrospective review of adenocarcinoma-in-situ and glandular atypia of the uterine cervix. Br J Obstet Gynaecol 94:699, 1987

26. Hopkins MP, Roberts JA, Schmidt RW: Cervical adenocarcinoma in situ. Obstet Gynecol 71:842, 1988

27. Jaworski RC, Pacey NF, Greenberg ML, Osborn RA: The histologic diagnosis of adenocarcinoma in situ and related lesions of the cervix uteri. Adenocarcinoma in situ. Cancer 61:1171, 1988

28. Tobon H, Dave H: Adenocarcinoma in situ of the cervix. Clinicopathologic observations of 11 cases. Int J Gynecol Pathol 7:139, 1988

29. Andersen ES, Arffmann E: Adenocarcinoma in situ of the uterine cervix: a clinicopathologic study of 36 cases. Gynecol Oncol 35:1, 1989

30. Matsukuma K, Tsukamoto N, Kaku T et al: Early adenocarcinoma of the uterine cervix—its histologic and immunohistologic study. Gynecol Oncol 35:38, 1989

31. Rollason TP, Cullimore J, Bradgate MG: A suggested columnar cell morphological equivalent of squamous carcinoma in situ with early stromal invasion. Int J Gynecol Pathol 8:230, 1989

32. Colgan TJ, Lickrish GM: The topography and invasive potential of cervical adenocarcinoma in situ, with and without associated squamous dysplasia. Gynecol Oncol 36:246, 1990

33. Muntz H, Lage J, Goff B et al: Adenocarcinoma-in-situ of the uterine cervix. Gynecol Oncol 45:89, 1992

34. Steiner G, Friedell GH: Adenosquamous carcinoma in situ of the cervix. Cancer 18:807, 1965

35. Lee KR, Belinson JL: Recurrence in noninvasive endometrial carcinoma. Relationship to uterine papillary serous carcinoma. Am J Surg Pathol 15:965, 1991

36. Littman P, Clement PB, Henriksen B et al: Glassy cell carcinoma of the cervix. Cancer 37:2238, 1976

37. Hasumi K, Ehrmann RL: Clear cell carcinoma of the uterine endocervix with an in situ component. Cancer 42:2435, 1978

38. Hurlimann J, Gloor E: Adenocarcinoma in situ and invasive adenocarcinoma of the uterine cervix. An immunohistologic study with antibodies specific for several epithelial markers. Cancer 54:103, 1984

39. Kluzak T, Kraus F: Adenocarcinoma in-situ of the uterine cervix (AIS): immunohistochemical staining for carcinoembryonic antigen (CEA) and human papillomavirus (HPV). Lab Invest 54:32A, 1986

40. Cooper P, Russell G, Wilson B: Adenocarcinoma of the endocervix—a histochemical study. Histopathology 11:1321, 1987

41. Nanbu Y, Fujii S, Konishi I et al: Immunohistochemical localizations of CA 125, carcinoembryonic antigen, and CA 19-9 in normal and neoplastic glandular cells of the uterine cervix. Cancer 62:2580, 1988

42. Joseph MG, Kontozoglou TE: Expression of ABH blood group antigens, carcinoembryonic, and other antigens in in situ and invasive adenocarcinoma of the cervix: an immunohistochemical study of 25 cases. Surg Pathol 3:259, 1990

43. Rollason TP, Byrne P, Williams A, Brown G: Expression of epithelial membrane and 3-fucosyl-N-acetyllactosamine antigens in cervix uteri with particular reference to adenocarcinoma in situ. J Clin Pathol 41:547, 1988

44. Griffin NR, Wells M, Fox H: Modulation of the antigenicity of amylase in cervical glandular atypia, adenocarcinoma in situ and invasive adenocarcinoma. Histopathology 15:267, 1989

45. Kudo R, Sasano H, Koizumi M et al: Immunohistochemical comparison of new monoclonal antibody IC5 and carcinoembryonic antigen in the differential diagnosis of adenocarcinoma of the uterine cervix. Int J Gynecol Pathol 9:325, 1990

46. Jaworski RC, Jones A: DNA ploidy in adenocarcinoma in situ of the uterine cervix. J Clin Pathol 43:435, 1990

47. Cullimore JE, Rollason TP, Marshall T: Nucleolar organiser regions in adenocarcinoma in situ of the endocervix. J Clin Pathol 42:1276, 1989

48. Darne JF, Polacarz SV, Sheridan E et al:

Nucleolar organiser regions in adenocarcinoma in situ and invasive adenocarcinoma of the cervix. J Clin Pathol 43:657, 1990

49. Kashimura M, Shinohara M, Oikawa K et al: An adenocarcinoma in situ of the uterine cervix that developed into invasive adenocarcinoma after 5 years. Gynecol Oncol 36:128, 1990

50. Yeh I-T, LiVolsi VA, Noumoff JS: Endocervical carcinoma. Pathol Res Pract 187:129, 1991

51. Burghardt E: Microinvasive carcinoma in gynaecological pathology. Clin Obstet Gynaecol 11:239, 1984

52. Yavner DL, Dwyer IM, Hancock WW, Ehrmann RL: Basement membrane of cervical adenocarcinoma: an immunoperoxidase study of laminin and Type IV collagen. Obstet Gynecol 76:1014, 1990

53. Berek JS, Hacker NF, Fu Y-S et al: Adenocarcinoma of the uterine cervix: histologic variables associated with lymph node metastasis and survival. Obstet Gynecol 65:46, 1985

54. Rosenthal DL, McLatchie C, Stern E et al: Endocervical columnar cell atypia coincident with cervical neoplasia characterized by digital image analysis. Acta Cytol 26:115, 1982

55. Brown LJR, Wells M: Cervical glandular atypia associated with squamous intraepithelial neoplasia: a premalignant lesion? J Clin Pathol 39:22, 1986

56. Brown LJR, Griffin NR, Wells M: Cytoplasmic reactivity with the monoclonal antibody HMFG1 as a marker of cervical glandular atypia. J Pathol 151:203, 1987

57. Alva J, Lauchlan SC: The histogenesis of mixed cervical carcinomas. The concept of endocervical columnar-cell dysplasia. Am J Clin Pathol 64:20, 1975

58. Abell MR, Gosling JRG: Gland cell carcinoma (adenocarcinoma) of the uterine cervix. Am J Obstet Gynecol 83:729, 1962

59. Gallup DG, Abell MR: Invasive adenocarcinoma of the uterine cervix. Obstet Gynecol 49:596, 1977

60. Hopkins MP, Sutton P, Roberts JA: Prognostic features and treatment of endocervical adenocarcinoma of the cervix. Gynecol Oncol 27:69, 1987

61. Brand E, Berek JS, Hacker NF: Controversies in the management of cervical adenocarcinoma. Obstet Gynecol 71:261, 1988

62. Silcocks PBS, Thornton-Jones H, Murphy M: Squamous and adenocarcinoma of the uterine cervix: a comparison using routine data. Br J Cancer 55:321, 1987

63. Vesterinen E, Forss M, Nieminen U: Increase of cervical adenocarcinoma: a report of 520 cases of cervical carcinoma including 112 tumors with glandular elements. Gynecol Oncol 33:49, 1989

64. Goodman HM, Buttlar CA, Niloff JM et al: Adenocarcinoma of the uterine cervix: prognostic factors and patterns of recurrence. Gynecol Oncol 33:241, 1989

65. Davis JR, Moon LB: Increased incidence of adenocarcinoma of uterine cervix. Obstet Gynecol 45:79, 1975

66. Greer BE, Figge DC, Tamimi HK, Cain JM: Stage IB adenocarcinoma of the cervix treated by radical hysterectomy and pelvic lymph node dissection. Am J Obstet Gynecol 160:1509, 1989

67. Wilczynski SP, Walker J, Liao S-Y et al: Adenocarcinoma of the cervix associated with human papillomavirus. Cancer 62:1331, 1988

68. Gordon AN, Bornstein J, Kaufman RH et al: Human papillomavirus associated with adenocarcinoma and adenosquamous carcinoma of the cervix: analysis by in situ hybridization. Gynecol Oncol 35:345, 1989

69. Dallenbach-Hellweg G: On the origin and histological structure of adenocarcinoma of the endocervix in women under 50 years of age. Pathol Res Pract 179:38, 1984

70. Brinton LA, Tashima KT, Lehman HF et al: Epidemiology of cervical cancer by cell type. Cancer Res 47:1706, 1987

71. Jones MW, Silverberg SG: Cervical adenocarcinoma in young women: possible relationship to microglandular hyperplasia and use of oral contraceptives. Obstet Gynecol 73:984, 1989

72. Takahashi M, Aoki K, Banham DG, McLean MR. Some effects of long-term use of oral contraceptives on cervical neoplasia. Int Cong Ser 644:21, 1984

73. Korhonen MO: Adenocarcinoma of the uterine cervix. Prognosis and prognostic significance of histology. Cancer 53:1760, 1984

74. Kilgore LC, Soong S-J, Gore H et al: Analysis of prognostic features in adenocarcinoma of the cervix. Gynecol Oncol 31:137, 1988
75. Saigo PE, Cain JM, Kim WS et al: Prognostic factors in adenocarcinoma of the uterine cervix. Cancer 57:1584, 1986
76. Hopkins MP, Schmidt RW, Roberts JA, Morley GW: The prognosis and treatment of stage I adenocarcinoma of the cervix. Obstet Gynecol 72:915, 1988
77. Angel C, Dubeshter B, Lin JY: Clinical presentation and management of Stage I cervical adenocarcinoma: a 25 year experience. Gynecol Oncol 44:71, 1992
78. Horowitz IR, Jacobson LP, Zucker PK et al: Epidemiology of adenocarcinoma of the cervix. Gynecol Oncol 31:25, 1988
79. Gusberg SB, Corscaden JA: The pathology and treatment of adenocarcinoma of the cervix. Cancer 4:1066, 1951
80. Hepler TK, Dockerty MB, Randall LM: Primary adenocarcinoma of the cervix. Am J Obstet Gynecol 63:800, 1952
81. Haggard JL, Cotten N, Dougherty CM, Mickal A: Primary adenocarcinoma of the cervix. Obstet Gynecol 24:183, 1964
82. Marcus SL, Marcus CC: Primary adenocarcinoma of the cervix uteri. Am J Obstet Gynecol 86:384, 1963
83. Rombaut RP, Charles D, Murphy A: Adenocarcinoma of the cervix. A clinicopathologic study of 47 cases. Cancer 19:891, 1966
84. Rutledge FN, Galakatos AE, Wharton JT, Smith JP: Adenocarcinoma of the uterine cervix. Am J Obstet Gynecol 122:236, 1975
85. Anderson MC, Fraser AC: Adenocarcinoma of the uterine cervix. A clinical and pathological appraisal. Br J Obstet Gynaecol 83:320, 1976
86. Hurt WG, Silverberg SG, Frable WJ et al: Adenocarcinoma of the cervix: histopathologic and clinical features. Am J Obstet Gynecol 129:304, 1977
87. Parker JC, Van Nagell JR, Bissig T: The histomorphologic spectrum of endocervical (Mullerian) adenocarcinoma—a potential prognostic indicator. J Surg Oncol 9:267, 1977
88. Korhonen MO: Adenocarcinoma of the uterine cervix. An evaluation of the available diagnostic methods. Acta Pathol Microbiol Scand [A] (suppl 264), 1978
89. Berek JS, Castaldo TW, Hacker NF et al: Adenocarcinoma of the uterine cervix. Cancer 48:2734, 1981
90. Shingleton HM, Gore H, Bradley DH, Soong SJ: Adenocarcinoma of the cervix. I. Clinical evaluation and pathologic features. Obstet Gynecol 139:799, 1981
91. Fu YS, Reagan JW, Hsiu JG et al: Adenocarcinoma and mixed carcinoma of the uterine cervix. 1. A clinicopathologic study. Cancer 49:2560, 1982
92. Ireland D, Hardiman P, Monaghan JM: Adenocarcinoma of the uterine cervix: a study of 73 cases. Obstet Gynecol 65:82, 1985
93. Deligdish L, Escay-Martinez, Cohen CJ: Endocervical carcinoma: a study of 23 patients with clinical-pathological correlation. Gynecol Oncol 18:326, 1984
94. Mober PJ, Einhorn N, Silfversward C, Soderberg G: Adenocarcinoma of the uterine cervix. Cancer 57:407, 1986
95. Berek JS, Hatcher NF, Fu YS et al: Adenocarcinoma of the uterine cervix: histologic variables associated with lymph node metastasis and survival. Obstet Gynecol 65:46, 1985
96. Hopkins MP, Schmidt RW, Roberts JA, Morley GW: Gland cell carcinoma (adenocarcinoma) of the cervix. Obstet Gynecol 72:789, 1988
97. LiVolsi VA, Merino MJ, Schwartz PE: Co-existent endocervical adenocarcinoma and mucinous adenocarcinoma of ovary: a clinico-pathologic study of four cases. Int J Gynecol Pathol 1:391, 1983
98. Kaminski PF, Norris HJ: Coexistence of ovarian neoplasms and endocervical adenocarcinoma. Obstet Gynecol 64:553, 1984
99. Young RH, Scully RE: Mucinous tumors of the ovary associated with mucinous adenocarcinomas of the cervix. A clinicopathologic analysis of 16 cases. Int J Gynecol Pathol 7:99, 1988
100. Young RH, Scully RE: Uterine carcinomas simulating microglandular hyperplasia. A report of six cases. Am J Surg Pathol 16:1092, 1992.
101. Collins RJ, Wong LC: Adenocarcinoma of the uterine cervix with -HCG production: a

case report and review of the literature. Gynecol Oncol 33:99, 1989

102. Husain AN, Gattuso P, Abraham K, Castelli MJ: Synchronous adenocarcinoma and carcinoid of the uterine cervix: immunohistochemical study of a case and review of literature. Gynecol Oncol 33:125, 1989

103. Silva EG, Gershenson D, Sneige N et al: Small cell carcinoma of the uterine cervix: "pathology and prognostic factors." Surg Pathol 2:105, 1989

104. Maier RC, Norris HJ: Coexistence of cervical intraepithelial neoplasia with primary adenocarcinoma of the endocervix. Obstet Gynecol 56:361, 1980

105. Choo YC, Naylor B: Coexistent squamous cell carcinoma and adenocarcinoma of the uterine cervix. Gynecol Oncol 17:168, 1984

106. Wahlstrom T, Korhonen M, Lindgren J, Seppala M: Distinction between endocervical and endometrial adenocarcinoma with immunoperoxidase staining of carcinoembryonic antigen in routine histologic tissue specimens. Lancet 2:1159, 1979

107. Azumi N, Jones M, Joyce J et al: Endometrial and endocervical adenocarcinomas: immunohistochemical studies and differentiating markers. Mod Pathol 4:54A, 1991

108. Van Nagell JR, Goldenberg DM: Carcinoembryonic antigen staining of endometrial and endocervical carcinomas. Lancet 1:213, 1980

109. Cohen C, Shulman G, Budgeon LR: Endocervical and endometrial adenocarcinoma. An immunoperoxidase and histochemical study. Am J Surg Pathol 6:151, 1982

110. Maes G, Fleuren GJ, Bara J, Nap M: The distribution of mucins, carcinoembryonic antigen, and mucus associated antigens in endocervical and endometrial adenocarcinomas. Int J Gynecol Pathol 7:112, 1988

111. McKelvey JL, Goodlin RR: Adenoma malignum of the cervix. Cancer 16:549, 1963

112. Silverberg SG, Hurt WG: Minimal deviation adenocarcinoma ("adenoma malignum") of the cervix. Am J Obstet Gynecol 123:971, 1975

113. Kaku T, Enjoji M: Extremely well-differentiated adenocarcinoma ("adenoma malignum") of the cervix. Int J Gynecol Pathol 2:28, 1983

114. Kaminski PF, Norris HJ: Minimal deviation carcinoma (adenoma malignum) of the cervix. Int J Gynecol Pathol 2:141, 1983

115. Michael H, Grawe L, Kraus FT: Minimal deviation endocervical adenocarcinoma: clinical and histologic features, immunohistochemical staining for carcinoembryonic antigen, and differentiation from confusing benign lesions. Int J Gynecol Pathol 3:261, 1984

116. Gilks CB, Young RH, Aguirre P et al: Adenoma malignum (minimal deviation adenocarcinoma) of the uterine cervix. A clinicopathological and immunohistochemical analysis of 26 cases. Am J Surg Pathol 13:717, 1989

117. Chen KTK: Female genital tract tumors in Peutz-Jeghers syndrome. Hum Pathol 17:856, 1986

118. Kaku T, Hachisuga T, Toyoshima S et al: Extremely well-differentiated adenocarcinoma ("adenoma malignum") of the cervix in a patient with Peutz-Jeghers syndrome. Int J Gynecol Pathol 4:266, 1985

119. McGowan L, Young RH, Scully RE: Peutz-Jeghers syndrome with "adenoma malignum" of the cervix. A report of two cases. Gynecol Oncol 10:125, 1980

120. Young RH, Welch WR, Dickersin GR, Scully RE: Ovarian sex cord tumor with annular tubules. Review of 74 cases including 27 with Peutz-Jeghers syndrome and four with adenoma malignum of the cervix. Cancer 50:1384, 1982

121. Szyfelbein WM, Young RH, Scully RE: Adenoma malignum of the cervix: cytologic findings. Acta Cytol 28:691, 1984

122. Fetissof F, Berger G, Dubois M et al: Female genital tract and Peutz-Jeghers syndrome: an immunohistochemical study. Int J Gynecol Pathol 4:219, 1985

123. Steeper TA, Wick MR: Minimal deviation adenocarcinoma of the uterine cervix ("Adenoma Malignum"). Cancer 58:1131, 1986

124. Bulmer JN, Griffin NR, Bates C et al: Minimal deviation adenocarcinoma (adenoma malignum) of the endocervix: histochemical and immunohistochemical study of two cases. Gynecol Oncol 36:139, 1990

125. Young RH, Scully RE: Villoglandular papillary adenocarcinoma of the uterine cer-

vix. A clinicopathological analysis of 13 cases. Cancer 63:1773, 1989

126. Hopson L, Jones MA, Boyce CR, Tarraza HM: Papillary villoglandular carcinoma of the cervix. Gynecol Oncol 39:221, 1990

127. Jones MW, Silverberg SG, Kurman RJ: Well differentiated villoglandular adenocarcinoma of uterine cervix: a clinico-pathological study of 24 cases. Int J Gynecol Pathol (in press)

128. Ulbright TM, Alexander RW, Kraus FT: Intramural papilloma of the vagina: evidence of mullerian histogenesis. Cancer 48:2260, 1981

129. Michael H, Sutton G, Hull MT, Roth LM: Villous adenoma of the uterine cervix associated with invasive adenocarcinoma: a histologic, ultrastructural, and immunohistochemical study. Int J Gynecol Pathol 5:163, 1986

130. Alvaro T, Nogales F: Villous adenoma and invasive adenocarcinoma of the cervix. Int J Gynecol Pathol 7:96, 1988

131. Chang SH, Maddox WA: Adenocarcinoma arising within cervical endometriosis and invading the adjacent vagina. Am J Obstet Gynecol 110:1015, 1971

132. Rahilly MA, Williams ARW, Al-Nafussi A: Minimal deviation endometrioid adenocarcinoma of cervix: a clinicopathological and immunohistochemical study of two cases. Histopathology 20:351, 1992

133. Scully RE, Welch WR: Pathology of the female genital tract after prenatal exposure to diethylstilbestrol. p. 26. In Herbst AL, Bern HA (eds): Developmental Effects of Diethylstilbestrol (DES) in Pregnancy. Thieme-Stratton, New York, 1981

134. Hart WR, Norris HJ: Mesonephric adenocarcinomas of the cervix. Cancer 29:106, 1972

135. Fawcett KJ, Dockerty MB, Hunt AB: Mesonephric carcinomas and adenocarcinomas of the cervix in children. J Pediatr 69:104, 1966

136. Kaminski PF, Maier RC: Clear cell adenocarcinoma of the cervix unrelated to diethylstilbestrol exposure. Obstet Gynecol 62:720, 1983

137. Clement PB, Young RH, Scully RE: Non-trophoblastic pathology of the female genital tract and peritoneum associated with pregnancy. Semin Diagn Pathol 6:372, 1989

138. Ferenczy A, Winkler B: Carcinoma and metastatic tumors of the cervix. p. 238. In Kurman RJ (ed): Blaustein's Pathology of the Female Genital Tract. 3rd Ed. Springer-Verlag, New York, 1987

139. Cary A, Free KE, Wright RG, Shield PW: Carcinoma of the cervix—recurrences in Queensland 1982–1986. Int J Gynecol Cancer 2:207, 1992

140. Dallenbach-Hellweg G, Poulsen H: Atlas of Histopathology of the Cervix Uteri. Springer-Verlag, Berlin, 1990

141. Gilks CB, Clement PB: Papillary serous adenocarcinoma of the uterine cervix. A report of three cases. Mod Pathol 5:426, 1992

142. Huffman JW: Mesonephric remnants in the cervix. Am J Obstet Gynecol 56:23, 1948

143. McGee CT, Cromer DW, Greene RR: Mesonephric carcinoma of the cervix-differentiation from endocervical adenocarcinoma. Am J Obstet Gynecol 84:358, 1962

144. Buntine DW: Adenocarcinoma of the uterine cervix of probable Wolffian origin. Pathology 11:713, 1979

145. Valente PT, Susin M: Cervical adenocarcinoma arising in florid mesonephric hyperplasia: report of a case with immunocytochemical studies. Gynecol Oncol 27:58, 1987

146. Ferry JA, Scully RE: Mesonephric remnants, hyperplasia and neoplasia in the uterine cervix: a study of 49 cases. Am J Surg Pathol 14:1100, 1990

147. Lang G, Dallenbach-Hellweg G: The histogenetic origin of cervical mesonephric hyperplasia and mesonephric adenocarcinoma of the uterine cervix studied with immunohistochemical methods. Int J Gynecol Pathol 9:145, 1990

148. Novak E, Woodruff JD, Novak ER: Probable mesonephric origin of certain female genital tumors. Am J Obstet Gynecol 68:1222, 1954

149. Azzopardi JG, Hou LT: Intestinal metaplasia with argentaffin cells in cervical adenocarcinoma. J Pathol 90:686, 1985

150. Lewis TLT. Colloid (mucus secreting) car-

cinoma of the cervix. J Obstet Gynaecol Br Common 78:1128, 1971

151. Fox H, Wells M, Harris et al: Enteric tumours of the lower female genital tract: a report of three cases. Histopathology 12:167, 1988

152. Lee KR, Trainer TD: Adenocarcinoma of the uterine cervix of intestinal type containing numerous Paneth cells. Arch Pathol Lab Med 114:731, 1990

153. Moll UM, Chumas JC, Mann WJ, Patsner B: Primary signet ring cell carcinoma of the uterine cervix. NY State J Med 90:559, 1990

154. De La Vega G: Signet ring cell carcinoma of the uterine cervix. Patologia 14:193, 1976

155. Kupryjanczyk J, Kujawa M: Signet-ring cells in squamous cell carcinoma of the cervix and in non-neoplastic ectocervical epithelium. Int J Gynecol Cancer 2:152, 1992

156. Dougherty CM, Cotten N. Mixed squamous cell and adenocarcinoma of the cervix. Cancer 17:1132, 1964

157. Glucksmann A, Cherry CP: Incidence, histology and response to radiation of mixed carcinomas (adenoacanthomas) of the uterine cervix. Cancer 9:971, 1956

158. Wheeless CR, Graham R, Graham JB: Prognosis and treatment of adenoepidermoid carcinoma of the cervix. Obstet Gynecol 35:928, 1970

159. Gallup DG, Harper RH, Stock RJ: Poor prognosis in patients with adenosquamous cell carcinoma of the cervix. Obstet Gynecol 65:416, 1985

160. Cherry CP, Glucksmann A: Histology of carcinomas of the uterine cervix and survival rates in pregnant and non-pregnant patients. Surg Gynecol Obstet 111:763, 1961

161. Hacker DF, Berek JS, Lagasse LD: Carcinoma of the cervix associated with pregnancy. Obstet Gynecol 59:735, 1982

162. Teshima K, Fukuda M, Ikeda M et al: A study on mixed carcinoma of the uterine cervix. Obstet Gynecol Surv 34:871, 1979

163. Ireland D, Cole S, Kelly P, Monaghan JM: Mucin production in cervical intraepithelial neoplasia and in stage IB carcinoma of

164. Yazigi R, Sandstad J, Munoz AK et al: Adenosquamous carcinoma of the cervix: prognosis in stage IB. Obstet Gynecol 75:1012, 1990

165. Lotocki RJ, Krepart GV, Paraskevas M et al: Glassy cell carcinoma of the cervix: a bimodal treatment strategy. Gynecol Oncol 44:254, 1992

166. Tamini HK, Ek M, Hesla et al: Glassy cell carcinoma of the cervix redefined. Obstet Gynecol 71:837, 1988

167. Talerman A, Alenghat E, Okagaki T: Glassy cell carcinoma of the uterine cervix. APMIS 23:119, 1991

168. Seltzer V, Sall S, Castadot MJ et al: Glassy cell cervical carcinoma. Gynecol Oncol 8:141, 1979

169. Maier RC, Norris HJ: Glassy cell carcinoma of the cervix. Obstet Gynecol 60:219, 1982

170. Ulbright TM, Gersell DJ: Glassy cell carcinoma of the uterine cervix. A light and electron microscopic study of five cases. Cancer 51:2255, 1983

171. Pak HY, Yokota SB, Paladugu RR, Agliozzo CM: Glassy cell carcinoma of the cervix. Cancer 52:307, 1983

172. Costa MJ, Kenny MB, Hewan-Lowe K, Judd R: Glassy cell features in adenosquamous carcinoma of the uterine cervix. Histologic, ultrastructural, immunohistochemical, and clinical findings. Am J Clin Pathol 96:520, 1991

173. Baggish MS, Woodruff JD: Adenoid-basal carcinoma of the cervix. Obstet Gynecol 28:213, 1966

174. Baggish MS, Woodruff JD: Adenoid basal lesions of the cervix. Obstet Gynecol 37:807, 1987

175. Daroca PJ, Dhurandhar HN: Basaloid carcinoma of the uterine cervix. Am J Surg Pathol 4:235, 1980

176. van Dinh T, Woodruff JD: Adenoid cystic and adenoid basal carcinomas of the cervix. Obstet Gynecol 65:705, 1985

177. Ferry JA, Scully RE: "Adenoid cystic" carcinoma and adenoid basal carcinoma of the uterine cervix. A study of 28 cases. Am J Surg Pathol 12:134, 1988

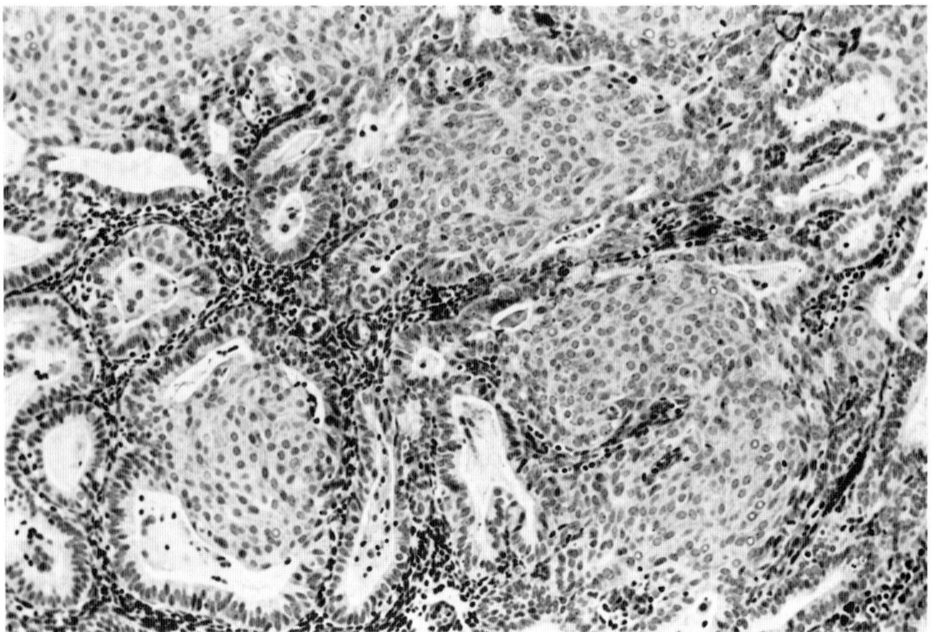

Fig. 4.1. Extensive squamous (morular) metaplasia accompanying simple hyperplasia ("adenoacanthosis"). Nests of immature squamous cells fill several gland lumens.

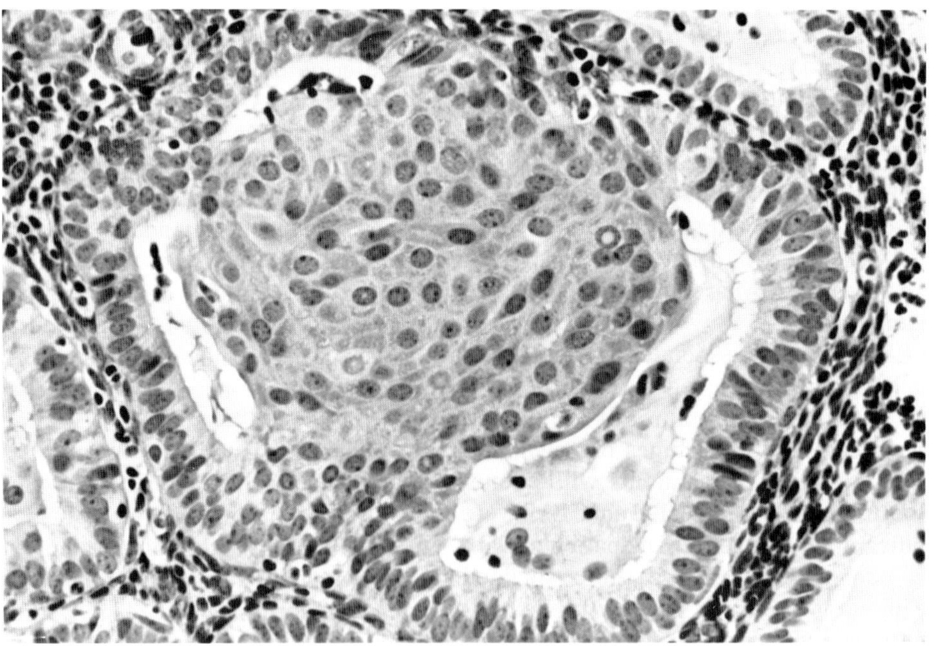

Fig. 4-2. Squamous (morular) metaplasia, higher power view of Fig. 4-1. Note the bland appearance of the nuclei.

ture squamous cells that have more abundant eosinophilic cytoplasm, intercellular bridges, and in some cases, keratin formation. Extensive replacement of the endometrium by mature keratinizing squamous epithelium has been referred to as *ichthyosis uteri*,[4] a lesion that is usually secondary to pyometra. The bland nuclear features, the mitotic inactivity, and lack of invasion exclude primary squamous cell carcinoma of the endometrium (see Ch. 5).

In *mucinous metaplasia*, endometrial glands are lined by columnar cells with mucin-rich cytoplasm[1,7] (Figs. 4-3 and 4-4). The cells typically mimic endocervical epithelium on routine and histochemical staining and ultrastructural examination but rarely the cells are of goblet type, including the presence of intestinal-type mucus with histochemical stains.[8] Rare cases may be accompanied by mucometra[9] or mucinous lesions elsewhere in the female genital tract; in one case, the patient also had bilateral borderline mucinous ovarian tumors, mucinous epithelial inclusions within pelvic lymph nodes, and papillary mucinous proliferations within endocervical glands.[10] When mucinous epithelium is atypical (Fig. 4-4), extensive, or both, there should be a high index of suspicion for mucinous adenocarcinoma (see Ch. 5), particularly in a postmenopausal patient.

Although small numbers of ciliated cells are found within the lining of normal proliferative endometrial glands, the term *ciliated metaplasia* refers to glands in which ciliated cells are the dominant or sole cell type (Figs. 4-5 and 4-6). Such glands are often variably cystic and individually disposed amongst nonmetaplastic glands. The ciliated cells have uniform round nuclei and often strikingly eosinophilic cytoplasm (Fig. 4-5). They usually line the gland as a single layer but occasionally stratify and form cribriform patterns. The absence of atypical nuclear features separates ciliated metaplasia from rare examples of atypical hyperplasia with a prominent component of ciliated cells (Fig. 4-6) and ciliated adenocarcinoma (see Ch. 5).

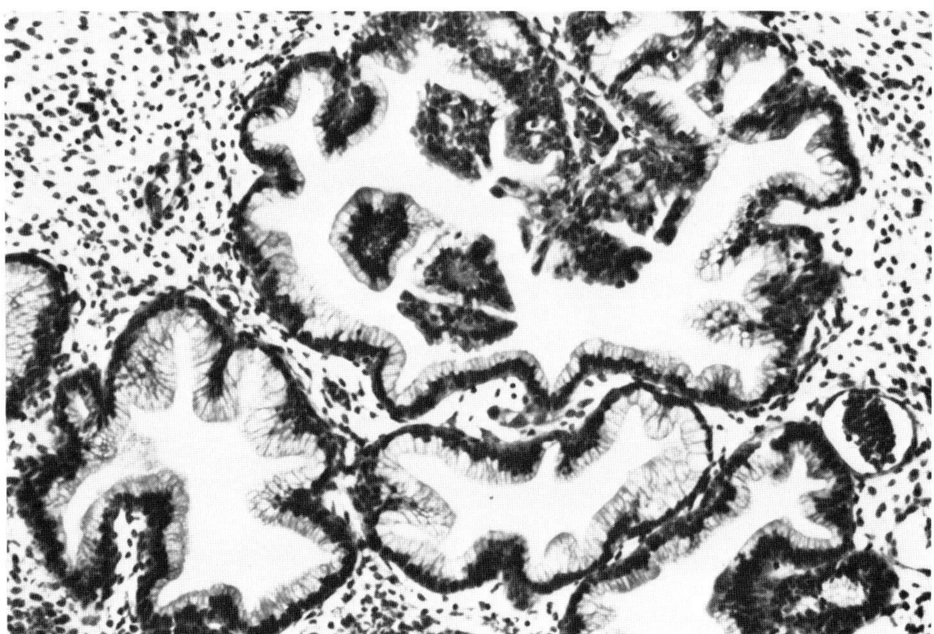

Fig. 4-3. Mucinous metaplasia. Benign-appearing endocervical-type cells line endometrial glands and intraglandular stromal papillae.

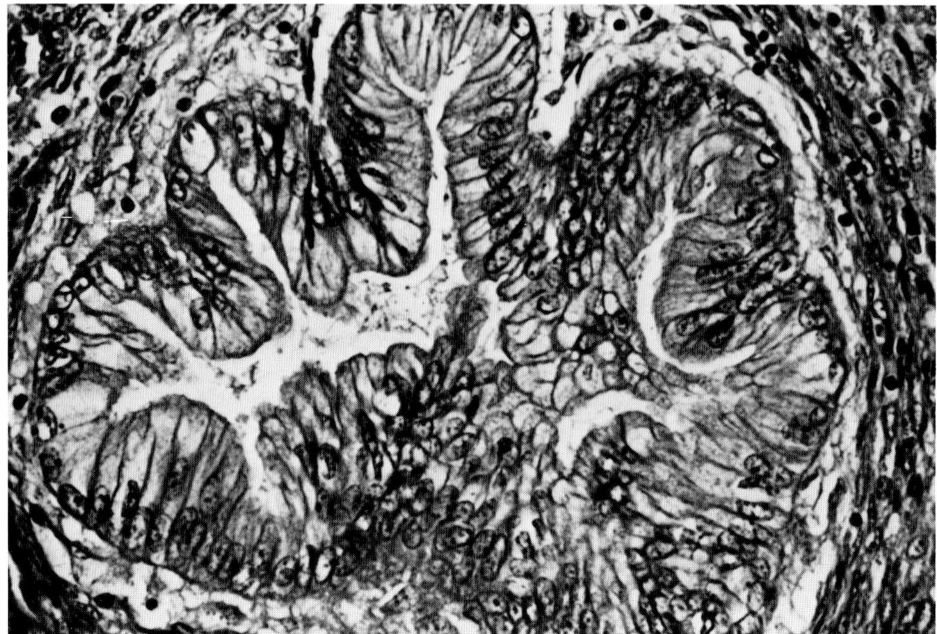

Fig. 4-4. Atypical mucinous metaplasia. Such glands were rare and individually disposed in this case. More extensive involvement of the endometrium by similar glands would raise the suspicion of a primary mucinous adenocarcinoma.

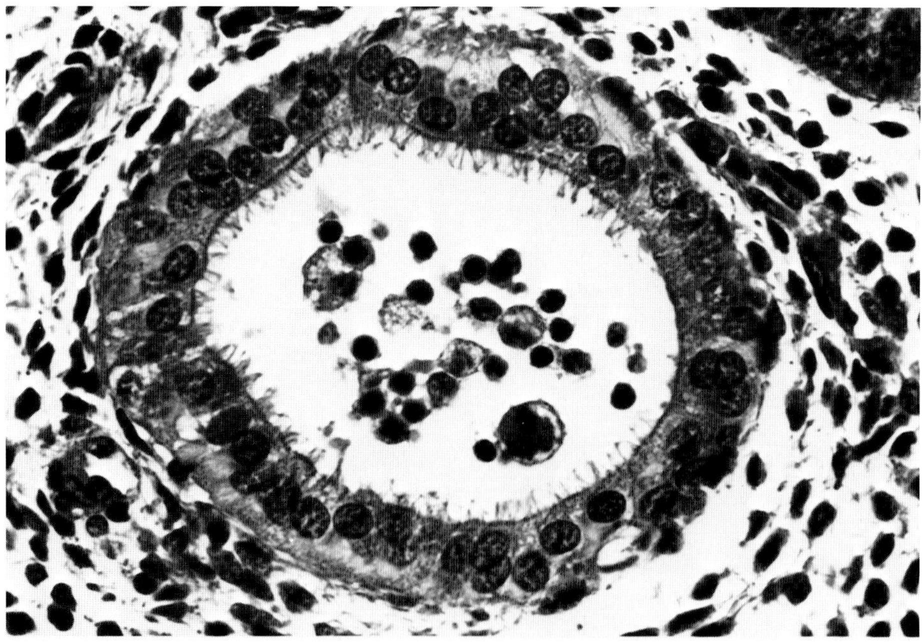

Fig. 4-5. Ciliated metaplasia.

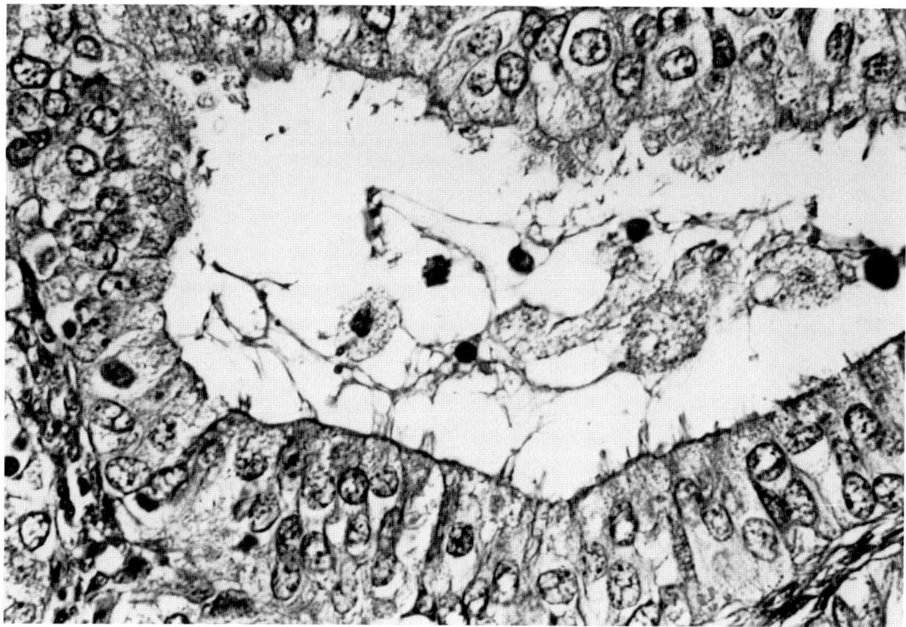

Fig. 4-6. Atypical endometrial hyperplasia with ciliated metaplasia.

In *eosinophilic metaplasia,* glands are lined by nonciliated cells with abundant eosinophilic cytoplasm[1] (Fig. 4-7). When the cytoplasm has a granular appearance, the term "oncocytic" metaplasia has been applied; in one such case, numerous mitochondria were found on ultrastructural examination.[11] The uniformity of the round central nuclei and paucity of mitotic figures distinguish this alteration from hyperplasia with atypia or occasional adenocarcinomas in which the cells have abundant eosinophilic cytoplasm.

Surface (papillary) syncytial metaplasia involves the endometrial surface epithelium and less commonly the superficial endometrial glands[1, 12] (Fig. 4-8). Cells with eosinophilic cytoplasm, indistinct cell borders, and bland nuclear features are arranged in cellular buds and papillae lacking stromal cores (Figs. 4-8 and 4-9). Occasionally, cells with similar features may grow in a nonpapillary sheetlike pattern. Infiltration by neutrophils is common. Syncytial metaplasia probably represents a regenerative phenomenon following ovulatory or anovulatory menstrual bleeding. It may be accompanied by other signs of recent bleeding, such as intraepithelial nuclear debris and aggregates of closely packed small stromal cells. Its microscopic size, usual confinement to the endometrial surface, and the benign appearance of its nuclei facilitate distinction from papillary carcinomas.

Rarely, endometrial glands exhibiting *hobnail cell* or *clear cell metaplasia* are an isolated finding with no apparent cause in a nonpregnant patient[1] (Fig. 4-10). Glands lined with the former cell type may occur following a curettage (see Fig. 4-34). The differential diagnosis of clear cell and hobnail cell metaplasia is with clear cell carcinoma, but the microscopic, focal nature of the metaplastic glands, as well as an absence of mitotic activity, should make misdiagnosis as carcinoma unlikely. Similar metaplastic changes occurring in pregnancy (Arias-Stella reaction) are discussed in the next section.

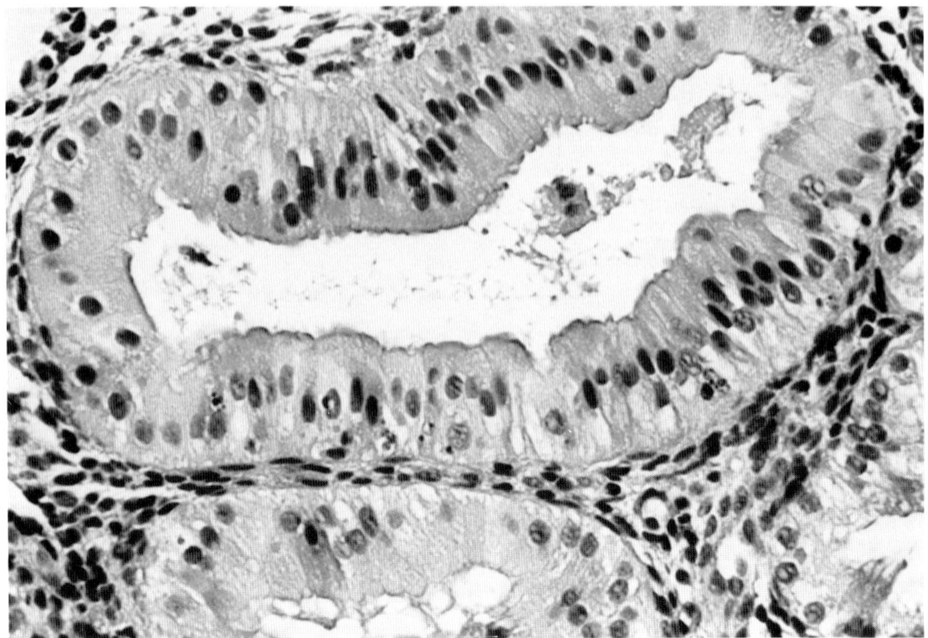

Fig. 4-7. Eosinophilic metaplasia. The glands are lined by nonciliated cells with abundant cytoplasm that was eosinophilic.

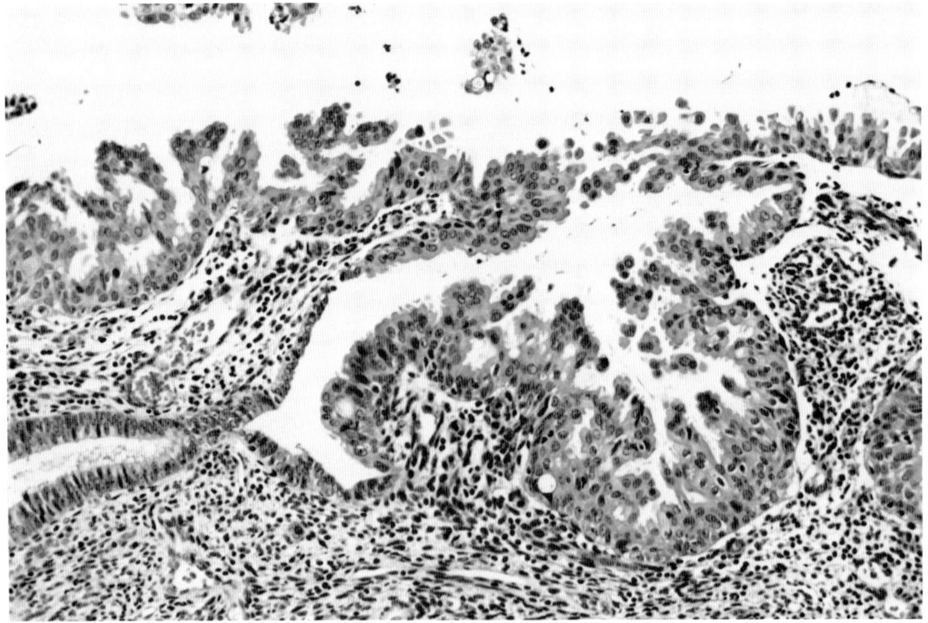

Fig. 4-8. Papillary syncytial metaplasia involving the endometrial surface and superficial glands.

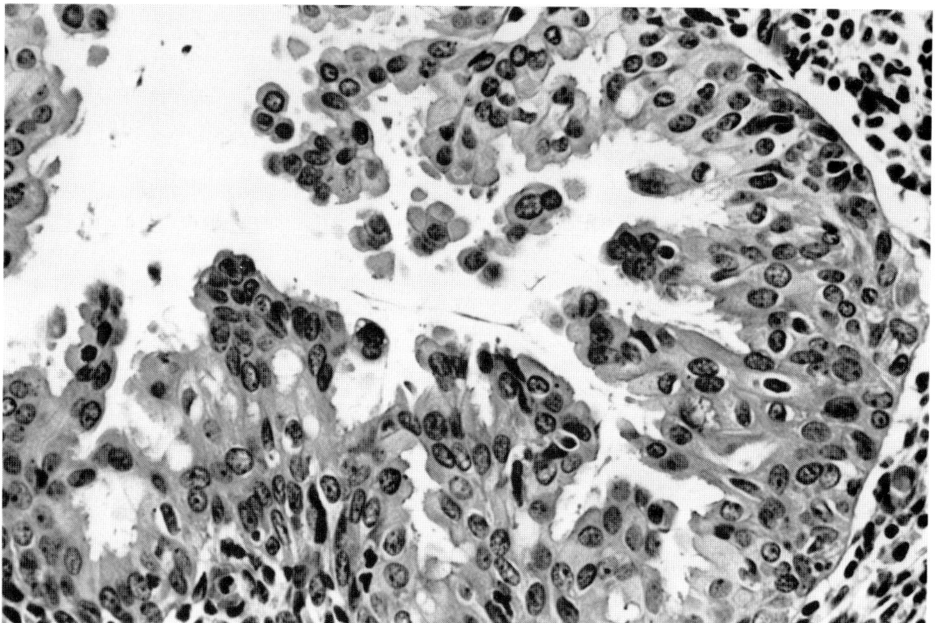

Fig. 4-9. Papillary syncytial metaplasia, higher power view of Fig. 4-8.

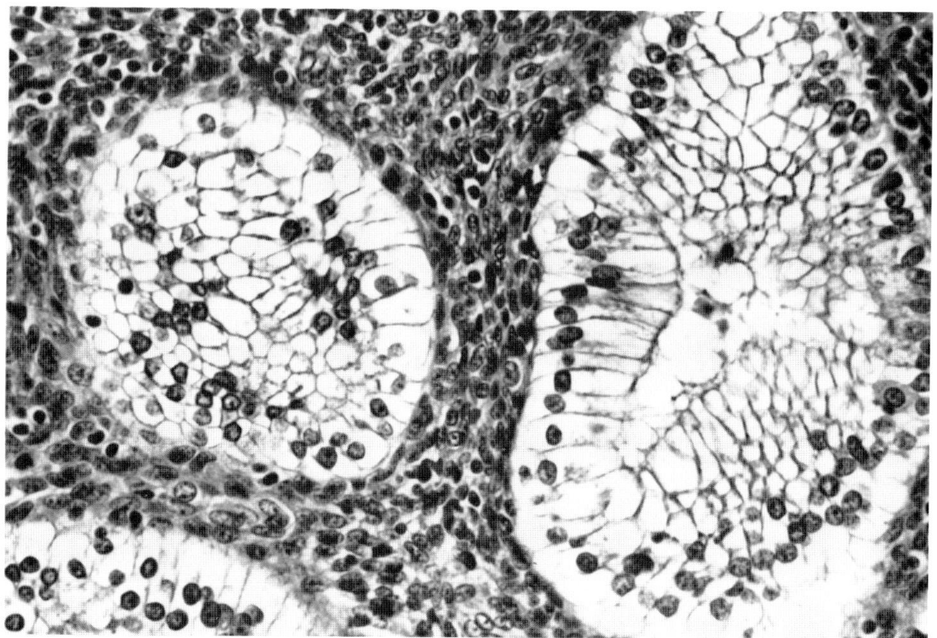

Fig. 4-10. Clear cell metaplasia in a nonpregnant patient.

PREGNANCY-RELATED AND HORMONAL CHANGES

A variety of pregnancy-related changes may be misinterpreted as neoplastic or preneoplastic, an error particularly likely to occur if the pathologist is unaware that the specimen is from a pregnant patient, if there is an absence of obvious trophoblastic tissue within the specimen, or the specimen is from a site in which pregnancy-related changes are uncommon, such as the endocervix (see Ch. 1). Similar findings may occasionally occur in patients receiving progestins, or even rarely in patients in whom there is no apparent cause. Normal postovulatory menstrual changes may also be misinterpreted as neoplastic or preneoplastic. Tumorlike trophoblastic lesions, such as exaggerated placental site and placental site nodule, are discussed in Chapter 9.

ARIAS-STELLA REACTION AND CLEAR CELL CHANGE

The Arias-Stella reaction (ASR) is a characteristic histologic finding within endometrial glands that occurs in association with intrauterine or extrauterine pregnancy and trophoblastic disease.[13–15] Similar, but less striking, changes may also occur in patients on hormonal medication. The ASR can occur in sites other than eutopic endometrium, including the glands of adenomyosis[16] and endometriosis,[16, 17] the epithelium of the fallopian tube,[16, 18] the endocervix (see Ch. 1), and in vaginal adenosis of the tuboendometrial type.[19]

The endometrial change, which is typically located in the spongiosa, may involve only a few glands or may be diffuse; the extent and intensity of the reaction do not correlate with the amount of trophoblast.[14] Regular papillary tufting is often present. The cells contain scanty cytoplasm and enlarged, pleomorphic, hyperchromatic nuclei, sometimes assuming a hobnail appearance (Fig. 4-11); in occasional cases, these nuclear changes may be particularly conspicuous (Fig. 4-12). The nuclei may be smudgy or optically clear (see below). Mitoses are absent or exceptionally rare. Familiarity with this lesion, its typical association with clinical or other histological evidence of pregnancy, and its mitotic inactivity facilitate its differentiation from endometrial adenocarcinoma. The hobnail cells should not be misinterpreted as cytomegalovirus endometritis; in the latter, only occasional cells are affected (with intervening normal cells), and the typical nuclear and cytoplasmic inclusions are present.

Another endometrial alteration related to pregnancy that may overlap with the ASR is the presence in the glandular epithelial cells of abundant clear, glycogen-rich cytoplasm (Figs. 4-11 and 4-13); nuclei similar to those of the ASR may or may not be present. These cells may exhibit regular papillary tufting or may proliferate to the extent that they almost obliterate the lumen. Although this clear cell change is often considered a component of the ASR, it was not emphasized by Arias-Stella in his original description of the lesion bearing his name[13] or in most of the subsequent literature.[15]

The ASR and clear cell change may be mistaken for in situ or, if extensive, invasive clear cell adenocarcinoma. These misdiagnoses are more likely to occur on examination of a biopsy or cytology specimen and when the pathologist is unaware that the specimen is from a pregnant patient. Clear cell carcinoma of the endometrium (see Ch. 5) usually occurs in perimenopausal or postmenopausal women and is typically associated with gross evidence suggestive of a tumor. Histologic examination may reveal one or more features inconsistent with the ASR, such as a tubulocystic pattern, mitotic activity and, in many cases, invasion. When papillae are encountered in clear cell adenocarcinoma, they are

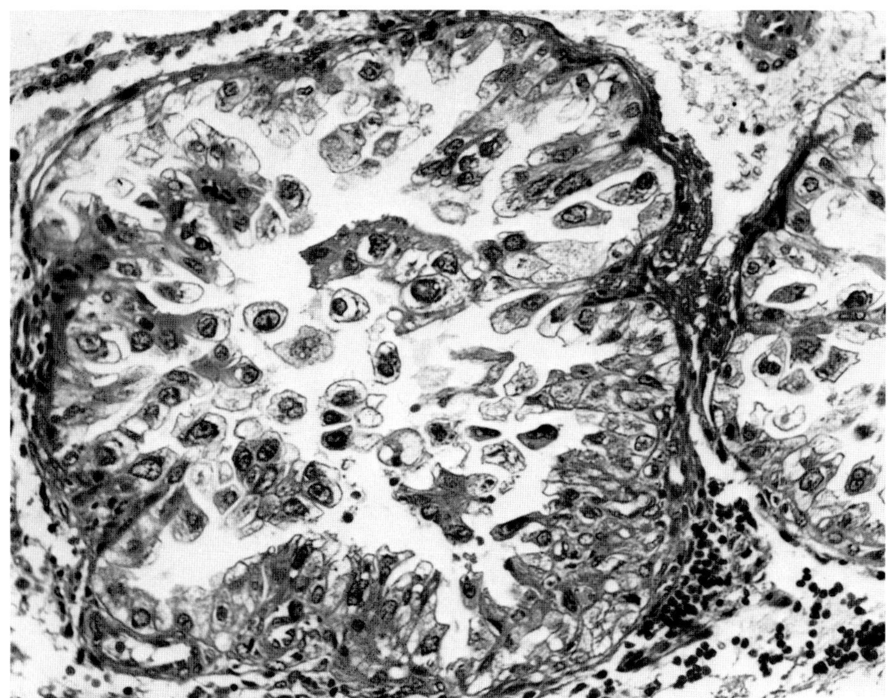

Fig. 4-11. Arias-Stella reaction.

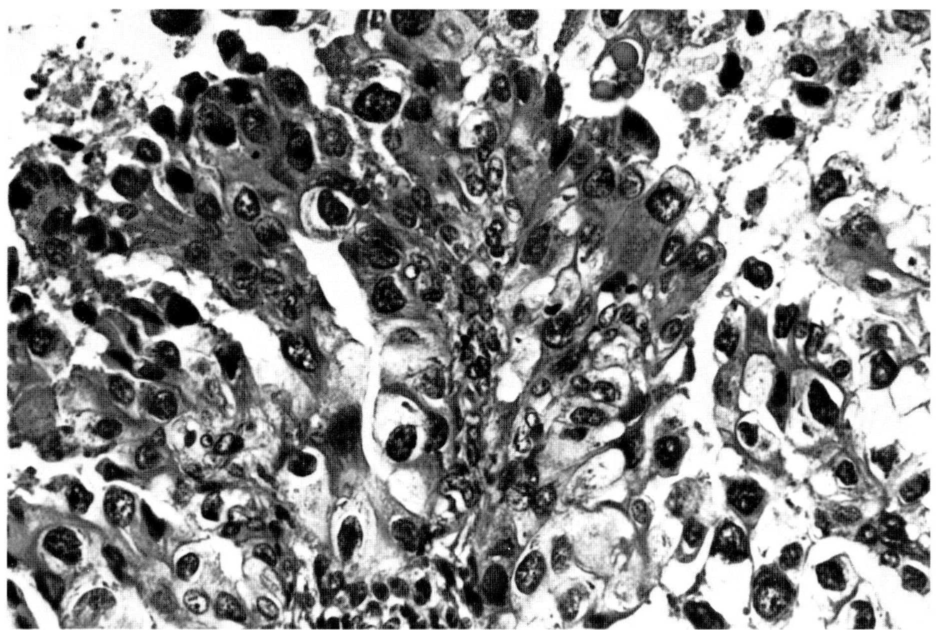

Fig. 4-12. Arias-Stella reaction with an unusual degree of cellular stratification and nuclear atypia.

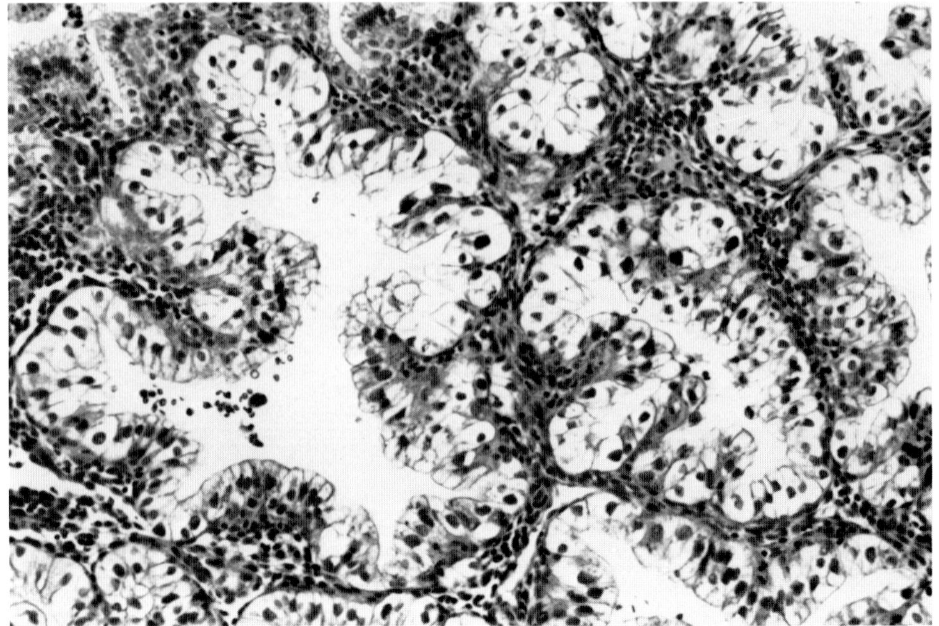

Fig. 4-13. Clear cell change of endometrial glands in a pregnant patient.

not of uniform size and shape, or regularly spaced as they are in the non-neoplastic endometrial glands of pregnancy, and frequently contain hyalinized cores. The presence of decidua in some cases is an additional clue to the diagnosis of a pregnancy-related change.

OPTICALLY CLEAR NUCLEI

Mazur and his associates drew attention to another distinctive pregnancy-related endometrial alteration,[20] that is, "optically clear nuclei" within endometrial glandular epithelium (Fig. 4-14) that in their experience was invariably associated with the presence of trophoblast. These nuclei were found in endometria from 7 percent of first-trimester abortion specimens, and less commonly within second-trimester abortion specimens and endometria associated with term pregnancies and gestational trophoblastic disease.[20] The change was often associated with the ASR. The appear-

ance of the nuclei resembled to some extent that of herpetic inclusions, but ultrastructural examination showed a network of fine filamentous material rather than herpes virus DNA.

DECIDUA

A fully developed decidual alteration of the endometrial stroma is almost invariably confined to pregnant women and those being treated with progestins; microscopic interpretation in such cases is usually straightforward. Diagnostic problems, however, may arise when the decidual reaction is encountered unexpectedly in a patient who is neither pregnant nor on any hormonal medication, when it has unusual histologic features, or when both features pertain. Nuclear pleomorphism and hyperchromasia of decidual cells have been described in patients on progestin therapy[21, 22] (Fig. 4-15). These changes, often associated with atrophy of the endometrial

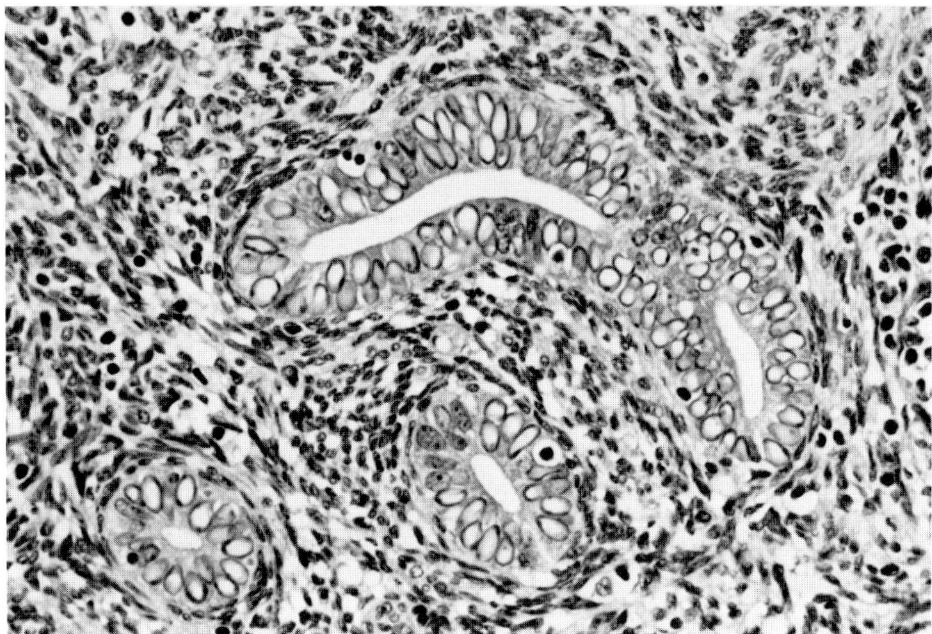

Fig. 4-14. Endometrial glands with optically clear nuclei in a pregnant patient.

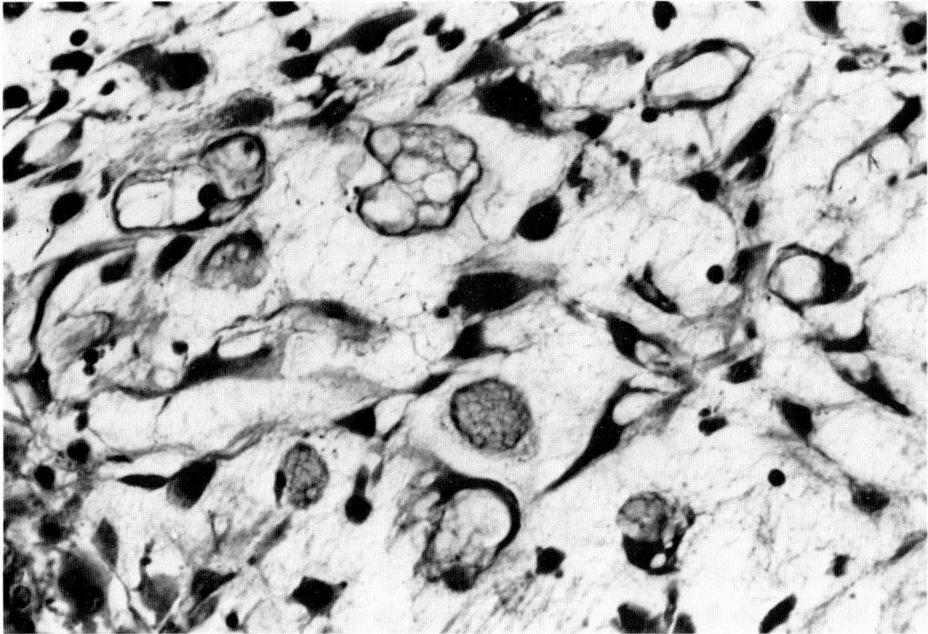

Fig. 4-15. Endometrial decidual reaction with signet-ring–like cells in a patient taking progestins. The decidual cells have atypical, hyperchromatic nuclei that are displaced by cytoplasmic vacuoles that contained acid mucin.

glands, may be misinterpreted as endometrial sarcoma.[21, 22] We have also seen occasional cases of decidual alteration in pregnant women or those on progestin therapy in which the decidual cells exhibit unusual degrees of cytoplasmic vacuolation (Fig. 4-15). In these cases, some of the decidual cells may be distended by one or more large cytoplasmic vacuoles that displace the nucleus, resulting in a signet-ring–like appearance (Fig. 4. 15). In contrast to a metastatic signet-ring adenocarcinoma (see Ch. 8), however, the vacuoles contain acid, rather than neutral mucin. This feature, the absence of obviously malignant nuclear features and mitotic figures, and the association with typical decidual cells should suggest the correct diagnosis in most cases.

An endometrial decidual reaction in the absence of evident progesterone stimulation is rare. Reinhart described such a case in a 25-year-old woman,[23] and Te Linde and Henriksen,[24] subsequently reported an additional 11 cases in premenopausal patients, 22 to 48 years of age. The patients typically presented with abnormal vaginal bleeding or discharge. None of the patients had received hormones, and the possibility of an intrauterine or extrauterine pregnancy was excluded or considered extremely unlikely. In some of the cases, the endometrium was grossly thickened and polypoid. The authors of these reports speculated that the decidual reaction in their patients was probably secondary to prolonged or excessive functioning of a corpus luteum.

Additionally, we have reported four cases of a florid idiopathic decidual reaction of the endometrium in postmenopausal women.[25] The patients, who were 53 to 73 years of age, presented with postmenopausal bleeding. None had received progestin therapy. Curettage in several of the cases yielded bulky, polypoid necrotic tissue suggestive of a neoplasm. Microscopic examination revealed diffuse decidual transformation of the endometrial stroma. The presence of nuclear pleomorphism and hyperchromasia, signet-ring-like cells (as noted above), focal necrosis, and focal glandular atypia, raised the question of a malignant tumor in two of the cases (Fig. 4-16).

HETEROTOPIC TISSUES

Heterotopic tissues, most commonly cartilage, bone, glia, and fat, are occasionally encountered within the endometrium and cervix, and less commonly, the myometrium.[26–52] This topic is considered here because implantation of fetal parts is the pathogenetic mechanism favored in the vast majority of cases. Most patients have a history of a therapeutic abortion or a spontaneous abortion that was followed by curettage; in some cases the heterotopic tissues have not been found until many years after the last known pregnancy. Cases in which there is no history of a curettage or an abortion[28] could be explained by the implantation of fetal tissues associated with an unrecognized spontaneous abortion. Some heterotopic tissues, however, may have other origins. The finding of nodules of hyaline cartilage in areas inconsistent with fetal origin, such as the subserosal myometrium, suggests a metaplastic origin or true heterotopia.[28] Bone occurring in the endometrium in cases of long-standing endometritis or pyometra may be dystrophic in origin.[32] Nodules of smooth muscle within the endometrium (*endometrial leiomyomas*)[51] (Fig. 4-17), likely derive from metaplasia of endometrial stromal cells.[53]

Hyaline Cartilage

In 1966, Roth and Taylor found 24 previously reported cases of hyaline cartilage within the uterus, and added nine of their own[28]; several subsequent examples have been described.[29, 35] The women, of reproductive age, typically have no clinical mani-

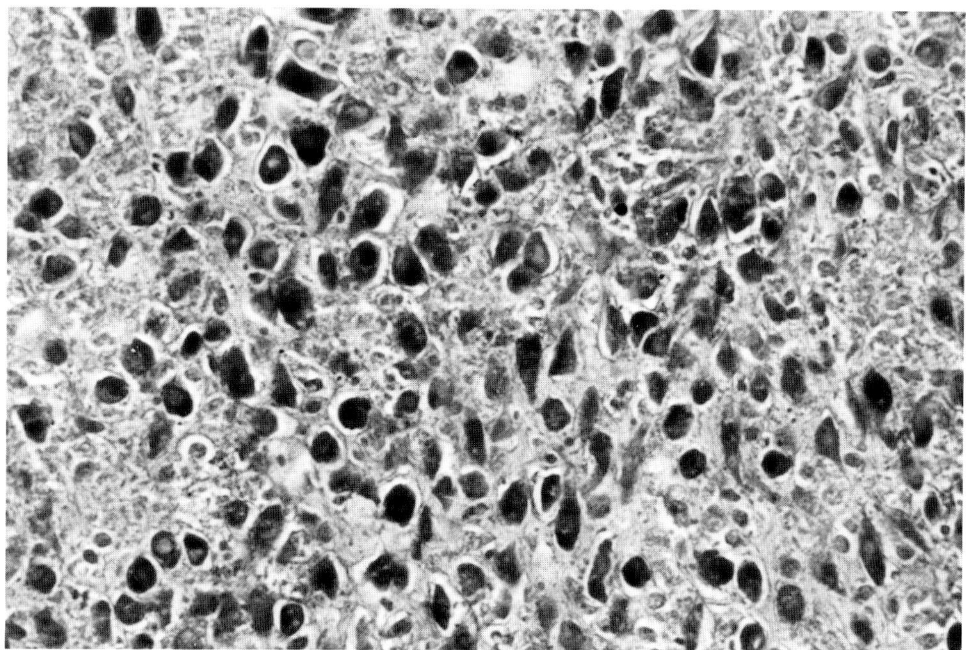

Fig. 4-16. Idiopathic decidual reaction in a postmenopausal woman. Most of the cells are necrotic and contain degenerating pyknotic nuclei.

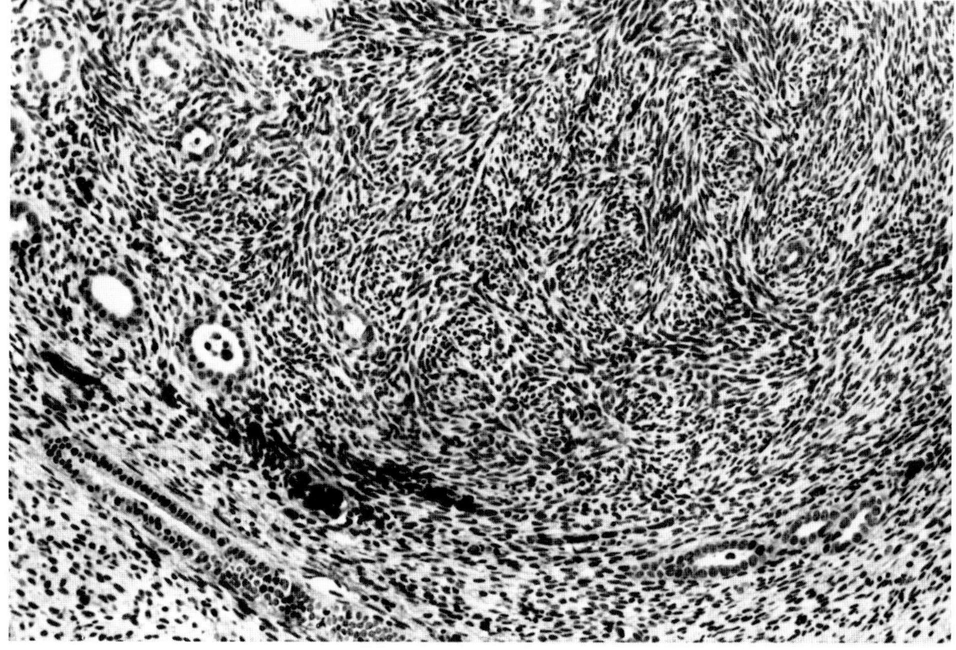

Fig. 4-17. Nodule of cellular smooth muscle within the endometrium; its border with the endometrial stroma (bottom) is well circumscribed. Occasional endometrial glands are entrapped within the lesion.

festations related to the cartilage, although in rare cases hard nodules have been palpated within the cervix or have been visible within the subserosal myometrium at laparotomy. When recognized on gross examination, one or multiple, well-circumscribed, round, oval, or fusiform, translucent structures less than 0.5 cm in maximum dimension (range, 0.1 to 5.5 cm) usually lie within the endometrium, superficial myometrium (Fig. 4-18), or endocervical stroma.[28] In rare cases, however, the cartilage has been found more deeply within the myometrium, or as noted above, has been subserosal. Most cases are recognized only on microscopic examination, the nodules consisting of fetal or mature hyaline cartilage without nuclear atypia or mitotic activity.[28, 29] Foci of calcification or bone are occasionally encountered within the nodules. There may be a chronic inflammatory infiltrate within the surrounding stroma.

Bone

More than 50 cases of heterotopic bone have been described within the uterus under a variety of designations, including endometrial or uterine "ossification," "osseus metaplasia," and "intrauterine retention of fetal bones."[26, 27, 29–32, 34, 35, 37–41, 44, 47–50] The patients have been of reproductive age, and have typically complained of abnormal vaginal bleeding or discharge, or less commonly pelvic pain or dysmenorrhea.[30, 50] Other women have had a history of repeated abortions or infertility[31, 39–41, 44, 48] or have passed bony tissue per vaginum.[27, 39] The bone has occasionally been visible on ultrasonographic or radiologic studies or at

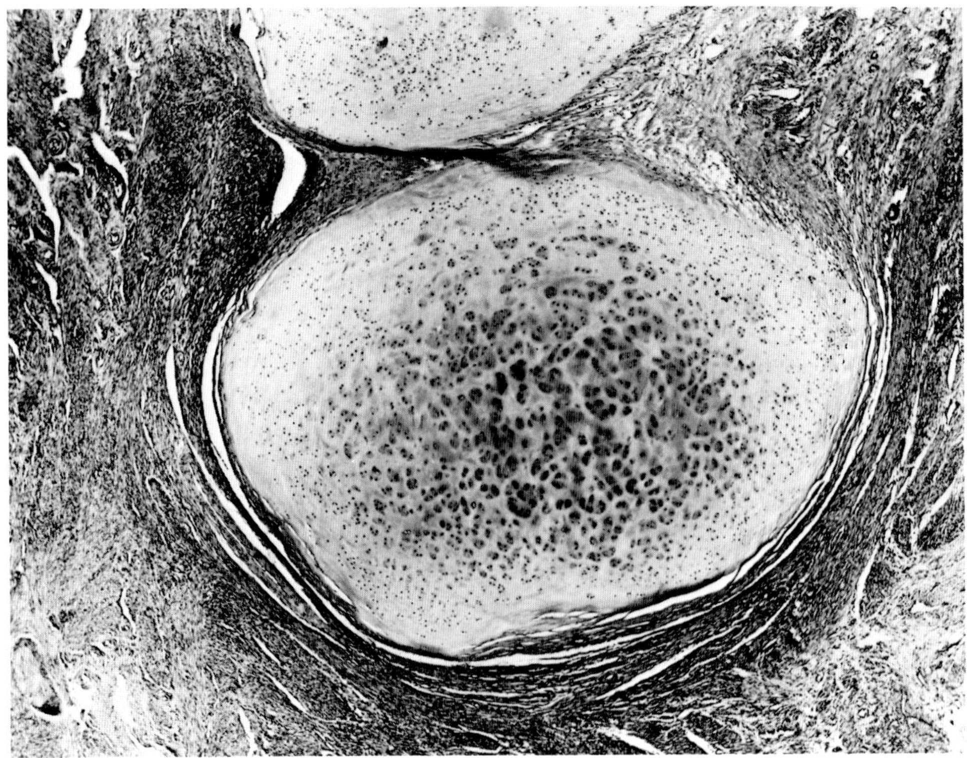

Fig. 4-18. Nodules of hyaline cartilage within the superficial myometrium.

hysteroscopy.[39, 40] Although often only a histologic finding, multiple bony spicules measuring up to 2.0 cm in size have been visible grossly in curettage, biopsy, or hysterectomy specimens, and in some cases, skeletal fragments, such as a tibia or clavicle, are recognizable.[27, 47, 50] In occasional patients, bone has been found in two or more specimens over periods of up to 3 years.[37] Histologic examination reveals spicules of viable or necrotic mature bone within the endometrial or endocervical stroma or myometrium (Fig. 4-19). Other heterotopic tissues, such as cartilage (see above) or glia (see below) have also been present in occasional cases. There may be an associated severe chronic endometritis.[27]

In many cases, the presenting symptoms have reversed following curettage or hysteroscopic removal of the bone. It has been suggested that in infertile patients, the bone may act as an intrauterine device (IUD).[40,41,44,49] Elevated menstrual fluid prostanoids were found in one case, a finding similar to that see in IUD users.[49] An associated endometritis, partial tubal occlusion, or both, found in some cases, may also contribute to the infertility.[49]

Glia and Other Neuroectodermal Tissues

In a literature review in 1973, Zettergren found 25 reported cases of mature glial tissue within the uterus and added four of his own[33]; a dozen additional examples have been described.[29, 34, 36, 42, 45, 46] The glial tissue is typically an incidental microscopic finding, but less commonly it forms a 1- to 2-cm, cervical or endometrial polyp that may be visible at the external os. In some cases, the polyps have been recurrent, probably secondary to incomplete removal.[36, 45] The glial tissue is typically confined to the endometrium or endocervical mucosa, but rare cases have penetrated some distance into the myometrium. The glial tissue, which may be multifocal, has

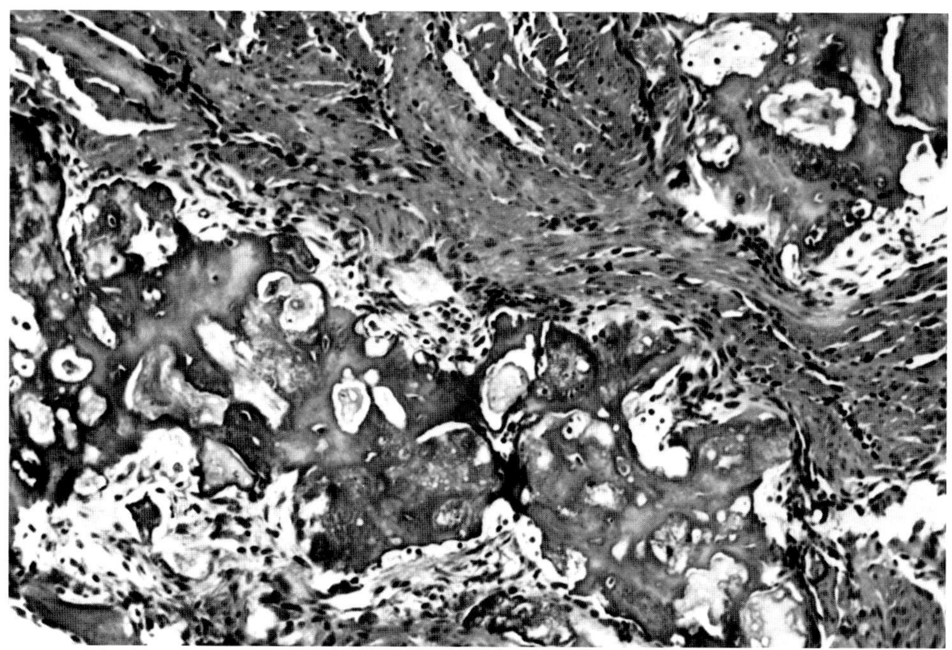

Fig. 4-19. Bone within the superficial myometrium.

an irregular, but usually well-demarcated, border with the indigenous stroma and may surround endocervical or endometrial glands. There may be an accompanying inflammatory response. Unusual additional findings have included gemistocytic glia, oligodendroglia, ganglion cells, ependyma-lined cavities, choroid plexus, myelinated nerve fibers, and psammoma bodies.[33] Immunoreactivity for glial fibrillary acidic protein (GFAP) has been observed in two recently studied cases.[45, 46]

Other Heterotopic Tissues

Small foci of mature adipose tissue may rarely be encountered within the endometrial stroma or myometrium. When associated with other heterotopic tissues,[35, 46] such foci are likely of fetal origin, whereas in other cases, they appear to be metaplastic.[52] Rare heterotopic tissues, probably of fetal origin, found within the endometrium have included renal, hepatic, and retinal tissue, skeletal muscle, and skin.[35, 43] In one unique case, a 19-year-old woman who underwent termination of pregnancy at 19 weeks of gestation required a hysterectomy shortly thereafter for uncontrollable bleeding.[54] Pathologic examination of the uterus revealed embolization of fetal tissue (liver, skeletal muscle) and placental tissue in the myometrial and parametrial veins.

Differential Diagnosis of Heterotopic Tissues

Heterotopic tissues, particularly cartilage or bone in a curettage specimen, may be confused with the heterologous elements of a malignant müllerian mixed tumor (MMMT) (see Ch. 7). Indeed, some patients have undergone unnecessary hysterectomy because a MMMT was suggested by the finding of cartilage in a curettage specimen.[28] In contrast to patients with he-

terotopic tissues, however, MMMTs typically occur in postmenopausal women who have an obvious intrauterine mass. Moreover, the heterologous elements are usually atypical or obviously malignant on histologic examination and are associated with carcinomatous and other sarcomatous elements. Benign-appearing bone and cartilage, however, may be rarely encountered within the stroma of otherwise typical endometrial adenocarcinomas (see Ch. 5). The frequently microscopic and multifocal nature of glial tissue, its histologic maturity, its occasional association with other heterotopic elements, and its typical association with a previous instrumental abortion, all aid in the distinction of the lesion from a neuroectodermal tumor of the uterus (see Ch. 8). Separate fragments of fat within a curettage specimen unassociated with other heterotopic tissues may originate from a uterine lipoma or lipoleiomyoma (see Ch. 6) or from traumatic uterine perforation.[55] In a unique case of the latter, implanted omental fat was found within the endometrial cavity 16 years after curettage-related uterine perforation.[55] When a variety of heterotopic tissues are present in the same specimen, the differential diagnosis is with a mature teratoma (see Ch. 8).

TUMORLIKE CHANGES ASSOCIATED
WITH MENSES

Normal menstrual changes may be misinterpreted as neoplastic or preneoplastic. The marked fragmentation and crowding of endometrial glands and surface epithelium that occur at the time of menses and that are accentuated by the curettage procedure have been confused with complex hyperplasia or even endometrial adenocarcinoma. The associated stromal changes (see below), the fragmented nature of the epithelium, the frequent presence of residual secretory changes within the epithelium, and the absence of nuclear atypicality mili-

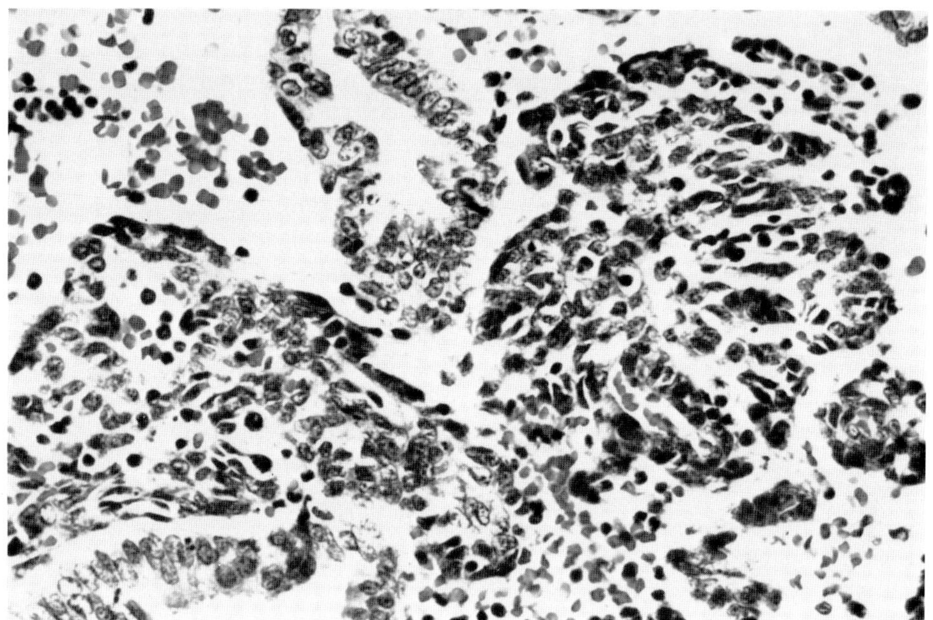

Fig. 4-20. Normal postovulatory menstrual endometrium. The degenerating stromal cells were initially misdiagnosed as representing an undifferentiated small cell carcinoma.

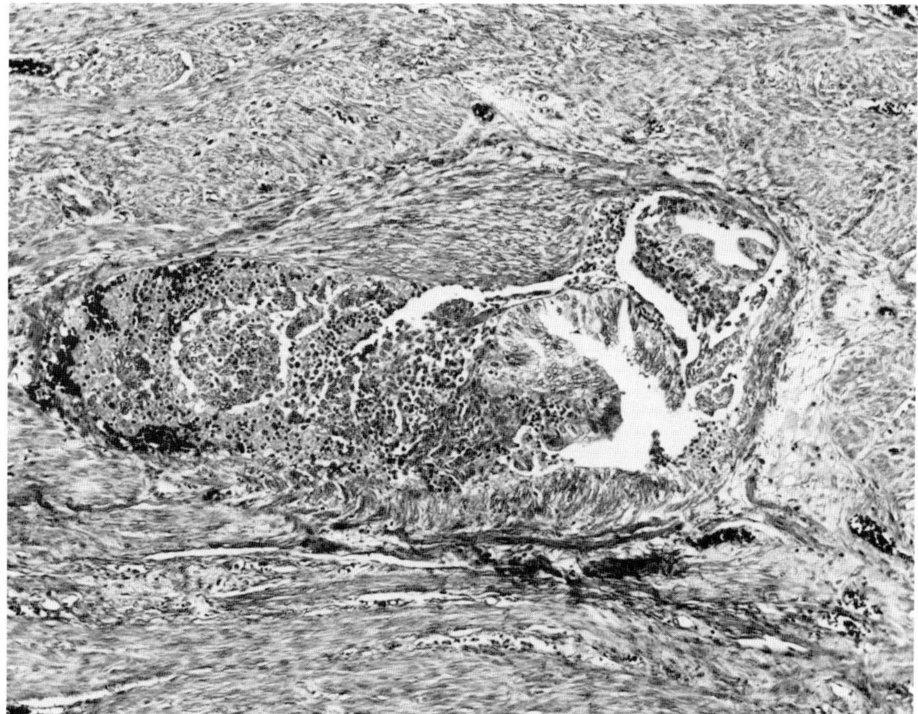

Fig. 4-21. Menstrual endometrium within a myometrial vein.

tate against a diagnosis of carcinoma or a precancerous lesion (Fig. 4-20). Another characteristic anovulatory or postovulatory menstrual change is the presence of compact, densely cellular nests of endometrial stromal cells.[56] The degenerating stromal cells have scanty cytoplasm and irregular, sometimes spindled, hyperchromatic nuclei (Fig. 4-20). The nests are often surrounded by larger epithelial cells; both cell types lack features of malignancy and mitotic activity. That these changes can create diagnostic problems is exemplified by a recently encountered consultation case of a normal postovulatory menstrual endometrium in which the menstrually altered endometrial stroma was initially misdiagnosed as an undifferentiated small cell carcinoma (Fig. 4-20). In other cases, the stromal cells may suggest the diagnosis of a stromal sarcoma. Awareness of this change and attention to the associated features noted above facilitate the correct diagnosis.

Menstrual endometrium may occasionally be found within uterine blood vessels (Fig. 4-21). In 1927, Sampson illustrated intravascular menstrual endometrium in two uteri from women who were menstruating at the time of hysterectomy.[57] More recently, Banks et al. have described a case in which numerous foci of menstrual endometrium were found within parametrial blood vessels of a hysterectomy specimen, the appearance simulating vascular invasion by a poorly differentiated malignant tumor.[58]

INFLAMMATORY AND REPARATIVE LESIONS

LYMPHOID INFILTRATES

Lymphoma-like Lesions

Inflammatory lesions of the endometrium are common and in the great majority of cases are obviously non-neoplastic and therefore do not pose a problem in differential diagnosis with lymphoma. For example, numerous lymphoid follicles may be found in the endometrial stroma in cases of severe chronic endometritis, especially those associated with *Chlamydia trachomatis* infection.[59, 60] Similar lymphoid follicles have been described within the myometrium in a patient with pelvic inflammatory disease and chronic endometritis[61]; some of the lymphoid follicles protruded into myometrial lymphatic spaces. In these cases, germinal centers within the follicles and a mixed inflammatory infiltrate that includes neutrophils and plasma cells within the endometrial stroma and epithelium indicate an inflammatory process rather than a follicular lymphoma. Such changes also facilitate distinction from endometria in which the only notable finding is an occasional lymphoid follicle, a finding that is considered normal.[62]

In contrast, reactive lymphoid infiltrates within the endometrium occasionally are sufficiently florid to be mistaken for lymphoma on microscopic examination. These lymphoma-like lesions are clinically and pathologically similar to their more common counterparts occurring within the cervix (see Ch. 1). Five of the 16 lymphoma-like lesions of the lower female genital tract reported by Young et al. involved the endometrium.[63] The patients ranged in age from 22 to 63 (mean, 40) years of age; only one was postmenopausal. The patients underwent endometrial curettage because of abnormal bleeding (three cases), bilateral adnexal masses interpreted as tubo-ovarian abscesses (one case), or at the time of cone biopsy for abnormal cytological smears (one case). None of the patients received any additional treatment. Two had uneventful follow-up periods of 9 months and 2 years duration; the other cases were recent or were lost to follow-up.

On microscopic examination, the specimens were characterized by the presence of variable numbers of large lymphoid cells, containing numerous mitotic figures, on a background of typical chronic endometritis (Figs. 4-22 and 4-23). In four cases, the large lymphoid cells formed focal, mostly ill-defined aggregates up to 2.5 mm in diameter (Fig. 4-22), whereas in the fifth case, the cells were diffusely distributed. Although the focal aggregates of large cells contained only rare plasma cells and polymorphonuclear leukocytes or were devoid of them, these cells were prominent at the periphery of the aggregates. The large cells included cleaved and noncleaved follicular center cells and immunoblasts (Fig. 4-23). In three cases, there was abundant nuclear debris, and in two of these cases there was a prominent starry-sky pattern of histiocytes containing phagocytosed debris. In one of the latter cases, this pattern resembled that of Burkitt's lymphoma. Most of the aggregates resembled reactive germinal centers, but they lacked a peripheral mantle of mature lymphocytes. In the case that lacked aggregates, the diffuse infiltrate was

composed of numerous immunoblasts admixed with smaller numbers of cleaved and noncleaved follicular center cells, many plasma cells, small lymphocytes, and polymorphonuclear leukocytes. The large lymphoid cells predominated in some areas. Most of the large lymphoid cells in the endometrial lymphoma-like lesions did not stain with anti-light chain antibodies.

Features useful in distinguishing endometrial lymphoma-like lesions from uterine lymphoma include an absence of a gross mass, reactive germinal centers within the lymphoid aggregates, a mixed inflammatory infiltrate at the periphery of the aggregates, and the presence of typical chronic endometritis elsewhere in the specimen. Although no lymphoma-like lesions of the corpus have been diagnosed in hysterectomy specimens, it would be expected that, as in the cervix, they would be confined to the endometrium (and possibly superficial myometrium), in contrast to the deep myometrial involvement that may occur in

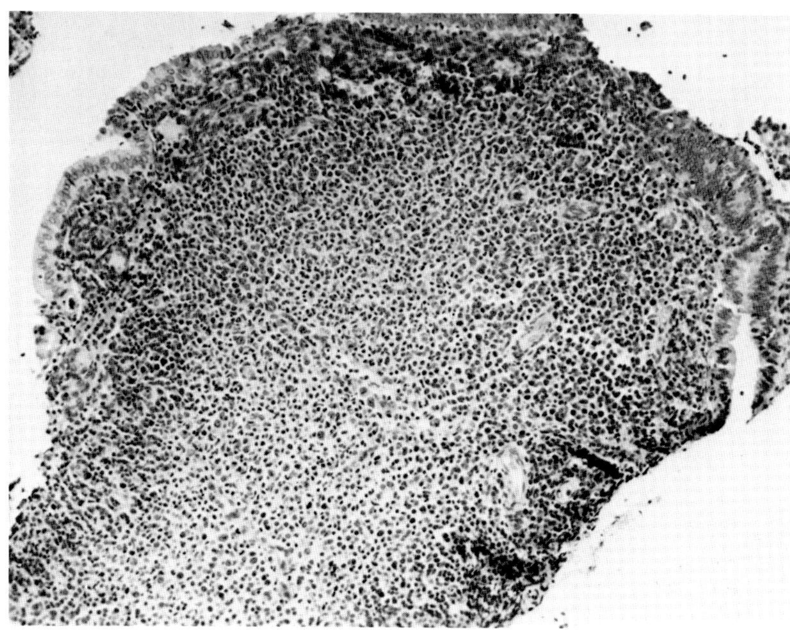

Fig. 4-22. Lymphoma-like lesion of the endometrium. A large aggregate composed predominantly of large lymphoid cells obscures the underlying endometrial stroma. (From Young et al.,[63] with permission.)

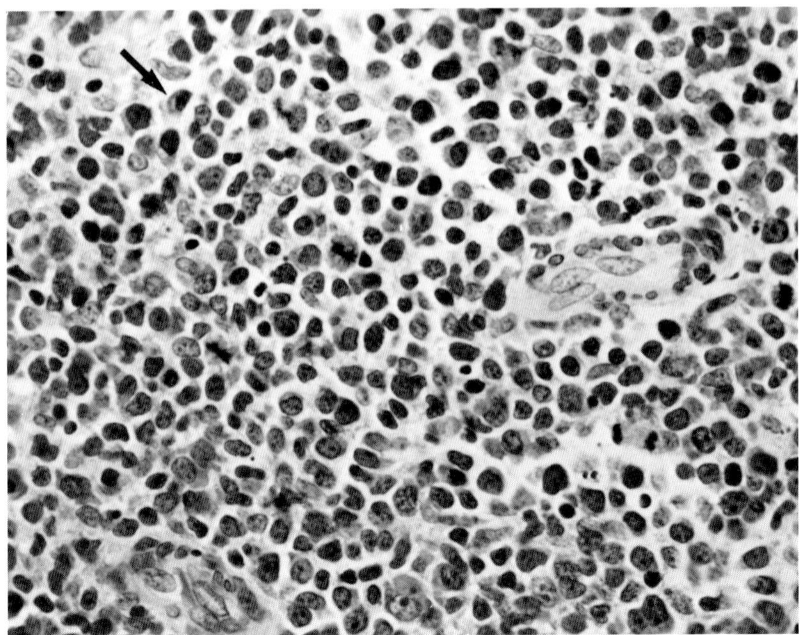

Fig. 4-23. Lymphoma-like lesion of the endometrium. Higher magnification of Fig. 4-22 shows cleaved and noncleaved follicular center cells and occasional immunoblasts. Scattered small lymphocytes and rare plasma cells (arrow) are also present. (From Young et al.,[63] with permission.)

uterine involvement by lymphomas (see Ch. 8).

Massive Lymphoid Infiltration in Leiomyomas

Ferry et al. have recently described seven uterine leiomyomas characterized by massive lymphoid infiltration.[64] The leiomyomas, which occurred in patients 35 to 50 years of age, ranged from 2 to 12 cm in greatest dimension, and contained a variably dense infiltrate of small lymphocytes with scattered larger lymphoid cells and occasionally, numerous plasma cells (Figs. 4-24 and 4-25). Germinal centers were identified in rare cases and ranged from large and florid to inconspicuous; rarely, eosinophils were present. Most of the tumors were focally to extensively sclerotic. In cases in which the adjacent myometrium was available for examination, the lymph-

oid infiltrate was confined to the leiomyoma (Fig. 4-24) or was present only to a minor extent in the adjacent myometrium. The polymorphous nature of the infiltrate and its confinement to the leiomyoma distinguish the lesion from malignant lymphoma.

HISTIOCYTIC INFILTRATES

Granulomatous endometritis, sometimes accompanied by granulomatous myometritis, is usually secondary to infection (tuberculous, fungal, parasitic), foreign material, or sarcoidosis, and in such cases, discrete granulomas are typically found.[65] Similarly, necrotizing granulomas, sometimes accompanied by palisading histiocytes, have been recently described following diathermy ablation of the endometrium.[66–68] Confusion with a neoplastic process in these granulomatous lesions is unlikely. By contrast, endometritis and

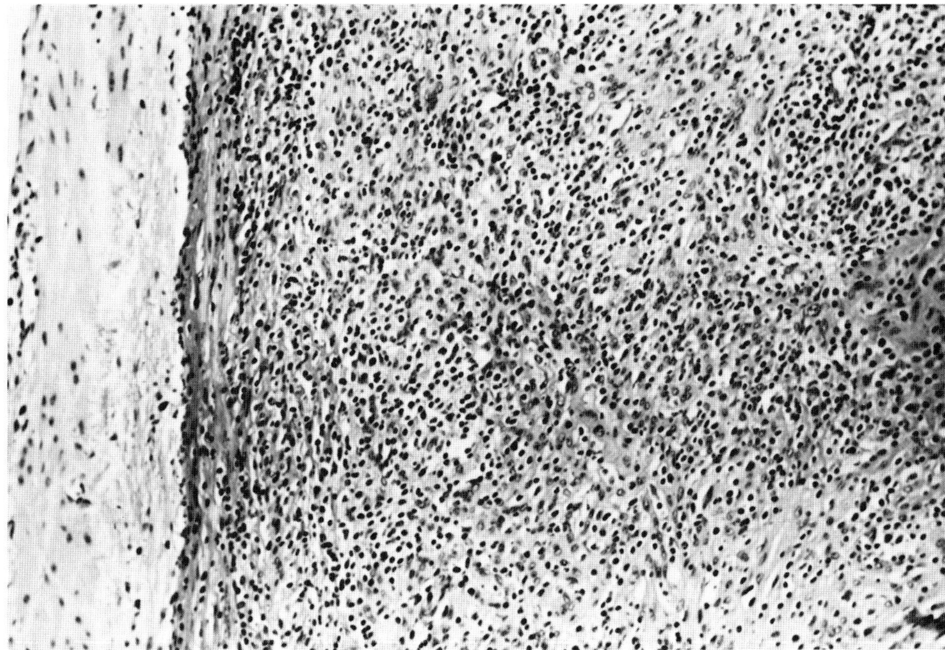

Fig. 4-24. Leiomyoma with massive lymphoid infiltrate. Note confinement of the infiltrate to the leiomyoma with sparing of the contiguous myometrium (extreme left).

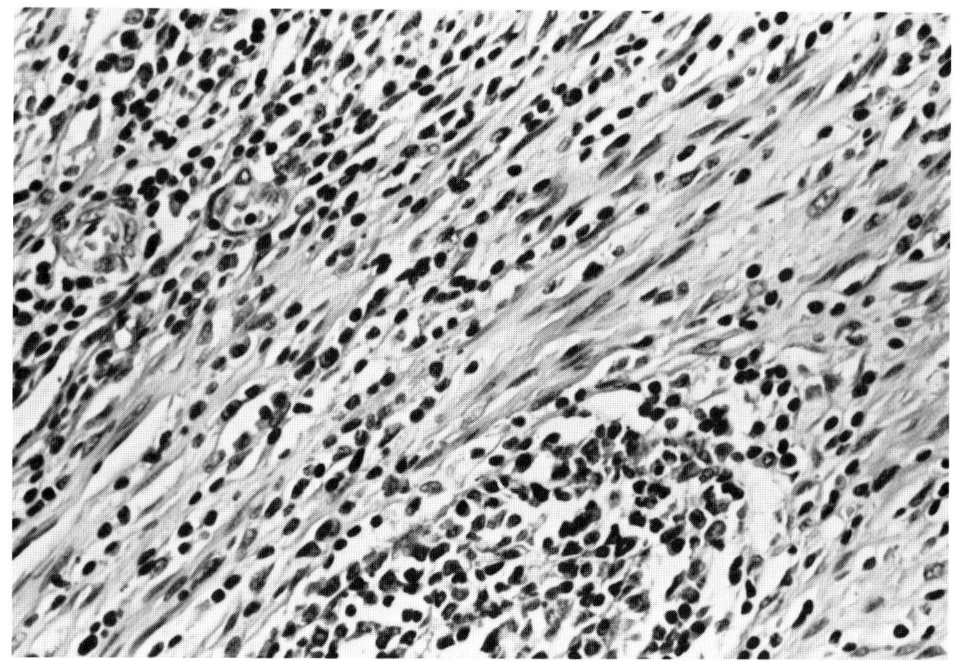

Fig. 4-25. Leiomyoma with massive lymphoid infiltrate. The infiltrate consists of mature lymphocytes and plasma cells.

myometritis can occasionally be characterized by a more diffuse infiltration of histiocytes that may cause a grossly evident tumorlike mass, and that on microscopic examination should be distinguished from uterine involvement by hematopoietic and histiocytic neoplasms (see Ch. 8).

Xanthogranulomatous Inflammation

As in other parts of the body, the endometrium can be the site of an inflammatory reaction characterized by striking numbers of foamy histiocytes; the myometrium is also involved in some cases. The designations *xanthogranulomatous* and *histiocytic* endometritis have been applied to this lesion.[69–73] In 1988, in a review of xanthogranulomatous inflammation of the female genital tract Ladefoged and Lorentzen,[69] found nine examples involving the corpus, and seven additional cases have been subsequently reported.[70, 71] The patients, all of

whom have been postmenopausal, have usually presented with vaginal bleeding or discharge; some had previously received radiation treatment for endometrial adenocarcinoma or squamous cell carcinoma of the cervix.[70, 72] Pelvic examination has revealed cervical stenosis or pyometra, or both, in most cases. In some patients, necrotic, friable, yellow-brown tissue within a curettage specimen or similar tissue lining the endometrial cavity in a hysterectomy specimen has erroneously suggested the presence of an endometrial carcinoma.[72, 73]

The cardinal histologic finding is the presence of sheets of histiocytes with abundant, eosinophilic, granular or foamy cytoplasm in the absence of Michaelis-Gutmann bodies (Fig. 4-26). The cytoplasm is typically rich in lipid and in some cases, ceroid pigment[71, 72]; cytoplasmic (periodic acid-Schiff (PAS)-positive material, at least some of which may be ceroid, has been present in some cases. The nuclei within the histiocytes are small, uniform, and oc-

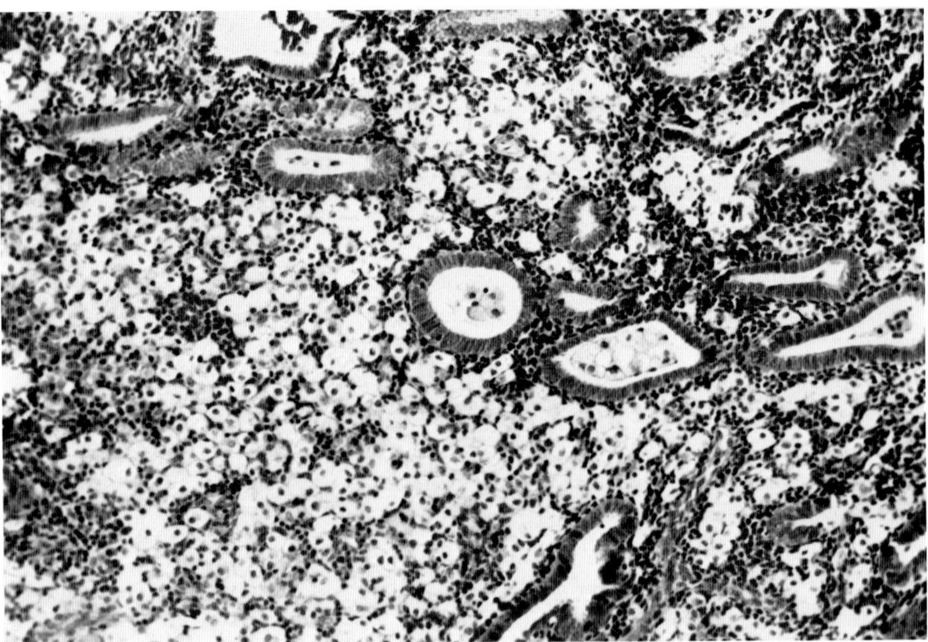

Fig. 4-26. Xanthogranulomatous endometritis. Numerous histiocytes with abundant foamy cytoplasm occupy the endometrial stroma. Other inflammatory cells, including lymphocytes and plasma cells, were also present.

casionally multiple; mitotic figures are typically absent. In florid cases, the histiocytes completely replace the endometrium and may infiltrate deep into the myometrium.[72] Large numbers of other inflammatory cells, including polymorphonuclear leukocytes, lymphocytes, plasma cells, hemosiderin-laden histiocytes, and foreign-body giant cells are also typically present. Cholesterol crystals, focal calcification, necrosis, and radiation-induced changes have been prominent in some cases. Organisms are not visible histologically but bacteria have been cultured in rare cases.[69]

The pathogenesis of xanthogranulomatous endometritis appears to be related to cervical obstruction resulting in pyometra, hematometra, endometrial necrosis, or combinations thereof. Radiation-induced tumor necrosis and bacterial infection may be additional factors in some cases.[70] The findings of xanthogranulomatous endometritis should be distinguished from malakoplakia (see below) as well as from endometrial stromal cells with abundant, foamy,

lipid-rich cytoplasm that are present in some cases of endometrial hyperplasia and carcinoma (see Ch. 5).

Malakoplakia

Seven cases of malakoplakia with endometrial involvement have been reported.[74–80] The patients were elderly (60 to 88 years of age) with the exception of one 40-year-old woman and presented with abnormal vaginal bleeding or spotting. A curettage was performed in each patient, followed in two by a hysterectomy. When the curetted tissue was described macroscopically, it was moderately abundant, soft, yellow to brown, and focally hemorrhagic. The endometrium was thick, soft, nodular, and gray-white in one hysterectomy specimen, and in the other, there was a polypoid lesion measuring 3 cm. On histologic examination (Fig. 4-27), the typical findings of malakoplakia were seen in each case, including sheets of histiocytes with copious

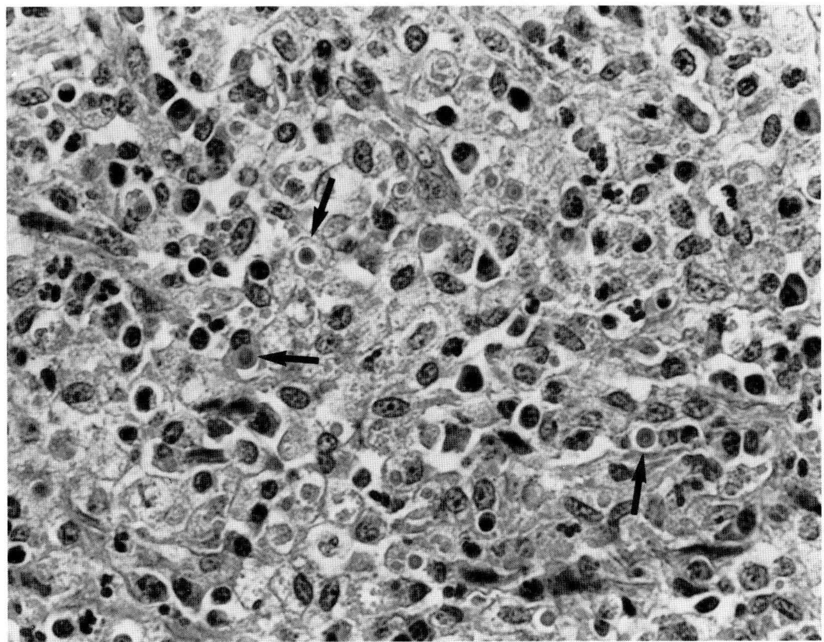

Fig. 4-27. Malakoplakia of the endometrium. Note Michaelis-Guttmann bodies (arrows). (Courtesy of Dr. W. Thomas, Jr., Chicago IL.)

granular cytoplasm (von Hansemann cells), Michaelis-Gutmann bodies, and intracellular bacilli; other inflammatory cells were also typically present. The myometrium was not involved in the two hysterectomy specimens, but in one other case the cervix was involved,[77] as was the broad ligament and inguinal region in another.[74] In one case, there was a synchronous endometrial adenocarcinoma.[78] Malakoplakia was found on repeated curettage in three of the patients 5 weeks to 8 months later.

Eosinophilic Infiltrates

Several studies have shown that the endometrium and the myometrium can occasionally be the sites of infiltration by prominent numbers of eosinophils that typically represent a response to a prior curettage.[81–83] In their series of cases of eosinophilic infiltration of the cervix or corpus, Bjersing and Borglin found four cases of eosinophilic myometritis.[81] Each patient had had a curettage performed 2 to 4 days prior to the hysterectomy. Several patients also had blood eosinophilia but it was not stated if the latter preceded or followed the curettage; one of the patients with peripheral eosinophilia also had a history of "allergic symptoms." In another study, Divack and Janovski found 25 cases of striking tissue eosinophilia in unselected gynecologic specimens that represented approximately 1 percent of their total number of specimens, and included eight cases of eosinophilic endomyometritis.[82] Only 8 of the 25 patients had undergone curettage or biopsy within the 6 months preceding hysterectomy.

The largest and most recent study of eosinophilic infiltrates within the uterine corpus was by Miko et al., who reviewed 2,619 hysterectomy specimens removed for noninflammatory and nonneoplastic disease[83]; all the patients had had a prior endometrial curettage performed. Patients known to

have any form of allergy, parasitic infestation, or significant blood eosinophilia were excluded from the study. Fifteen cases of severe eosinophilic endomyometritis and 93 cases with milder degrees of eosinophilic infiltration were found. In the severe cases, the curettage had antedated the hysterectomy by periods of 18 hours to 21 days (mean, 9 days). There were no clinical signs or symptoms that could be correlated with the eosinophilic endomyometritis. The distribution of the eosinophils was variable, but focally they formed dense aggregates within the endometrial stroma and myometrium; in the latter site, they were found within perivascular connective tissue and between the muscle bundles (Fig. 4-28). In some cases, the eosinophils extended as far as the parametrium. Occasional other inflammatory cells, especially lymphocytes, were admixed with the eosinophils. The degree of eosinophilic endomyometritis appeared to correlate with the extent of injury from the prior curettage, and in the severe cases, there was circumferential mucosal injury, myometrial damage, and an occluding blood clot at the internal os. It was suggested that the eosinophilic infiltrates were caused by the release of eosinophil chemotactic substances liberated from myometrial mast cells and from the degrading blood clot within the endometrial cavity.

The differential diagnosis of eosinophilic endomyometritis is with uterine involvement by hypereosinophilic syndrome and chronic myelogenous leukemia (CML) with a prominent component of eosinophils. The former disorder is characterized by striking degrees of blood eosinophilia and other systemic manifestations not found in cases of eosinophilic endomyometritis. The exclusively mature nature of the eosinophils with an absence of blast cells and other myeloid precursors, as well as an absence of the characteristic findings of CML in the marrow and peripheral blood, should render confusion between eosinophilic endomyometritis and CML unlikely.

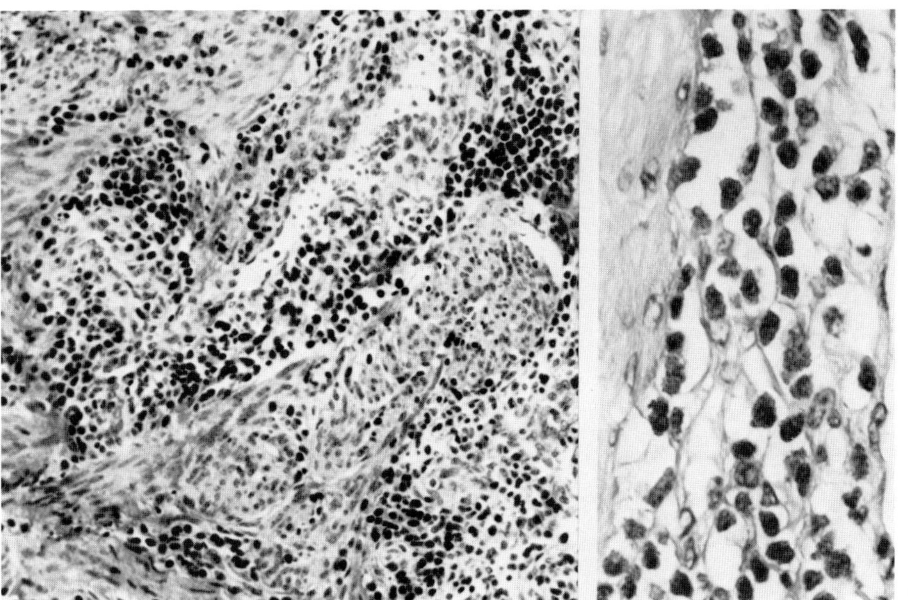

Fig. 4-28. Eosinophilic myometritis. **(A)** Numerous eosinophils are present between the smooth muscle bundles of the myometrium. **(B)** Mature eosinophils are seen at high-power magnification.

MAST CELL INFILTRATES

Crow et al. recently studied the distribution of mast cells in the female genital tract, including the endometrium and myometrium, using tissues from routine hysterectomy specimens fixed with basic lead acetate and stained with the Long toluidine-blue technique.[84] They found that small to moderate numbers of mast cells are present normally in the endometrium and myometrium and that occasionally their numbers could be striking. There was a clear trend for lower numbers of mast cells in both the endometrium and myometrium with advancing age, with a significant drop after the menopause. In none of the patients in their study was there any evidence of systemic manifestations or mastocytosis.

Within the endometrium, the highest counts were found within the stroma of endometrial polyps, especially those with a dense fibrous core (as many as 185/mm²) or in those containing areas of hyperplastic glands (114/mm²). In the myometrium and within leiomyomas, the mast cells were randomly distributed, and the range of counts in the myometrium varied from 8 to 128/mm². Although the density of mast cells in leiomyomas was generally lower than that within the rest of the myometrium, some leiomyomas contained as many as 87/mm², and one leiomyoma in a patient treated with luteinizing hormone-releasing hormone (LH-RM) analogue contained a massive 312/mm². Smaller leiomyomas tended to have higher counts than those of larger tumors. High endometrial and myometrial counts were also found in patients with an IUD in place or in patients who had had an IUD removed in the preceding few years.

INFLAMMATORY PSEUDOTUMOR

This lesion, which is considered reactive, has also been referred to as *plasma cell granuloma* and more recently, as *inflam-*

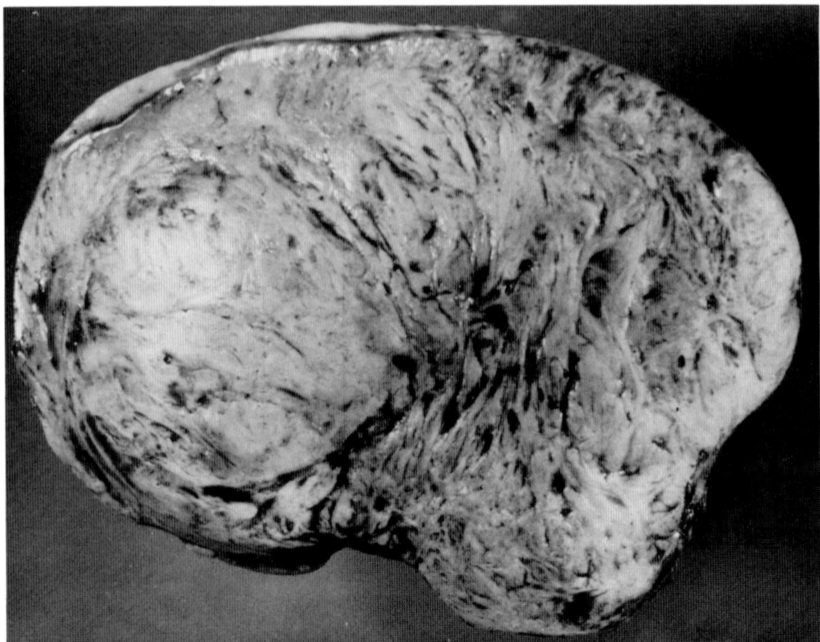

Fig. 4-29. Inflammatory pseudotumor of the uterus (sectioned surface). The whorled mass completely replaces the myometrium in this view. (From Gilks et al.,[86] with permission.)

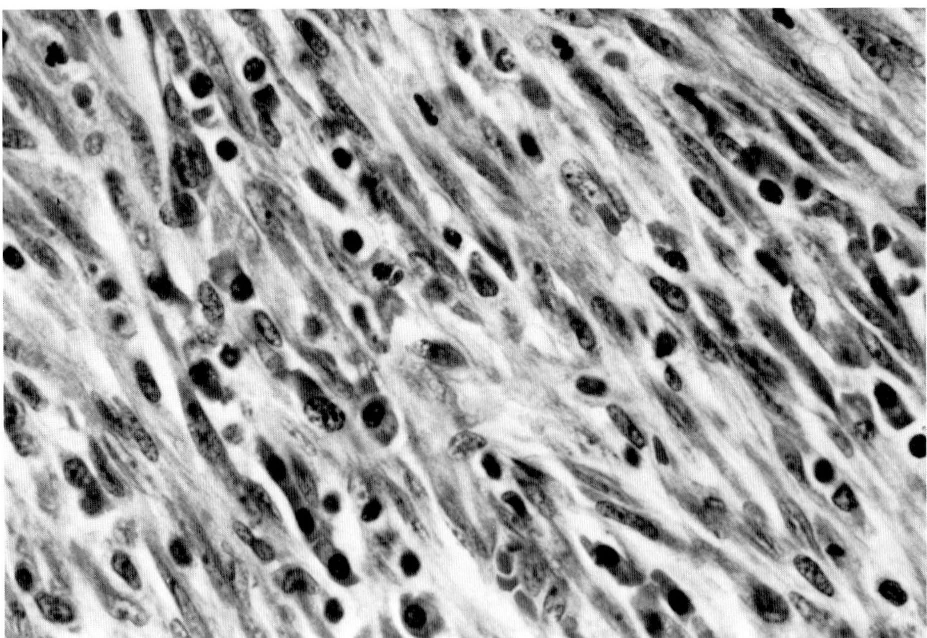

Fig. 4-30. Inflammatory pseudotumor of the uterus. Note admixture of benign-appearing spindle cells of myofibroblastic type, lymphocytes, and plasma cells. (From Gilks et al.,[86] with permission.)

matory myofibroblastic tumor[85]. It is most common in the lung, but has also been encountered in a variety of sites. Two typical examples involving the uterine corpus have been described.[86] In one of these cases, a 6-year-old girl presented with abdominal pain, distention, had a suprapubic mass on physical examination, and underwent hysterectomy. The other lesion was an incidental finding in a 30-year-old woman at the time of vaginal hysterectomy for uterine prolapse. In both cases, solitary, well circumscribed, leiomyoma-like masses, 12.5 and 4.5 cm in maximum diameter, focally replaced the myometrium (Fig. 4-29); in one case the process extended to the overlying endometrium. Microscopic examination revealed that the lesions were composed of an admixture of uniform, mitotically inactive spindle cells and a mixed inflammatory infiltrate rich in plasma cells (Fig. 4-30). The spindle cells were immunoreactive for actin and in one case exhibited the ultrastructural features of myofi-

broblasts. Both patients had uneventful follow-up intervals of approximately 5 years.

POSTOPERATIVE SPINDLE CELL NODULE

This characteristic reparative lesion, first described in 1984 by Proppe et al., is most common in the vagina, prostatic urethra, and urinary bladder[87]; only one example has been described in the endometrium.[88] A 75-year-old woman, who presented with postmenopausal bleeding, underwent an endometrial curettage; a well-differentiated endometrial adenocarcinoma was diagnosed on microscopic examination; $2\frac{1}{2}$ weeks later, a hysterectomy was performed. Within the endometrium and superficial myometrium was a 1.0-cm (at maximum dimension) lesion that consisted of a densely cellular proliferation of mitotically active spindle cells, small blood vessels,

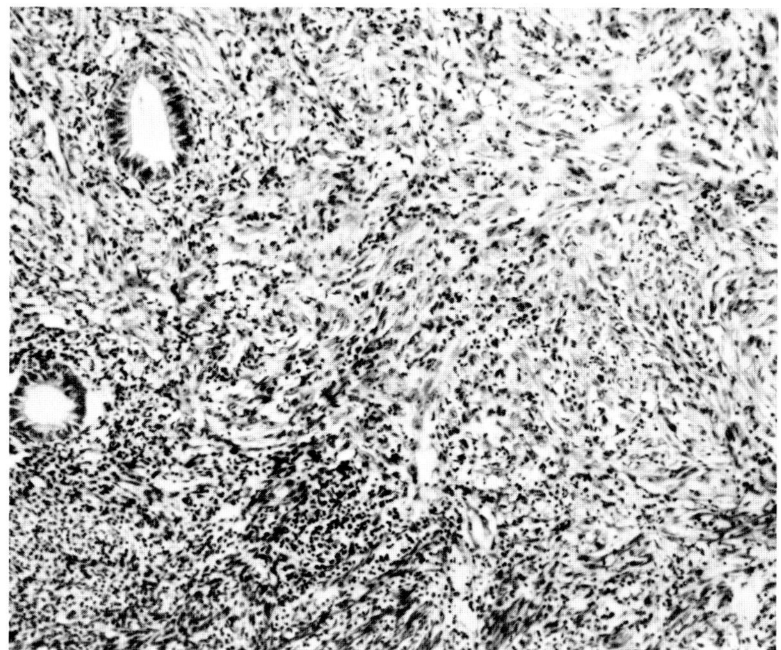

Fig. 4-31. Postoperative spindle-cell nodule of endometrium. The lesion partially surrounds two endometrial glands (left) and abuts the endometrial stroma (lower left).

and a sprinkling of inflammatory cells (Fig. 4-31). Although the lesion was initially misinterpreted as a sarcoma, its resemblance to previously described postoperative spindle cell nodules, including the history of a prior operation in the same site, its small size, and the lack of significant nuclear atypicality, indicated that it was reactive in nature. Because the lesional cells of a postoperative spindle cell nodule can be immunoreactive for cytokeratin, the lesion may also be misdiagnosed as a spindle cell carcinoma.[89]

VIRAL LESIONS

Human papilloma virus (HPV)[90, 91] herpes simplex virus (HSV),[92, 93] and cytomegalovirus (CMV),[94–97] the only viruses known to infect the endometrium,[65] may be associated with changes that could be interpreted as neoplastic or preneoplastic. Two cases of endometrial condyloma have been reported as either "diffuse viral papillomatosis" or "condylomatous atypia" of the endometrial cavity. In one case,[90] a 46-year-old woman, who underwent hysterectomy because of a 13-year history of cervical condyloma, had a thickened and gray-white endometrium. Histologic examination revealed that the entire endometrial cavity was lined by condyloma. In the other case,[91] a 46-year-old woman underwent hysterectomy for cervical condyloma and severe dysplasia. Macroscopic examination revealed that the entire endometrial cavity was thickened, white, and warty; the endometrial lesion had the typical appearance of condyloma acuminatum on microscopic examination (Fig. 4-32). As in other sites, endometrial condylomata should be distinguished from the rare verrucous carcinomas[98, 99] and other well-differentiated squamous carcinomas that may occur at this site (see Ch. 5), a differential that might be difficult on a small biopsy specimen. Features favoring the former diagnosis include premenopausal age, associated cervical condyloma, prominent koilocytosis, and prominent papillomatosis with central fibrovascular cores. The two endometrial verrucous carcinomas, in contrast, occurred in elderly women, lacked the

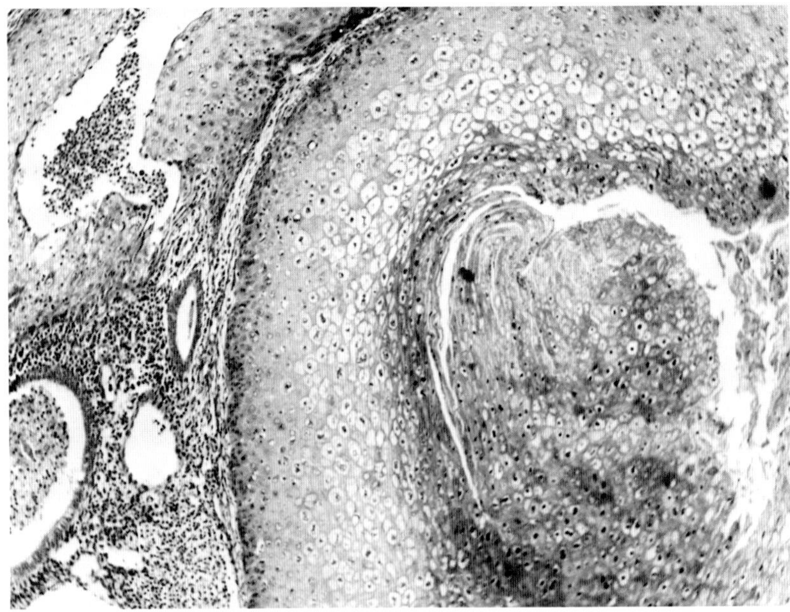

Fig. 4-32. Condyloma acuminatum of endometrium (residual endometrial glands are visible at extreme left). (Case courtesy of Dr. P. F. Roberts, Norwich, England.)

aforementioned features, exhibited prominent hyperkeratosis, and invaded the myometrium.

Herpetic endometritis is rare and is usually associated with herpetic cervicitis suggesting an ascending infection[92, 93]; some cases, however, have been found at autopsy in patients with disseminated infection. The typical histologic features, as in other sites, include extensive necrosis and acute inflammation, multinucleated giant cells, and ground-glass nuclei with intranuclear inclusions. Stromal, epithelial, and endothelial cells may be immunoreactive for HSV.[93] The differential diagnosis includes glands lined by optically clear nuclei, a pregnancy-related change (see p. 146).

Although CMV infection is relatively common in pregnant women and their infants, and may be a significant cause of fetal mortality and morbidity,[100] CMV endometritis is only rarely encountered on microscopic examination.[94–96] As has been noted in the endocervix (see Ch. 1), the characteristic intranuclear inclusion bodies in occasional cells lining otherwise benign endometrial glands should render confusion with atypical hyperplasia or adenocarcinoma unlikely. The surrounding endometrial stroma may contain prominent numbers of lymphocytes, lymphoid follicles with germinal centers, and plasma cells. In one recently described case of a 32-year-old woman with histologically diagnosed CMV cervicitis, there was an associated granulomatous endometritis but no other findings to suggest CMV endometritis.[97] CMV, however, was identified by polymerase chain reaction in DNA extracted from a paraffin section.

POSTCURETTAGE REPARATIVE CHANGES

Regenerative and reparative endometrial changes within uteri removed shortly after a dilation and curettage (D&C) should not be confused with a cancerous or precancer-

ous lesion. Such changes are characterized by epithelial atypia, which may be striking, typically confined to the surface epithelium and superficial glands, and include focal nuclear enlargement, hyperchromasia, and prominent nucleoli; some of the cells may have a hobnail appearance (Figs. 4-33 and 4-34). Papillary syncytial metaplasia (Figs. 4-8 and 4-9) may also represent a postcurettage reparative response. Awareness of a recent curettage, the superfical location of the changes, an absence of significant architectural changes in the underlying glands, and in some cases, inflammatory changes in the stroma, will facilitate the diagnosis.

RADIATION-INDUCED CHANGES

Radiation-induced changes in the uterine corpus are similar to those occurring elsewhere, including the cervix[101] (see Ch. 1). Adenomyotic glands may also exhibit radiation-induced atypia.[102] Awareness of the history, combined with the typical histological findings, should facilitate distinction from preneoplastic or neoplastic changes. In this differential, it is noteworthy that Silverberg and DeGiorgi found that the microscopic appearance of endometrial carcinomas is typically not altered, or altered to only a minimal degree, by radiotherapy.[102] They concluded that in postradiation hysterectomy specimens, glands lined by cells with bizarre nuclear features were almost always benign.[102]

Mazur and Kraus studied the microscopic and ultrastructural features of the myometrium from two hysterectomy specimen removed approximately 6 weeks after intracavitary radiation for endometrial cancer.[103] In these cases, enlarged cells with granular or foamy vacuolated cytoplasm were scattered singly or in small groups among the relatively normal appearing smooth muscle of the inner 5 mm of the myometrium. Their close association with intact smooth muscle cells and their ultrastructural features suggested that these

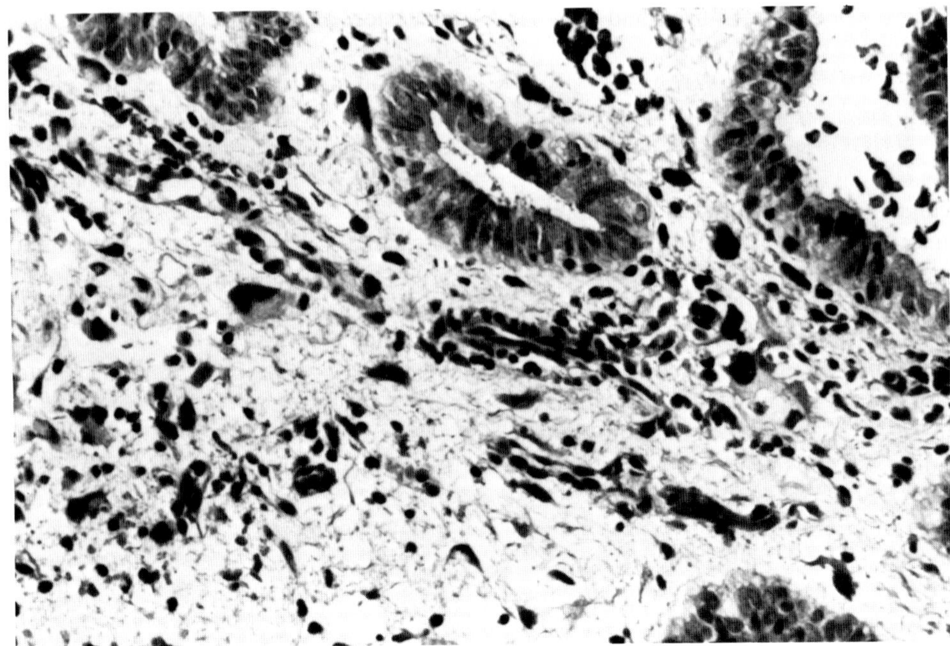

Fig. 4-36. Stromal cells with atypical hyperchromatic nuclei within an endometrial polyp that was otherwise typical. Some of the nuclei are multilobed or multinucleated.

nomas of usual[108] and unusual (serous, clear cell) types,[109, 110] and malignant müllerian mixed tumors (see Ch. 7). Several recent reports have found an association between chronic tamoxifen therapy and endometrial polyps.[111–113] In such cases, the polyps have typically contained foci of endometrial hyperplasia (Fig. 4-35) or even adenocarcinoma; in two cases, there were also foci of stromal decidual cells within the polyp.[112]

A rare pseudoneoplastic endometrial lesion that we have seen in otherwise typical endometrial polyps but not elsewhere in the endometrium is the presence of atypical, frequently multinucleated stromal giant cells (Fig. 4-36). These benign cells are identical to their more common counterparts occurring in fibroepithelial polyps of the lower female genital tract, including the cervix (see Ch. 1). Endometrial polyps with atypical stromal giant cells should not be misinterpreted as müllerian adenosarcoma, which in contrast, are characterized by marked, typically periglandular, stromal

cellularity and stromal mitotic figures (see Ch. 7).

ADENOMYOSIS AND TYPICAL ADENOMYOMAS

Adenomyosis is a common disorder that may cause tumorlike enlargement of the uterus on clinical examination. Gross examination in such cases typically reveals a focally or diffusely thickened, trabeculated myometrium (Fig. 4-37). Blood-filled cysts, usually less than 0.5 cm in diameter but occasionally larger,[114] may occasionally be grossly visible within the lesions. When the process forms a discrete, leiomyoma-like mural mass, the designation adenomyoma is used and when a polypoid mass projects into the endometrial cavity, the lesion is referred to as a polypoid adenomyoma (Figs. 4-38 and 4-39). Whether these adenomyomas represent circumscribed adenomyosis or benign mixed neoplasms is not clear.

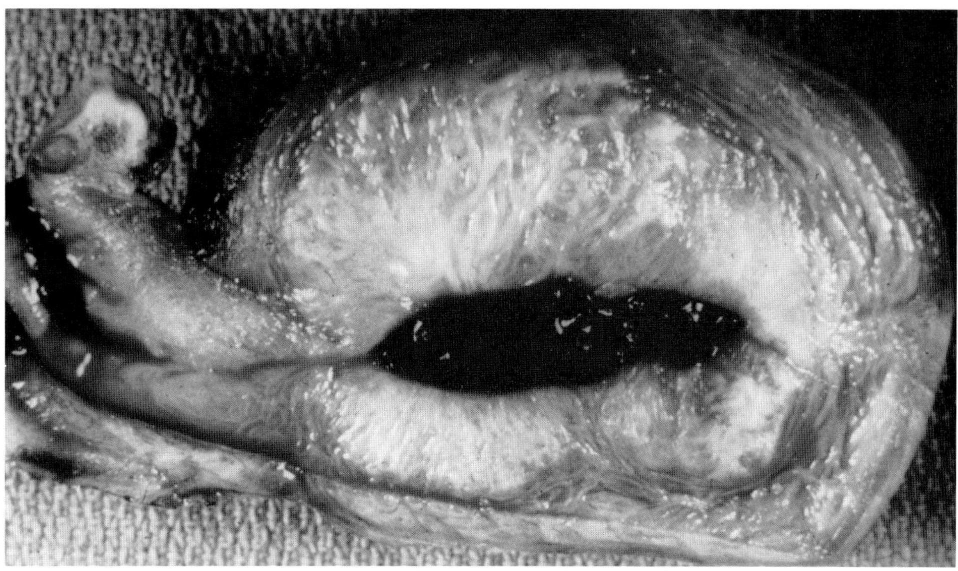

Fig. 4-37. Adenomyosis, sectioned surface. Note the thickened and trabeculated myometrium.

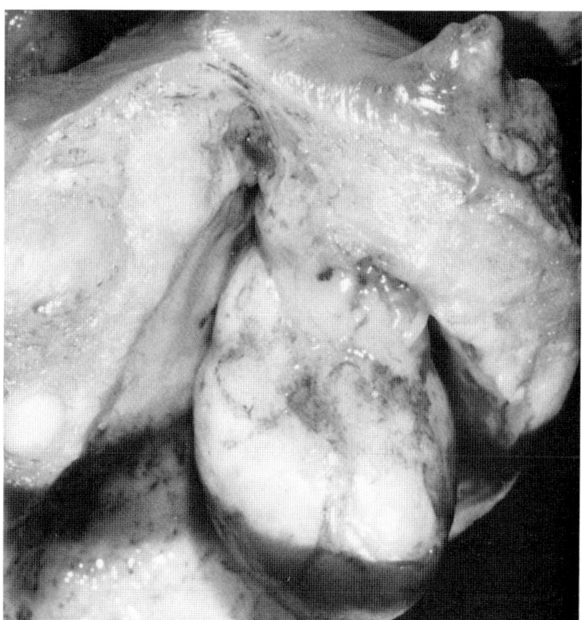

Fig. 4-38. Polypoid adenomyoma.

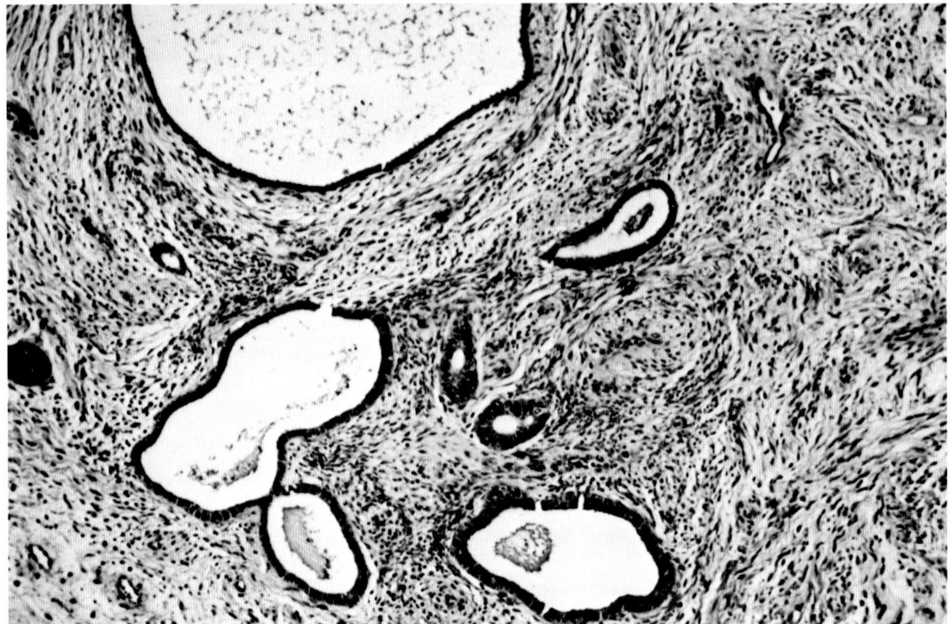

Fig. 4-39. Polypoid adenomyoma, microscopic appearance of the lesion in Figure 4-38. Well-separated benign-appearing endometrial glands are separated by smooth muscle.

Polypoid adenomyomas usually resemble typical adenomyosis microscopically (Fig. 4-39), but when they have atypical histologic features, including an atypical glandular component, the designation *atypical polypoid adenomyoma* is used (see Ch. 7). A polypoid adenomyoma that was cystic[115] and another with mature adipose tissue within its stroma (*adenomyolipoma*) have been recently reported.[116]

The usual, admittedly arbitrary, criterion for the diagnosis of adenomyosis is the presence of endometrial tissue within the myometrium at least one ×100 microscopic field below the endomyometrial junction. The adenomyotic foci typically consist of endometrial glands and stroma, surrounded by hyperplastic myometrium. In cases in which the eutopic endometrial glands are hyperplastic or carcinomatous, the latter processes may also involve or replace the adenomyotic glands (see Ch. 5).

In occasional otherwise typical cases of adenomyosis, especially in postmenopausal women, the glandular or the stromal component may be focally inconspicuous or absent (Figs. 4-40 and 4-41). In the former circumstance, the appearance should not be misinterpreted as a low-grade endometrial stromal sarcoma (Fig. 4-40). Conversely, when the stromal component is atrophic, glands deep within the myometrium are surrounded directly by hyperplastic smooth muscle (Fig. 4-41), a finding that should not be misinterpreted as invasive adenocarcinoma. The atrophic appearance of the adenomyotic stroma or glands, the lack of mitotic activity, the association with more typical adenomyosis elsewhere in the myometrium, and the lack of an endometrial neoplasm facilitate the diagnosis.

Another pseudoneoplastic finding in otherwise typical adenomyosis is intravascular endometrium (Figs. 4-42 and 4-43). Sahin et al.[117] recently demonstrated the latter in 5 percent of hysterectomy specimens from nonmenstruating women, all of whom had adenomyosis; approximately 18 percent of women with adenomyosis had intravascular endometrium. The adenomyosis in such

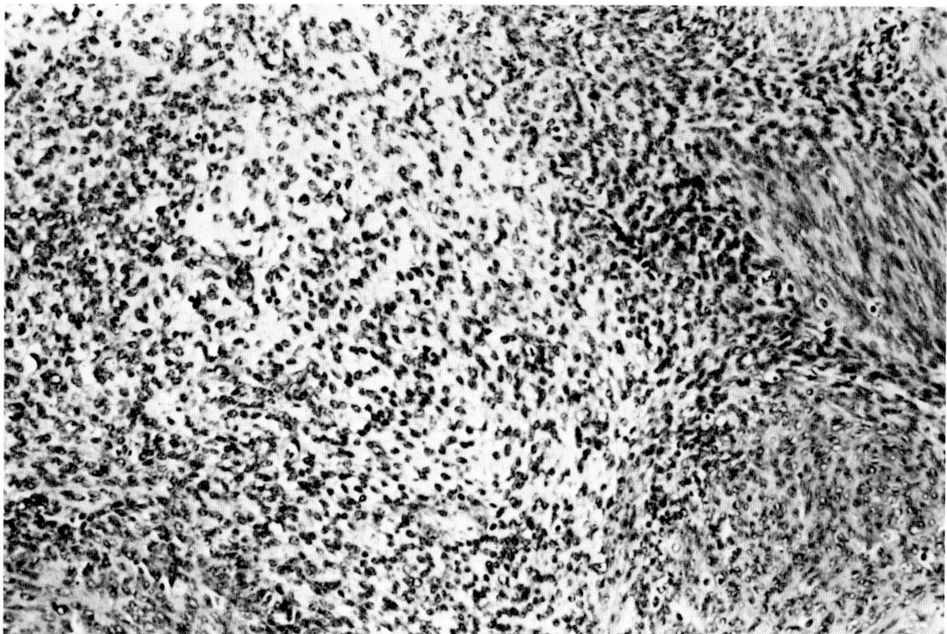

Fig. 4-40. Focus of adenomyosis consisting only of endometrial stroma.

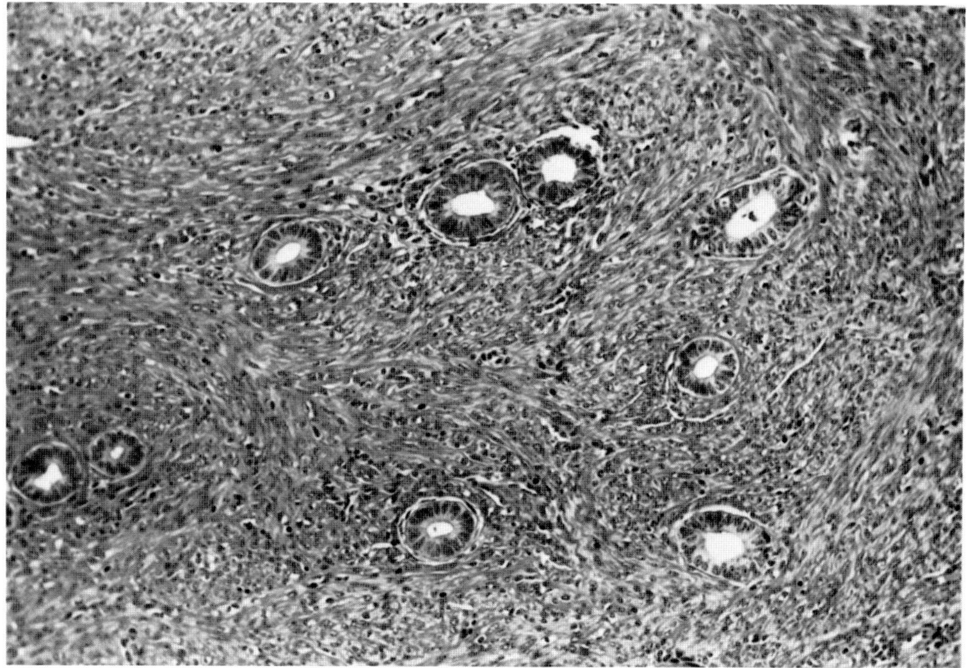

Fig. 4-41. Focus of adenomyosis within the myometrium consisting only of glands in an elderly patient. The stromal component has atrophied. Typical adenomyosis was present in adjacent fields.

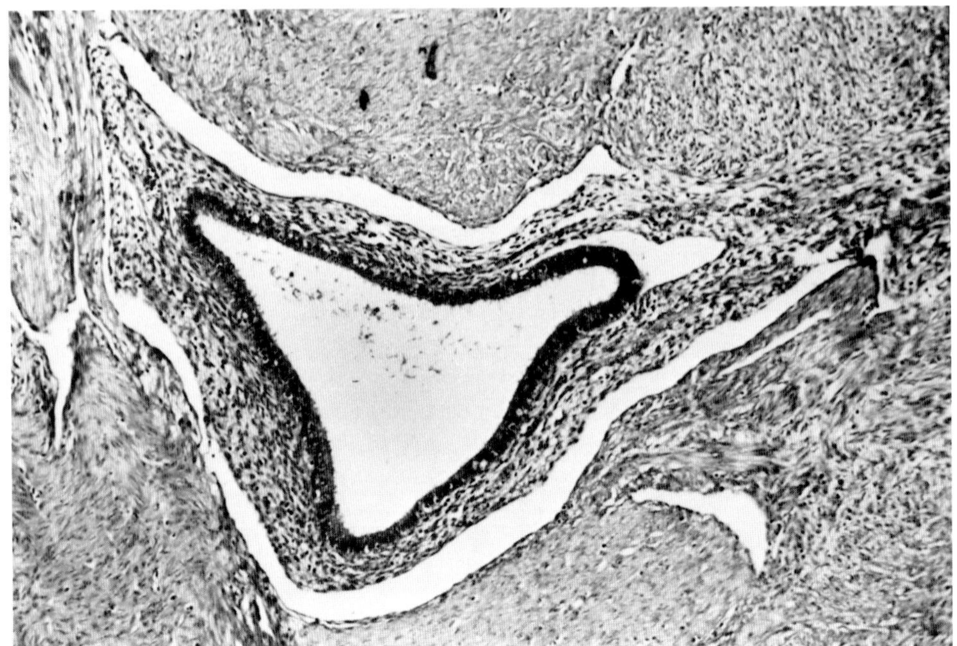

Fig. 4-42. Intravascular endometrium (gland and stroma) within the myometrium in a patient with adenomyosis.

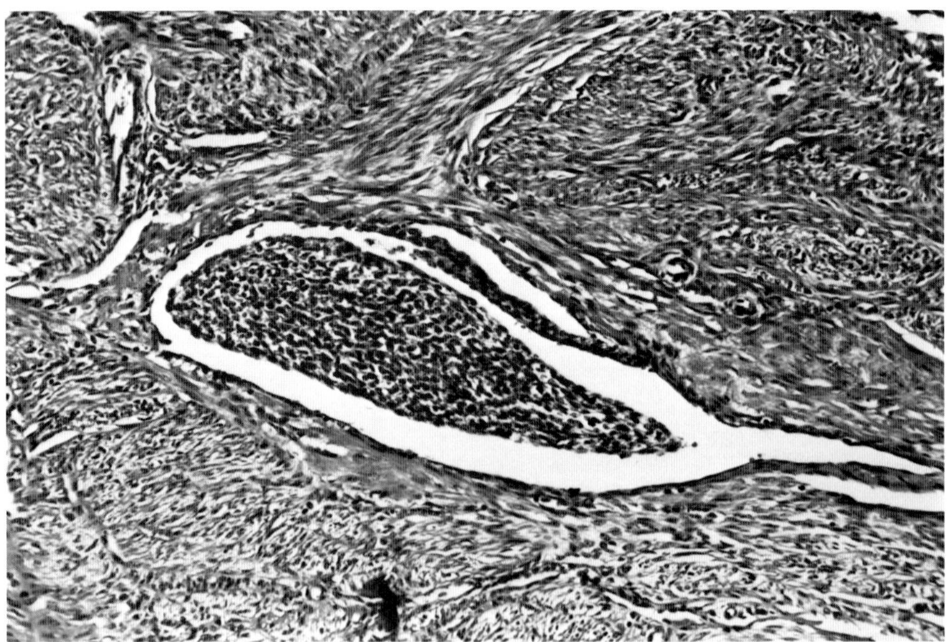

Fig. 4-43. Intravascular endometrial stroma within the myometrium in patient with adenomyosis.

cases was extensive and usually present in multiple foci. In eight of the 14 cases with intravascular endometrium, the latter was composed of endometrial stroma only (Fig. 4-43); in the remaining cases, both glands and stroma were present (Fig. 4-42). In 9 cases, the vessels containing endometrial tissue were closely associated with the foci of adenomyosis, whereas in the other 5 cases, the involved vessels were at a distance from the adenomyosis. The number of vessels containing endometrium averaged two per section, with a range of one to four. In the majority of cases, the myometrial vessels containing endometrium were thin-walled, and varied from slitlike to dilated. The authors of this report speculated that the observed findings were due to perivascular adenomyotic tissue that proliferates and protrudes into vascular spaces, eventually becoming ensheathed by endothelial cells. This finding appears to have no clinical significance other than providing a potential explanation for endometriosis in distant sites.

MYOMETRIAL HYPERTROPHY

Idiopathic or primary myometrial hypertrophy is a rarely diagnosed lesion that has been arbitrarily defined as a uterine weight of more than 120 g in the absence of any other myometrial lesion.[118] The frequency of this finding was 5.7 percent in one series of 1,000 consecutive hysterectomy specimens.[118] The uterus is typically only moderately enlarged, with the heaviest uterus in the aforementioned series weighing 230 g. Gross examination typically reveals a symmetrically enlarged uterus with a diffusely thickened myometrium potentially mimicking adenomyosis; the micronodularity of diffuse leiomyomatosis (see Ch. 6) is absent. On histologic examination, the myometrium appears normal but the smooth muscle fibers are hypertrophied as evidenced by a decrease in the number of muscle fibers within an arbitrarily defined unit area.[118] In the study by Lewis et al., uteri weighing more than 120 g had an average of 83 fibers per unit in contrast to 121 fibers per unit in the group weighing less than 120 g. In the same study, there was no evident difference between the two groups in the amount of fibrous tissue present. The finding of myometrial hypertrophy is of uncertain clinical significance, although 74 percent of patients in the above series complained of excessive menstrual bleeding.[118]

CYSTS

Excluding adenomyotic cysts (see above), cystic neoplasms (adenomatoid tumor, lymphangioma; see Ch. 8), and cystic degeneration of uterine neoplasms (most commonly leiomyomas; see Ch. 6), myometrial cysts are rare. Most of them are congenital in origin.[119–121] Women with congenital cysts are typically of reproductive age and usually present with symptoms relating to uterine enlargement; some of the cysts have enlarged the uterus to the size of a term pregnancy. The cysts are typically unilocular and filled with clear to amber fluid, and surrounded by myometrium. The majority are of müllerian type, and these are usually located in the midline of the anterior or posterior uterine wall. The lining is usually composed of a single layer of columnar cells that may also line intracystic papillae with fibrous cores. The epithelium is most commonly ciliated (tubal-like), less commonly, it is endometrial or endocervical in appearance. There may be an underlying connective tissue layer, but the endometrial stroma of an adenomyotic cyst is absent. Myometrial cysts of mesonephric origin are situated in the lateral walls of the corpus (usually below the insertion of the round ligaments) or cervix. They are lined by mucin-free, typically nonciliated, columnar or cuboidal epithelium resembling that of mesonephric cysts elsewhere in the female genital tract, such as Gartner's cyst in the vagina. Rare primary echinococcal cysts of the uterus have been reported.[122] Uterine cysts of tubal origin are discussed below.

CALCIFICATION, LITHIASIS, AND PIGMENTATION

Although uterine calcification is most commonly associated with a neoplasm (dystrophic calcification in leiomyomas, psammoma bodies in papillary serous carcinomas), endometrial calcification occasionally occurs in the absence of a tumor, such as in association with heterotopic bone (page 150), chronic endometritis, an IUD,[123] and intrauterine adhesions (Asherman's syndrome).[124] In addition, two cases of psammomatous endometrial calcification associated with the use of exogenous hormones have been reported.[125, 126] In one case , a 46-year-old woman taking combination oral contraceptives was found to have psammoma bodies on a routine cervicovaginal smear, and a subsequent endometrial biopsy revealed psammoma bodies in the glandular lumina and stroma.[125] In the other case, a 28-year-old woman, who had a history of oral contraceptive use and clomiphene treatment, underwent an endometrial curettage.[126] Psammoma bodies were found in the endometrial stroma and glands, and a similar finding was present in a specimen obtained by a repeated curettage performed 5 months later.

Alpert et al. have recently reported a unique case of uterine lithiasis in a 73-year-old woman who underwent vaginal hysterectomy for prolapse.[127] The endometrial cavity contained ten white, starlike calcified structures that each measured 0.5 cm in maximum dimension. Chemical analysis showed the concretions to be composed of calcite, a crystalline form of calcium carbonate.

Siboni et al.[128] reported a unique case of

striking dark brown pigmentation of the myometrium in a 37-year-old woman with Friedrich's ataxia and the brown bowel syndrome. On microscopic examination, large numbers of brown granules were seen in the cytoplasm of smooth muscle cells of the myometrium, the stromal cells of the basal endometrium, and macrophages. Special stains confirmed the pigment to be lipofuschin.

LESIONS OF TUBAL ORIGIN

Occasionally, disorders of the fallopian tube may present as tumorlike lesions of the uterine corpus. In one case, massive hydrosalpinx of the intrauterine portion of the tube created a myometrial cyst that contained 750 ml of clear watery fluid.[129] Two examples of a fallopian tube prolapsing through a defect in the fundal myometrium have been reported.[130, 131] In one case, an intrauterine polypoid mass was found,[131] whereas in the other, continued prolapse of the tube through the cervix resulted in an intravaginal mass.[130]

PERITONEAL LESIONS

Although beyond the scope of this review, it should be remembered that tumorlike lesions of the pelvic peritoneum may involve the uterine serosa, and less commonly, the subserosal myometrium. These lesions, including mesothelial hyperplasia, endosalpingiosis, and peritoneal inclusion cysts, have recently been discussed elsewhere.[132,133]

REFERENCES

1. Hendrickson MR, Kempson RL: Endometrial epithelial metaplasias: proliferations frequently misdiagnosed as adenocarcinoma. Report of 89 cases and proposed

classification. Am J Surg Pathol 4:525, 1980

2. Hendrickson MR, Kempson RL: The differential diagnosis of endometrial adenocarcinoma. Some viewpoints concerning a common diagnostic problem. Pathology 12:35, 1980

3. Andersen WA, Taylor PT, Jr, Fechner RE, Pinkerton JV: Endometrial metaplasia associated with endometrial adenocarcinoma. Am J Obstet Gynecol 157:597, 1987

4. Baggish MS, Woodruff JD: The occurrence of squamous epithelium in the endometrium. Obstet Gynecol Surv 22:69, 1967

5. Crum CP, Richart RM, Fenoglio CM: Adenoacanthosis of the endometrium. A clinicopathologic study in premenopausal women. Am J Surg Pathol 5:15-20, 1981

6. Blaustein A: Morular metaplasia misdiagnosed as adenoacanthoma in young women with polycystic ovarian disease. Am J Surg Pathol 6:223, 1982

7. Demopoulos RI, Greco MA: Mucinous metaplasia of the endometrium: ultrastructural and histochemical characteristics. Int J Gynecol Pathol 1:383, 1983

8. Wells M, Tiltman A: Intestinal metaplasia of the endometrium. Histopathology 15:431, 1989

9. Honore LH: Benign obstructive myxometra: report of a case. Am J Obstet Gynecol 133:227, 1979

10. Baird DB, Reddick RL: Extraovarian mucinous metaplasia in a patient with bilateral mucinous borderline ovarian tumors: a case report. Int J Gynecol Pathol 10:96, 1991

11. Bergeron C, Ferenczy A: Oncocytic metaplasia in endometrial hyperplasia and carcinoma. Int J Gynecol Pathol 7:93, 1988

12. Rorat E, Wallach RC: Papillary metaplasia of the endometrium: clinical and histopathologic considerations. Obstet Gynecol 64:90S, 1984

13. Arias-Stella J: Atypical endometrial changes associated with the presence of chorionic tissue. Arch Pathol Lab Med 58:112, 1954

14. Arias-Stella J: A topographic study of uterine epithelial atypia associated with chorionic tissue: demonstration of alteration in the endocervix. Cancer 12:782, 1959

15. Clement PB, Young RH, Scully RE: Nontrophoblastic pathology of the female genital tract and peritoneum associated with pregnancy. Semin Diagn Pathol 6:372, 1989

16. Birch HW, Collins CG: Atypical changes of genital epithelium associated with ectopic pregnancy. Am J Obstet Gynecol 81:1198, 1961

17. Moller NE: The Arias-Stella phenomenon in endometriosis. Acta Obstet Gynecol Scand 38:271, 1959

18. Milchgrub S, Sandstad J: Arias-Stella reaction in fallopian tube epithelium. Am J Clin Pathol 95:892, 1991

19. Sedlis A, Robboy SJ: Diseases of the vagina. p. 97. In Kurman RJ (ed): Blaustein's Pathology of the Female Genital Tract. 3rd Ed. Springer-Verlag, New York, 1987

20. Mazur MT, Hendrickson MR, Kempson RL: Optically clear nuclei. An alteration of endometrial epithelium in the presence of trophoblast. Am J Surg Pathol 7:415, 1983

21. Dockerty MB, Smith RA, Symmonds RE: Pseudomalignant endometrial changes induced by administration of new synthetic progestins. Mayo Clin Proc 34:321, 1959

22. Cruz-Aquino M, Shenker L, Blaustein A: Pseudosarcoma of the endometrium. Obstet Gynecol 29:93, 1967

23. Reinhart HL: Diffuse decidual hyperplasia of the endometrium in the absence of pregnancy. Am J Clin Pathol 5:365, 1935

24. Te Linde RW, Henriksen E: Decidualike changes in the endometrium without pregnancy. Am J Obstet Gynecol 39:733, 1940

25. Clement PB, Scully RE: Idiopathic postmenopausal decidual reaction of the endometrium: a clinicopathologic analysis of four cases. Int J Gynecol Pathol 7:152, 1988

26. Ganem KJ, Parsons L, Friedell GH: Endometrial ossification. Am J Obstet Gynecol 83:1592, 1962

27. Courpas AS, Morris JD, Woodruff JD: Osteoid tissue in utero. Report of 3 cases. Obstet Gynecol 24:636, 1964

28. Roth E, Taylor HB: Heterotopic cartilage in the uterus. Obstet Gynecol 27:838, 1966

29. Newton CW III, Abell MR: Iatrogenic fetal implants. Obstet Gynecol 40:686, 1972

30. Hsu C: Endometrial ossification. Br J Obstet Gynaecol 82:836, 1975

31. Dutt S: Endometrial ossification associated with secondary infertility. Br J Obstet Gynaecol 85:787, 1978

32. Waxman M, Moussouris HF: Endometrial ossification following an abortion. Am J Obstet Gynecol 130:587, 1978

33. Zettergren L: Glial tissue in the uterus. Am J Pathol 71:419, 1983

34. Slavutin L: Uterine gliosis and ossification. Am J Diagn Obstet Gynecol 1:351, 1979

35. Tyagi SP, Saxena K, Rizvi R, Langley FA: Foetal remnants in the uterus and their relation to other uterine heterotopia. Histopathology 3:339, 1979

36. Roca AN, Guajardo M, Estrada WJ: Glial polyp of the cervix and endometrium: report of a case and review of the literature. Am J Clin Pathol 73:718, 1980

37. Ceccacci L, Clancy G: Endometrial ossification: Report of an additional case. Am J Obstet Gynecol 141:103, 1981

38. Bhatia NN, Hoshiko MG: Uterine osseous metaplasia. Obstet Gynecol 60:256, 1982

39. Chervenak FA, Amin HK, Neuwirth RS: Symptomatic intrauterine retention of fetal bones. Obstet Gynecol 59:58S, 1982

40. Dawood YM, Jarrett JC III: Prolonged intrauterine retention of fetal bones after abortion causing infertility. Am J Obstet Gynecol 143:715, 1982

41. Degani S, Gonen R, de Vries K, Sharf M: Endometrial ossification associated with repeated abortions. Acta Obstet Gynecol Scand 62:281, 1983

42. Gronroos M, Meurman L, Kahra K: Proliferating glia and other heterotopic tissues in the uterus: fetal homografts? Obstet Gynecol 61:261, 1983

43. Taylor RN, Welch KL, Sklar DM et al: Heterotopic skin in the uterus: a report of an unusual case. J Reprod Med 29:837, 1984

44. Dajani YF, Khalaf SM: Intrauterine bone contraceptive device: an accident of nature. Fertil Steril 43:149, 1985

45. Luevano-Flores E, Sotelo J, Tena-Suck M: Glial polyp (glioma) of the uterine cervix. Report of a case with demonstration of glial fibrillary acidic protein. Gynecol Oncol 21:385, 1985

46. Brown LJR, Wells M: Heterotopic adipose and glial tissue in the endometrium with staining for glial fibrillary acidic protein. Case report. Br J Obstet Gynaecol 93:637, 1986

47. Igerslev HJ, Kristensen IB: Fetal tibia retained in uterine cavity for eight years after legal abortion. Acta Obstet Gynecol Scand 65:371, 1986

48. Ombelet W: Endometrial ossification, an unusual finding in an infertility clinic. A case report. J Reprod Med 34:303, 1989

49. Lewis V, Khan-Dawood F, King M et al: Retention of intrauterine fetal bone increases menstrual prostaglandins. Obstet Gynecol 75:561, 1990

50. Melius FA, Julian TM, Nagel TC: Prolonged retention of fetal bones. Obstet Gynecol 78:919, 1991

51. Hendrickson MR, Kempson RL: Non-neoplastic metaplasias—epithelial and mesenchymal musical chairs. p. 211. In Surgical Pathology of the Uterine Corpus. WB Saunders, Philadelphia, 1980

52. Nogales FF, Pavcovich M, Medina MT, Palomino M: Fatty change in the endometrium. Histopathology 20:362, 1992

53. Scully RE: Smooth-muscle differentiation in genital tract disorders. Arch Pathol Lab Med 105:505, 1981

54. Saltzman R, Miranda P, Jerez E: Fetal parts embolization during termination of pregnancy: report of a case. Hum Pathol 21:117, 1990

55. Armin A, Moradi A, Winters G: Posttraumatic intrauterine omental implantation mimicking lipomatous lesion 16 years later. Int J Gynecol Pathol 6:89, 1987

56. Picoff RC, Luginbuhl WH: The significance of foci of dense stromal cellularity in the endometrium. Am J Obstet Gynecol 94:820, 1966

57. Sampson JA: Metastatic or embolic endometriosis, due to the menstrual dissemination of endometrial tissue into the venous circulation. Am J Pathol 3:93, 1927

58. Banks ER, Mills SE, Frierson HF, Jr: Uterine intravascular menstrual endometrium simulating malignancy. Am J Surg Pathol 15:407, 1991

59. Winkler B, Gallo L, Reumann W et al: Chlamydial endometritis: a histological and immunohistochemical analysis. Am J Surg Pathol 8:771, 1984

60. Kiviat NB, Wolner-Hanssen P, Eschenbach DA et al: Endometrial histopathology in patients with culture-proven upper genital tract infection and laparoscopically diagnosed acute salpingitis. Am J Surg Pathol 14:167, 1990

61. Ismail SM: Follicular myometritis: a previously undescribed component of pelvic inflammatory disease. Histopathology 16:91, 1990

62. Payan H, Daino J, Kish M: Lymphoid follicles in endometrium. Obstet Gynecol 23:570, 1964

63. Young RH, Harris NL, Scully RE: Lymphoma-like lesions of the lower female genital tract: a report of 16 cases. Int J Gynecol Pathol 4:289, 1985

64. Ferry JA, Harris NL, Scully RE: Uterine leiomyomas with lymphoid infiltration simulating lymphoma. A report of seven cases. Int J Gynecol Pathol 8:263, 1989

65. Kurman RJ, Mazur MT: Benign diseases of the endometrium. p. 292. In Kurman RJ (ed): Blaustein's Pathology of the Female Genital Tract. 3rd Ed. Springer-Verlag, New York, 1987

66. Ashworth MT, Moss CI, Kenyon WE: Granulomatous endometritis following hysteroscopic resection of the endometrium. Histopathology 18:185, 1991

67. Thurrell W, Reid P, Kennedy A, Smith JHF: Necrotizing granulomas of the peritoneum (Letter). Histopathology 18:190, 1991

68. Clark IW: Necrotizing granulomatous inflammation of the uterine body following diathermy ablation of the endometrium. Pathology 24:32, 1992

69. Ladefoged C, Lorentzen M: Xanthogranulomatous inflammation of the female genital tract. Histopathology 13:541, 1988

70. Russack V, Lammers RJ: Xanthogranulomatous endometritis: report of six cases and a proposed mechanism for development. Arch Pathol Lab Med 114:929, 1990

71. Shintaku M, Sasaki M, Baba Y: Ceroid-containing histiocytic granuloma of the endometrium. Histopathology 18:169, 1991

72. Buckley CH, Fox H: Histiocytic endometritis. Histopathology 4:105, 1980

73. Budny NN: Pyometra with massive foam cell reaction: a case report. Am J Obstet Gynecol 112:126, 1972

74. Rao NR: Malacoplakia of broad ligament, inguinal region, and endometrium. Arch Pathol 88:85, 1969

75. Thomas W, Jr, Sadeghieh B, Fresco R et al: Malacoplakia of the endometrium, a probable cause of postmenopausal bleeding. Am J Clin Pathol 69:637, 1978

76. Molnar JJ, Poliak A: Recurrent endometrial malakoplakia. Am J Clin Pathol 80:762, 1983

77. Willen R, Stendahl U, Willen H, Trope C: Malacoplakia of the cervix and corpus uteri: a light microscopic, electron microscopic, and X-Ray microprobe analysis of a case. Int J Gynecol Pathol 2:201, 1983

78. Tesluk H, Munn RJ: Malacoplakia of the uterus (letter). Arch Pathol Lab Med 108:692, 1984

79. Chadha S, Vuzevski VD, ten Kate FJW: Malakoplakia of the endometrium: a rare cause of postmenopausal bleeding. Eur J Obstet Gynecol Reprod Biol 20:181, 1985

80. Kawai K, Fukuda K, Tsuchiyama H: Malacoplakia of the endometrium: An unusual case studied by electron microscopy and a review of the literature. Acta Pathol Jpn 38:531, 1988

81. Bjersing L, Borglin NA: Eosinophilia in the myometrium of the human uterus. Acta Pathol Microbiol Scand 54:353, 1962

82. Divack DM, Janovski NA: Eosinophilia encountered in female genital organs. Am J Obstet Gynecol 84:761, 1962

83. Miko TL, Lampe LG, Thomazy VA et al: Eosinophilic endomyometritis associated with diagnostic curettage. Int J Gynecol Pathol 7:162, 1988

84. Crow J, Wilkins M, Howe S et al: Mast cells in the female genital tract. Int J Gynecol Pathol 10:230, 1991

85. Pettinato G, Manivel C, De Rosa N, Dehner LP: Inflammatory myofibroblastic tumor (plasma cell granuloma). Clinicopathologic study of 20 cases with immunohistochemical and ultrastructural observations. Am J Clin Pathol 94:538, 1990

86. Gilks CB, Taylor GP, Clement PB: Inflammatory pseudotumor of the uterus. Int J Gynecol Pathol 6:275, 1987

87. Proppe KH, Scully RE, Rosai J: Postoper-

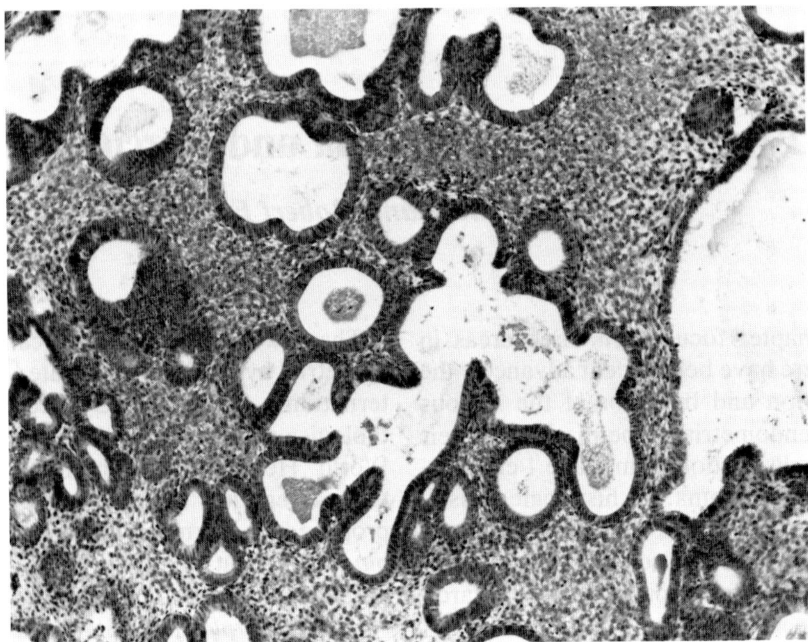

Fig. 5-1. Simple hyperplasia (mild "adenomatous hyperplasia") (mild architectural atypicality).

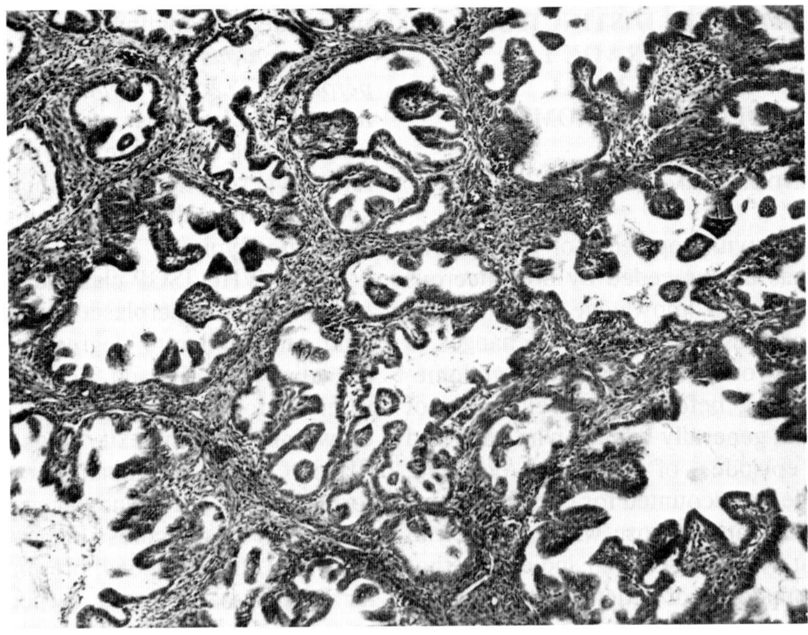

Fig. 5-2. Simple hyperplasia (moderate architectural atypicality with intraluminal papillae).

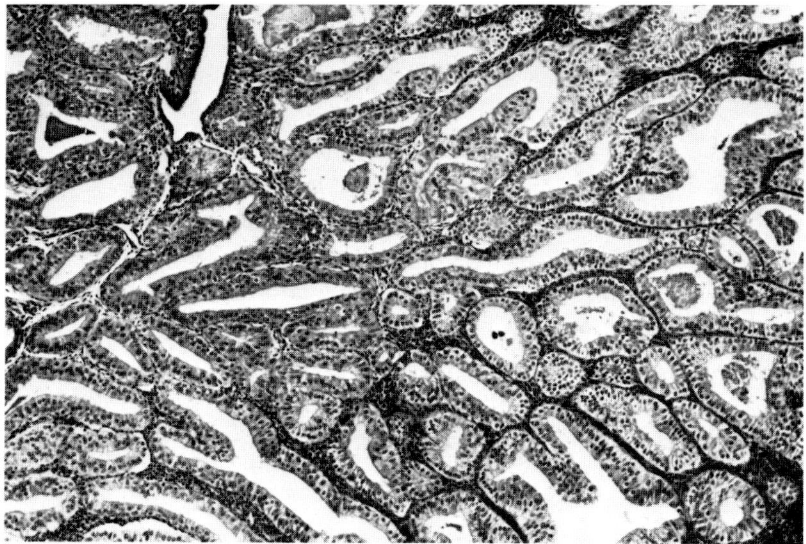

Fig. 5-3. Complex hyperplasia.

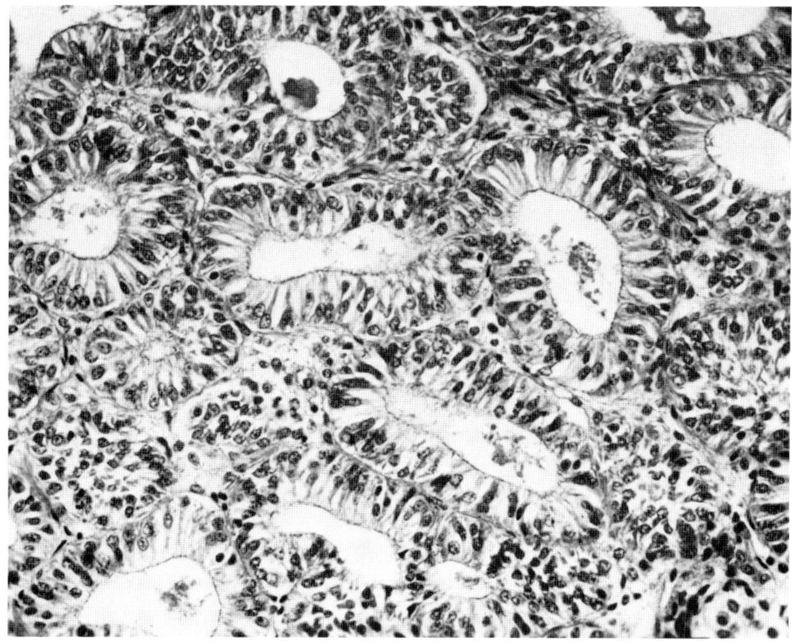

Fig. 5-4. Complex hyperplasia with moderate cytologic atypia.

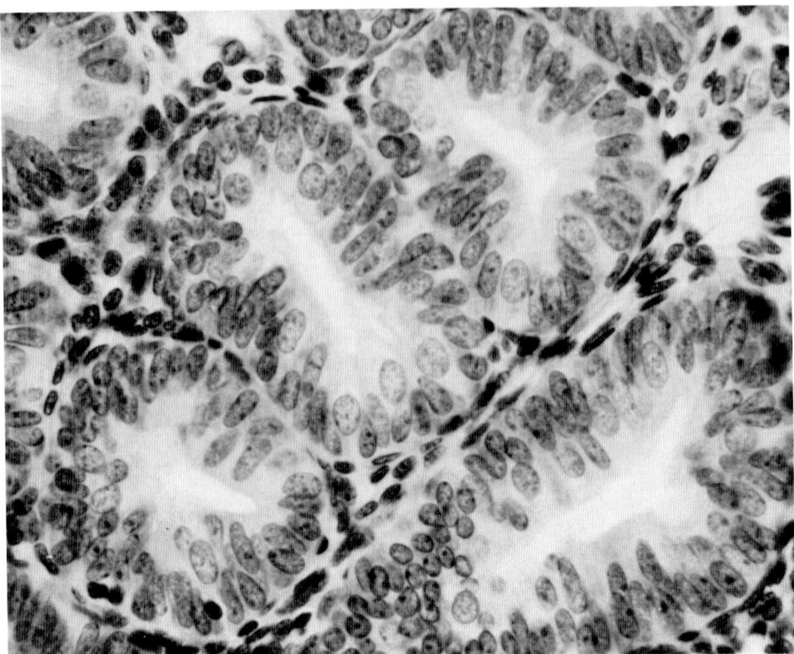

Fig. 5-5. Complex hyperplasia with moderate cytologic atypia.

of their polarity (Figs. 5-4 to 5-8). Additionally, the atypical cells often have increased amounts of eosinophilic cytoplasm. Cellular stratification, which may be characterized by cellular buds (Fig. 5-6), intraglandular bridges (Fig. 5-8), or even obliteration of the glandular lumen, may accompany any type of hyperplasia but most often accompanies cytologic atypia. A cribriform pattern (Fig. 5-8) may be encountered in occasional hyperplastic glands, but when numerous glands with a cribriform pattern as well as significant cytologic atypia are present, a diagnosis of grade 1 adenocarcinoma is warranted (see below).

In the study by Kurman et al.,[3] atypia proved the most important feature in identifying a significant frequency of progression to carcinoma. Carcinoma developed in only 2 of 122 patients (1.6 percent) with SH and CH compared with 11 of 48 patients (22 percent) of patients with atypia (ASH or ACH). These observations are consistent with those from a number of studies published predominantly in the older literature[4–9] and summarized elsewhere[10–13]; the conclusions of several such studies, however, were obfuscated by the inclusion of some patients who had been treated by pelvic radiation (a known carcinogen) before the appearance of the carcinoma.[2, 5] A more recent study by Huang et al.[13] also confirmed the prognostic significance of cytologic atypia: 24 percent of the hyperplasias accompanied by nuclear atypia progressed to carcinoma, whereas progression was seen in only 2.9 percent of hyperplasias lacking nuclear atypia.

Kurman et al.[3] found that progression to carcinoma occurred in 1 of 93 patients (1 percent) with SH after an 11-year interval, in 1 of 29 patients (3 percent) with CH after an 8.3-year interval, in 1 of 13 patients (8 percent) with ASH, and in 10 of 35 patients (29 percent) with ACH. The interval between the diagnosis of ASH or ACH and carcinoma ranged from 1 to 11 years (mean, 4.1 years). This study therefore suggests

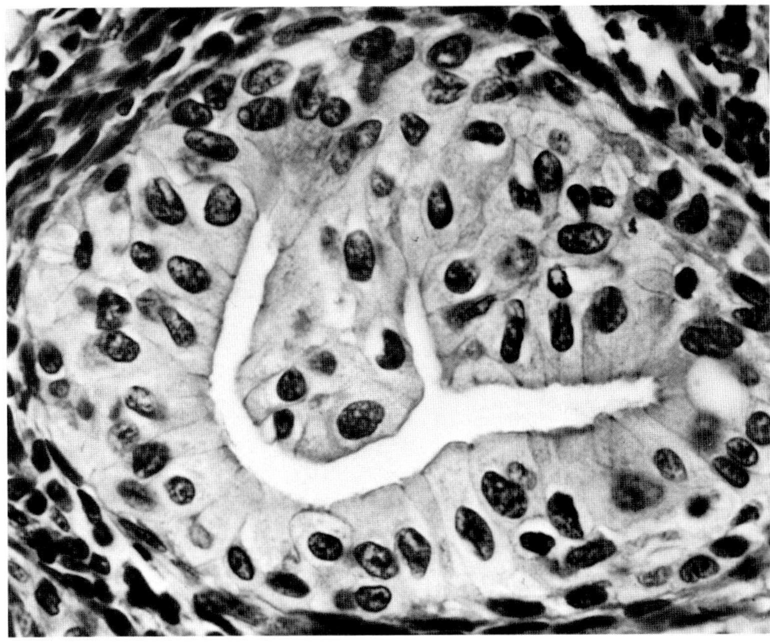

Fig. 5-6. Moderate cytologic atypia. Note cellular stratification, intraluminal papilla, and hyperchromatic nuclei that vary in size and shape.

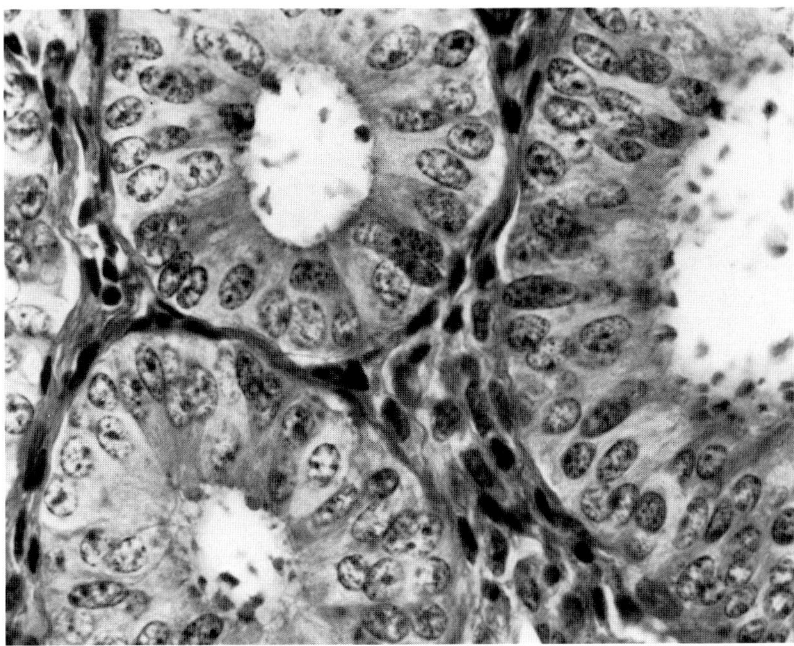

Fig. 5-7. Severe cytologic atypia. Note rounding of nuclei, clumped chromatin, and moderate amounts of (eosinophilic) cytoplasm.

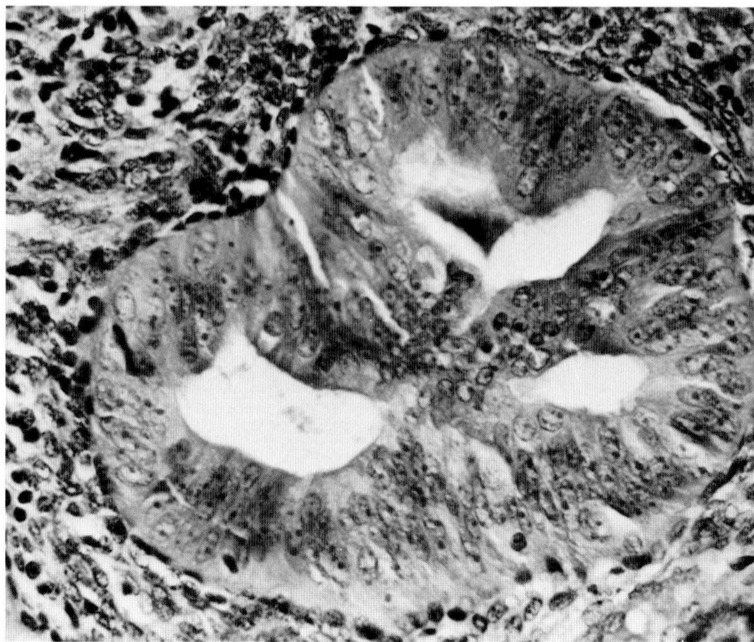

Fig. 5-8. Severe cytologic atypia and intraluminal bridges creating a cribriform pattern.

that SH and CH are not obviously precancerous, whereas complex hyperplasia with cytologic atypia is significantly precancerous. The difference in progression rates between ASH and ACH (8 versus 29 percent), however, was not statistically significant because of the small number of patients in the group with ASH. The precancerous potential of ASH, therefore, requires study of a larger cohort of patients.

There are several problems with the new classification of endometrial hyperplasia. First, although complex hyperplasia is often equated with the older designations "adenomatous hyperplasia" and "architectural atypicality," it is apparent that mild and even some moderate degrees of adenomatous and architectural abnormalities are regarded as simple hyperplasia in the new classification, and interconversion of the traditional and the new terminology is not possible. Another problem exists in the sharp separation between typical and atypical hyperplasia. There are degrees of nuclear atypicality acknowledged in the older terminologies as mild, moderate, and severe (Figs. 5-4 to 5-8). It is biologically most probable that mild atypicality is not as serious a change as severe atypicality in which the glandular epithelium has a fully malignant appearance. Finally, there is no provision in the new terminology for distinguishing small foci of various forms of hyperplasia from extensive areas of involvement. In our laboratories, we provide gynecologists with information about the degree and extent of the different types of hyperplasia on the assumption that such information will be of value to the clinician in therapeutic decision-making. Obviously, whatever terminology is used by the pathologist should be clearly understood by the gynecologist; close communication between the two is essential in this difficult area of interpretation.

With one exception, the carcinomas that developed in the patients studied by Kurman et al.[3] were well differentiated and

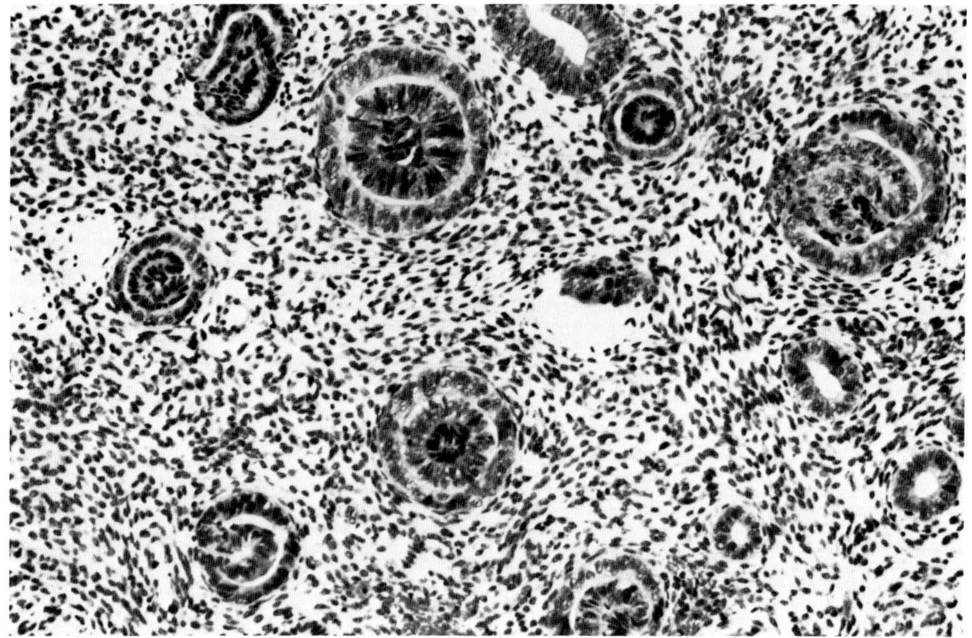

Fig. 5-12. Artifactual telescoping of endometrial glands.

ous hyperplasia might be due to an end-organ abnormality, such as a deficiency of progesterone receptors, permitting estrogens to act alone on the abnormal glands.

There appears to be considerable individual variation in the response of the endometrium to abnormal estrogenic stimulation. This is illustrated by the finding of several investigators that the administration of estrogens to a series of women leads to precancerous hyperplasia in only a minority of cases.[22] No explanation is available for this lack of uniformity of response. If estrogens are a cause of precancerous hyperplasia, the question arises as to what subtypes of the latter are reversible by withdrawal of the abnormal estrogen stimulation, restoration of progesterone stimulation, or both. This question is impossible to answer with certainty, since the diagnosis of precancerous hyperplasia presupposes endometrial curettage or biopsy, which may in itself remove the lesion being studied. Taking into account the possible contribution of surgical excision, one can conclude that lesions

up to and including severe ACH (and even grade 1 adenocarcinoma in young women) are sometimes reversible by curettage, cessation of estrogen therapy, the induction of ovulation (in patients with polycystic ovarian disease), and the institution of progesterone therapy, alone or in combination. In the study cited earlier by Kurman et al.,[3] cessation of estrogen therapy in women with endometrial hyperplasia, including those with cytologic atypia, resulted in regression of the lesion in 90 percent of the cases. Similarly, Kistner[23] and Wentz[7] found that all types of endometrial hyperplasia, including lesions that were classified as "carcinoma in situ," may be successfully treated with progestin therapy and curettage. Moreover, Tavassoli and Kraus suggested that even lesions classified as grade 1 adenocarcinoma are consistently reversed by progesterone when they are associated with precancerous hyperplasia in perimenopausal women exposed to estrogen.[9] By contrast, Gal et al.[24] found that 10 percent of women had persistent or progressive endometrial hyperplasia during progestin therapy. More strikingly, Ferenczy and Gelfand[25] determined that although none of 65 patients with endometrial hyperplasia lacking cytologic atypia subsequently had carcinoma while receiving progestogen therapy, 5 of 20 similarly treated patients who had cytologically atypical lesions had carcinoma 2 to 7 years (mean, 5.5 years) after starting progesterone therapy.

DISTINCTION OF ATYPICAL ENDOMETRIAL HYPERPLASIA FROM GRADE 1 ENDOMETRIAL ADENOCARCINOMA

The histologic distinction between severely atypical precancerous hyperplasia (ACH) and grade 1 endometrial adenocarcinoma remains difficult and controversial, as reflected in the numerous publications that have addressed this issue during the past 15 years.[9, 15, 26–32] Although low-grade carcinoma is clearly recognizable in most sites because malignant-appearing cells have invaded the stroma or follow-up examination has indicated a potential for spread, low-grade adenocarcinoma of the endometrium is typically characterized by a close approximation of glands lined by atypical epithelial cells, usually without the stromal reaction characteristic of invasion in other sites. Also, the cure rate of a low-grade adenocarcinoma confined to the endometrium is so high that it is difficult to distinguish from severely atypical hyperplasia on the basis of follow-up data alone. Recent studies have evaluated this problem in differential diagnosis by accepting as well-differentiated adenocarcinomas only lesions that have invaded the myometrium as evaluated in hysterectomy specimens and contrasting them with highly atypical lesions not proved to be carcinoma by myometrial invasion in the hysterectomy specimen. The two groups of investigators who have utilized this approach, however, have formulated criteria for the differential diagnosis that differ significantly. The criteria of Hendrickson et al.[26, 29] are more subjective than those of Kurman and Norris,[28] and include a number of architectural and cytologic features, some of which may be absent in individual cases, leaving the final judgment to the pathologist evaluating all the features and weighing their cumulative significance. Kurman and Norris, in contrast, emphasize architecture, stromal characteristics, and quantitative features, proposing strict criteria for the diagnosis of carcinoma.[28]

The architectural and cytological features of grade 1 endometrial adenocarcinoma are illustrated in Figures 5-13 to 5-21. The architectural features for this diagnosis proposed by Hendrickson et al.[26, 29] include a complex or confluent gland pattern (Figs. 5-13 to 5-15) exhibiting one or more of the following features: a back-to-back arrangement without intervening stroma (Fig. 5-14), a gland-within-gland pattern, villoglandular areas, papillary infolding into the glands (Fig. 5-15), as well as epithelial stratification and bridging (Fig. 5-19 and 5-20). In their experience, a true cribriform pattern (Figs. 5-16 and 5-17) is rare in grade 1 adenocarcinoma but is characteristic of grade 2 adenocarcinoma.[29] Cytologic criteria include nuclear abnormalities (Figs. 5-20 and 5-21), specifically nuclear enlargement and loss of polarity, chromatin clearing (Fig. 5-21) and clumping, prominent nucleoli (Fig. 5-21), and mitotic figures, including abnormal forms; luminal neutrophils, karyorrhectic debris, and necrosis are also commonly present (Fig. 5-13). These investigators found that invasion of the endometrial stroma, per se, was not a useful criterion for grade 1 adenocarcinoma; indeed, they state that "endometrial stromal invasion . . . was not identified frequently" in grade 1 cases.[29] Although some of the architectural and cytological criteria may be absent in individual cases, these authors generally require marked architectural atypia combined with moderate to marked cytologic

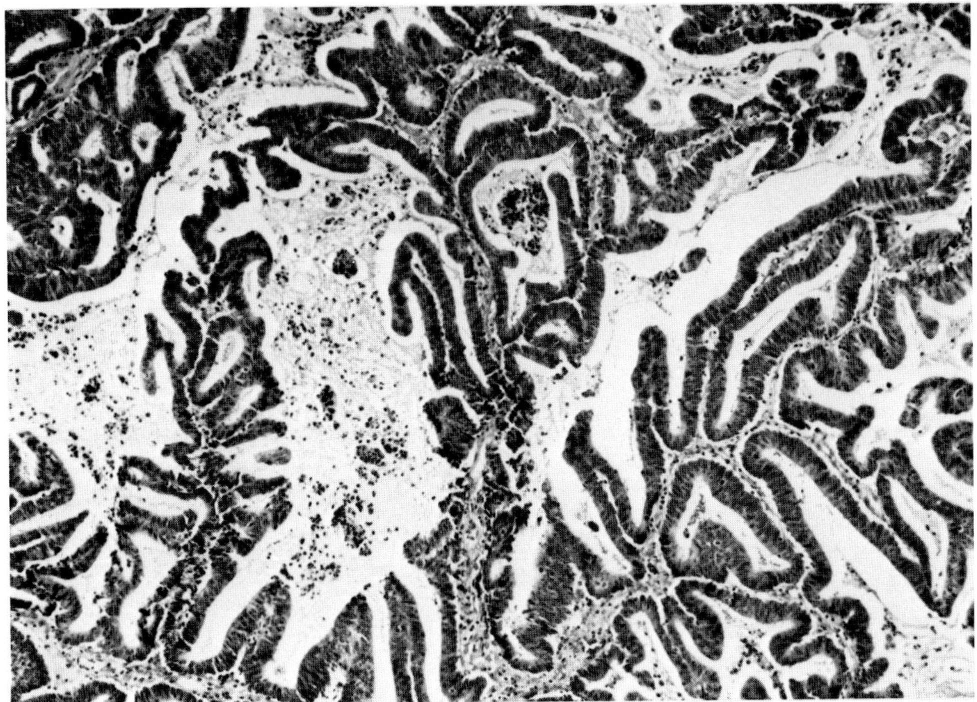

Fig. 5-13. Grade 1 endometrial (endometrioid) adenocarcinoma with confluent villoglandular pattern and interconnecting gland lumens; the latter contain necrotic debris and inflammatory cells.

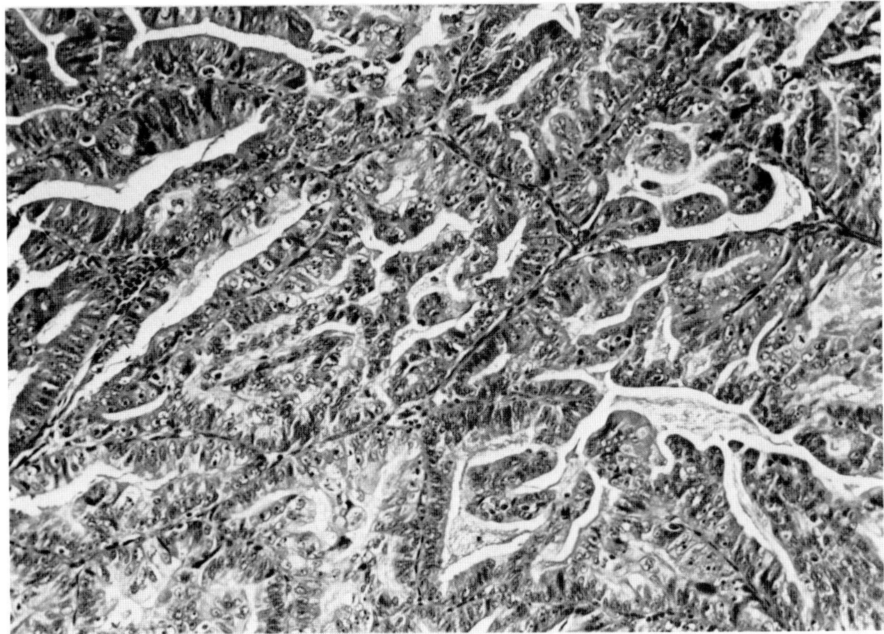

Fig. 5-14. Grade 1 endometrial (endometrioid) adenocarcinoma. Note complex haphazard gland pattern with papillary infoldings.

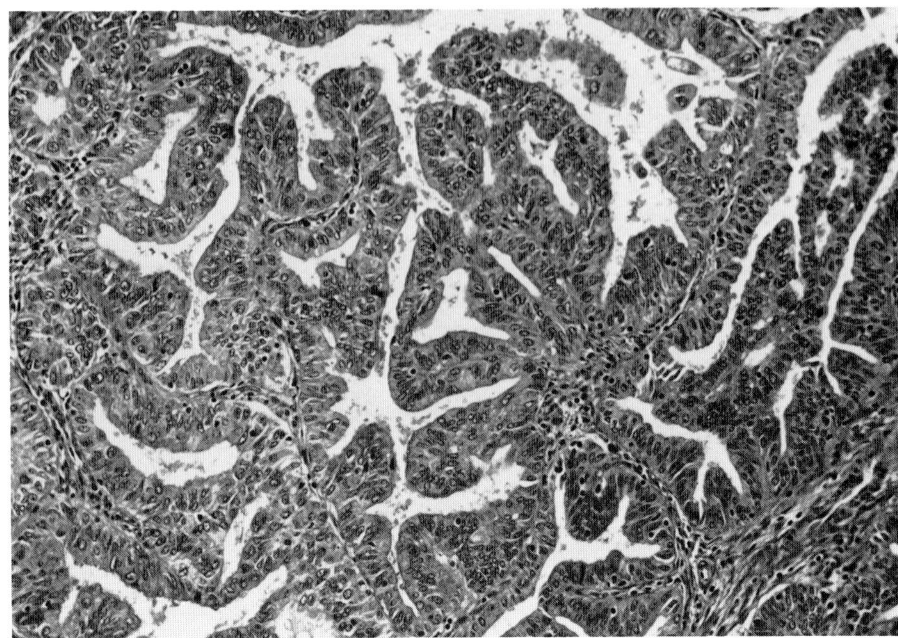

Fig. 5-15. Grade 1 endometrial (endometrioid) adenocarcinoma. Note confluent glands and papillary infoldings, which contain scant connective tissue cores.

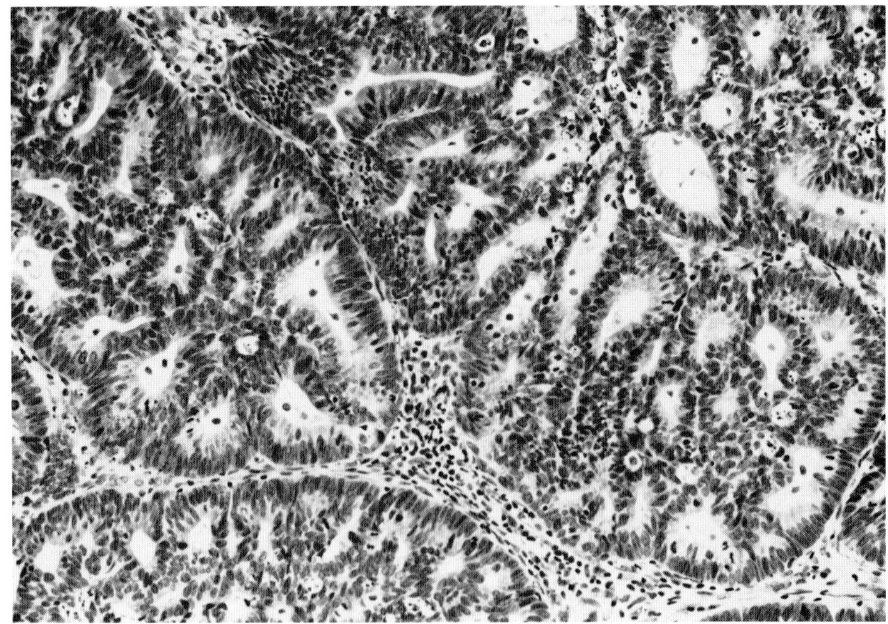

Fig. 5-16. Grade 1 endometrial (endometrioid) adenocarcinoma with a cribriform pattern.

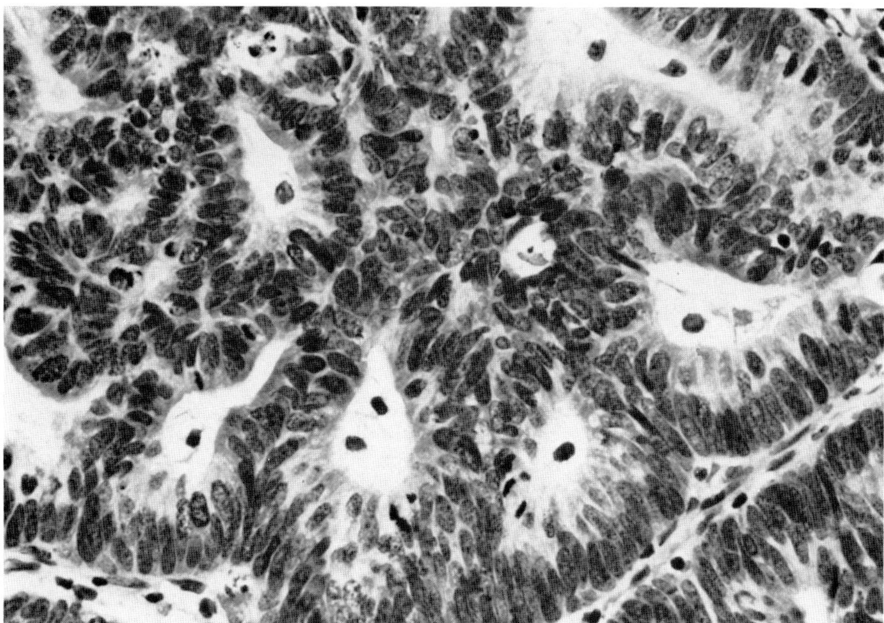

Fig. 5-17. Grade 1 endometrial (endometrioid) adenocarcinoma. Higher power of tumor illustrated in Figure 5-16, showing a cribriform pattern.

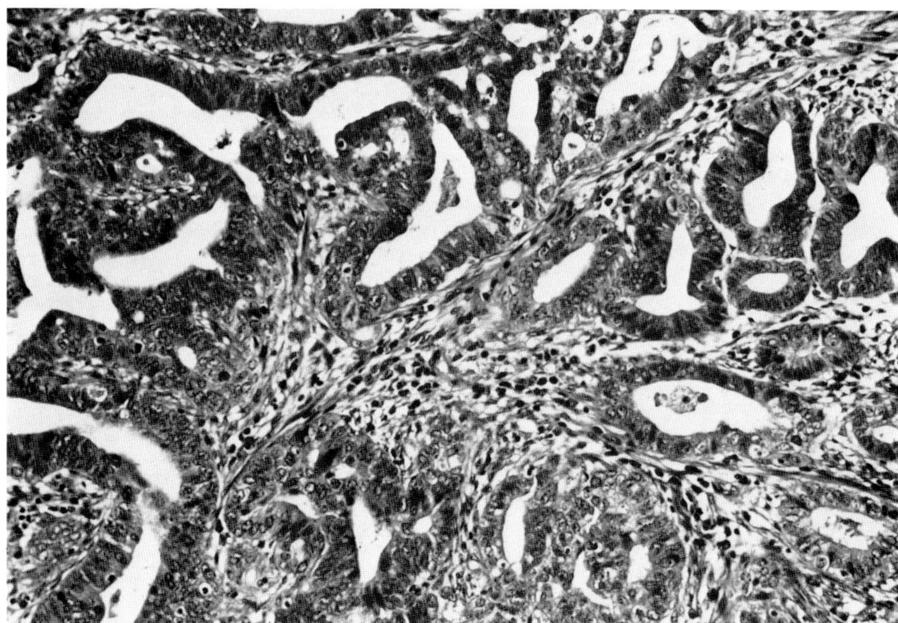

Fig. 5-18. Grade 1 endometrial (endometrioid) adenocarcinoma with irregular glands surrounded by a reactive fibroblastic stroma.

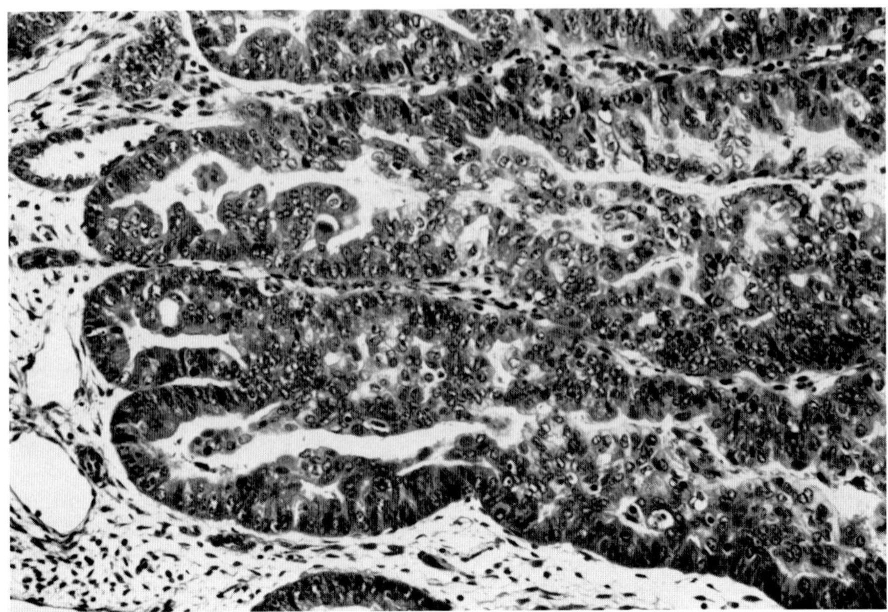

Fig. 5-19. Grade 1 endometrial (endometrioid) adenocarcinoma Note marked cellular stratification and bridging.

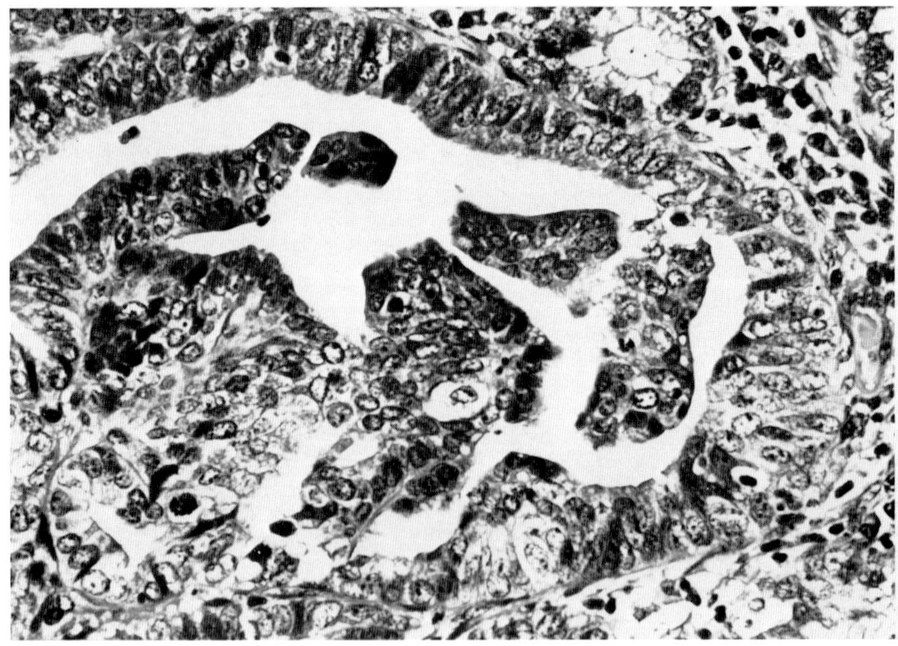

Fig. 5-20. Grade 1 endometrial (endometrioid) adenocarcinoma. Note cellular stratification, cellular papillae, nuclear enlargement, and chromatin clumping.

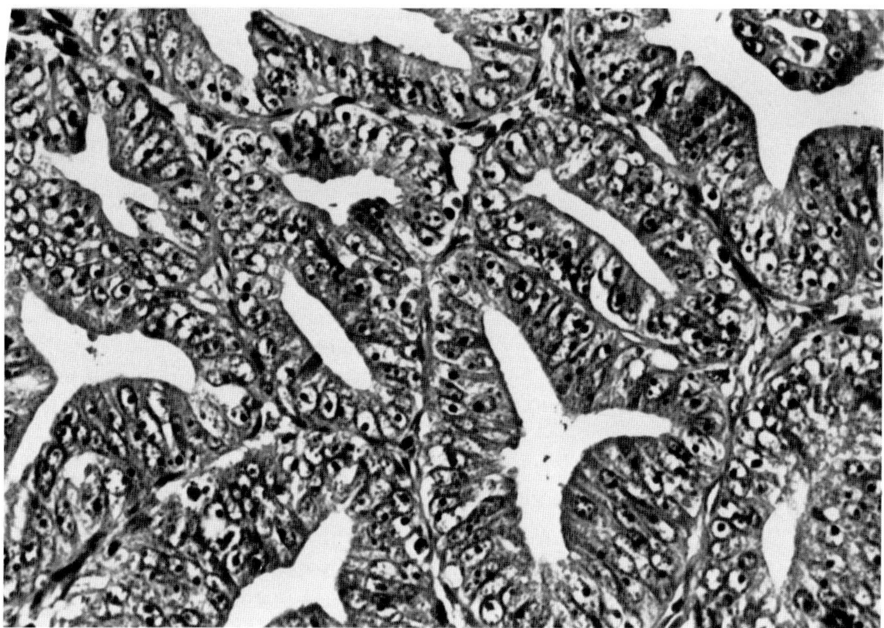

Fig. 5-21. Grade 1 endometrial (endometrioid) adenocarcinoma. Note clearing of chromatin and prominent nucleoli.

atypia in most cases, although only mild cytologic atypia may be present in rare cases.

By contrast, Kurman and Norris use as their primary criterion for carcinoma the presence of "stromal invasion," which they define arbitrarily as the presence of at least one of the following findings: (1) an irregular infiltration of glands that elicit a desmoplastic stromal response (Fig. 5-18); (2) a confluent glandular pattern in which individual glands are uninterrupted by stroma and merge to form a cribriform pattern (Figs. 5-13 to 5-17); (3) an extensive papillary pattern; and (4) replacement of the stroma by masses of squamous cells.[15, 28, 30] To qualify as invasion, the last three changes are required to occupy at least half of a low-power microscopic field 4.2 mm in diameter.

The criteria of Kurman and Norris were found useful but not infallible in predicting the presence or absence of myometrial invasion in their study and in a subsequent study by King et al.[33] When "stromal inva-

sion," as defined, was present in the curettings, residual carcinoma, which was moderately to poorly differentiated in one-third of cases, was present in the uterus in 50 percent of cases, invaded the myometrium in 36 percent of cases, and involved the middle or outer one-third of the myometrium in 12 percent of cases.[28] When stromal invasion was absent in the curettings, carcinoma was present in the uterus in 17 percent[28] to 28 percent[33] of cases, and invaded the myometrium in 8 to 16 percent of cases.[28, 33] While these "unsuspected" adenocarcinomas were well differentiated and only superficially invasive in one study,[28] some tumors in this category invaded into the deep myometrium in the other series.[33]

The criteria of Hendrickson et al. are less precise than those of Kurman and Norris, reflecting the great difficulty differentiating severe ACH and grade 1 adenoacarcinoma.[26, 29] The diagnostic criteria of Kurman and Norris, while helpful, are more precise than warranted by available evidence. Fulfillment of quantitative criteria for the diagnosis of carcinoma depends on complete sampling of the endometrial cavity, which is seldom if ever achieved in biopsy or curettage specimens. Also, in our experience and those of others,[29] a desmoplastic stroma is uncommon in endometrial carcinomas; when it is present, the diagnosis is usually obvious for other reasons. Also, a desmoplastic stroma is occasionally present in reparative processes and endometrial polyps.[29]

In practice, the differential diagnosis of severely atypical hyperplasia and low-grade adenocarcinoma is usually not of great clinical importance if the gynecologist is aware of their close similarity and the frequent difficulty of distinguishing them on histological examination of biopsy or curettage specimens. It is important for the pathologist to be extremely vigilant in excluding carcinoma on examination of abundant atypical endometrial tissue in postmenopausal women and, conversely, conservative in the interpretation of atypical endometria in young women.[14]

Special techniques have also been used in an attempt to distinguish atypical endometrial hyperplasia from grade 1 adenocarcinoma. A variety of immunohistochemical studies have shown differences in staining between the two lesions for a variety of antigens, including carcinoembryonic antigen (CEA),[34, 35] epithelial membrane antigen,[36, 37] TAG-72,[38] human milk fat globule,[39] ferritin,[35] lectins,[40] sialyl-Tn,[41] and basement membrane components.[42, 43] Similarly, a variety of quantitative techniques have been applied in an attempt to provide more objective means of distinguishing precancerous hyperplasias from grade 1 adenocarcinoma. They include cytomorphometry and cytophotometry,[44–46] flow cytometry,[47] and counts of nucleolar organizer regions.[48–51] These techniques, although claimed to be objective, depend on the subjective selection of tissue for analysis; present experience with them in this differential diagnosis is too limited to permit conclusions about their ultimate value in routine practice, and the final diagnosis remains dependent on the interpretation of routinely prepared microscopic sections.

SUBTYPES OF ENDOMETRIAL CARCINOMA

The new ISGP/WHO classification of endometrial carcinomas is based primarily on the cell type of the tumor (Table 5-1). The various histologic subtypes are discussed separately, but two or more of them are often admixed in the same specimen. In these mixed carcinomas, the histologic composition of the tumor should be specifically noted in the pathology report, as the prognosis and treatment may be determined by the presence of a minor focus of an aggressive histologic subtype. Several rare subtypes of primary carcinomas (small cell undifferentiated carcinomas, transitional cell carcinomas) and metastatic carcinomas involving the endometrium are discussed in Chapter 8.

The various subtypes of endometrial carcinoma are essentially indistinguishable from each other on gross examination, and may occasionally be macroscopically mimicked by other lesions, including mesenchy-

**Table 5-1. WHO/ISGP Classification of
Endometrial Carcinoma**

Endometrioid
  Typical
  Variants
    With squamous differentiation
    Secretory
    Ciliated
Serous papillary adenocarcinoma
Clear cell adenocarcinoma
Mucinous adenocarcinoma
Squamous cell carcinoma
Undifferentiated carcinoma[a]
Mixed carcinoma[b]

[a] Small cell undifferentiated carcinomas are discussed in Chapter 8.

[b] A carcinoma containing greater than 10 percent of a second cell type.

mal (see Ch. 6) or mixed epithelial–mesenchymal tumors (see Ch. 7). Endometrial carcinomas vary from sessile polypoid masses that may fill the endometrial cavity (Fig. 5-22), to irregular thickened areas that may be diffuse or localized; occasional examples of the latter type are confined to the lower uterine segment.[52] The neoplastic tissue typically has a pale tan to white opaque appearance and is fleshy, firm, or gritty; foci of hemorrhage and yellow foci of necrosis are often visible, especially in poorly differentiated tumors; the appearance typically differs from the translucent gray appearance of the normal proliferative and secretory endometrium. The surface of the carcinoma typically has a more irregular or shaggy appearance (Fig. 5-22) than that of a tumor containing sarcomatous elements, which characteristically has a smooth surface. Some or all of the carcinoma may have been removed by a prehysterectomy curettage, and there may be little or no grossly visible tumor within the endometrial cavity. Myometrial invasion usually appears as a well or sometimes poorly demarcated extension of firm, gray-white tissue, but microscopic examination of a grossly normal myometrium may also reveal invasive tumor, especially if it is confined to vascular spaces. The gross description of the tumor in the pathology report should include a measurement of the estimated size of the tumor; the depth of myometrial invasion, if present; the location of the tumor within the uterus; and the presence or absence of cervical involvement. These findings, as well as the presence or absence of an ovarian tumor of a similar or different histologic type, may have prognostic significance, as discussed later in this chapter.

ENDOMETRIOID CARCINOMA

Approximately 80 percent of endometrial adenocarcinomas are of endometrioid type.[53] These tumors are composed in whole or in part of tubular glands lined exclusively or predominantly by pseudostratified or stratified columnar cells; cytoplasmic mucin is either absent or sparse and confined to the luminal tips of the cells (Figs. 5-13 to 5-21). Occasional otherwise typical endometrioid carcinomas that con-

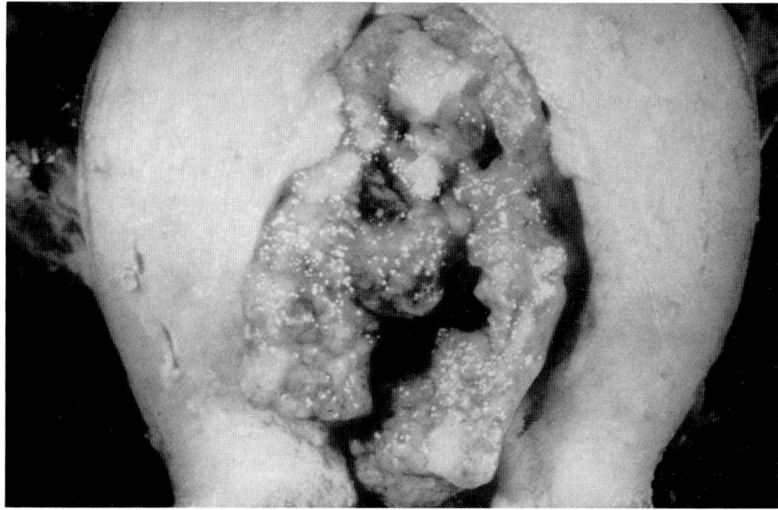

Fig. 5-22. Endometrial adenocarcinoma, endometrioid type. A polypoid fleshy mass with an irregular surface fills the endometrial cavity.

tain prominent amounts of luminal mucin ("mucin-rich" endometrioid carcinomas) (Fig. 5-23) should not be regarded as mucinous adenocarcinomas.[54] The proportion of the tumor that is composed of solid versus glandular areas is used in assessing the histologic grade of the tumor (see grading, page 233). Rare otherwise typical endometrioid carcinomas may have focal sertoliform tubular patterns[55] (Fig. 5-24), patterns resembling adenoid cystic carcinoma,[56, 57] or foci simulating microglandular hyperplasia. Because the last pattern is more commonly associated with mucinous carcinomas, it is discussed in the section dealing with the latter tumors. Rare otherwise typical endometrioid carcinomas may contain cells with abundant oxyphilic cytoplasm (Fig. 5-25) or clear or foamy lipid-rich cytoplasm.[58] A variety of histologic variants of endometrioid adenocarcinoma (not all of which are included in the ISGP/WHO classification) are discussed below.

Some endometrial carcinomas, usually of endometrioid type, have stromal changes that may be a striking finding. Stromal cells characterized by abundant spongy lipid-rich cytoplasm and small shrunken nuclei, similar to those occasionally found in association with endometrial hyperplasia, also occur in endometrioid adenocarcinomas (Fig. 5-26). The presence of these cells in a curettage or biopsy specimen should therefore alert the pathologist to the possibility of an associated carcinoma or precancerous lesion. Foam cells have been found in 3 to 43 percent of endometrial adenocarcinoma[59–64]; Dawagne and Silverberg calculated an average figure of 15 percent from the literature.[64] The cells are more common in well-differentiated tumors,[59] and they may also be more common in women being treated with estrogens.[62] Although the foam cells are indistinguishable on microscopic examination from foamy macrophages, Fechner et al.[62] showed by ultrastructural examination that most such cells are altered endometrial stromal cells; only a minority

of them have ultrastructural features of macrophages. When they are present, the differential diagnosis includes xanthogranulomatous endometritis, a lesion characterized by benign-appearing glands admixed with foamy macrophages typically accompanied by a variety of other inflammatory cells (see Ch. 4). Foam cells of endometrial stromal origin should also be distinguished from mucin-containing macrophages that have been encountered in occasional endometrial polyps.[60] Nogales and associates[65] reported two cases of endometrial adenocarcinoma (one endometrioid, one clear cell) that contained benign mesenchymal elements (fat, osteoid) within their stroma. The heterologous tissues were interpreted as metaplastic rather than neoplastic. Such tumors should not be misinterpreted as heterologous malignant müllerian mixed tumors. Additionally, we have encountered carcinomas in which foci of well-differentiated endometrial stromal neoplasia, sometimes associated with sex cord-like differentiation, have been present (see Fig. 7-6). Such foci should not be misinterpreted as undifferentiated carcinoma or lead the pathologist to a diagnosis of carcinosarcoma of the usual type.

Villoglandular Endometrioid Carcinoma

Some endometrioid carcinomas, which are typically well differentiated, have a villoglandular pattern characterized by villuslike papillae with typically thin fibrovascular cores, admixed with a variable proportion of endometrioid glands[66–71] (Figs. 5-27 and 5-28). These tumors (VGECs), also referred to as papillary endometrioid carcinomas, accounted for 2.5 to 2.8 percent of endometrial carcinomas in three series,[67, 68, 71] and a surprisingly high 22 percent in a fourth series.[70] Chen et al.[67] found that patients with VGECs were a decade younger than patients with serous papillary

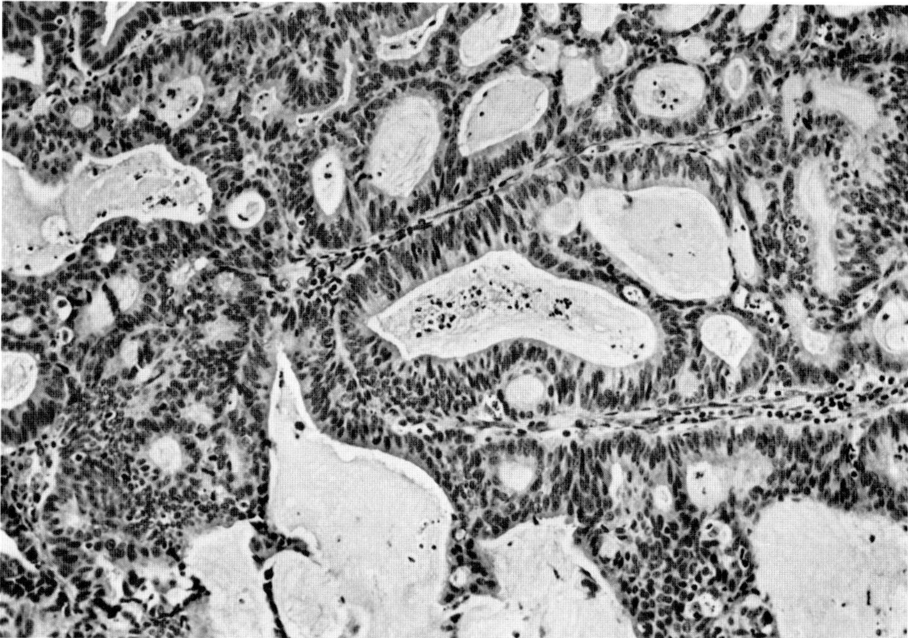

Fig. 5-23. Endometrial (endometrioid) adenocarcinoma of "mucin-rich" type. The glandular lumens contain abundant mucin.

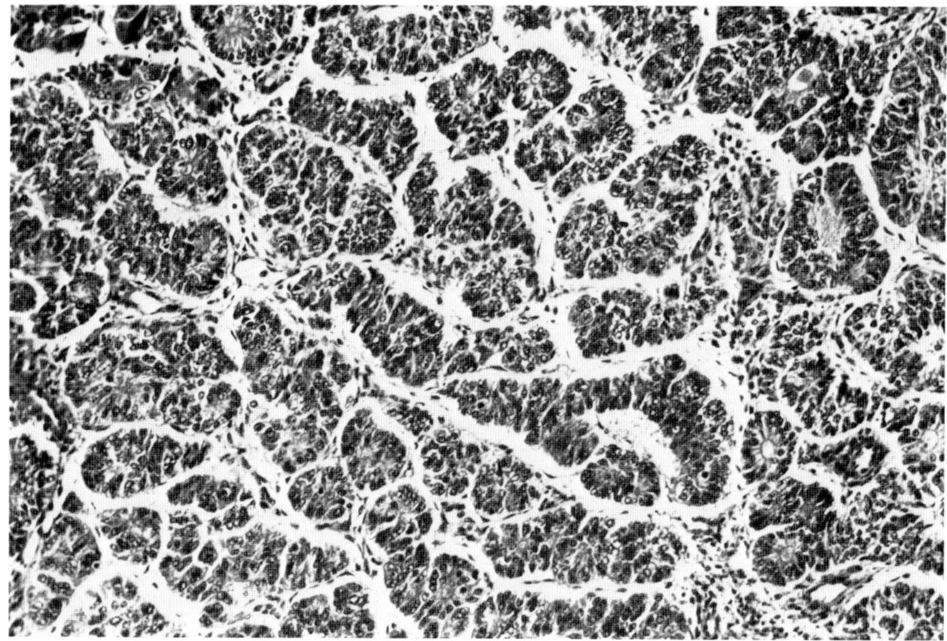

Fig. 5-24. Endometrioid endometrial adenocarcinoma with a solid tubular (sertoliform) pattern.

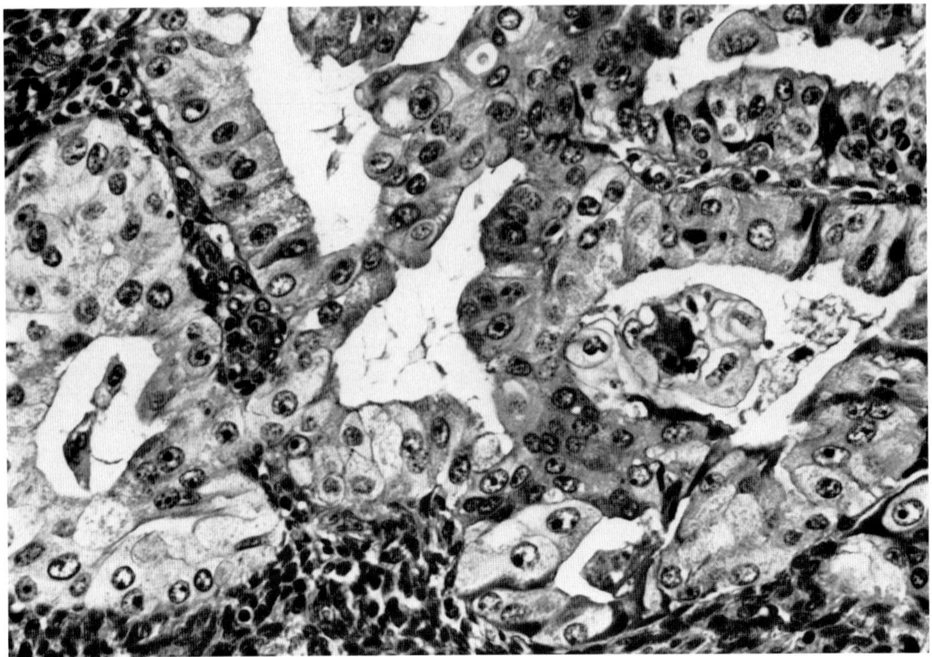

Fig. 5-25. Endometrioid adenocarcinoma containing oxyphil cells.

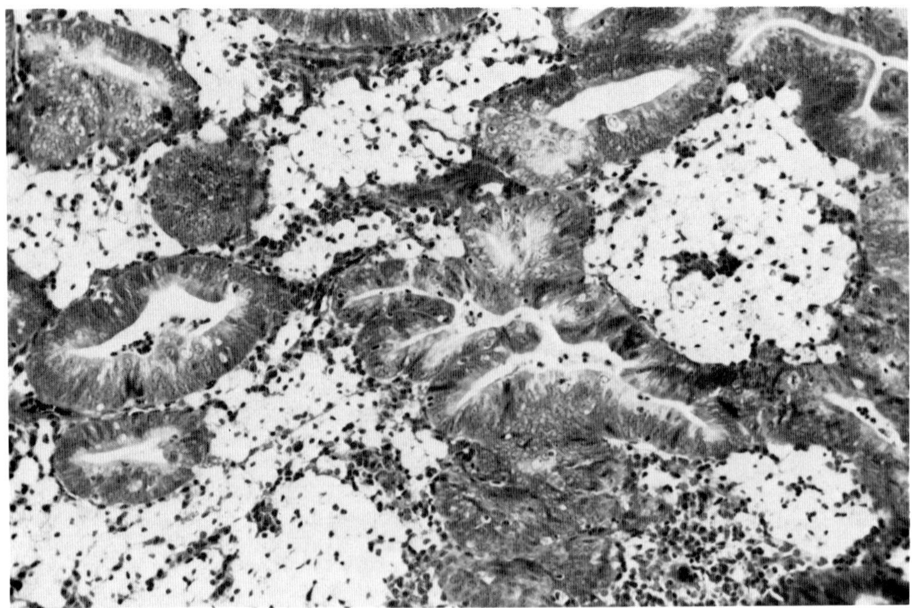

Fig. 5-26. Endometrial adenocarcinoma with prominent collections of stromal foam cells.

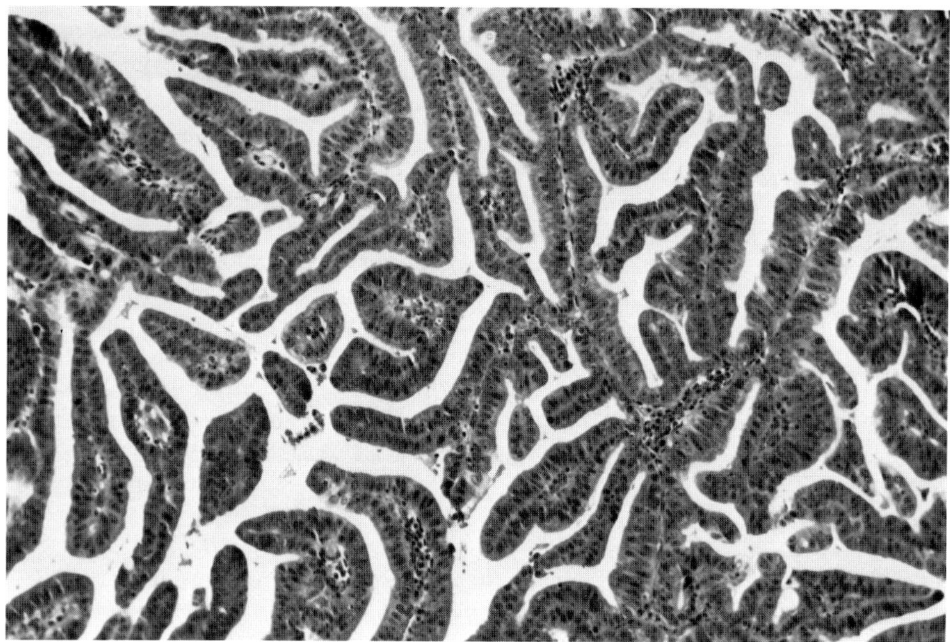

Fig. 5-27. Villoglandular endometrioid adenocarcinoma.

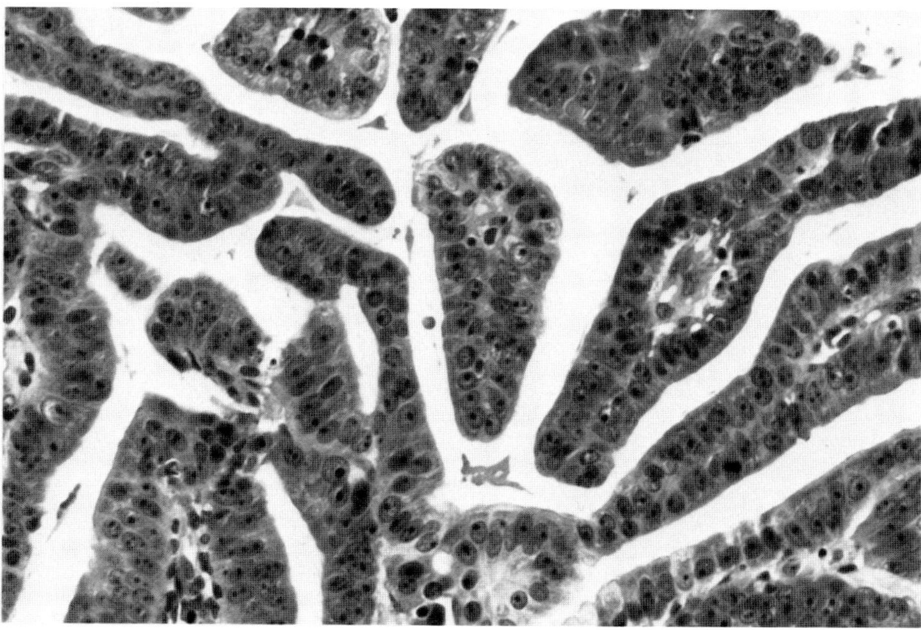

Fig. 5-28. Villoglandular endometrioid adenocarcinoma. Note lack of high-grade cytological atypia, in contrast to serous papillary carcinoma.

carcinomas (SPECs), but in three other series.[68, 70, 71] there was no significant difference in the mean ages of the patients in the two groups. Most studies have found that VGECs have a behavior similar to that of other endometrioid adenocarcinomas of the same grade,[66–68, 71] whereas the studies by Burke et al.[69] and O'Hanlan et al.[70] concluded that the behavior of VGECs was intermediate between that of typical endometrioid carcinomas and SPECs. Eighty percent of VGECs in the latter study,[70] however, had grade 2 or grade 3 nuclear features, suggesting the possible inclusion of some tumors with a component of SPEC. Because of the difference in behavior and treatment between VGECs and SPECs, these tumors should be clearly distinguished on histologic examination; the term *"papillary adenocarcinoma"* without designation of its cell type is inadequate for indicating the prognosis of the patient and her optimal therapy. The differential features of these two types of carcinoma are discussed in the section dealing with SPECs.

Secretory Adenocarcinoma

The term *"secretory carcinoma"* has been applied to rare well-differentiated endometrioid carcinomas in which glycogen vacuoles (subnuclear or supranuclear, or both) are present within the neoplastic cells (Fig. 5-29). These tumors account for approximately 1 percent of endometrial carcinomas; less than 30 examples have been reported in detail.[72–74] In the only two series of secretory carcinomas, two-thirds of the patients were postmenopausal, with an age range of 35 to 79 years (mean, 57 years).[72, 73] In some cases, the vacuoles appear to represent a transitory response to an endogenous or exogenous progestational stimulus; in such cases, a secretory pattern within an adenocarcinoma obtained by curettage may not be present within the tumor at the time of hysterectomy or vice versa. In cases encountered in premenopausal women who are not on hormone therapy, a corpus luteum has typically been present when the ovaries have been available for histological examination.[75] The adjacent uninvolved en-

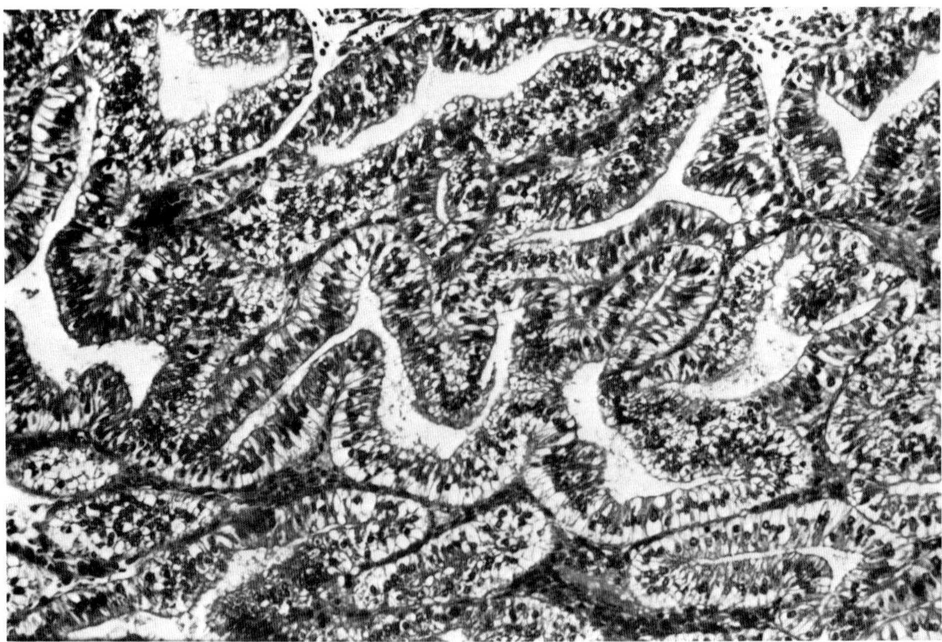

Fig. 5-29. Secretory adenocarcinoma.

dometrium in such cases usually has a secretory pattern more advanced than that of a 17-day secretory endometrium.[75] Additionally, a disproportionate number of secretory carcinomas were encountered during the 1970s among adenocarcinomas occurring in young women using Oracon, a sequential oral contraceptive agent with a large estrogen and relatively small progesterone content.[76, 77] In other cases, a secretory pattern is encountered in endometrial adenocarcinomas during the course of treatment with progestins. Most cases of secretory carcinoma, however, have occurred in women in whom there is no known source of excess progesterone. The tumors have a behavior similar to that of other well-differentiated endometrioid adenocarcinomas; only 3 of 24 patients in the two series cited above died of tumor.[72, 73] Secretory carcinomas should be distinguished on histological examination from clear cell adenocarcinomas, which, in contrast, typically have an aggressive behavior (p. 219).

Ciliated Adenocarcinoma

The designation *"ciliated carcinoma"* is appropriate for rare, otherwise typical endometrioid adenocarcinomas, in which the glands are lined predominantly by ciliated cells[78, 79] (Fig. 5-30). The presence of such cells appears to be more common in endometrioid carcinomas encountered in women on estrogen therapy.[80] In contrast to the rarity of ciliated carcinomas on routine microscopic examination, cilia are observed commonly on ultrastructural examination of typical endometrioid adenocarcinomas.[81]

In the only series of ciliated carcinomas in the literature, reported by Hendrickson and Kempson,[78] the neoplasms had distinctive features in addition to the ciliation of the tumor cells. The tumors accounted for approximately 2.5 percent of endometrial carcinomas in their material. All their patients were postmenopausal (range, 42 to 79 years; mean, 65 years) and presented with vaginal bleeding. Four patients were re-

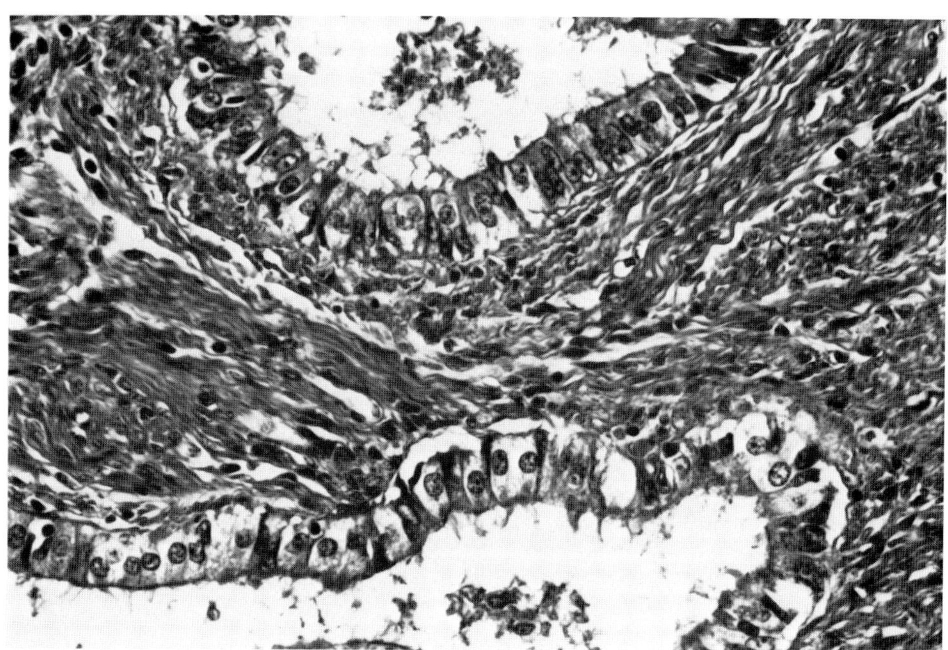

Fig. 5-30. Ciliated adenocarcinoma invading myometrium.

ceiving estrogens. The tumors were characterized by sheets of cells punctured by extracellular lumina that imparted a cribriform appearance (Figs. 5-31 and 5-32). The neoplastic cells had eosinophilic cytoplasm and nuclear features of low grade malignancy, and were arranged around lumina into which cilia projected. Some of the cells not in contact with an extracellular lumen contained an intracytoplasmic lumen containing numerous cilia. Nine of the tumors were mixed with nonciliated endometrioid carcinoma; in two such cases, there were also focal areas of mucinous carcinoma. In 5 of the 10 hysterectomy specimens, the ciliated carcinomas invaded the myometrium; in 1 of these cases, the invasion was deep, and the myometrial lymphatics also contained tumor. None of the eight patients with follow-up data died of tumor.

Endometrioid Carcinomas With Squamous Differentiation

Squamous differentiation occurs in approximately 25 percent of endometrioid adenocarcinomas (Figs. 5-33 to 5-35), and its significance has been controversial for decades. Two decades ago, Ng[82, 83] proposed the designation *"mixed"* or *"mixed adenosquamous"* carcinoma for endometrioid adenocarcinomas with cytologically malignant and invasive squamous elements (Fig. 5-34), reserving the term *"adenoacanthoma"* for endometrioid adenocarcinomas that contain benign-appearing noninvasive squamous elements (Fig. 5-33). A number of studies over the subsequent 20 years confirmed the findings of Ng and associates that adenosquamous carcinomas were associated with a significantly worse prognosis than were adenoacanthomas and endo-

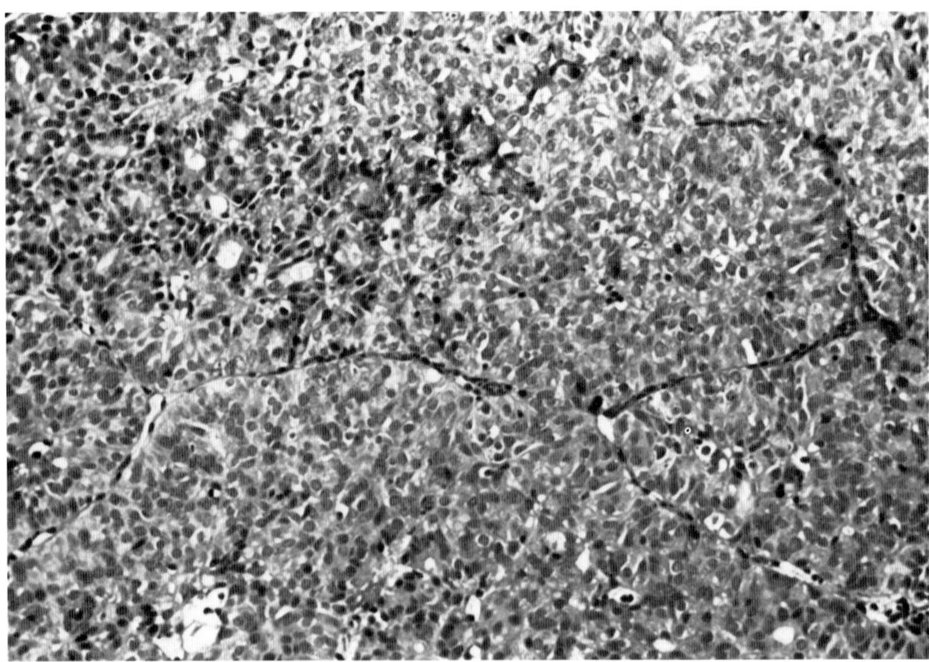

Fig. 5-31. Ciliated adenocarcinoma of distinctive type described by Hendrickson and Kempson. The tumor has a sheetlike growth pattern punctured by small lumina. (Case courtesy of Dr. M. R. Hendrickson.)

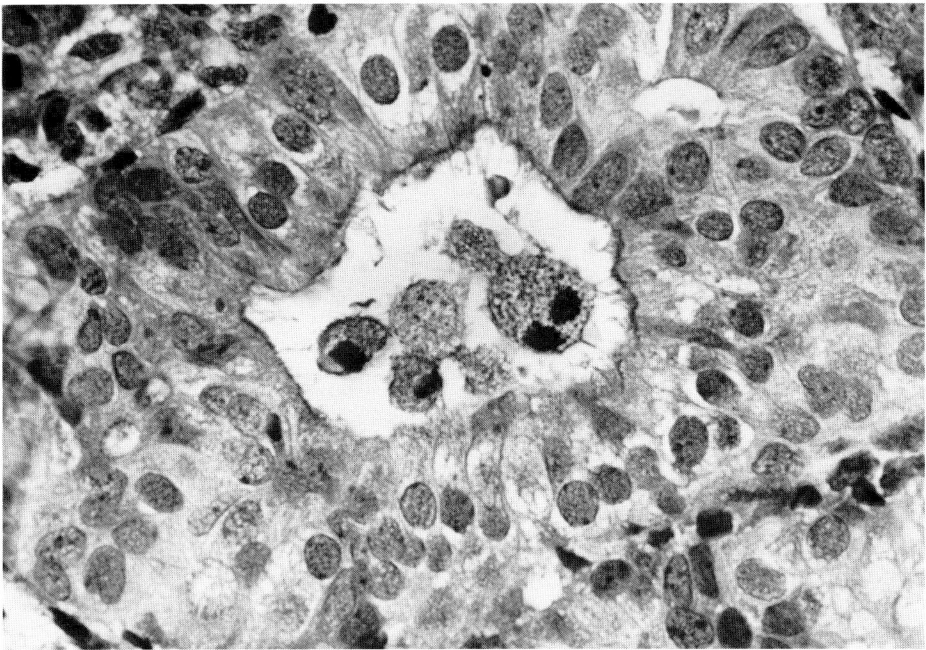

Fig. 5-32. Ciliated adenocarcinoma, higher-power view of tumor illustrated in Figure 5-31. Note cilia lining gland lumen, which also contains several foamy macrophages.

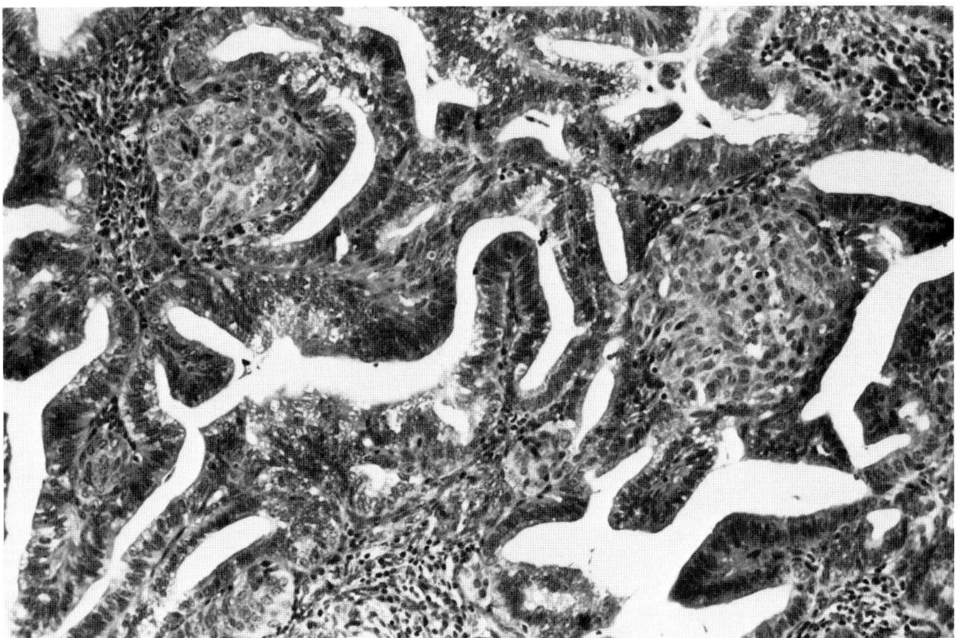

Fig. 5-33. Endometrioid adenocarcinoma, grade 1, with squamous differentiation ("adenoacanthoma"). The latter consists of well-circumscribed morules of immature squamous cells with bland nuclear features.

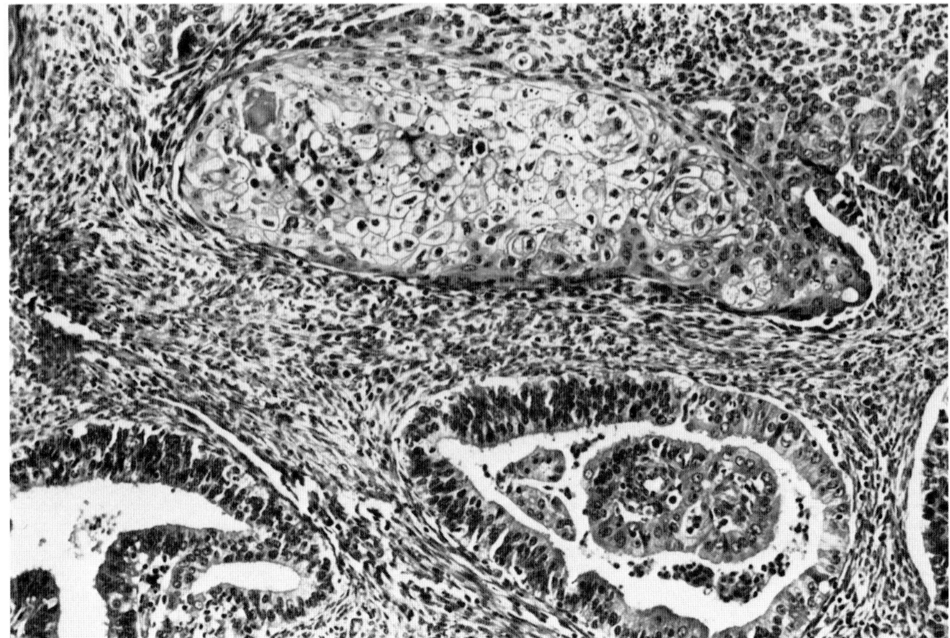

Fig. 5-34. Endometrioid adenocarcinoma with squamous differentiation (''adenosquamous carcinoma''). Both the glandular and squamous elements are invading the myometrium and are surrounded by a reactive stroma. The squamous component has malignant cytologic features.

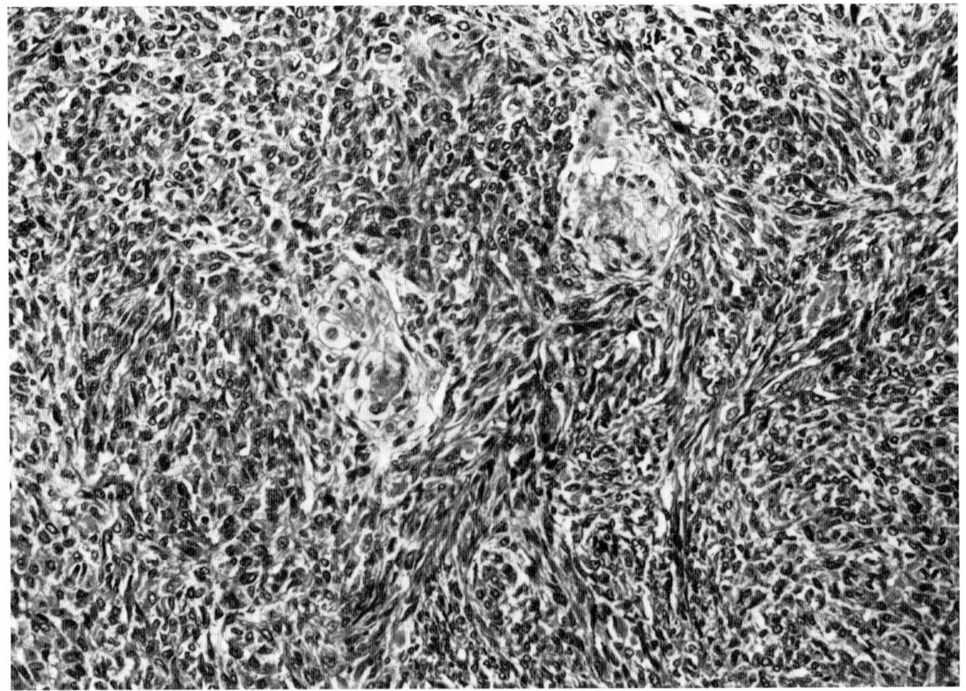

Fig. 5-35. Endometrioid adenocarcinoma with squamous differentiation (''adenosquamous carcinoma''). Only the squamous elements are depicted here, most of which are malignant spindle cells. The latter focally merge with nests of more typical squamous cell carcinoma.

metrioid adenocarcinomas of the same grade lacking squamous differentiation.[84–87] The poor prognosis of the adenosquamous carcinomas was usually ascribed specifically to the presence of cytologically malignant squamous cells and not to the grade of the glandular component of the tumor. In some of these studies, adenoacanthomas had a significantly better prognosis than did endometrioid carcinomas of the same grade without squamous elements.[17, 84, 86, 87] Other studies, however, found no significant differences in the prognosis of adenocarcinomas, adenoacanthomas, and adenosquamous carcinomas[88] or concluded that the poorer prognosis of adenosquamous carcinomas was a function of the less well-differentiated glandular component typically found in these tumors.[84]

Recently, the ISGP/WHO committee chose the term *"adenocarcinoma with squamous differentiation"* (grade 1 to 3 based on the degree of differentiation of the glandular component) over *"adenoacanthoma"* and *"adenosquamous carcinoma,"* but permitted the latter terms as alternative designations. This change was a result of problems encountered in the classification of tumors in which the squamous component is neither clearly benign or malignant from a cytologic viewpoint, as well as recent studies that have shown that the behavior of adenocarcinomas with squamous foci is largely dependent on the grade of the glandular component.[89–91] In one of these studies (based on Gynecologic Oncology Group data), Zaino et al.[90] found that the differentiation of the squamous component parallels that of the glandular component in most tumors. Specifically, benign-appearing squamous elements usually accompany adenocarcinomas with a low-grade glandular component, whereas cytologically malignant squamous elements usually accompany adenocarcinomas with a high-grade glandular component. Pure adenocarcinomas and those with squamous elements had a similar frequency of nodal metastases at each level of invasion, al-

though surprisingly, the risk of death for women whose tumors contained squamous elements was only one-half of that for women with pure adenocarcinomas. It was concluded that the grade (architectural or nuclear, or combined) of the glandular component in adenocarcinomas with squamous elements, as well as the depth of invasion, provided prognostic information (frequency of lymph node metastases, recurrence at three years) that was superior to that provided by dividing the tumors into the categories of pure adenocarcinoma, adenoacanthoma, and adenosquamous carcinoma.[90] Identical conclusions were reached in a similar study of 255 cases of endometrial carcinomas with squamous differentiation by Abeler and Kjorstad.[91] The conclusions of these studies[90, 91] are therefore at variance with those from the older literature cited above.[83, 85–87] Until these differences are resolved with additional investigation, the significance of squamous elements in endometrial adenocarcinomas will remain controversial.

Rare variants of endometrioid adenocarcinomas in the mixed glandular and squamous category include glassy cell carcinoma and those in which the malignant squamous elements consist of a prominent population of clear or spindle cells.[92] Indeed, we have seen examples of endometrioid adenocarcinoma with a predominant component of malignant spindle squamous cells in which a malignant müllerian mixed tumor (MMMT) was a serious diagnostic consideration (Fig. 5-35). A similar case has been documented in the literature.[93] In contrast to MMMTs, however, the spindle cells in such cases merge almost imperceptibly with foci of more obvious squamous differentiation (Fig. 5-35). Eight examples of glassy cell carcinoma of the endometrium, considered poorly differentiated adenosquamous carcinomas similar to those encountered more commonly in the cervix (see Ch. 3), have been reported.[94–97] Although five of the eight tumors behaved aggressively (including one with pulmonary metastases[96]), the number of cases is too small to determine if this histological pattern has an adverse prognostic effect independent of that attributable to the high grade of these tumors.

An unusual complication of endometrial (and ovarian) adenocarcinomas with squamous differentiation is the presence of keratin granulomas on the peritoneum.[98, 99] Although these lesions are usually incidental microscopic findings, in some cases they have been recognizable grossly as granules, flecks, or small yellow-white nodules[99] (Fig. 5-36). The involved sites include, in descending order of frequency, the ovaries (Fig. 5-36), the fallopian tubes, the uterus, the omentum, the extragenital parietal peritoneum, the appendix, the sigmoid colon, the small bowel, and the cul-de-sac.[99] On histologic examination, the granulomas consist of keratin or shadows of necrotic squamous cells, or both, surrounded by a foreign-body granulomatous response (Fig. 5-37), and in some cases, by a florid proliferation of mesothelial cells. These keratin granulomas are likely due to transtubal spread of keratin and necrotic cells that exfoliate from the surfaces of the carcinomas; the finding of keratin within the lumina of the fallopian tubes in occasional cases supports this interpretation.[98, 99] In the reported series of cases, the presence of keratin granulomas appears to have had no adverse prognostic significance. The prognostic significance of these lesions, however, has not been established with complete certainty because of the short follow-up intervals in some cases, and because some of the patients have received postoperative radiation therapy or chemotherapy, or both, that might have influenced the postoperative course of any residual peritoneal lesions.[99] Keratin granulomas, if visible, should be extensively biopsied by the surgeon and carefully examined microscopically by the pathologist to exclude the additional presence of viable carcinoma cells.

Endometrioid Carcinomas With Trophoblastic Differentiation

Rare endometrioid adenocarcinomas exhibit focal trophoblastic differentiation, which in its fullest expression may include foci histologically indistinguishable from choriocarcinoma. Four endometrioid carcinomas with focal trophoblastic differentiation have been reported in women 48 to 78 years of age.[100, 101] Each tumor was characterized by the focal presence of syncytiotrophoblastic cells that were immunoreactive for human chorionic gonadotropin (hCG). The high serum level of hCG in the three cases in which it was determined dropped significantly after treatment. All patients had an unusually rapid clinical course; three patients died from tumor within 15 months of presentation and the fourth was alive with pulmonary metastases at the time of reporting. In one case, biopsy of the metastases revealed pure choriocarcinoma.[100] An additional case of an hCG-secreting endometrial adenocarcinoma in the literature was described as "highly anaplastic," but the presence of syncytiotrophoblastic elements was not specifically noted.[102] We have also seen endometrial carcinomas with trophoblastic differentiation, including a poorly differentiated endometrioid adenocarcinoma with squamous differentiation in a 63-year-old woman that contained extensive areas of typical choriocarcinoma (Fig. 5-38).

Endometrioid Carcinomas With Giant Cell Carcinoma or Osteoclast-Like Giant Cells

Recently, Jones et al.[103] reported six high-grade endometrial adenocarcinomas with a malignant giant cell component in women 43 to 85 years (mean, 65) of age. The giant cell component of the tumors (five of which were otherwise typical endometrioid carcinomas, and one, a clear cell adenocarcinoma) was composed of poorly

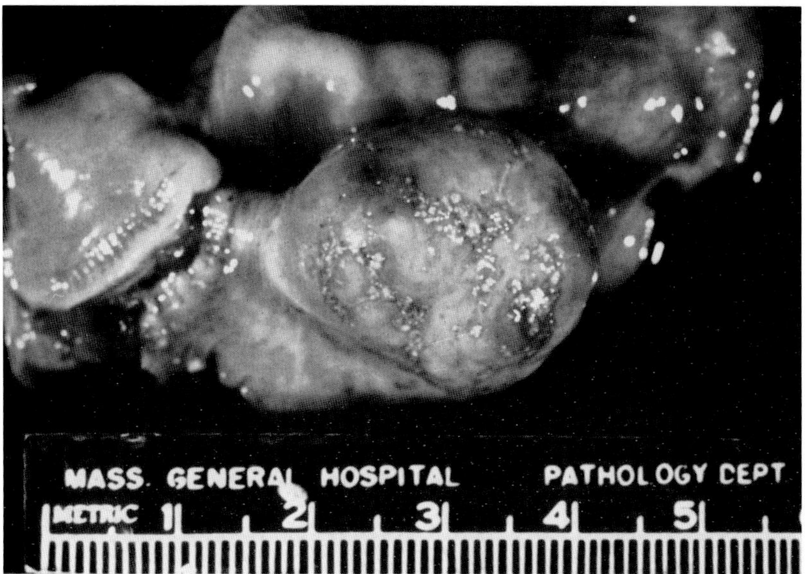

Fig. 5-36. Keratin granulomas on ovarian surface in patient with an endometrial endometrioid adenocarcinoma with squamous differentiation.

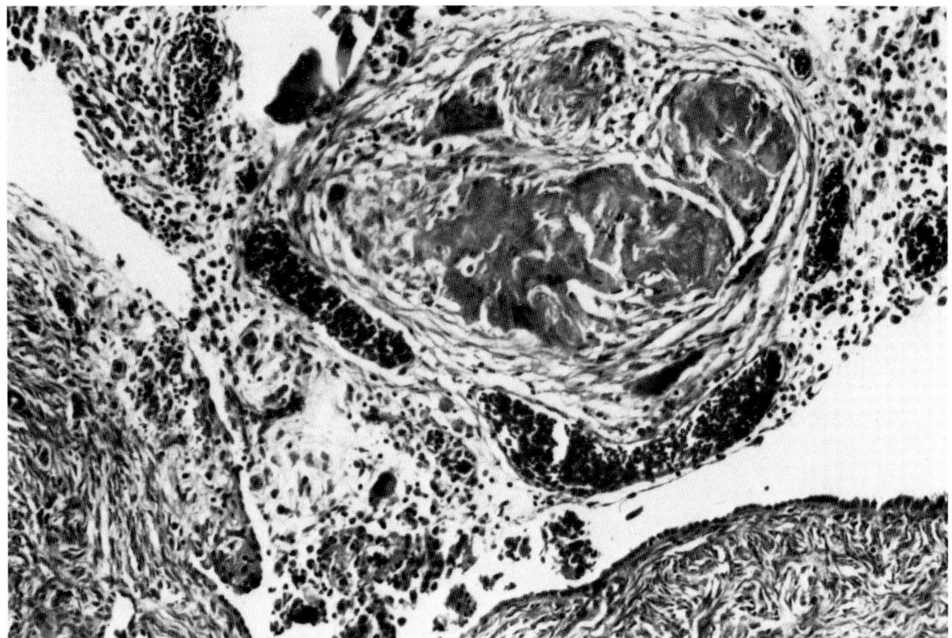

Fig. 5-37. Keratin granuloma on ovarian surface. A central mass of keratin is surrounded by foreign-body-type giant cells and a fibrotic reaction.

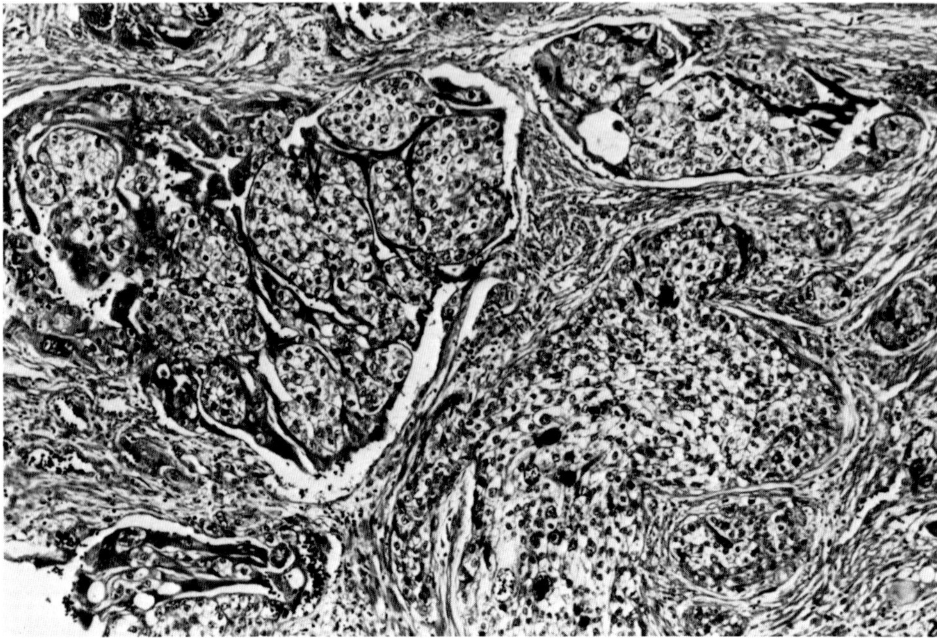

Fig. 5-38. Choriocarcinomatous differentiation in an endometrial adenocarcinoma in a 63-year-old woman; the neoplastic cells were immunoreactive for hCG. Elsewhere the tumor had the appearance of a poorly differentiated endometrioid adenocarcinoma.

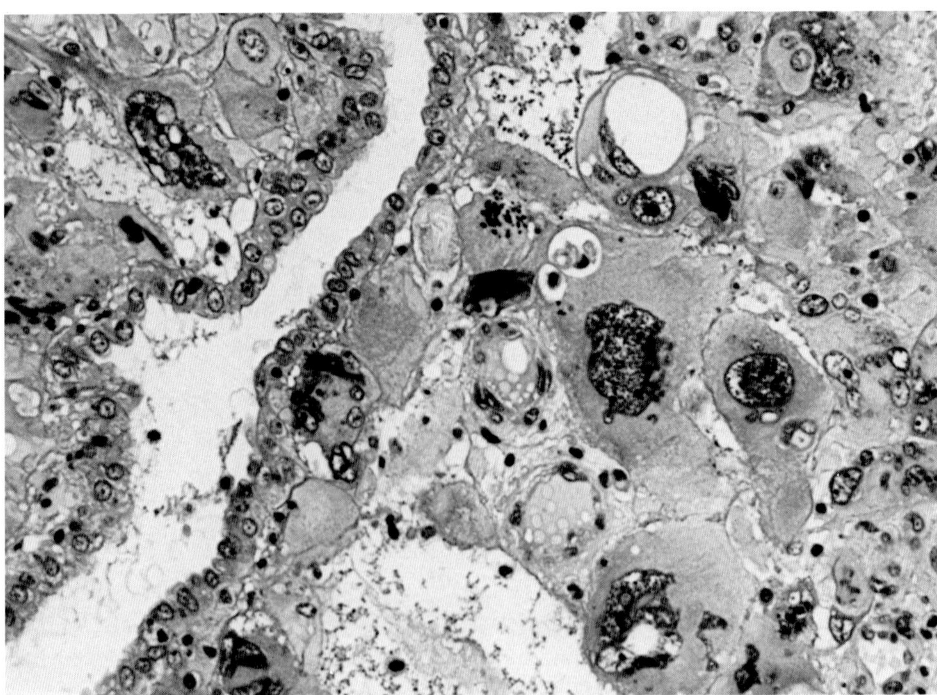

Fig. 5-39. Endometrial carcinoma with a component of malignant giant cells; in this field, the giant cells surround a benign gland.

cohesive sheets and nests of bizarre multi-nucleated giant cells (Figs. 5-39) admixed with an approximately equal number of mononucleate tumor cells. A sarcomatoid pattern and a marked inflammatory infiltrate were present in three cases. Occasional malignant giant cells were immunoreactive for cytokeratins, and epithelial membrane antigen (EMA) was present in the neoplastic giant cells in all three tumors tested. Osteoclast-like giant cells were not present. Three tumors were stage I, one was stage III, and two were stage IV. Two of the patients with stage I disease (each with superficial myometrial invasion) were alive and well 2 and 6 years later. Of the remaining four patients, three died of disease 5 months, 6 months, and 2.5 years after presentation, and one was alive with extensive abdominal disease after 1 year. Endometrial carcinomas with malignant giant cells are usually aggressive tumors that should be distinguished from other endometrial tumors with a prominent giant cell component, including trophoblastic tumors, certain primary sarcomas, and MMMTs. It is also obviously imperative that malignant giant cells and non-neoplastic giant cells not be confused.

These tumors should also be distinguished from carcinomas characterized by the presence of large numbers of cytologically benign multinucleated osteoclast-like giant cells.[104] In two tumors of this type, "a larger component of atypical stromal cells, including malignant-appearing giant cells" was also present. Those cells were described as larger and more atypical than the osteoclast-like giant cells and, unlike them, were positive for cytokeratins, EMA, and vimentin.

SEROUS PAPILLARY
ADENOCARCINOMA

Clinical Features. Although papillary carcinomas of the endometrium resembling serous carcinomas of the ovary had been described sporadically in the literature over the past 25 years, it was not until 1981 and 1982 that Lauchlan[105] and Hendrickson et al.,[66] respectively, drew major attention to these tumors (SPECs). SPECs accounted for 10 percent of pathologic stage I carcinomas in the series of the latter investigators, although some tumors in that study might have been interpreted as papillary clear cell carcinomas by other authorities.[66] At other centers, the frequency has varied from 1.1 to 7.8 percent.[67–69, 71, 106–108]

The presenting clinical features of the patients with SPECs are in general similar to those with typical endometrial carcinoma, although some differences have been noted.[66–71, 105–131] The patients tend to be a decade older (mean age late sixties to early seventies) than are patients with typical endometrial carcinoma,[66, 67, 106, 108, 117] are less apt to have a history of estrogen use,[66, 119] and are more likely to have an abnormal Papanicolaou smear, which may contain psammoma bodies.[66, 70, 107, 126] One study has noted a higher frequency in blacks.[67] The patients typically present with postmenopausal bleeding, but occasionally a serous or serosanguinous vaginal discharge is the initial manifestation of the disease.[105, 110] Some tumors may be a late complication of pelvic radiation: in one study, three of eight cases of postradiation endometrial carcinomas were SPECs.[119] In another series of six postradiation SPECs, the mean interval between the radiation and the development of the SPEC was 16.1 years (range 4 to 25 years).[129]

Patients with SPEC frequently present with high-stage disease: in some of the earlier studies, as many as 25 percent had clinical stage III or IV tumors at the time of diagnosis,[67] with this figure rising to as high as 75 percent if intraoperative findings are considered (surgicopathological stage).[67, 68, 71, 106, 110, 114, 115, 119, 131] When lymph node dissections are performed, the pelvic and para-aortic lymph nodes are involved in 25 to 57 percent of the cases.[109, 111, 117, 118] Intraoperative peritoneal washings contain malignant cells in 35 to 75 percent of cases.[71, 106, 107, 117, 118] The serum CA 125 level may be elevated at presentation and may be useful in monitoring the effects of therapy.[70, 121] Elevations of serum carcinoembryonic antigen (CEA),[116] α-fetoprotein (AFP),[127] NB/70K,[121] and lipid-associated sialic acid[121] have also been reported.

Pathologic Features. On gross examination, SPECs do not differ significantly from typical endometrial carcinoma except that the uterus may be small and atrophic in the presence of extensive myometrial and myometrial lymphatic involvement[66] (Fig. 5-40). On histologic examination, SPECs resemble ovarian serous carcinomas, and are characterized by a complex papillary pattern composed of papillae with thin (or rarely broad) fibrovascular stalks covered by stratified epithelial cells associated with cellular buds (Figs. 5-41 to 5-44). The tumor cells and cellular buds may also line irregular slit-like glandular spaces, and occasionally such a pattern may predominate (Fig. 5-42). The tumor cells are usually high grade with nuclear pleomorphism, hyperchromasia, macronucleoli, and frequent mitotic figures (Figs. 5-42 and 5-43). Hobnail-type cells (Fig. 5-42) and giant cells with bizarre nuclear features may be present.

Psammoma bodies (Fig. 5-44) have been observed in 10 to 59 percent of cases.[66, 131] Tumor necrosis is frequent. In occasional cases, SPECs appear to arise within an endometrial polyp (Figs. 5-45 and 5-46), and may be confined to it or invade the underlying myometrium[123, 128, 131] (Fig. 5-45). SPECs may be admixed with other types of endometrial carcinoma, including endometrioid (typical and villoglandular forms) and clear cell carcinoma.[128, 131] In contrast to endometrioid adenocarcinomas, which are frequently associated with endometrial hyperplasia elsewhere in the same uterus, the endometrium uninvolved by SPEC was atrophic in more than 90 percent of the cases in one study.[131]

Microscopic examination reveals a high frequency of local invasion, or metastasis, or both, manifested by deep myometrial invasion in 40 to 70 percent of cases[66, 70, 106, 117] and permeation of myometrial lymphatics in 37 to 87 percent of cases[66, 70, 114] (Fig. 5-44). The lower uterine segment, cervix, adnexa, and peritoneal surfaces are more commonly involved than by endometrioid carcinomas.[66] Cervical and adnexal involvement is often within lymphatics and inapparent grossly. The papillary pattern is typically preserved in

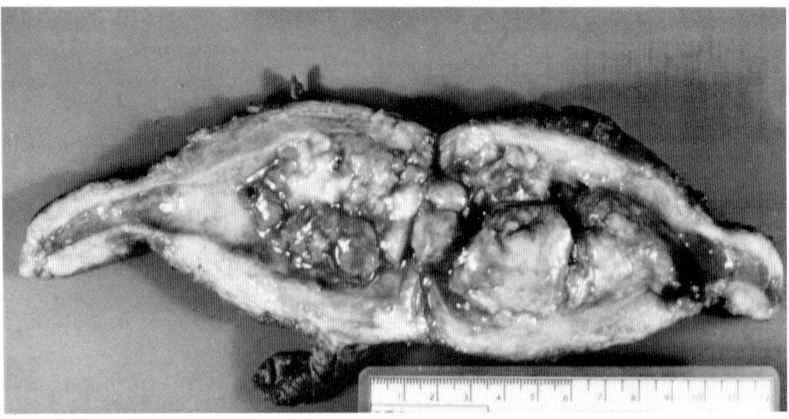

Fig. 5-40. Serous papillary adenocarcinoma of endometrium. An exophytic mass fills the endometrial cavity. The myometrium appears grossly normal, but the myometrial lymphatics were extensively involved on microscopic examination (see Fig. 5-44).

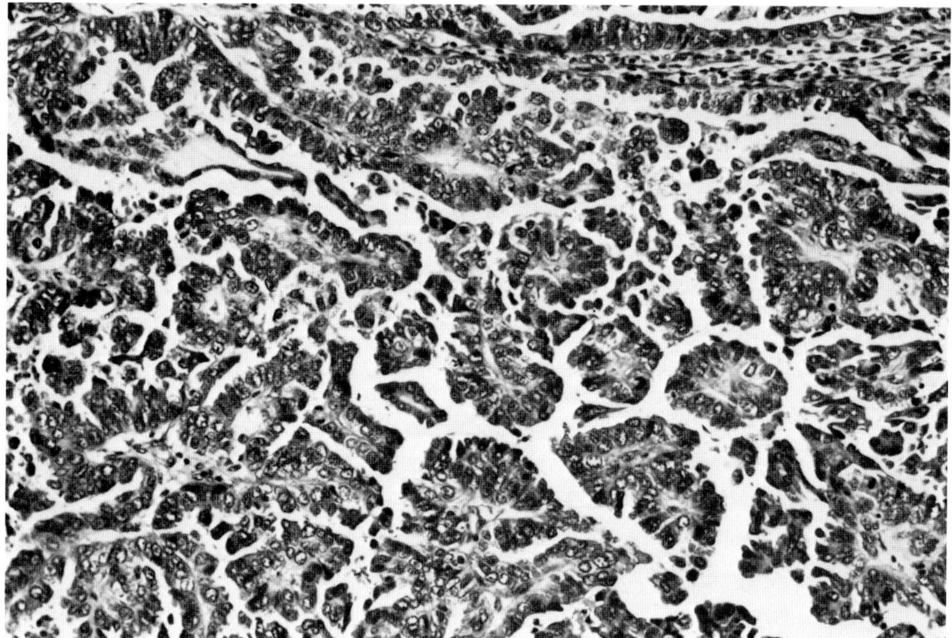

Fig. 5-41. Serous papillary adenocarcinoma.

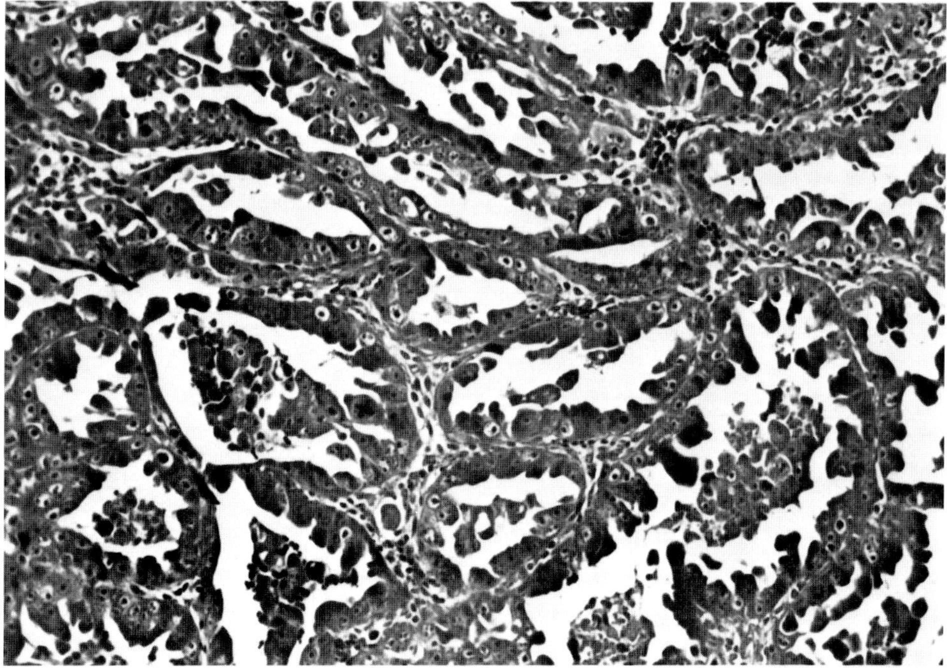

Fig. 5-42. Serous papillary adenocarcinoma. The predominant pattern in this field is that of glands and slitlike spaces lined by anaplastic tumor cells, some of hobnail type, that form intraluminal buds and papillae.

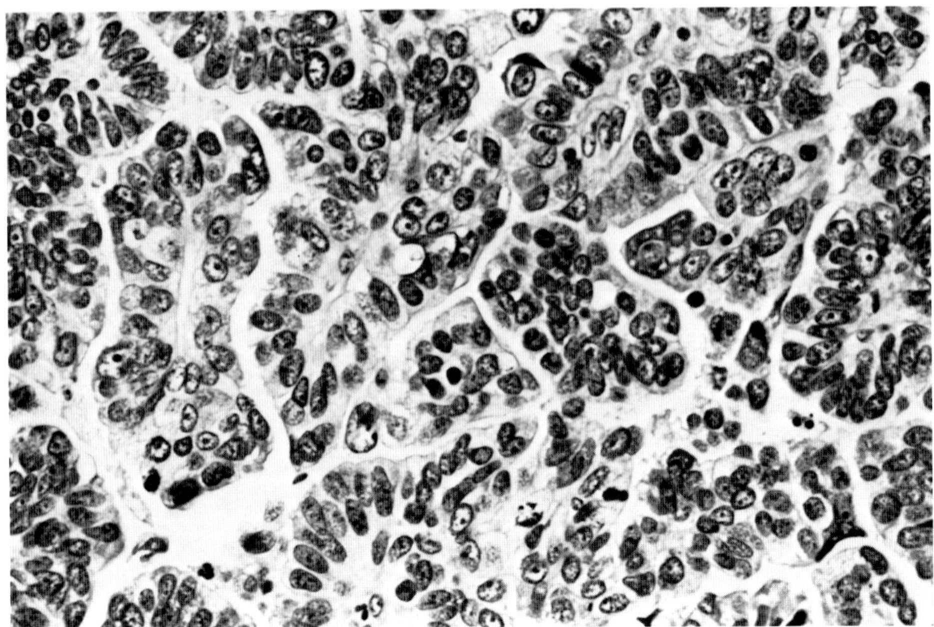

Fig. 5-43. Serous papillary adenocarcinoma. Note marked cellular stratification, cellular buds, and moderate to high-grade nuclear features.

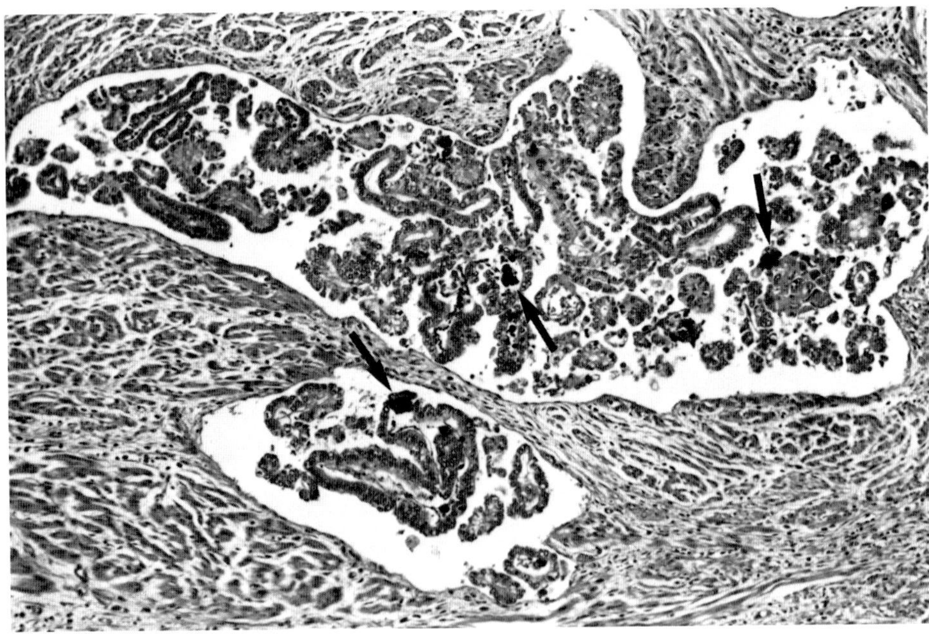

Fig. 5-44. Serous papillary adenocarcinoma invading myometrial lymphatics (same tumor as illustrated in Fig. 5-40). Note psammoma bodies (arrows).

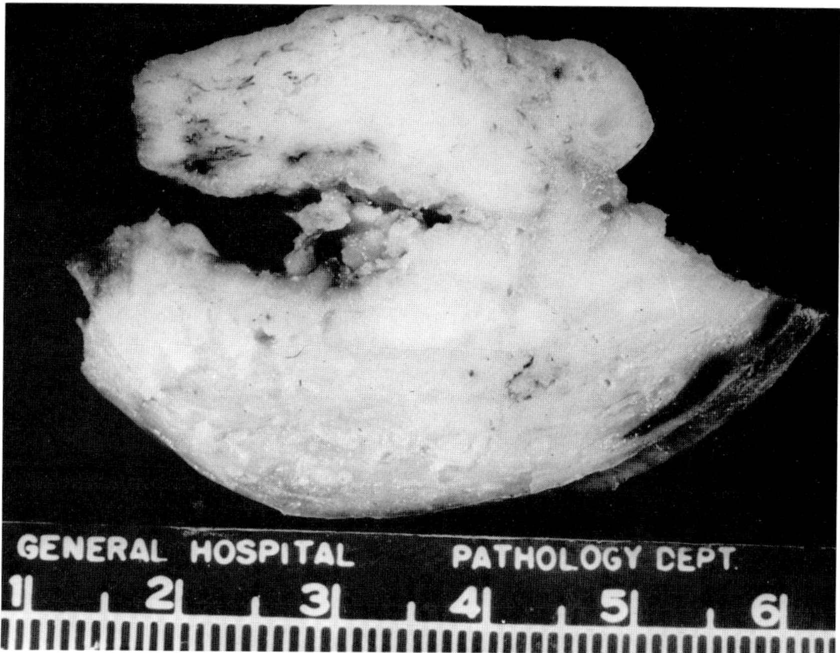

Fig. 5-45. Serous papillary adenocarcinoma involving an endometrial polyp and invading the underlying myometrium.

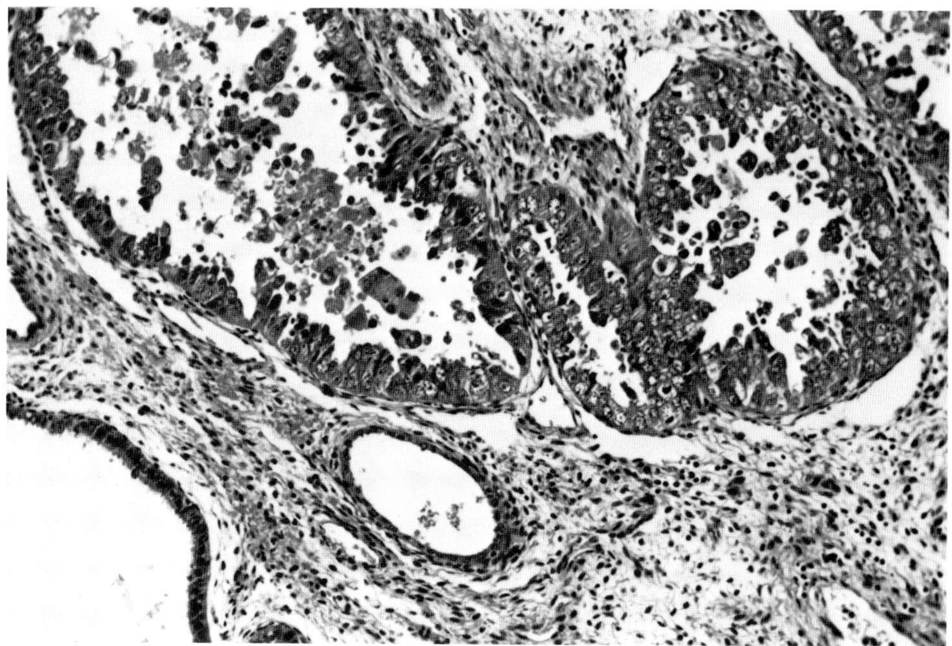

Fig. 5-46. Serous papillary adenocarcinoma involving an endometrial polyp. The fibrotic stroma of the polyp and part of a residual atrophic gland (lower left) are also seen.

the invasive (Fig. 5-44) and metastatic tumor. Changes suggestive of in situ serous papillary carcinoma have been noted on the surface of the endometrium, endocervix, endosalpinx, omentum and ovary,[66, 110, 118, 123, 128, 131, 131a] although it is unclear whether these findings reflect luminal and peritoneal spread of exfoliated tumor cells or multicentric neoplasia. Because of the high frequency of microscopic involvement of the myometrium, cervix, and adnexa, extensive pathologic sampling of these areas should be performed.

SPECs do not differ significantly from other endometrial carcinomas on immunohistochemical examination[130] and do not have distinctive ultrastructural features.[112] A high frequency of aneuploidy,[122, 131b] C-*myc* amplification,[122] and p53 expression (p. 250) have been found in SPECs.

Behavior and Management. SPECs have a much worse prognosis than that of typical endometrial carcinoma and are more aggressive than even poorly differentiated and deeply invasive examples of the latter. In the series of Hendrickson et al., 50 percent of the patients with surgical stage I tumor had a relapse, a frequency five times that of patients with endometrioid endometrial adenocarcinoma.[66] Although SPECs accounted for only 10 percent of the surgical stage I endometrial carcinomas in that study, they accounted for 50 percent of the cases with relapse, and for 6 of 7 cases with relapse in the upper abdomen. Only 15 percent of patients with higher-stage disease were alive with no evidence of tumor at the time of the last follow-up examination. In another series of SPECs,[108] the 5- and 10-year survival rates were 27 percent and 14 percent, respectively. In additional series, overall survival rates have been 27 percent[106] and 34 percent,[71] and for surgical stage I tumors, 33 percent[114] and 47 percent.[71] One study found that when a SPEC is admixed with another histologic subtype and accounts for at least 25 percent of the tumor, the tumor

typically behaves as a pure SPEC.[131] However, we have seen occasional otherwise typical or villoglandular endometrioid adenocarcinomas that contained only microscopic foci of SPEC in which the latter component extensively invaded myometrial lymphatics, and therefore suspect that any component of SPEC in a mixed carcinoma may adversely affect the prognosis. Although an absence of myometrial invasion has been a good prognostic factor in some series,[66, 119] tumors that were apparently confined to the endometrium or an endometrial polyp were associated with peritoneal spread in other studies.[123, 128, 131, 131a] These observations may reflect multicentric origin of tumor or metastases from transtubal spread of tumor. In the study by Sherman et al., tumors with vascular invasion were more commonly associated with extrauterine dissemination than tumors lacking this feature (84 percent versus 56 percent).[131] Occasional patients with clinical or pathologic stage I disease may have a recurrence outside the pelvis and abdomen.[115, 119]

Because SPECs exhibit a propensity to spread transperitoneally in a manner similar to that of surface epithelial carcinomas of the ovary, it has been recommended that if the diagnosis is made by curettage, peritoneal washings, inspection of the peritoneum including that of the upper abdomen, biopsy of suspicious lesions, sampling of para-aortic lymph nodes (which may harbor microscopic tumor in the absence of grossly evident extrauterine tumor[106]), and omentectomy should be performed at the time of hysterectomy. Grossly evident extrauterine disease should be resected as completely as possible. Current postoperative treatment recommendations include adjuvant abdominopelvic irradiation for stage I cases with any degree of myometrial invasion. One recent study[125] has suggested that irradiation also be given to the vaginal apex, in an effort to decrease the risk of recurrence at this site. In some centers, chemotherapy is also added to the treatment regimen.[119] Complete, but often only temporary, remission after combination chemotherapy has been observed in some patients with higher stage disease.[113, 116] As noted, even patients with no demonstrable myometrial invasion may experience recurrence, but much less commonly than patients with myometrial invasion, suggesting a possible role for similarly aggressive treatment in these patients.

Differential Diagnosis. Involvement of the uterine corpus by a serous carcinoma arising at other sites, especially the ovary and fallopian tube, should be excluded before rendering a diagnosis of SPEC. With respect to cases with synchronous ovarian involvement, the tumor was considered a SPEC in the Stanford series only when the dominant disease was in the uterus and the ovarian involvement was confined to lymphatics within the hilus or was limited to microscopic disease within the cortex as part of widespread peritoneal disease.[66] The differential diagnosis of SPEC also includes villoglandular endometrioid carcinoma. VGECs are characterized by an orderly pattern composed of villus-like papillae and glands lined by a pseudostratified layer of columnar cells that usually have low-grade nuclear features and form few or no cellular buds. The complex papillarity, the marked cellular stratification, and the high-grade nuclear features of SPECs are absent. Clear cell carcinomas (see below) may be papillary, and when accompanied by high-grade nuclear features, have an appearance that overlaps with that of SPECs. Indeed, one-third of the SPECs in two series contained foci of clear cells,[66, 131] and the authors of one of these studies[66] indicated that some of these tumors would be regarded as clear cell carcinomas by other investigators. The presence of papillae with hyalinized cores, a tubulocystic pattern, and a prominent component of clear cells or hobnail cells, or combinations thereof, strongly support or are diagnostic of a diagnosis of clear cell carcinoma. Psammoma bodies may occur in both tumors, but are more common in SPECs. In some cases, the distinction between the two tumors may be arbitrary. As both tumors have a similar behavior, their histologic distinction is not crucial. Finally, SPECs should be distinguished from "papillary syncytial metaplasia" (see Ch. 4). This distinction should not be problematic, as this type of metaplasia is typically a microscopic finding confined to the endometrial surface, and is characterized by the presence of cytologically bland cells, and is generally considered a regenerative phenomenon in a late menstrual or postcurettage endometrium.

CLEAR CELL ADENOCARCINOMA

Clear cell adenocarcinomas of the endometrium (CCCEs), as noted above, overlap to some extent both clinically and histologically with serous papillary carcinomas, and account for 1 to 6.6 percent of endometrial carcinomas.[69, 72, 75, 124, 128, 132–142] At one institution their frequency declined over a 30-year period from 6 (1955 to 1969) to 3 percent (1970 to 1984) of endometrial adenocarcinomas.[140] Patients with CCCE tend to be slightly older than those with endometrioid adenocarcinomas[72, 136, 141]; the mean ages of those with the former tumors in four large series were 63 years,[142] 65 years,[141] 66 years,[137] and 68 years.[75] In another study,[72] the median age was 67 years, 7 years older than the age of patients with all types of endometrial carcinoma combined. Two tumors have occurred in women in their third decade, although in one case the tumor occupied the lower uterine segment and was in contact with the upper endocervix from which it could have arisen.[75, 138] In several series, the tumors were more common in black patients.[72, 136] In one study,[72] 16 percent of patients had a history of pelvic irradiation 10 to 44 years prior to the diagnosis of the carcinoma. There has been no association between

CCCEs and in utero exposure to diethylstilbestrol. The presenting clinical manifestations do not differ significantly from those of patients with typical endometrial adenocarcinoma. In the largest series of cases,[141] 30 percent of the patients were surgicopathologic stage II or higher.

CCCEs have no characteristic gross features (Fig. 5-47). On microscopic and ultrastructural examination, the tumors resemble clear cell carcinomas of ovarian, vaginal, and cervical origin, being composed of one or more of the following cell types and patterns: polygonal cells with abundant, clear, glycogen-rich cytoplasm and generally eccentric nuclei, hobnail cells, and flattened cells; these cells may be arranged in tubulocystic, papillary, or solid patterns, or in a combination of these patterns (Figs. 5-48 to 5-52). Solid areas are typically composed mainly of clear cells (Fig. 5-48); tubules and papillae are typically lined by clear or hobnail cells (Figs. 5-49 to 5-52); and cystic spaces are lined by flattened or hobnail cells (Figs. 5-49, 5-51, and 5-52). In occasional cases, some tumor cells have abundant oxyphilic cytoplasm

(Fig. 5-52). Intraluminal mucin is typically present and eosinophilic hyaline mucin droplets in intracytoplasmic vacuoles producing signet-ring-like or "targetoid" cells are present focally in up to one-half of cases.[72, 142] The tumor cells typically have grade 2 or grade 3 nuclear features.[72, 142] Prominent stromal hyalinization resulting from the deposition of basement membrane material may be present, especially within the cores of the papillae (Figs. 5-49 and 5-50). Psammoma bodies are identifiable in approximately 10 percent of the cases, usually in association with a papillary pattern.[72, 75, 136] The stroma frequently contains a lymphoplasmocytic infiltrate.[142] The tumor may involve, or occasionally be confined to, endometrial polyps.[75, 128, 142] In the largest series in the literature,[141] 17 percent of the tumors were intramucosal, 50 percent invaded the inner half of the myometrium, and 22 percent extended into the outer half. Invasion of myometrial blood vessels or lymphatics was present in 23 percent of cases and was typically associated with deep myometrial invasion.

The distinction of CCCEs from serous

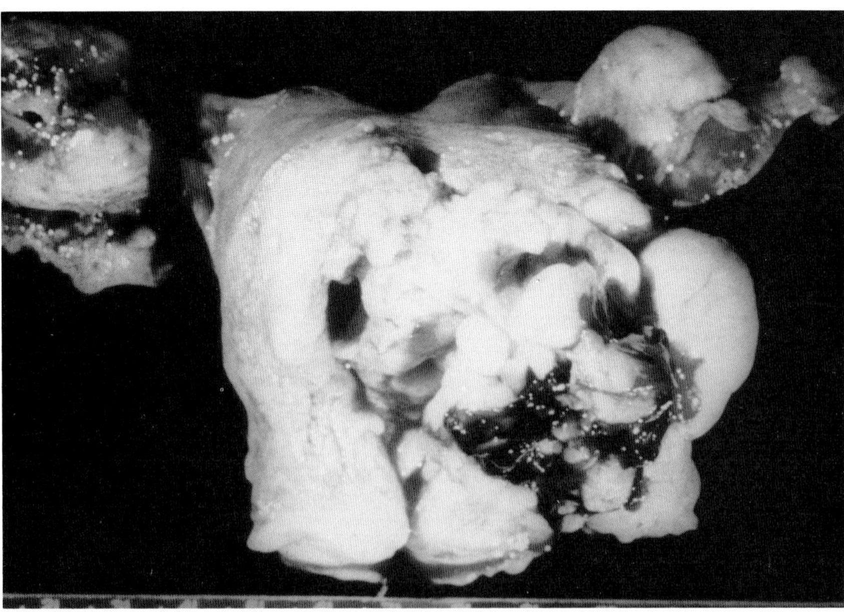

Fig. 5-47. Clear cell adenocarcinoma of endometrium. A polypoid mass fills the endometrial cavity.

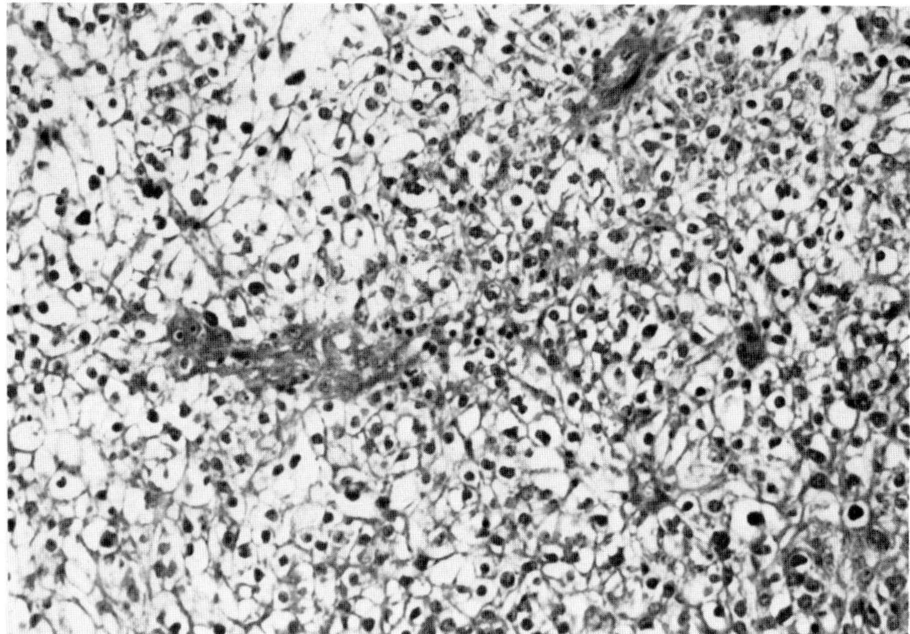

Fig. 5-48. Clear cell adenocarcinoma of endometrium, solid pattern of polygonal cells with clear cytoplasm and eccentric nuclei.

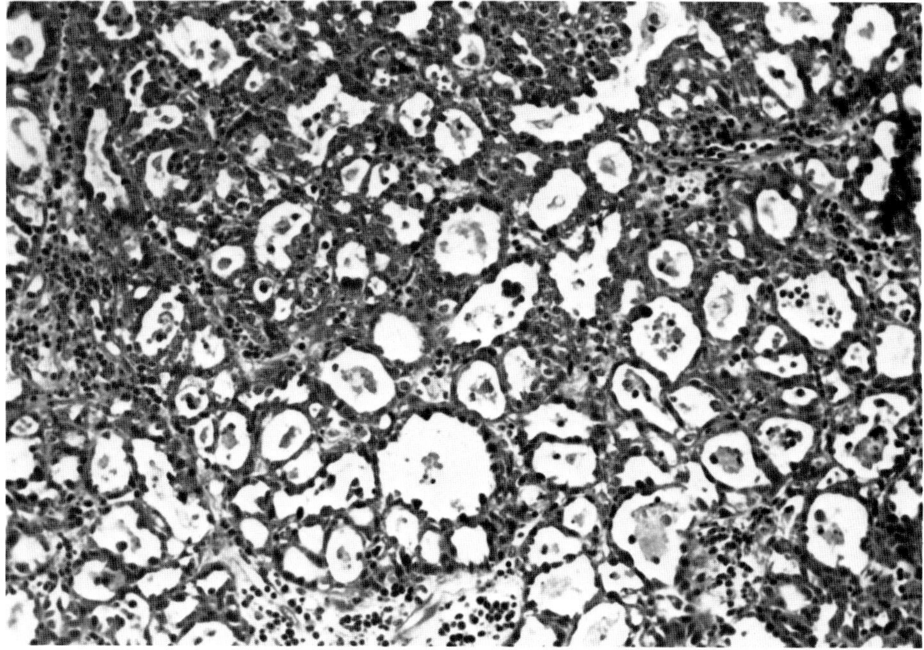

Fig. 5-49. Clear cell adenocarcinoma of endometrium, tubulocystic pattern. The tubules and cysts are lined by flattened, cuboidal, and hobnail cells.

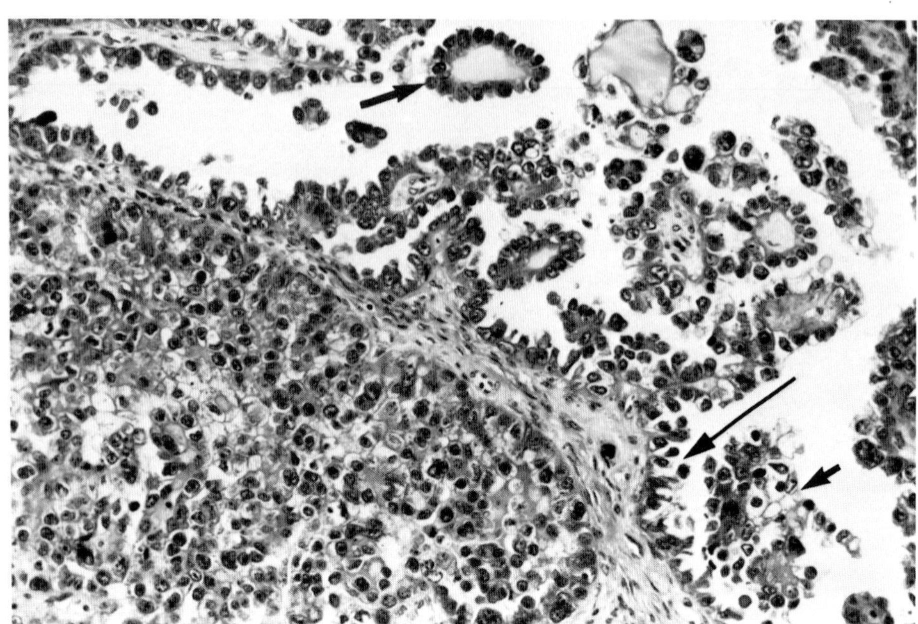

Fig. 5-50. Clear cell adenocarcinoma of endometrium solid and papillary patterns. Note papillae with hyalinized cores (medium arrow), clear cells (short arrow), and hobnail cells (long arrow).

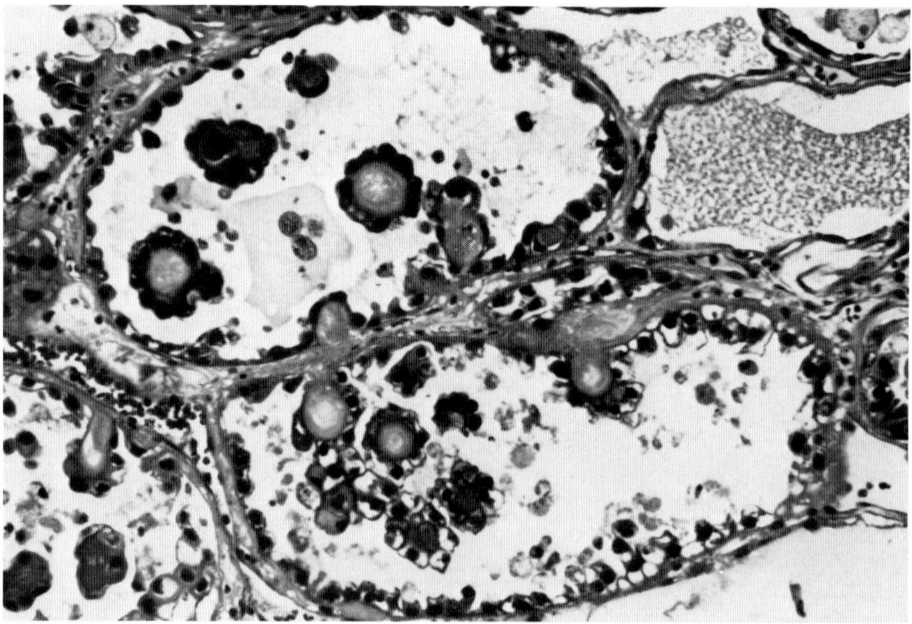

Fig. 5-51. Clear cell adenocarcinoma of endometrium, tubulocystic pattern with intraluminal papillae. Note papillae with hyalinized cores, clear cells, and hobnail cells.

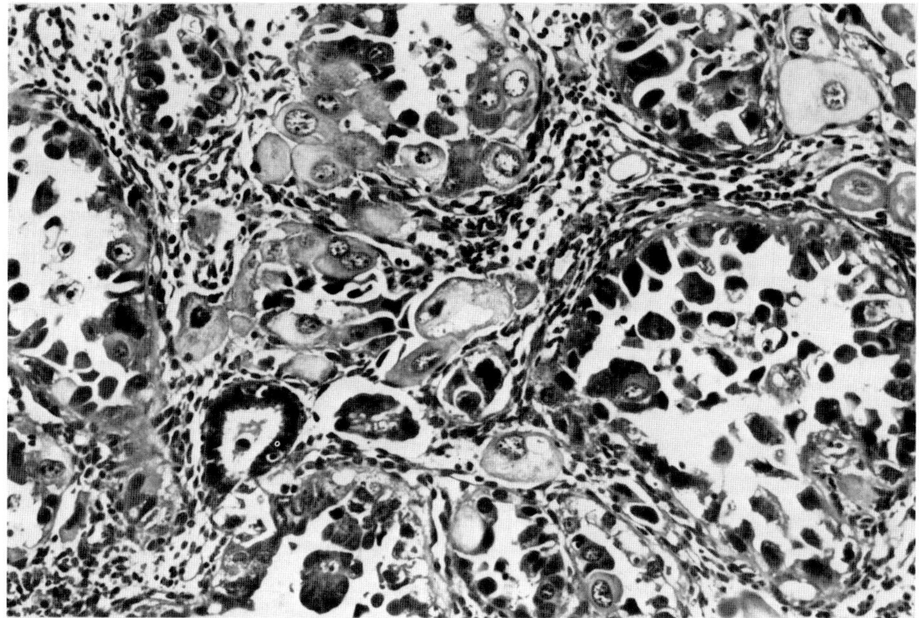

Fig. 5-52. Clear cell adenocarcinoma of endometrium, tubulocystic pattern. In addition to hobnail cells, some of the cells lining the tubules and cysts have abundant oxyphilic cytoplasm.

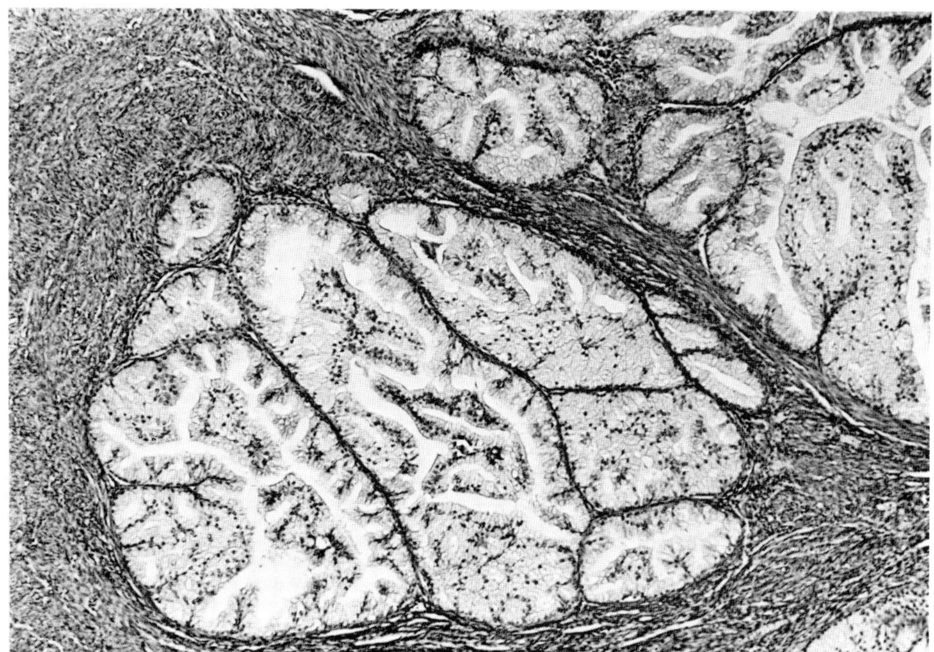

Fig. 5-53. Mucinous adenocarcinoma, grade 1, invading the myometrium.

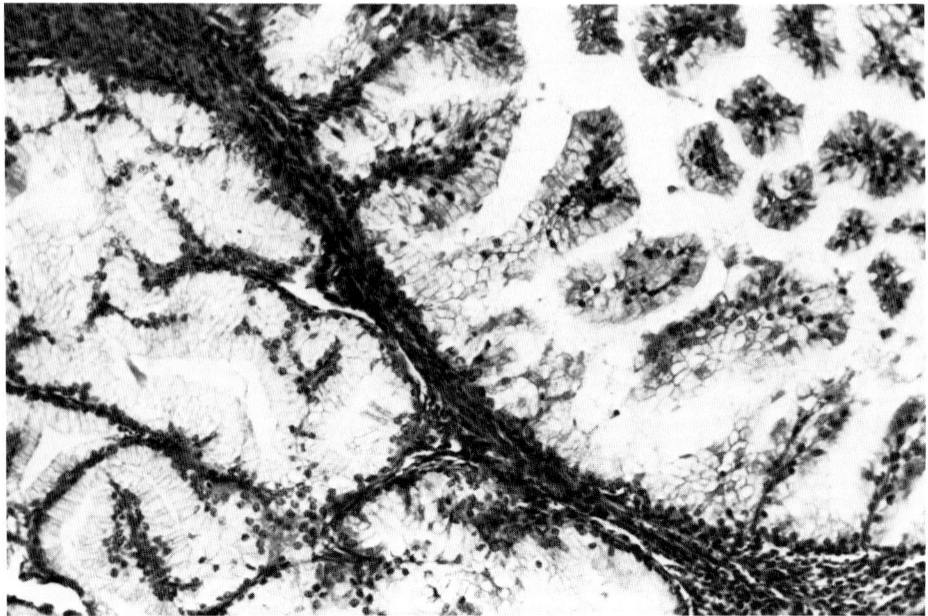

Fig. 5-54. Mucinous adenocarcinoma, grade 1, invading the myometrium, higher-power view of tumor illustrated in Figure 5-53. Note villoglandular pattern.

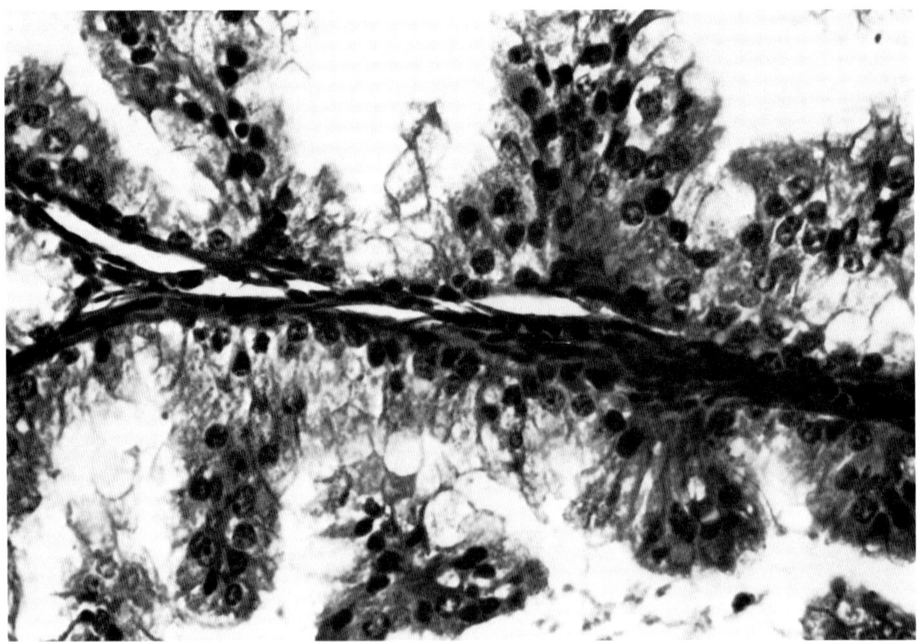

Fig. 5-55. Mucinous adenocarcinoma, higher-power view of tumor illustrated in Figure 5-53. Note stratified mucin-rich cells with relatively bland nuclear features.

papillary carcinomas has been discussed above. Secretory carcinomas have sometimes been grouped with CCCEs[132] and rare CCCEs contain foci of secretory carcinoma,[75] but as already noted the latter tumors are more appropriately considered a variant of endometrioid endometrial adenocarcinoma. Secretory carcinomas, in contrast to CCCEs, are characterized by a purely or predominantly glandular pattern, columnar cells with subnuclear vacuoles, and low-grade nuclear features.

CCCEs are aggressive tumors. In some studies, their prognosis has been similar to that of SPECs. In four large recent series, the 5-year survival rates (5YSR) have been 34 percent,[72] 42 percent,[141] 64 percent,[140] and 75 percent.[142] The higher survival rates in some series likely reflect a greater proportion of patients with stage I tumors, including those confined to the endometrium,[142] as stage and the presence or absence of myometrial invasion are the two most important prognostic parameters.[72, 75, 141] For example, in one study in which the overall 5YSR was 42 percent, it was 59 percent for stage 1 tumors and 90 percent for those with no myometrial invasion. By contrast, tumors that deeply invaded the myometrium were associated with a 15 percent 5YSR.[141] In the same study, invasion of endothelium-lined spaces was also an important prognostic parameter: this feature was associated with a 17 percent 5YSR compared to 49 percent in its absence. Five-year survival rates may underestimate the malignant potential of CCCEs. In one study, the 5YSR was 64 percent, but the 10YSR was only 35 percent.[140]

Mucinous Adenocarcinoma

This tumor is characterized by a predominant component of endocervical-type cells with mucin-rich cytoplasm; less than 75 cases have been reported in detail.[143–146] The diagnostic criterion in the series of Ross et al. was the presence of abundant periodic acid-Schiff (PAS) positive diastase-resistant intracytoplasmic material in more than 50 percent of the neoplastic cells; there was considerable variability in mucin content and distribution, however, between the cases and even within an individual case.[145] More than 70 percent of neoplastic cells were required to have mucin-rich cytoplasm for inclusion in the study of mucinous carcinomas of the endometrium (MCEs) by Melhem and Tobon.[146] In the study by Ross et al.,[145] mucinous carcinomas accounted for 9 percent of pathologic stage I endometrial carcinomas, a figure that corresponds closely to that of 10 percent[147] obtained from the older literature. In contrast to the relative rarity of MCEs as just defined, minor foci of mucinous differentiation occur in almost 40 percent of otherwise typical endometrioid carcinomas.[145] The presenting features of patients with MCEs do not differ significantly from those of patients with endometrioid adenocarcinomas. The age range in one study was 47 to 89 (mean, 60.2 years).[146] The patients almost invariably have tumor confined to the uterus at presentation.

Most MCEs are well or moderately differentiated tumors with architecturally complex glandular, villoglandular, or villous patterns (Figs. 5-53 to 5-55). In the study by Ross et al., 80 percent of the tumors had at least a focal villoglandular or villous architecture.[145] In the same study, cribriform patterns, cystically dilated mucin-filled glands, and neutrophils within the luminal mucin or within intracellular mucin-filled spaces were also frequent findings.[145] Rare MCEs have a focal pattern simulating that of microglandular hyperplasia (see below). Zones of epithelial stratification (Fig. 5-55) and loss of nuclear polarity were present in all but one of the cases reported by Ross et al., although such changes were often very focal. All tumors had foci of cells with moderate nuclear atypia, but in more than 60 percent of cases, there were areas in which the nuclear atypia was only mild (Fig. 5-55), and 50 percent of the tumors contained small foci of mucinous epithelium that resembled normal endocervical epithelium.[145] Only 20 percent of the tumors had focal marked atypia. Using a combined architectural and cytologic grading system, the authors of this study graded the tumors as 1, 2, and 3 in 43 percent, 52 percent, and 5 percent of cases, respectively. Mitotic figures were not a prominent finding in any case. In the study by Melhem and Tobon, the tumors were graded 1, 2, and 3 in 72 percent, 17 percent, and 11 percent of the cases, respectively.[146] In occasional cases, the endometrium distant from the tumor may exhibit mucinous metaplasia.[146] The neoplastic cells in one study were immunoreactive for CEA in all cases, although there was considerable variability in the staining intensity.[146] Ross et al. found that the frequency of myometrial invasion in MCEs (50 percent), as well as the post-hysterectomy relapse rate, did not differ significantly from those of endometrioid carcinomas with minor mucinous differentiation or endometrioid carcinomas devoid of mucinous differentiation.[145]

Five endometrial adenocarcinomas characterized by focal histologic patterns that simulated microglandular hyperplasia on low-power examination of the curettage or biopsy specimens have been recently reported.[148] All the patients were postmenopausal, and two of them were receiving, or had received, Premarin and Provera and two patients, only Premarin. In the microglandular areas (Figs. 5-56 and 5-57), gland lumens typically contained eosinophilic mucinous secretion and numerous acute inflammatory cells, which were also characteristically prominent in the stroma. High-power examination, however, showed more cytologic atypia (Fig. 5-57) than acceptable for microglandular hyperplasia, and subsequent hysterectomy specimens contained residual adenocarcinoma

with more typical features; three were mucinous carcinomas and two, mixed mucinous and endometrioid carcinomas. These cases illustrate that microglandular hyperplasia should be diagnosed with caution in a postmenopausal patient if the lesional tissue is obtained from the endometrial cavity.

It is obviously important to differentiate MCEs from mucinous metaplasia, both typical and atypical (see Ch. 4); histologic distinction between the two lesions may be difficult, especially in a biopsy or curettage specimen. Features strongly favoring a diagnosis of MCE, as noted in the series by Ross et al., include architectural complexity, epithelial stratification, loss of nuclear polarity, and moderate nuclear atypia, although the last feature may be only focal.[145] Lesions not fulfilling these criteria are regarded as typical or atypical mucinous metaplasias (see Ch. 4). Because the evolution of untreated atypical mucinous metaplasia is unknown, Ross et al. recommend a hysterectomy when that diagnosis is made.[145]

When a mucinous carcinoma is found in a curettage or biopsy specimen, it is important to determine whether the tumor arose within the endocervix or endometrium because of differences in management of endocervical and endometrial adenocarcinomas; this differential diagnosis is discussed in Chapter 3. Colposcopy, hysteroscopy, and examination of both specimens from a fractional curettage with close attention to the nature of any non-neoplastic glands and stroma contiguous to the carcinoma establish the diagnosis in most cases. No histochemical or immunohistochemical methods are reliable in this distinction.[144, 145] Although the immunoprofile of most endometrial carcinomas (vimentin +, CEA−) differs from that of most endocervical adenocarcinomas (CEA +, vimentin −),[149–151] the typical CEA-immunoreactivity of MCEs noted above is an exception to these observations. In the study by Azumi et al., however, seven of

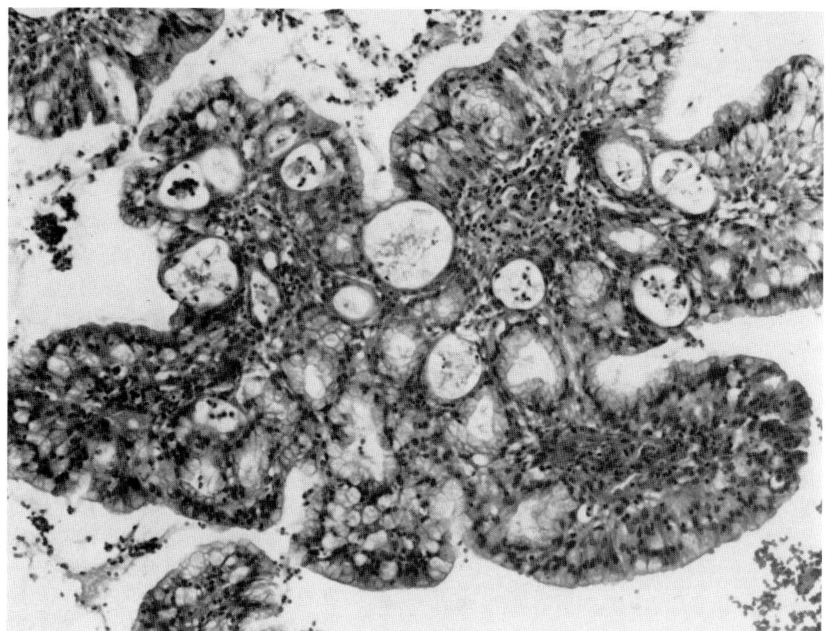

Fig. 5-56. Mucinous adenocarcinoma with focal microglandular pattern.

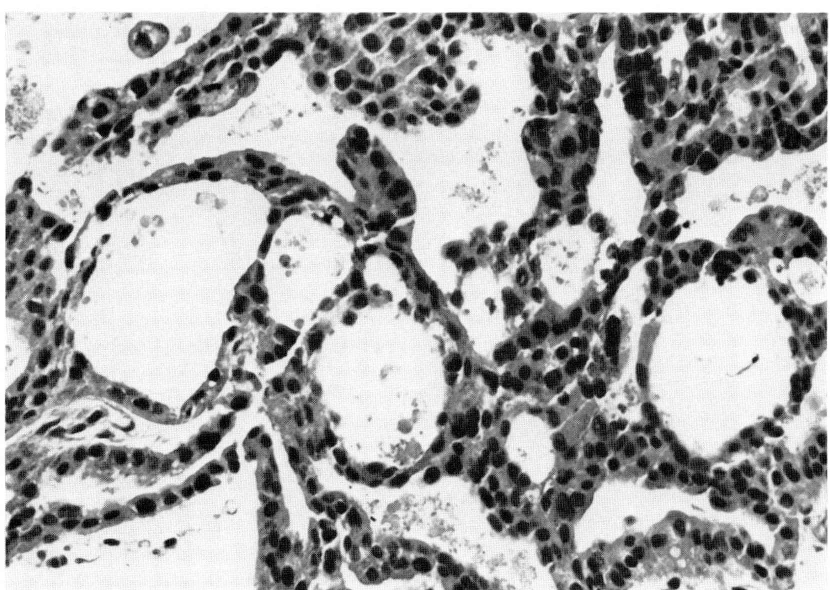

Fig. 5-57. Endometrial adenocarcinoma with focal microglandular pattern. Note hyperchromatic, focally pleomorphic nuclei.

seven MCEs, in contrast to only one of 12 endocervical adenocarcinomas, were immunoreactive for vimentin, suggesting that immunoreactivity for this marker favors a diagnosis of MCE over that of endocervical adenocarcinoma (Azumi N: personal communication).

SQUAMOUS CELL CARCINOMA

In contrast to the frequency of squamous elements within endometrioid adenocarcinomas, pure squamous cell carcinoma of the endometrium (ESCCs) is one of the rarest subtypes of endometrial carcinoma. Approximately 40 cases have been reported.[152–159] Criteria for ESCCs[152, 155] include an absence of coexisting adenocarcinoma, a lack of contiguity between the tumor and the cervical squamous epithelium, and an absence of an invasive cervical squamous cell carcinoma; if an in situ cervical squamous carcinoma exists, there must be no connection between it and the endometrial carcinoma as in situ squamous cell carcinoma of the cervix may spread to and line the entire endometrial cavity.[160, 161] The age of women with ESCCs has not differed significantly from those with other types of endometrial adenocarcinoma (range, 47 to 85 years; mean, 62.7 years).[152] Potentially predisposing factors that have been present in a minority of cases have included cervical stenosis, pyometra, and extensive endometrial squamous metaplasia. Approximately 50 percent of the tumors have spread beyond the uterus at the time of presentation (pathologic stage III or IV). ESCCs have a poor prognosis. In a review of the cases in the literature, Abeler and Kjorstad found that 40 percent of patients with pathologic stage I tumors died of their disease within 36 months.[152]

ESCCs may resemble endometrioid carcinomas on gross examination, although occasionally they have a condylomatous appearance (Fig. 5-58). Some ESCCs are obviously malignant on histologic examination, but occasional nonverrucous ESCCs are extremely well differentiated. In two such cases that we have encountered, endometrial curettage specimens in a postmenopausal woman yielded fragments of normal appearing, glycogenated squamous epithelium devoid of cellular atypia. Examination of the subsequent hysterectomy specimen disclosed a squamous cell carcinoma of the endometrium composed of

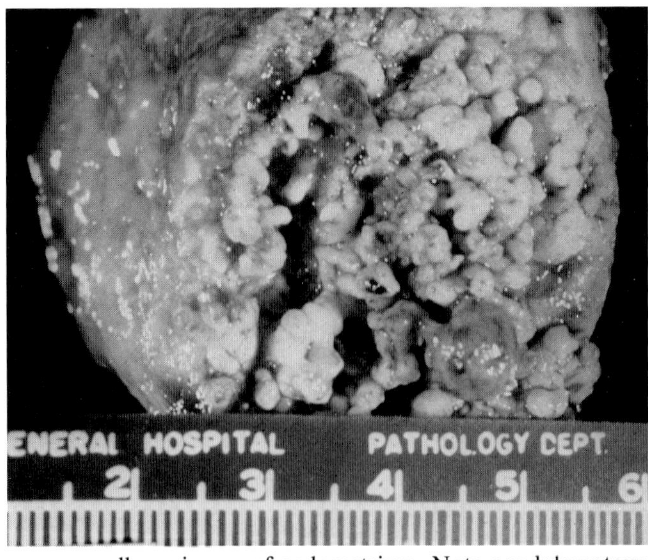

Fig. 5-58. Squamous cell carcinoma of endometrium. Note condylomatous appearance.

squamous epithelium identical to that within the curettage specimens (Fig. 5-59). Both tumors invaded the myometrium (Fig. 5-59) and one metastasized to several pelvic lymph nodes. Additional diagnostic problems can be encountered when an otherwise typical ESCC becomes infected by the human papillomavirus. In such cases, the virus can induce a condylomatous appearance with koilocytosis within, but more commonly on the surface of, the tumor.

Two cases of endometrial carcinoma that resembled verrucous carcinomas in other sites have been reported in women 61 and 64 years of age.[162, 163] In one case, the diagnosis was delayed 3 years because a curettage specimen at the time of presentation had been misinterpreted as a squamous papilloma.[163] Both tumors invaded the myometrium within the hysterectomy specimens, with one tumor extending almost to the serosa. The patients had uneventful follow-up periods of 2.5 and 6 years.

UNDIFFERENTIATED CARCINOMAS

Endometrial carcinomas that are too poorly differentiated to be categorized as one of the subtypes discussed above are unusual. In the only series of such tumors in the literature, undifferentiated carcinomas accounted for 1.6 percent of endometrial carcinomas.[164] In that study, approximately one-half of the tumors were of large cell type (Fig. 5-60), and the remainder of intermediate or small cell type; the latter tumors are considered in Chapter 8.

In the series cited above, patients with undifferentiated carcinomas (all cases) ranged in age from 45 to 86 years (mean, 63.9 years); the mean age of patients with large and intermediate cell tumors was older (66.2 years) than those with small cell tumors (58.3 years). One-third of the large cell tumors were associated with extrauterine spread (surgical stage III or IV). On microscopic examination, 78 percent of the large cell tumors invaded into the outer half of the myometrium, and 62 percent invaded lymphatics or blood vessels. All the large cell tumors were immunoreactive for cytokeratin, and less frequently vimentin (64 percent), CEA (18 percent), and NSE (36 percent). Occasional tumors that were immunoreactive for NSE also stained for Leu-7, bombesin, β-endorphin, or S-100. The 5- and 10-year survival rates for the large cell tumors were 54 percent and 39 percent, respectively. In another recent study, only one of five patients with undifferentiated carcinoma survived 5 years.[124]

ENDOMETRIAL CARCINOMAS WITH ARGYROPHIL CELLS

Up to 70 percent[165–167] of otherwise typical endometrioid endometrial adenocarcinomas contain cells that are positive on argyrophil staining; other studies report lower frequencies (22 to 53 percent).[168–171] Argyrophilia may also be encountered in other subtypes of endometrial adenocarcinoma, especially in small cell undifferentiated (neuroendocrine) carcinomas. Aguirre et al.[169] found that 14 of 48 endometrioid endometrial carcinomas (29 percent) were argyrophilic; five nonendometrioid carcinomas (three SPECs and two CCCEs) were not argyrophilic. The argyrophilia was present in the apical region of glandular cells or throughout the cytoplasm of glandular or squamous cells in eight of the cases. These patterns of argyrophilia were related to the presence of apical cytoplasmic mucin and glycogen granules, respectively; in a subsequent study, it was found that the apical mucin granules were immunoreactive for chromogranin.[166] In the remaining six cases in the series of Aguirre et al. (12.5 percent of the total),[169] the argyrophil cells resembled enterochromaffin cells (EC) of the intestinal tract; a similar frequency (10 percent) of EC-like cells was found in a study by Inoue et al.[167] EC-like

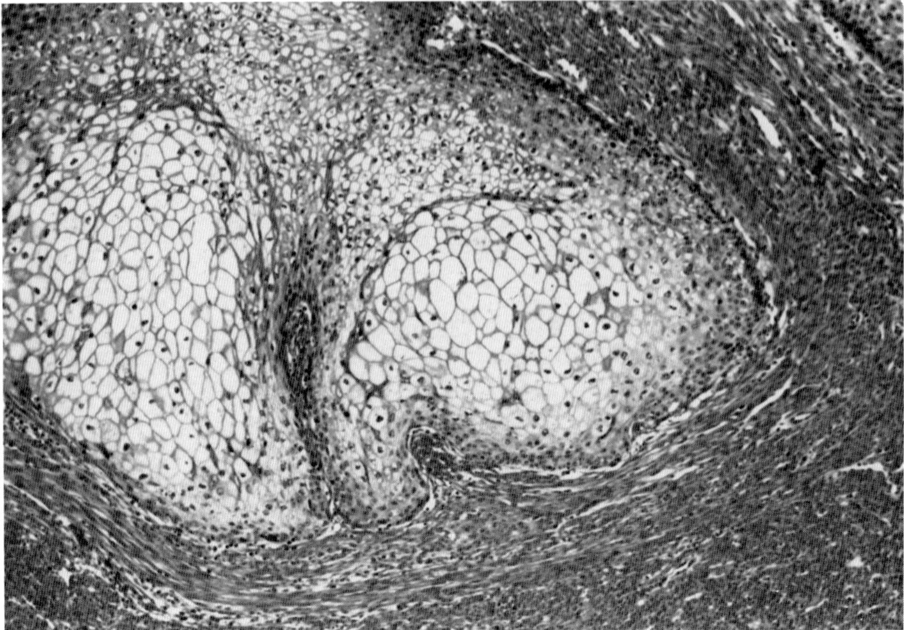

Fig. 5-59. Extremely well-differentiated squamous cell carcinoma of endometrium. In this field, the tumor is deeply invading the myometrium.

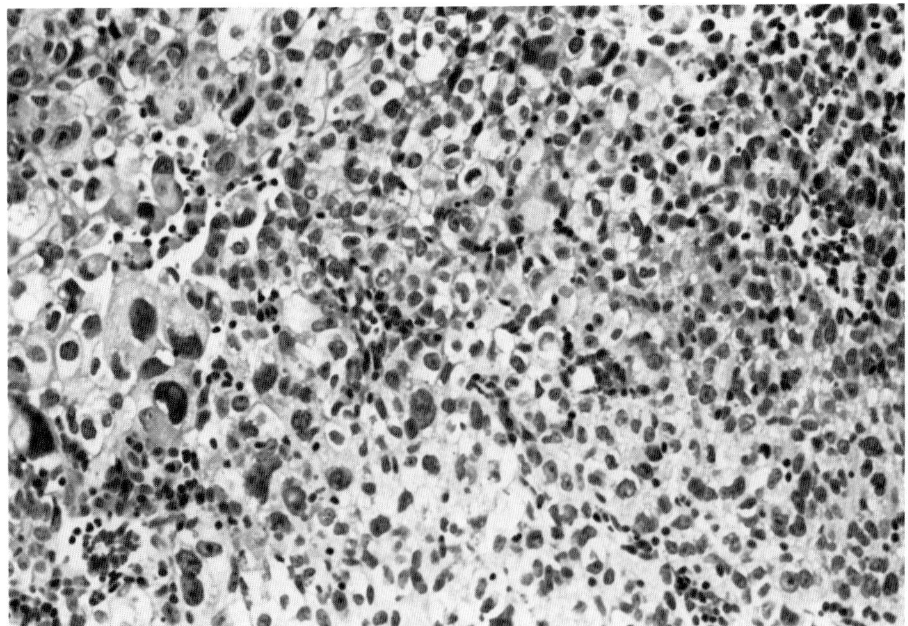

Fig. 5-60. Undifferentiated large cell carcinoma of endometrium.

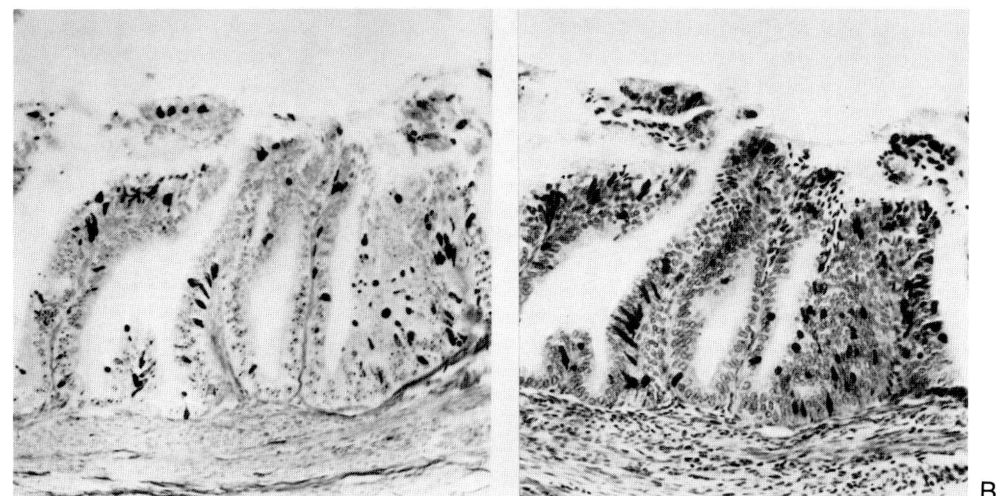

Fig. 5-61. Endometrial adenocarcinoma with argyrophilic cells of enterochromaffin type. **(A)** Grimelius stain. **(B)** Chromogranin stain.

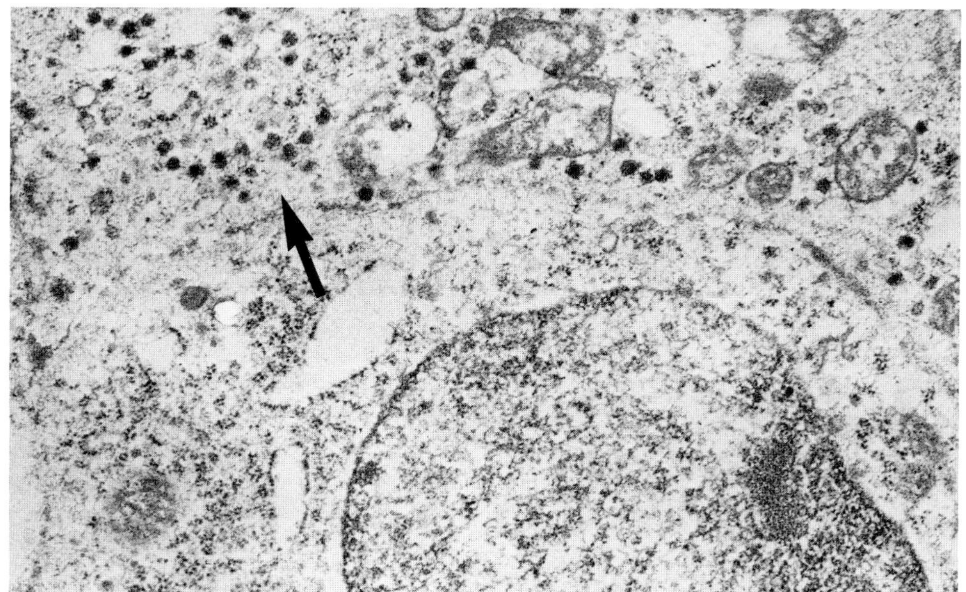

Fig. 5-62. Endometrial adenocarcinoma with argyrophilic cells of enterochromaffin type. Electron micrograph of tissue retrieved from paraffin. Collections of dense secretory granules (arrow) are present within the cytoplasm. (From Aguirre et al.,[169] with permission.)

cells appear as round, ovoid, or flask-shaped cells individually disposed within the glandular epithelium; occasional cells contain long cytoplasmic processes (Fig. 5-61). The cells may be vertically disposed (extending from the base of the gland to its lumen), in the midportion of the stratified neoplastic epithelium (without reaching the base or lumen in the plane of section), or horizontal along the base of the epithelium.[169] The EC-like argyrophil cells are typically immunoreactive for chromogranin (Fig. 5-61),[168, 172] serotonin,[169] and occasionally, one or more polypeptide hormones, including calcitonin, somatostatin, and ACTH.[165, 167, 169] Ultrastructural examination of these cells has disclosed granules 80 nm in diameter[169] (Fig. 5-62).

None of the patients with argyrophilic endometrioid carcinomas have had any associated endocrine manfestations. Apart from the tendency for argyrophil cells to be more common in well-differentiated carcinomas, most studies have found that their presence has had no apparent influence on tumor behavior.[165, 169, 170] Sato et al.,

however, found that grade 1 endometrial carcinomas with EC-like cells were associated with deeper myometrial invasion, a higher frequency of lymph node metastases, and a decreased survival.[171] Because of the widespread finding of argyrophilia in endometrial carcinomas of various types and because of its questionable clinical significance, the designation *"argyrophil cell carcinoma"* does not appear to be justified for clinical usage at the present time.

Berger et al. have reported an endometrial carcinoma that contained a variety of intestinal type cells.[173] The tumor had the appearance of a villoglandular endometrioid adenocarcinoma, but contained goblet cells and cells resembling Paneth cells. Histochemical and immunohistochemical stains revealed numerous argyrophilic EC-like cells, argentaffin cells, and cells that were immunoreactive for CEA, serotonin, gastrin, and somatostatin. We have also seen an otherwise typical endometrioid adenocarcinoma that contained prominent numbers of goblet cells (Fig. 5-63).

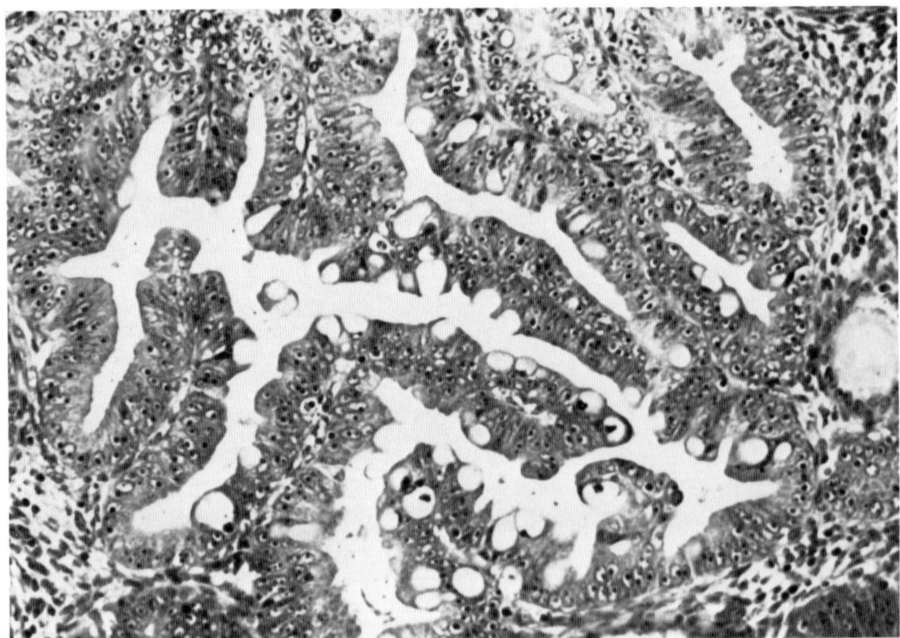

Fig. 5-63. Endometrial endometrioid adenocarcinoma with prominent goblet cells.

PROGNOSTIC FACTORS IN ENDOMETRIAL CARCINOMA

Aside from determining the histologic subtype of an endometrial carcinoma, the pathologist plays an important role in assessing a variety of other prognostic factors, some of which are used to determine the FIGO stage of the tumor (Table 5-2). Additionally, at some centers, the preoperative or intraoperative assessment of some of these features may play a role in determining the advisability of sampling retroperitoneal lymph nodes. Prognostic factors in endometrial carcinoma include tumor size, grade, depth of myometrial invasion, presence or absence of vascular invasion, cervical invasion, lymph node metastases, adnexal involvement, peritoneal cytologic findings, DNA and steroid receptor content, and oncogene expression, as well as nontumor prognostic factors.

Histologic Grade

The FIGO grading system for endometrial carcinoma adopted in 1971[174] was based solely on the architecture of the tumor, specifically the relative proportion of solid to glandular areas within the tumor.

Table 5-2. FIGO Surgical Staging for Endometrial Carcinoma

Stage	Description
Ia (G123)	Tumor limited to endometrium
Ib (G123)	Invasion to <1/2 myometrium
Ic (G123)	Invasion to >1/2 myometrium
IIa (G123)	Endocervical glandular involvement only
IIb (G123)	Cervical stromal invasion
IIIa (G123)	Tumor invades serosa and/or adnexa and/or positive peritoneal cytology
IIIb (G123)	Vaginal metastases
IIIc (G123)	Metastases to pelvic and/or para-aortic lymph nodes
IVa (G123)	Tumor invasion of bladder and/or bowel mucosa
IVb (G123)	Distant metastases (including intra-abdominal) and/or inguinal lymph node metastases

Numerous studies disclosed a strong correlation between this architectural grading system and survival.[53, 69, 175–178] In the largest study of endometrioid carcinomas in the literature (1,566 cases),[53] the 5- (and 10-year) survival rates for grades 1, 2, and 3 carcinomas were 86.8 (78.3) percent, 75.0 (61.0) percent, and 58.3 (46.2) percent, respectively. In a large Gynecologic Oncology Group (GOG) study of endometrioid carcinomas (895 cases), the most accurate determinant of recurrence in pathologic stage I tumors was a grade of 3.[178] Other studies, however, found that survival correlated better with the nuclear grade or the nuclear grade combined with the architectural grade than with the architectural grade alone.[17, 179–181] Accordingly, the revised FIGO (ISGP/WHO) histologic grading system[182] is based on the relative amounts of solid and glandular areas and the degree of nuclear atypicality. In grade 1 carcinoma, 5 percent or less of the tumor is composed of solid nonsquamous neoplastic tissue, whereas the latter accounts for 6 to 50 percent in grade 2 carcinomas and for more than 50 percent in grade 3 carcinomas. Nuclear atypicality exceeding that expected for grade 1 or grade 2 carcinoma raises the grade by one. Adenocarcinomas with squamous differentiation are graded according to the grade of the glandular component. Serous, clear cell, and pure squamous carcinomas are graded only by nuclear features. In the case of a mixed carcinoma (Table 5-1), the grade of each component should be specified separately.

In opposition to the above approach, two recent studies have cast doubt on the reproducibility and utility of nuclear grading of endometrial carcinomas. Nielsen et al. applied the 1988 FIGO grading system to 47 endometrial carcinomas and found that intraobserver and interobserver reproducibility of nuclear grade was poor, in contrast to that of architectural grade.[183] These observers also found a lack of uniformity between various studies in the literature on the criteria used in determining nuclear grade. Alone or in combination, such criteria include, nuclear/cytoplasmic ratio, size, shape, chromatin, nucleoli, and mitotic activity.[183] Similarly problematic, as noted by these investigators, is the absence of a definition for an "inappropriate" nuclear grade for grade 1 or 2 architectural grade. Nielsen et al. concluded that the utility of the revised FIGO grading system is due primarily to the architectural grade and doubted that the incorporation of nuclear grade will prove of additional prognostic value, as long as there is a lack of concensus on the criteria for nuclear grading. In a GOG study, Zaino et al., compared a three-level architectural grading system with a two-level nuclear grading system.[184] They found that both systems had moderate reproducibility and similar prognostic utility, with survival rates of 84, 72, and 52 percent for architectural grades 1, 2, and 3, respectively, and survival rates of 80 percent and 62 percent for low and high nuclear grades, respectively; the assessment of nuclear grade, however, was more tedious than that of architectural grade. They recommended continued use of a three level architectural grading system for endometrial adenocarcinoma. Similarly, Ambros and Kurman found in a recent study that architectural grade correlated more closely with survival than nuclear grade or architectural grade combined with nuclear grade.[185]

Two recent studies have shown that mitotic activity has prognostic significance in endometrial carcinoma. In the study by Mittal et al. of clinical stage I tumors,[181] 6 percent of patients with tumors that contained less than 10 mitotic figures per 10 high-power-fields (MF/10HPF) died of disease, whereas 20 percent of tumors with more than 10MF/HPF were fatal. Tornos et al.[185a] found that 10 percent of their patients with stage I grade 1 endometrial carcinoma died of recurrent disease; the fatal cases were characterized by two or more of the following adverse prognostic factors: 8 or

more MF/10HPF, and, as discussed below, deep myometrial invasion, vascular invasion, and absence of progesterone receptors.

The grading of tumors is difficult to standardize, but when based on general pathological principles remains a valuable prognostic indicator as evidenced by the results of studies by the Surveillance, Epidemiology, and End Results Program involving large numbers of participating pathologists who analyzed a variety of malignant tumors without being assigned specific criteria for grading.[186] Consequently, all of the grading systems are considered prognostically useful, with grade 3 tumors (architectural grade, nuclear grade, or combined architectural-nuclear grade) belonging in a "high-risk" group with a relatively high risk of lymph node metastases. In the GOG study by Creasman et al., for example, the frequency of pelvic lymph node metastases was 3, 9, and 18 percent for grade 1, 2, and 3 tumors; the corresponding figures for para-aortic lymph node involvement were 2, 5, and 11 percent, respectively.[187] In another study, in which para-aortic nodes were assessed in clinical stage I patients, Piver et al. found that these nodes were involved in 0, 13.6, and 37.5 percent of patients with grade 1, 2, and 3 tumors, respectively.[188] A correlation also exists between tumor grade and other prognostic parameters, as noted in the following sections.

MYOMETRIAL INVASION

Numerous studies have shown that myometrial invasion is an important prognostic parameter in patients with endometrial adenocarcinoma.[17, 53, 175, 176, 178–180, 181, 185, 185a, 189] In a Stanford study, for example, the relapse rates for 173 patients with pathologic stage I endometrial carcinomas (excluding SPECs and CCCEs) without myometrial invasion, with invasion limited to the inner half of the myometrium, and with invasion into the outer half of the myometrium were less than 1, 7, and 30 percent, respectively.[179] Similarly, death rates in another study of 164 patients were 4, 15, and 33 percent for the three groups.[181] In an even larger study from the University of Louisville, 5-year survival rates for patients with tumors confined to the endometrium, with invasion of the inner third, the middle third, and the outer third of the myometrium, were 100, 88.7, 71.4, and 47.8 percent, respectively.[17] Only 2.9 percent and 2.8 percent of patients with superficial myometrial invasion (inner third) died of tumor at five and ten years, respectively.[180] In the largest study of endometrioid adenocarcinomas in the literature (1,566 cases),[53] patients with tumors invading into the inner half of the myometrium fared only slightly worse (85.3 versus 88.7 percent 5-year survival) than those with tumors confined to the endometrium. The corresponding figures for tumors with invasion into the outer half of the myometrium and for tumors extending to the serosa were 63.5 and 46.9 percent, respectively.[53] Uterine serosal involvement (stage IIIa disease) was also shown by multivariate analysis to be a significant predictor of local failure by Grigsby et al.[190]

Many studies have noted a direct correlation between the depth of invasion and the grade of the tumor. In the study of 1,566 endometrioid carcinomas cited above, grade 1, 2, and 3 tumors invaded the outer half of the myometrium in 8, 23, and 35 percent of cases, respectively.[53] In a GOG study of 621 patients, grade 1, 2, and 3 tumors invaded into the outer third of the myometrium in 10, 20, and 42 percent of cases, respectively.[187] Deep myometrial invasion also correlates with the frequency of vascular invasion (see below)[185] and the risk of lymph node spread.[178, 187, 188] For example, the risk of lymph node involvement was 0, 9, and 15 percent in patients with invasion involving the inner, mid, and outer

thirds of the myometrium, respectively, in one series,[176] and 5, 6, and 25 percent in another.[187] Piver et al. found the frequency of para-aortic nodal metastases to be 0, 4.5, and 45.5 percent in patients with tumor confined to the endometrium, superficial myometrial invasion, and invasion of the outer half of the myometrium, respectively.[188] Two recent studies[190, 190a] using the 1988 FIGO staging system determined that the survival of patients with stage Ic disease (deep myometrial invasion but negative lymph nodes and negative peritoneal washings) was not statistically different from that of patients with stage Ia or Ib disease. These findings need to be confirmed in additional studies but may indicate that the depth of myometrial invasion in pathologic stage I tumors may be less important than the presence or absence of other prognostic variables such as histologic subtype, grade, vascular invasion, etc.

The pathology report should include not only the depth of invasion as measured from the endomyometrial junction (nearest to the tumor) to the point of deepest tumor invasion (excluding intravascular tumor), but also the depth of uninvolved myometrium beneath the tumor. The latter measurement may have independent prognostic significance[191]; one study showed that tumor extending to within less than 5 mm of the uterine serosa was an adverse prognostic factor independent of the proportion of myometrium involved by tumor.[192] A number of recent studies have shown that intraoperative pathologic assessment of myometrial invasion by careful gross examination and selective frozen sections can be accurate and useful in determining the need for lymph node sampling.[193–197a]

Histopathologic recognition of myometrial invasion by endometrial carcinomas is straightforward when irregularly shaped glands surrounded by a desmoplastic stroma have an infiltrative border with the myometrium. Other growth patterns of the tumors, however, may create problems in determining the presence and depth of myometrial invasion. A carcinoma filling the endometrium but not invading the myometrium may accentuate the normally irregular endomyometrial junction. In such cases, well-circumscribed rounded nests of tumor appear to bulge into the superficial myometrium (Fig. 5-64), an appearance that should not be misinterpreted as superficial myometrial invasion. Awareness of this appearance, the presence of occasional noncancerous endometrial glands or foci of endometrial stroma between the tumor and the myometrium (Fig. 5-65) and the absence of a reactive stroma facilitate the correct interpretation. Some endometrial carcinomas are exophytic and fill the endometrial cavity but do not invade the myometrium or do so only superficially; obviously the thickness of the exophytic part of the tumor (that part above the endomyometrial junction) should not be included in the measurement of tumor depth.

In other cases, the invasive tumor has a circumscribed "pushing" border with the myometrium, and in such cases the myometrial invasion may not be recognizable if the normal endomyometrial junction is not included in the tissue section. Occasionally the invasive tumor has a deceptively bland appearance, in which deeply invasive glands have rounded regular contours and evoke no discernible stromal reaction[29]; if the tumor is well differentiated, this pattern may be mistaken for adenomyosis. Mittal and Barwick recently described an unusual pattern of invasion which they refer to as "diffusely infiltrating," in which the predominant pattern of invasive tumor occurs as individually disposed glands widely scattered through the myometrium (Figs. 5-66 and 5-67)[198].

When an endometrial carcinoma and adenomyosis coexist in the same uterus, the latter process is involved by the carcinoma in 20 to 30 percent of cases.[199, 200] In some of these cases, the adenomyotic in-

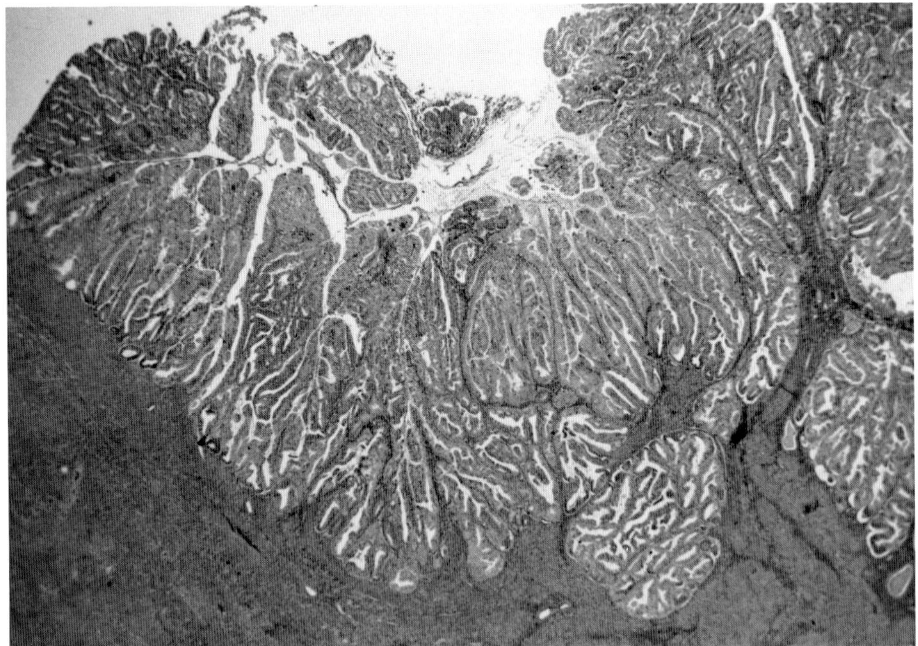

Fig. 5-64. Endometrial carcinoma confined to the endometrium. Note the normal irregularity of the endomyometrial junction.

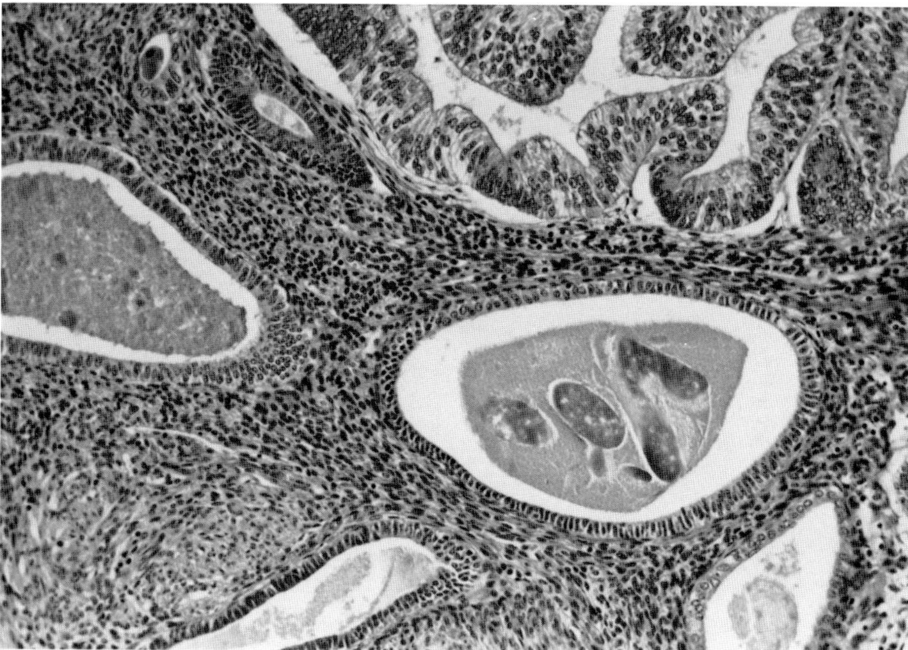

Fig. 5-65. Endometrial carcinoma confined to the endometrium. Higher-power view of Figure 5-66, showing residual benign glands and endometrial stroma separating the tumor from the underlying myometrium, indicating an absence of myometrial invasion in this area.

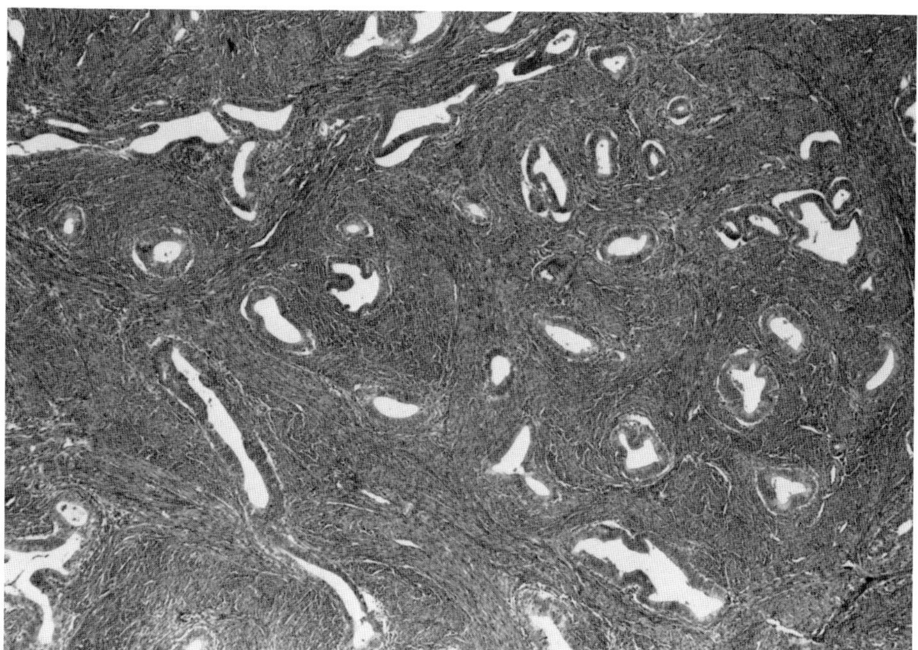

Fig. 5-66. Endometrial adenocarcinoma invading the myometrium with a ''diffusely infiltrating'' pattern.

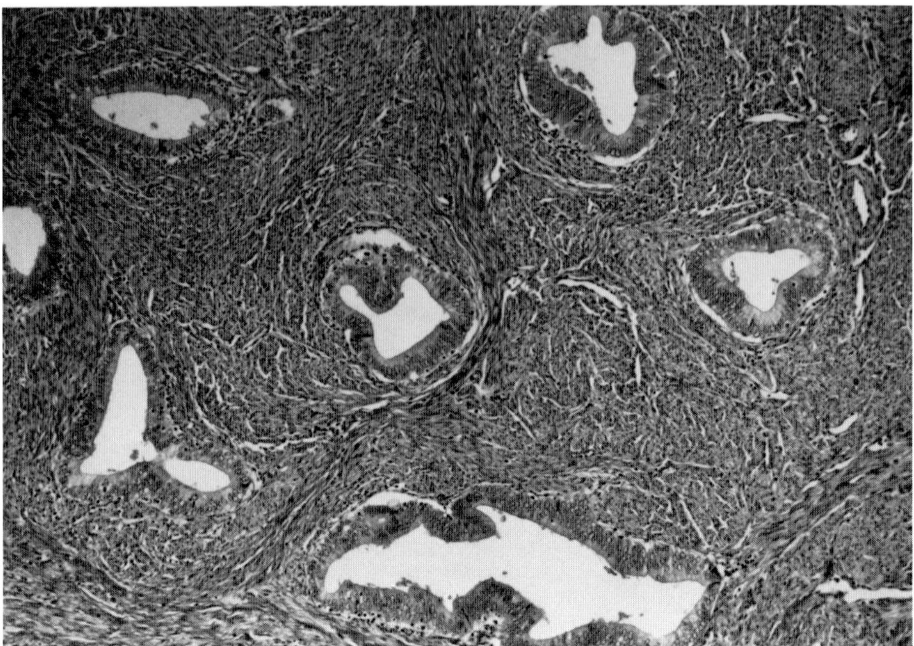

Fig. 5-67. Endometrial adenocarcinoma invading the myometrium with a "diffusely infiltrating" pattern, higher-power of tumor illustrated in Figure 5-66. Note absence of a stromal response around the glands.

volvement may represent multifocal origin of the carcinoma, and in other cases, direct invasion by the endometrial carcinoma. That some carcinomas arise from adenomyotic glands is suggested by the rare confinement of the adenocarcinoma to adenomyosis[201] or an adenomyoma,[202] or more often, by the finding of precancerous changes within adenomyotic glands next to foci of adenocarcinoma. A number of studies have found that the prognosis of an endometrial adenocarcinoma is not adversely affected when the myometrial involvement by the carcinoma is confined to the adenomyosis.[199, 200, 203, 204] It should be noted, however, that these studies contained only a small number of cases of carcinomatous involvement of deep adenomyotic foci; a larger group of patients with this depth of involvement therefore requires study. In any case, the pathologist should distinguish between carcinomatous involvement of ad-

enomyosis and true myometrial invasion. Jacques and Lawrence found one or more features useful in identifying involvement of adenomyotic foci by carcinoma, including the presence of a smooth rounded contour with the surrounding myometrium, the presence of non-neoplastic glands or endometrial-type stroma within the foci in question (Fig. 5-68), the absence of desmoplasia or an inflammatory response, and the presence of adacent uninvolved islands of adenomyosis.[204] Problems in interpretation may persist, however, in older women in whom the adenomyotic stroma is frequently atrophic. In such cases, it may be difficult or impossible to determine whether the malignant glands are in direct contact with the myometrium or are surrounded by thin wisps of atrophic stroma. In difficult cases, serial sections and connective tissue stains may be useful in reaching the correct diagnosis.

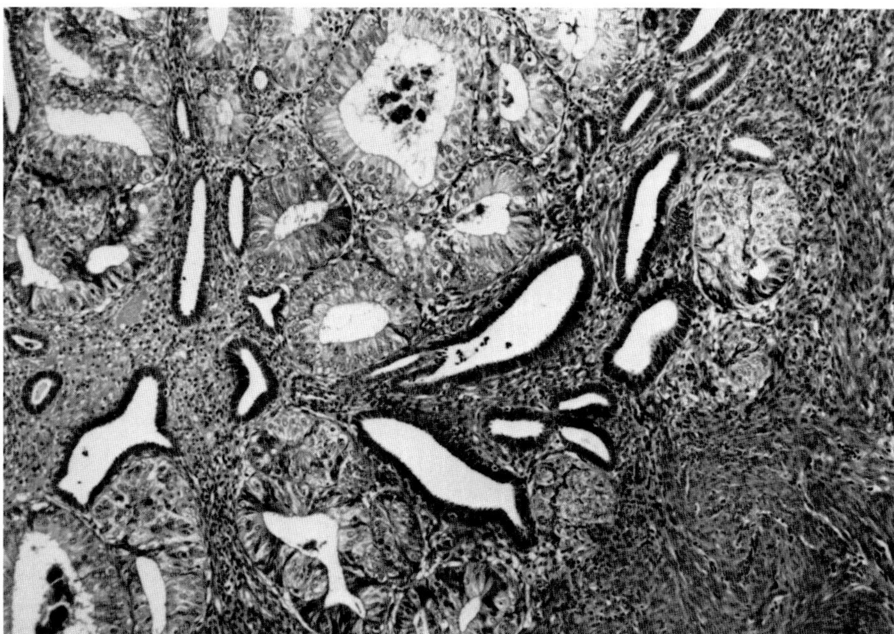

Fig. 5-68. Endometrial adenocarcinoma involving a focus of adenomyosis. Note benign glands and stroma.

LYMPHATIC AND VASCULAR INVASION

Eight recent studies have shown that vascular invasion is a major adverse prognostic factor in cases of endometrial carcinoma.[53, 181, 185, 185a, 189, 205–207] In these studies, "vascular" or "lymphvascular" invasion was considered present if tumor cells were present within myometrial spaces lined by endothelial cells; no attempt was made to differentiate between blood vessels and lymphatic channels. Only one of these studies confirmed the presence of vascular invasion with immunohistochemical stains for endothelial antigens[185]; these stains, however, did not detect vascular invasion that was not suspected on routinely stained slides. In four series, only clinical stage I tumors were considered[181, 185, 189, 205]; in one of them, only endometrioid adenocarcinomas were included to eliminate the possible confounding effect of the high frequency of vascular invasion in serous papillary carcinomas.[185] Another study was confined to pathologic stage I grade 1 tumors.[185a]

The frequency of vascular invasion in four studies of stage I tumors was 4, 14, 14, and 16 percent,[181, 185, 189, 205] in contrast to 48 percent in stage II to IV tumors in one study that included higher stage tumors.[207] In the largest study of endometrioid carcinomas (all stages), 22.4 percent of tumors were associated with vascular invasion.[53] Ambros and Kurman found that vascular invasion was frequently associated with perivascular lymphocytic infiltrates adjacent to or at a distance from the tumor, and the presence of one or both findings were grouped together as "vascular invasion-associated changes."[185, 208] In another study, Spiegel found an increased frequency of vascular invasion (44 versus 13 percent) in grade 1 and 2 endometrial adenocarcinomas when pools of mucin were found within the myometrium ("free mucin") adjacent to degenerating or ruptured neoplastic glands.[209]

The presence of vascular invasion was an important independent adverse prognostic indicator in seven of the studies cited above, and was one of four adverse prognostic parameters in the eighth study (which included only pathologic stage I grade 1 tumors).[185a] Hanson et al. found[205] that tumor recurred in 44 percent of cases with vascular invasion, in contrast to only 2 percent of those without this feature. Five-year survival rates from other studies for patients with and without vascular invasion were 18 and 82 percent (figures approximate),[206] 40 and 100 percent,[189] 33 and 94 percent,[181] 66 and 83 percent,[53] and 42 and 60 percent[207] (the last two series included stage II to IV tumors). The finding of "vascular invasion-associated changes" was the most important prognostic parameter in the series of clinical stage I tumors reported by Ambros and Kurman.[185] In these and other studies, the frequency of vascular invasion was significantly associated with other adverse prognostic parameters, including high tumor grade,[53, 185, 189, 205] deep myometrial invasion,[53, 185, 189, 205, 207] lymph node involvement,[178, 187, 189] positive peritoneal cytology,[189] aneuploidy,[208] and advanced stage[207]; in one of these studies, vascular invasion was also associated with squamous differentiation.[185] Ambros and Kurman postulated that the highly predictive value of vascular invasion as a prognostic factor in Stage I endometrial carcinoma suggests that it is the mechanism by which occult metastases develop in patients whose disease progresses after hysterectomy.[185] They further suggested that other variables correlating with recurrence, such as deep myometrial invasion and high tumor grade, may act by increasing the probability of vascular invasion.

CERVICAL INVOLVEMENT

Cervical involvement in endometrial carcinoma[210–233] is usually a result of direct surface or stromal extension, although occa-sionally it may be secondary to implantation (see below) or lymphatic spread.[218] In the 1971 FIGO staging system, endometrial carcinomas were considered stage II if the cervix was judged to be involved by tumor on clinical examination or if tumor was present within an endocervical curettage specimen. The 5-year survival reported by FIGO from 131 institutions was 52 percent for clinical stage II tumors, compared with 75 percent for stage I disease.[226] This difference in prognosis was largely due to the increased frequency of lymph node involvement in patients with clinical stage II disease, which in one study was 35.5 percent, compared with only 10.6 percent for women with clinical stage I tumors.[210] In another study, involvement of the isthmus or cervix increased the frequency of pelvic lymph node metastases from 8 to 16 percent, and para-aortic node metastases from 4 to 14 percent.[187] As in stage I tumors, histologic grade, depth of invasion, and serous or clear cell histology were prognostically significant in clinical stage II carcinoma.[213, 216, 217, 221, 223, 225, 228, 229] The extent of cervical involvement (gross versus occult or microscopic involvement) was found to be an important prognostic parameter in some studies[213, 216, 217, 219] but not others.[211, 214, 215, 224, 229] The behavior of endometrial carcinomas extending into[187, 214] or arising within[52] the lower uterine segment appeared to be similar to that of stage II tumors.

A number of studies focusing on the problems associated with the microscopic interpretation of endocervical curettage specimens (ECSs), which was an integral part of the 1971 FIGO staging system, found that ECSs are often artifactually contaminated by tumor from the endometrial cavity.[218, 223, 227, 230] One study found that serous and clear cell carcinomas, because of their papillary architecture and tendency to desquamate, are particularly likely to contaminate an ECS.[230] Artifactual contamination most commonly takes the form of tumor fragments unattached to stroma (free-floating tumor) admixed with normal endocervical tissue. Abeler and Kjorstad reviewed 278 ECSs initially considered positive for involvement by endometrial carcinoma, and concluded that only 24 percent of them represented unequivocal stage II disease, as indicated by the presence of stromal invasion in tissue fragments that were covered by normal squamous or endocervical glandular epithelium.[53] An absence of histologically confirmed stromal invasion in several studies, however, did not exclude cervical involvement in the hysterectomy specimen. Weiner et al. and Frauenhoffer et al., for example, found that the presence of free-floating tumor in an ECS predicted cervical involvement in the hysterectomy specimen in one-fourth to one-third of cases.[223, 227] Moreover, Kadar et al. found that the exclusive presence of tumor in an ECS (with no normal endocervical tissue present) was associated with a prognosis similar to that associated with cervical stromal invasion.[218] Additionally, Bigelow et al. could find no correlation between the type of tumor involvement in the ECS (tumor continuous with endocervical tissue, tumor separate from endocervical tissue, pure tumor) with the pattern of cervical involvement in the hysterectomy specimen (surface tumor only, surface and stromal tumor, stromal tumor only).[220] It should also be remembered that rarely the deep cervical stroma may be involved by endometrial carcinoma in the absence of any superficial involvement, a pattern not diagnosable by ECC.[218, 220]

Because the diagnosis of stage II disease in the 1988 FIGO staging system is based on the pathological findings within the hysterectomy specimen, the potential errors in staging arising from the problems in the pathological interpretation of ECSs have been eliminated. Applying the new FIGO staging system, Fanning et al.[231] found that none of 12 patients with stage IIa disease (endocervical glandular involvement only) had recurrent tumor; in contrast, tumor recurred in 5 of 8 patients (63 percent) with stage IIb disease (endocervical stromal involvement). All five recurrences were extrapelvic (abdomen, lung, bone). Five-year survival rates reported from a similar study by Bigelow et al. were 80 percent (stage IIa) and 50 percent (stage IIb).[220] These investigators found that stage IIa tumors tended to be lower grade and had less myometrial invasion than stage IIb tumors. Similar differences in survival in stage II tumors with and without cervical stromal invasion can be found in other studies: 47 versus 74 percent 3-year survival (Surwit et al.[213]), 46 versus 86 percent 5-year survival (Resinger et al.[232]) and 62 versus 88 percent (Grigsby et al.[222]). By contrast, Lurain et al. found that surgical stage IIb was not an adverse prognostic parameter; there were no recurrences in seven such patients in their study.[233] A recent GOG study suggested that cervical involvement per se may not diminish survival and that the poorer prognosis in these patients is due to the greater tendency for tumors that are high grade and deeply invasive to involve the cervix.[178] Reisinger et al. reached a similar conclusion in their study of stage II tumors in which a grade of 3 was a more significant adverse prognostic factor than stage IIb disease.[232] Sixty-three percent of their grade 3 stage II tumors were associated with distant metastases.

Fanning et al. identified a pattern of cervical involvement, so-called "implantation metastasis," that is equivalent in prognosis to stage IIa tumors.[234] This finding was present in 5 percent of hysterectomy specimens removed for endometrial carcinoma in patients who had undergone a fractional curettage. The implantation metastases were considered to be secondary to implantation of endometrial carcinoma in the denuded endocervix after fractional dilatation and curettage (D&C). Criteria for this diagnosis include (1) tumor embedded in the endocervial epithelium or superficial stroma surrounded by inflammatory cells and granulation tissue; (2) cervical tumor similar histologically to that within the endometrial cavity; (3) cervical tumor separate from the endometrial tumor with no evidence of direct extension; and (4) cervical tumor surrounded by non-neoplastic endocervical glands with no transition between the two.[234]

Lymph Node Involvement

Involvement of pelvic and para-aortic lymph nodes is one of the most important prognostic factors in patients with endometrial carcinoma. In one study of clinical stage I tumors, the recurrence rate was 47.6 percent with positive lymph nodes (45 percent with positive pelvic nodes, 64 percent with positive para-aortic nodes) compared with 8.3 percent for patients with negative lymph nodes.[233] In the same study, the 5-year disease-free survival rate for patients with nodal metastases was 54 percent, compared with 90 percent for patients without nodal metastases; corresponding figures from another series were 33 and 94 percent.[189] In another study of clinical stage I to IV endometrial carcinomas,[235] survival at 48 months was 76 percent for patients with negative para-aortic nodes, in contrast to 26 percent when these nodes were involved. A more recent GOG study, however, found that the prognosis for patients with pelvic node metastases in the absence of other adverse prognostic factors was good: only 5 of 18 such patients experienced a recurrence.[178]

Retroperitoneal nodal metastases have been documented in a significant proportion of cases of clinical stage I endometrial carcinoma. In a large GOG study of such tumors,[187] 11 percent of patients had metastases to either pelvic nodes or para-aortic nodes, or both; 3 percent had involvement of both nodal groups; and 2 percent had metastases to aortic nodes only. As already discussed, however, the frequency of nodal involvement in an individual patient is highly dependent on the histologic grade and the depth of myometrial invasion, as well as the presence or absence of vascular invasion and cervical involvement.[178, 187, 236] Additionally, a recent GOG study found that cases associated with grossly positive pelvic nodes, gross adnexal metastases, and outer third myometrial invasion, alone or in combination, accounted for 98 percent of cases with para-aortic nodal metastases.[178]

Tumor size also affects the frequency of lymph node spread. Schink et al.[237, 238] found that only 4 percent of patients with tumors less than or equal to 2 cm had lymph node metastases; the frequency increased to 15 percent for tumors larger than 2 cm, and to 35 percent when the entire uterine cavity was involved. Corresponding 5-year survival rates for the three groups were 98, 84, and 64 percent.[238] Schink et al. noted that although patients with grade 2 tumors and invasion confined to the inner half of the myometrium are often considered to have a risk of lymph node metastases too low to justify adjuvant pelvic irradiation, this group is better defined by including tumor size as a prognostic factor. Patients in this group had no lymph node metastases when their tumors were less than 2 cm, but 18 percent had nodal disease when the tumors were larger than 2 cm. Thus hysteroscopic or intraoperative assessment of tumor size may be an additional factor of value in determining the need for lymph node sampling in patients with endometrial carcinoma.

Adnexal Involvement

As many as 8 percent of endometrial carcinomas are accompanied by a simultaneous ovarian carcinoma[239–244] (Fig. 5-69). In most such cases, both tumors are of similar histologic subtype, most commonly, endometrioid; in these cases, determination as to whether the tumors are independent primary tumors or metastatic one to the

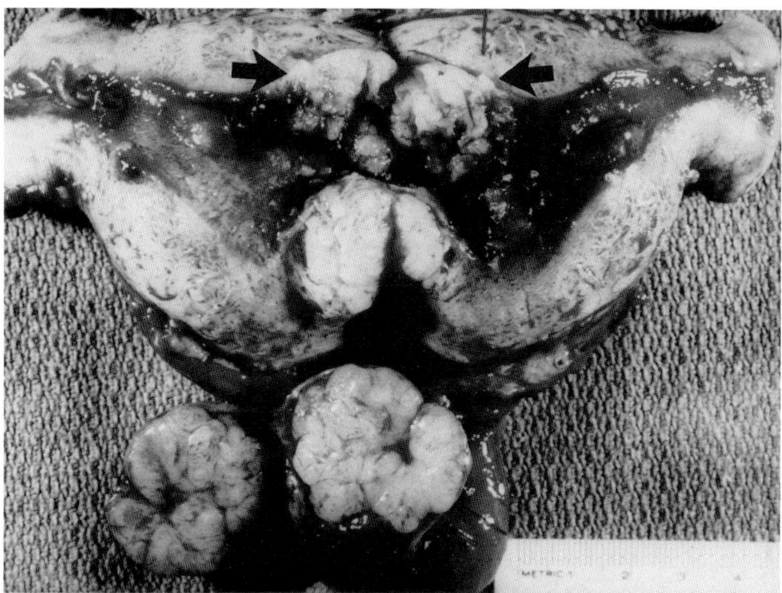

Fig. 5-69. Endometrioid carcinoma involving uterine corpus (between arrows) and one ovary (bottom of figure), which has been bisected. The circumscribed mass within the myometrium opposite the carcinoma is a leiomyoma.

other may be a problem. In the remaining cases, the ovarian and endometrial tumors are of different histology, favoring an independent origin in most such cases.[240, 243]

In three recent series, the percentage of cases in which the endometrial and ovarian carcinomas of similar histologic type were judged to be independent primary tumors was 35,[241] 50[244] and 55 percent.[239] The patients with these tumors were often younger than the usual patients with endometrial or ovarian carcinoma.[239, 241] and usually had an excellent prognosis, consistent with the presence of two stage I neoplasms.[239, 241, 242] The ovarian tumors in these cases are occasionally associated with, and in such cases likely arise from, ovarian endometriosis.[241] The ovarian tumors in almost all of the remaining cases in the three series cited above were considered metastatic from the endometrial carcinoma; not surprisingly, these patients had a significantly worse prognosis than the patients with independent primary tumors.[239] In only very rare cases was the endometrial carcinoma diagnosed as metastatic from the ovarian carcinoma.[241, 244] The patients considered to have endometrial primary tumors with ovarian metastases as well as those with independent primary tumors both had a high frequency of associated endometrial hyperplasia, supporting the belief that the endometrium was a primary site in both groups.[239, 241]

As with metastatic involvement of the ovaries in general, a variety of features of the ovarian tumor favor metastatic spread from an endometrial carcinoma when the two tumors coexist in the same patient (Table 5-3). These include a smaller size of the ovarian tumor(s) than the endometrial tumors, bilateral involvement, a multinodular growth pattern, the presence of multiple surface implants, and prominent lymphatic or vascular invasion within the ovarian stroma.[241, 245] Additional features, including grade 3 endometrioid carcinoma, the presence of malignant squamous elements, a nonendometrioid histologic subtype (particularly serous or clear cell), deep myome-

Table 5-3. Criteria for Interpretation of Nature of Concomitant Uterine Corpus and Ovarian Carcinomas

Corpus Primary Ovarian Metastasis	Ovarian Primary Corpus Metastasis	Ovarian Primary Corpus Primary	Ovarian Metastasis Corpus Metastasis Primary Tumor Elsewhere	Uncertain Primary
Direct extension to ovary from large corpus tumor	Direct extension to corpus from large ovarian tumor	No direct extension of either tumor	Usually no direct extension of tumors	Massive involvement of both organs or inconclusive findings listed in first four columns
Deep myometrial invasion from endometrium	Myometrial invasion from serosal surface	Myometrial invasion usually absent or superficial	Tumor characteristically in endometrial stroma; myometrial invasion may be present	
Lymphatic or blood vessel invasion in corpus or ovary, or both	Lymphatic or blood vessel invasion in corpus or ovary, or both	No lymphatic or blood vessel invasion	Lymphatic or blood vessel invasion frequent, in ovary and corpus	
Atypical hyperplasia of endometrium frequent	Atypical hyperplasia of endometrium usually absent	Atypical hyperplasia of endometrium frequent	Atypical hyperplasia of endometrium absent	
Tumor present in fallopian tube	Tumor present on peritoneal surfaces and sometimes in fallopian tube	Usually both tumors confined to primary sites or have spread minimally	Tumor usually evident outside female genital tract	
Tumor predominant on surface of ovary	Tumor predominant within ovary	Tumor predominant within ovary and endometrium	Ovarian tumor usually bilateral–ovarian surface involvement frequent	
Usually no endometriosis in ovary	Endometriosis sometimes present in ovary	Endometriosis sometimes present in ovary	Endometriosis absent	
Histologic types uniform and consistent with corpus primary	Histologic types uniform and consistent with ovarian primary	Histologic types uniform or dissimilar	Type of tumor inconsistent with, or unusual for, either organ	

trial invasion, myometrial vascular invasion, and involvement of the tubal lumen and other pelvic tissues, have been present more commonly in the cases in which the ovarian tumors were considered metastatic.[239, 241] No single feature, however, is diagnostic, and the differential diagnosis depends on evaluation of a constellation of features (Table 5-3). In one study, for example, the ovarian tumors were bilateral in seven of 16 patients considered to have independent uterine and ovarian tumors.[239] In two of the 16 cases, a unilateral grade 3 ovarian tumor coexisted with a grade 3 endometrial carcinoma.[239] Similarly, Ulbright and Roth included examples of serous and clear cell carcinomas in their group of tumors considered independent primaries.[241] Prat et al.[244] found that the immunoprofiles of the endometrial and ovarian tumors were similar in only two of the nine cases with independent primary tumors, whereas four of the nine cases with metastases had similar staining characteristics. In the same study, five of the seven cases with independent primary tumors exhibited different aneuploid stemlines, in contrast to one of six cases with this finding in the metastatic group.[244] It was concluded that, although these techniques may be of some value, the distinction between metastatic and independent primary tumors must rely largely on conventional clinicopathologic findings. The criteria for interpretation of the nature of concomitant uterine corpus and ovarian carcinomas are summarized in Table 5-3.

PERITONEAL CYTOLOGY

During the past decade, a number of studies have focused on the prognostic significance of malignant cells in peritoneal washings performed at the time of hysterectomy in patients with endometrial carcinoma.[177, 178, 189, 190, 233, 246–252a] The cytopathologic features of these specimens, including lesions in the differential diagnosis (mesothelial hyperplasia, endosalpingiosis), have been recently reviewed by Sidaway and Silverberg.[92] Most studies have found that positive peritoneal cytology (PPC) is an adverse prognostic parameter in patients with clinical or pathologic stage I endometrial carcinoma.[178, 190, 246–248] In at least some of these studies, PPC had independent prognostic significance. In the first major such study of clinical stage I patients Creasman et al found that 15.5 percent of patients had PPC; recurrence developed in 34 percent of these patients, in contrast to only 9.9 percent of those with negative peritoneal cytology (NPC).[246] Of patients with PPC, survival rates were similar in those with and without extrauterine disease at operation: 46 percent and 54 percent. In a study published the same year, Szpak et al. found that, not only the presence of malignant cells, but also their concentration in peritoneal fluid, was of prognostic significance in pathologic stage I cases.[249] Two of eight patients with PPC and low concentrations of malignant cells (less than 1,000 cells/100 ml) had a recurrence, whereas four of four patients with PPC and more than 1,000 cells/100 ml had a recurrence; in contrast, all 42 patients with NPC had an uneventful follow-up.

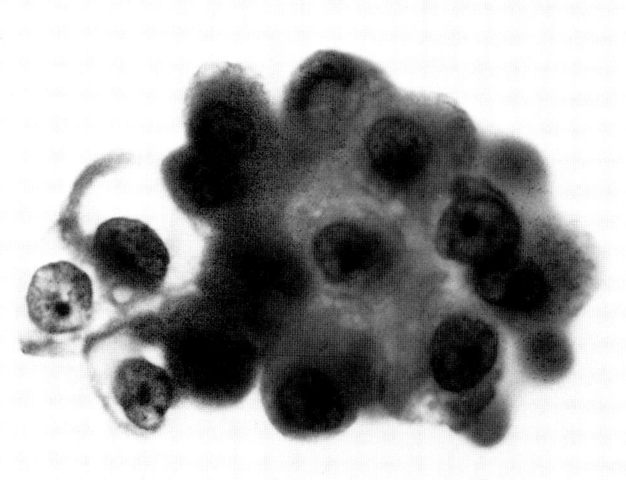

Fig. 5-70. Positive peritoneal cytologic specimen in a patient with serous papillary carcinoma of the endometrium, showing an aggregate of epithelial cells with malignant nuclear features.

More recently, in a study of patients with clinical stage I disease, Harouny et al.[247] found that 17 percent had PPC; the corresponding figures for patients with stage II, III, and IV disease were 19.5, 68.7, and 85.7, percent, respectively. In the clinical stage I group, the frequency of PPC increased with increasing grade, depth of myometrial invasion, and adnexal spread. Recurrent tumor developed in 29 percent of stage I patients with PPC, compared to only 2.9 percent of those with NPC. Intra-abdominal recurrences were more common among clinical and surgical stage I patients with PPC than in those with NPC.[247] In the recent study by Turner et al. of surgical stage I cases,[248] 4.9 percent of patients had PPC; recurrent tumor developed in 32 percent of these patients, compared with only 8.6 percent of those with NPC. The 5-year survival rates were 84 and 96 percent for the two groups. Multivariate analysis revealed that PPC remained significant for both survival rate and progression-free survival. Similarly, in a recent GOG study, 29 percent of patients with PPC had a regional or distant recurrence, compared with only 18.5 percent of those with NPC.[178] Multivariate analysis determined that PPC was a significant prognostic variable that predicted both local failure and distant metastases in the study by Grigsby et al.[190] PPC has been considered a significant adverse prognostic parameter in a number of other studies.[177, 189, 250b, 250c]

In contrast to the foregoing observations, other studies have found that PPC is not a prognostic factor in stage I endometrial cancer. In a study of 93 patients by Yazigi et al.[250] 89 percent of women had NPC and 11 percent had PPC; all patients were followed for a minimum of 10 years or until dead from cancer or intercurrent disease and no patients received treatment for PPC. There was no significant difference in actuarial survival between patients with PPC and those with NPC. Similarly, in a study of 235 patients, Hirai et al.[251] found no differences in 5- and 10-year survival rates in

stage I patients with PPC compared with those with NPC. Lurain et al.[233] found that PPC was significantly associated with disease recurrence in univariate analysis but was not an independent variable in multivariate analysis. Grigsby et al.[252] and Kadar et al.[252a] found that PPC did not influence survival when tumor was confined to the uterus (surgical stage I). In the latter study, however, PPC had a significant adverse affect on survival in patients with adnexal, nodal, or peritoneal spread, reducing 5-year survival from 73 to 13 percent; all recurrences were at distant sites.[252a] Similar observations were made in the study by Imachi et al.[250b] In an editorial accompanying the study of Kadar et al., Lurain[252b] concluded that in the absence of disease outside the uterus, other poor prognostic factors, or both, PPC probably has no significant effect on survival and adjuvant treatment is unnecessary. On the other hand, PPC associated with extrauterine disease or other poor prognostic factors increases the likelihood of intra-abdominal recurrence and distant metastases, and decreases survival; systemic therapy should therefore be administered to such patients.[252a, 252b]

DNA PLOIDY

Cell cycle parameters obtained from flow cytometry have been investigated as prognostic indicators in endometrial carcinomas. Aneuploid endometrial carcinomas, which have accounted for 12 to 56 percent of these tumors,[47, 131b, 253–270] have been significantly more aggressive than diploid tumors in most studies. Three of three aneuploid tumors, but none of 16 diploid tumors, recurred or were fatal in the study by Naus et al.[253] Iverson found that patients with aneuploid tumors, compared to those with diploid tumors, had higher recurrence rates, shorter disease-free intervals, higher death rates, and shorter median survivals.[255] Similarly, there was a higher proportion of deaths in patients with aneuploid tumors compared with those with diploid tumors (26 versus 7 percent) in the study by Stendahl et al.[260] In patients with stage I or II carcinoma, aneuploidy was a stronger prognostic variable than grade in one study,[270a] and a better prognosticator than grade, depth of myometrial invasion, or hormone receptor status in another.[257] Quillamor et al. found that well-differentiated tumors, both diploid and aneuploid, had a favorable prognosis, but diploid tumors that were moderately or poorly differentiated had a better prognosis than aneuploid tumors with the same degree of differentiation.[258] In another study, Iverson et al. determined that although ploidy, receptor status, histologic grade, surgical stage, and myometrial invasion were of significant prognostic value, multivariate analysis found that ploidy was the best predictor of survival.[261] In a large series (256 cases), Britton and co-workers found that 10 percent of patients with diploid tumors had relapses compared with 39 percent of those with nondiploid (aneuploid and tetraploid) tumors.[262, 263] Four-year progression-free survival rates were 88 and 57 percent for patients with diploid and nondiploid tumors, respectively.[263] Stage, grade, depth of myometrial invasion, histologic subtype, peritoneal cytology, and ploidy all had independent prognostic significance in this study, but only histologic subtype and ploidy maintained significant prognostic power after multivariate analysis.[263] In the study by Newbury et al.,[264] a DNA index of greater than 1.4 strongly predicted death from disease in patients with endometrioid and serous papillary carcinomas, independent of stage or grade.[264] Similarly, Symonds found that a DNA index of greater than 1.5 had a strong association with metastasizing endometrial cancers.[265] Only 31 percent of nonmetastasizing carcinomas were aneuploid, whereas 89 percent of the metastasizing tumors were aneuploid.[265] In the same study, twice as many aneuploid as diploid nuclear grade 2 endometrioid carci-

nomas metastasized. A similar relationship was found with deep myometrial invasion.[265] Recently, Ambros and Kurman determined by multivariate analysis of pathologic stage I endometrioid carcinoma that only DNA ploidy, depth of invasion, and "vascular invasion associated changes" (p. 239) correlated significantly with survival.[208]

Aneuploidy has been associated with other adverse prognostic parameters in some studies, including adverse histologic type (serous, clear cell),[131b, 262–264] increasing grade,[131b, 259–261, 264, 267] deep myometrial invasion,[264, 269] high stage,[256] and receptor negativity.[261, 267] Some studies, however, have found that most aneuploid tumors are well differentiated[47, 256, 261] and that even some examples of endometrial hyperplasia lacking cytologic atypia may be aneuploid.[47]

In contrast to the foregoing, Sorbe et al.[270] concluded that DNA ploidy did not add significant prognostic information to that determined by nuclear grade, depth of myometrial invasion, and stage. Similarly, Stendahl et al.[260] and Wagenius et al.[259] found that the DNA content was prognostically insignificant, but that the S-phase fraction was, next to clinical stage III and IV, the strongest predictor of outcome. Konski et al.[268] found that a high percentage of S-phase cells may identify diploid tumors with a poorer prognosis. Patients with diploid tumors and less than 3.7 percent S-phase cells had a median survival of 75 months, in contrast to only 48 months for patients with diploid tumors and more than 3.7 percent S-phase cells.[268] Similarly, Rosenberg et al.[131b] found that 93 percent of patients with an S-phase fraction of less than 5 percent survived 5 years, compared to only 51 percent of those in whom the S-phase fraction was more than 10 percent. In other studies, elevated S-phase rates (or S-phase fraction) have also correlated with increasing grade,[256, 260, 269] stage II to IV disease,[260] and tumor recurrence.[260]

Despite conflicting data, some of which

may be related to differing methodologies (e.g., using fresh versus paraffin-embedded tissue), DNA ploidy appears to be a significant prognostic and therapeutic determinant for surgical stage I endometrial carcinoma. The ploidy status, combined with other prognostic parameters such as histologic subtype and grade, may identify patients who are at increased risk of recurrence and who would potentially benefit from adjuvant therapy.[262–264] Symonds concluded that DNA analysis appears to be most useful when histologic studies are inconclusive in predicting a high risk of recurrence.[265]

Steroid Hormone Receptors

Numerous studies[271–303] have shown that the steroid hormone receptor content of the tumor is of prognostic significance in patients with endometrial carcinoma; this subject has been recently well reviewed elsewhere.[301–303] In the earlier studies, the receptors were measured biochemically, but more recently it has been shown that their immunohistochemical determination may provide similar or even superior prognostic information.[282–284, 290, 291, 295, 296, 300] The latter method also allows for recognition of receptors present within the tumor stroma or within admixed benign tissue in cases in which the neoplastic glands may be receptor negative.[279, 290, 294, 298] The immunohistochemical technique can also be applied to small specimens and archival material.

Increased survival times have been found for patients with tumors that are rich in estrogen receptors (ERs)[274, 275, 278, 280, 281, 286, 287, 296] progesterone receptors (PRs),[275, 278, 280, 285–287, 289, 293, 296, 297] or both ERs and PRs,[273, 275, 280, 281, 292] as compared with tumors with low levels of these receptors. There have been considerable differences among studies, however, in the biochemical methods used and the threshold con-

centration of receptors required to consider tumors receptor positive. The threshold concentration chosen in each study may affect which clinicopathologic features (see below) are significantly associated with the hormone receptor status.[303] Palmer et al. recently suggested that maximum prognostic information is obtained by using levels that are much higher (70 fmol/mg protein for ERs, 30 fmol/mg protein for PRs) than those traditionally accepted.[288]

Although receptor-rich tumors, in comparison to receptor-poor tumors, are more commonly endometrioid in type,[295] well differentiated,[272, 273, 275, 278, 281, 286, 290, 295] not deeply invasive,[273, 277] not angioinvasive,[278] and of low stage,[273, 286, 290] the receptor content of the tumors, in at least some studies, has provided prognostic information independent of such variables.[274, 275, 286] Creasman et al. found by multivariate analysis that ER-positive, PR-positive, and combined ER–PR-positive status were each independent predictors of survival.[275] Similarly, multivariate analysis in the series by Chambers et al. determined that ER status was a better predictor of survival than grade.[286] Ingram et al. found that PR level was the single most important prognostic indicator of 3-year disease-free survival,[293] and in the above cited study by Palmer et al., stage, age, and an ER level of greater than 70 fmol/mg, combined with a PR content of greater than 30 fmol/mg, were independently associated with survival.[288] As noted elsewhere (p. 234), PR-negativity was one of four adverse prognostic factors in patients with stage I grade 1 endometrial carcinomas in the study by Tornos et al.[185a]

Determination of steroid receptors also has therapeutic implications. Receptor-rich recurrent or metastatic endometrial carcinomas are more likely to respond to progestational therapy.[272, 276, 280, 287] Conversely, Kaupilla et al. found that in patients with advanced or recurrent endometrial carcinoma, receptor-poor tumors are more likely to respond to cytotoxic chemotherapy than receptor-rich tumors.[271] In this study, however, all patients had previously received progestin therapy (which lowers the receptor protein levels), so that this observation needs to be confirmed in patients with no prior hormonal therapy.[303]

Richardson and MacLaughlin concluded that performing receptor assays on all endometrial carcinomas is not cost effective, because most tumors are receptor-rich and have a good prognosis without adjuvant hormonal treatment.[301] They suggest that tumor tissue could be stored at -70°C until other prognostic factors such as grade and extent of disease have been assessed. If a patient is considered at high risk of recurrence, the tissue could then be analyzed for receptors, and adjuvant hormonal therapy offered to patients with receptor-rich tumors.[301]

ONCOGENES

Activation of a number of oncogenes has recently been reported in endometrial carcinoma. Although some of these investigations, as summarized in this section, have prognostic implications, the significance of these findings require clarification and confirmation by additional studies.

Bauknecht et al.[304] found *erb*B-1 (EGFR) expression in 15 of 26 (58 percent) of endometrial adenocarcinomas using an EGF binding assay; the number of binding sites was greater than observed in breast or ovarian carcinomas. Berchuk et al.[305] demonstrated EGFR expression immunohistochemically in normal endometrial glands and stroma as well as in 67.5 percent of endometrial carcinomas. There was no correlation between tumor expression of EGFR and grade, depth of invasion, ER or PR status, the presence of metastases, or recurrent disease.

Expression of *erb*B-2 (*neu*, HER-2) has also been observed in endometrial carcinomas. In a brief communication, Garuti and Genazzani documented by Northern blot

assays specific 4.6-kb *erb*B-2-related RNA in five endometrial adenocarcinomas (60 percent of the cases studied); no *erb*B-2 transcription was found in normal endometrium.[306] In a study using Southern blot analysis Borst et al.[307] found *erb*B-2 amplification in 11 of 16 endometrial carcinomas; 4 of the 11 patients died of disease an average of 16 months after diagnosis. In contrast, all 5 of the patients without *erb*B-2 amplification had no evidence of recurrent tumor at an average follow-up interval of 31.2 months. Brumm et al.[308] studied immunohistochemically 11 endometrial carcinomas, and found enhanced *erb*B-2 translation in 2 tumors, both of which were poorly differentiated and stage IV. Nine stage I tumors (as well as 13 normal endometria and 4 cases of endometrial hyperplasia) had translation activity at or below baseline levels.[308] Similarly, Berchuk et al.[309] found that 9 of 95 endometrial carcinomas overexpressed the *erb*B-2 product and that this feature was associated with an absence of ERs, a higher frequency of metastases, and decreased survival. In another study, by Bigsby et al.,[310] 7 of 49 endometrial carcinomas exhibited *erb*B-2 immunoreactivity in excess of normal endometrial tissue; all 7 of the tumors were grade 1 or 2 and stage I. In the same study,[310] an inverse relationship between *erb*B-2 expression and the presence of progesterone receptors was demonstrated.

In one of the studies cited above, Borst et al.[307] found c-*myc* amplification in 10 of 15 endometrial carcinomas; 5 of the 10 patients died of tumor at an average of 13.4 months after diagnosis. Six of 16 tumor specimens exhibited amplification of both the c-*myc* and *erb*B-2 genes, and four of these patients died of recurrent disease. A high frequency of c-*myc* amplification has also been found, as noted earlier, in serous papillary carcinomas of the endometrium.[122]

Agnantis et al.[311] found immunohistochemical overexpression of *ras* p21 in 17 of 17 endometrial adenocarcinomas and in 6 of

12 cases of "hyperplastic endometrial lesions." In another immunohistochemical study, Long et al.[312] documented *ras* p21 in 95 percent of grade 2 and 3 endometrial carcinomas, in contrast to only 18 percent of grade 1 tumors. The p21 protein was localized not only to the neoplastic epithelial cells, but also within the stromal cells of high-grade carcinomas. Using DNA sequencing, Enomoto et al.[313, 314] found point mutations of *ras* genes in 7 of 19 endometrial carcinomas; six involved Ki-*ras* and one N-*ras*. In one of the cancers, tumor cells with point mutations in Ki-*ras* were predominantly localized to a part of the tumor that had "a more aggressive histological pattern." Similar mutations were found in 2 of 16 endometrial hyperplasias with cytologic atypia, but in none of 18 cases of hyperplasias lacking atypia.[314] In a recent study, Mizuuchi et al. found mutations in codon 12 or 13 of K-*ras* in six cases of endometrial carcinoma (12 percent of their cases), five of which were endometrioid and one of which was clear cell.[314a] The presence of K-*ras* mutations appeared to be an unfavorable prognostic factor: 3 of 6 patients with the mutation, compared to only 3 of 43 patients without the mutation, died during the follow-up period. Multivariate analysis showed that K-*ras* mutation was an independent risk factor in this study.[314a]

In a study utilizing in situ hybridization techniques, Kacinski et al.[315] found significantly higher levels of *fms* mRNA in endometrial carcinomas compared to those found in proliferative endometria and endometrial hyperplasia. These higher levels of mRNA were significantly associated with high grade, deep myometrial invasion, and high stage. It is noteworthy that in another study, Azuma et al.[316] found that exogenous sex-steroids could induce *fms* transcription in nonpregnant women.

In recent immunohistochemical studies, Bur et al.[317] and Kohler et al.[318] found p53 expression (associated with gene mutation) in endometrial cancers. Strong and diffuse staining for p53 was seen in 21 percent[318] and 50 percent[317] of carcinomas. p53 overexpression was more frequent with nonendometrioid (including serous) tumors, PPC, extrauterine metastases, negative PR status, stage III to IV disease, tumor recurrence, and death from disease.[317, 318]

NONTUMOR FACTORS

Aside from features of the tumor itself, a variety of other parameters have been shown to have prognostic significance in endometrial carcinoma. Numerous studies have found that older women (over 50 years of age) have a worse prognosis than that of younger women.[17, 53, 175, 177, 180, 185, 233] Beckner et al.[16] found that women in this age group, as well as postmenopausal women of any age, had less favorable histologic features, higher stage of their tumors, and a lower survival. Black women also tend to have higher grade tumors, higher stage tumors, and poorer survival rates than white women.[16, 17, 180] Several studies have found that endometrial carcinomas occurring in women who have used estrogen tend to be associated with endometrial hyperplasia, well differentiated, of a favorable histologic subtype, noninvasive or only superficially invasive of the myometrium, and of low stage.[18, 176, 319] Consequently, such tumors are almost always associated with a good prognosis compared to tumors in women who have not used estrogens. Beckner et al. found that the presence of an associated endometrial hyperplasia was the single most important nontumor prognostic factor in patients with endometrial carcinoma.[16] Patients with this finding survived 5 years more frequently than did patients without an associated hyperplasia. This improved survival persisted after correction for age and race. For this reason, as noted elsewhere in this chapter (p. 188), the presence or absence of an associated endometrial hyperplasia should be noted specifically in the pathology report in cases of endometrial carcinomas.[16]

On the basis of these observations, it has been suggested that there may be two types of endometrial carcinoma: (1) a prognostically favorable one arising on a background of hyperplasia predominantly in premenopausal women, and (2) a prognostically unfavorable one occurring principally in postmenopausal women without an associated hyperplasia.[16, 320]

REFERENCES

1. Beutler HK, Dockerty MB, Randall LM: Precancerous lesions of the endometrium. Am J Obstet Gynecol 86:433, 1963
2. Hertig AT, Sommers SC: Genesis of endometrial carcinoma. I. Study of prior biopsies. Cancer 2:946, 1949
3. Kurman RJ, Kaminski PF, Norris HJ: The behavior of endometrial hyperplasia. A long-term study of "untreated" hyperplasia in 170 patients. Cancer 56:403, 1985
4. McBride JM: Pre-menopausal cystic hyperplasia and endometrial carcinoma. J Obstet Gynaecol Br Emp 66:288, 1959
5. Gusberg SB, Kaplan AL: Precursors of corpus cancer. IV. Adenomatous hyperplasia as stage 0 carcinoma of the endometrium. Am J Obstet Gynecol 87:662, 1963
6. Chamlian DL, Taylor HB: Endometrial hyperplasia in young women. Obstet Gynecol 36:659, 1970
7. Wentz WB: Progestin therapy in endometrial hyperplasia. Gynecol Oncol 2:362, 1974
8. Sherman AI, Brown S: The precursors of endometrial carcinoma. Am J Obstet Gynecol 135:947, 1979
9. Tavassoli F, Kraus FT: Endometrial lesions in uteri resected for atypical endometrial hyperplasia. Am J Clin Pathol 70:770, 1978
10. Welch WR, Scully RE: Precancerous lesions of the endometrium. Hum Pathol 8:503, 1977
11. Scully RE: Definitions of precursors in gynecologic cancer. Cancer 48:531, 1981
12. Scully RE: Definition of endometrial carcinoma precursors. Clin Obstet Gynecol 25:39, 1982
13. Huang SJ, Amparo EG, Fu YS: Endometrial hyperplasia: histologic classification and behavior. Surg Pathol 1:215, 1988
14. Lee KR, Scully RE: Complex endometrial hyperplasia and carcinoma in adolescents and young women 15 to 20 years of age. A report of 10 cases. Int J Gynecol Pathol 8:201, 1989
15. Norris HJ, Connor MP, Kurman RJ: Preinvasive lesions of the endometrium. Clin Obstet Gynaecol 13:725, 1986
16. Beckner ME, Mori T, Silverberg SG: Endometrial carcinoma: nontumor factors in prognosis. Int J Gynecol Pathol 4:131, 1985
17. Connelly PJ, Alberhasky RC, Christopherson WM: Carcinoma of the endometrium. III. Analysis of 865 cases of adenocarcinoma and adenoacanthoma. Obstet Gynecol 59:569, 1982
18. Deligdisch L, Cohen CJ: Histologic correlates and virulence implications of endometrial carcinoma associated with adenomatous hyperplasia. Cancer 56:1452, 1985
19. Gray LA, Robertson RW, Jr, Christopherson WM: Atypical endometrial changes associated with carcinoma. Gynecol Oncol 2:93, 1974
20. Winkler B, Alvarez S, Richart RM, Crum CP: Pitfalls in the diagnosis of endometrial neoplasia. Obstet Gynecol 64:185, 1984
21. Hendrickson MR, Kempson RL: Endometrial hyperplasia. p. 308. In: Surgical Pathology of the Uterine Corpus. WB Saunders, Philadelphia, 1980
22. Whitehead MI, McQueen J, Minardi J et al: Progestogen modification of estrogen-induced endometrial proliferation in climacteric women. In Pasetto N, Paoletti R, Ambrus JL (eds): The Menopause and Postmenopause. MTP Press Limited, Lancaster, England, 1980
23. Kistner RW: Endometrial alterations associated with estrogen and estrogen-progestin combinations. In Norris HJ, Hertig AT, Abell MR (eds): The Uterus. Williams & Wilkins, Baltimore, 1973
24. Gal D, Edman CD, Vellios F, Forney JP: Long-term effect of megestrol acetate in

the treatment of endometrial hyperplasia. Am J Obstet Gynecol 146:316, 1983

25. Ferenczy A, Gelfand M: The biologic significance of cytologic atypia in progestogen-treated endometrial hyperplasia. Am J Obstet Gynecol 160:126, 1989

26. Hendrickson MR, Kempson RL: The differential diagnosis of endometrial adenocarcinoma. Some viewpoints concerning a common diagnostic problem. Pathology 12:35, 1980

27. Fox H, Buckley CH: The endometrial hyperplasias and their relationship to endometrial neoplasia. Histopathol 6:493, 1982

28. Kurman RJ, Norris HJ: Evaluation of criteria for distinguishing atypical endometrial hyperplasia from well-differentiated carcinoma. Cancer 49:2547, 1982

29. Hendrickson MR, Ross JC, Kempson RL: Toward the development of morphologic criteria for well-differentiated adenocarcinoma of the endometrium. Am J Surg Pathol 7:819, 1983

30. Norris HJ, Tavassoli FA, Kurman RJ: Endometrial hyperplasia and carcinoma. Diagnostic considerations. Am J Surg Pathol 7:839, 1983

31. Kraus FT: High-risk and premalignant lesions of the endometrium. Am J Surg Pathol 9:31, 1985

32. Silverberg SG: Hyperplasia and carcinoma of the endometrium. Semin Diagn Pathol 5:135, 1988

33. King A, Seraj IM, Wagner RJ: Stromal invasion in endometrial adenocarcinoma. Am J Obstet Gynecol 149:10, 1984

34. Hustin J: Immunohistochemical demonstration of several tumour markers in neoplastic and preneoplastic states of the uterine mucosa. Gynecol Obstet Invest 9:3, 1978

35. Tsionou C, Minaretzis D, Papageorgiou I et al: Expression of carcinoembryonic antigen and ferritin in normal, hyperplastic, and neoplastic epithelium. Gynecol Oncol 41:193, 1991

36. Morse AR, Curran GJ: Distribution of epithelial membrane antigen in normal and abnormal endometrial tissue. Br J Obstet Gynaecol 92:1286, 1985

37. Nakopoulou L, Minaretzis D, Tsionou C, Mastrominas M: Value of immunohisto-chemical demonstration of several epithelial markers in hyperplastic and neoplastic endometrium. Gynecol Oncol 37:346,1990

38. Thor A, Viglione MJ, Muraro R et al: Monoclonal antibody B72.3 reactivity with human endometrium: A study of normal and malignant tissues. Int J Gynecol Pathol 6:235, 1987

39. Morris WPR, Griffin NR, Wells M: Patterns of reactivity with the monoclonal antibodies HMFG1 and HMFG2 in normal endometrium, endometrial hyperplasia and adenocarcinoma. Histopathology 15:179, 1989

40. Soderstrom K: Lectin binding into human endometrial hyperplasias and adenocarcinoma. Int J Gynecol Pathol 6:356, 1987

41. Inoue M, Ogawa H, Tanizawa O et al: Immunodetection of sialyl-Tn antigen in normal, hyperplastic and cancerous tissues of the uterine endometrium. Virchows Arch A 418:157, 1991

42. Furness PN, Lam EWH: Patterns of basement membrane deposition in benign, premalignant, and malignant endometrium. J Clin Pathol 40:1320, 1987

43. Bulletti C, Galassi A, Jasonni VM et al: Basement membrane components in normal hyperplastic and neoplastic endometrium. Cancer 62:142, 1988

44. Colgan TJ, Norris HJ, Foster W et al: Predicting the outcome of endometrial hyperplasia by quantitative analysis of nuclear features using a linear discriminant function. Int J Gynecol Pathol 1:347, 1983

45. Baak JPA: The use and disuse of morphometry in the diagnosis of endometrial hyperplasia and carcinoma. Pathol Res Pract 179:20, 1984

46. Norris HJ, Becker RL, Mikel UV: A comparative morphometric and cytophotometric study of endometrial hyperplasia, atypical hyperplasia, and endometrial carcinoma. Hum Pathol 20:219, 1989

47. Thornton JG, Quirke P, Wells M: Flow cytometry of normal, hyperplastic, and malignant human endometrium. Am J Obstet Gynecol 161:487, 1989

48. Wilkinson N, Buckley CH, Chawner L, Fox H: Nucleolar organiser regions in normal, hyperplastic, and neoplastic endometria. Int J Gynecol Pathol 9:55, 1990

49. Coumbe A, Mills BP, Brown CL: Nucleolar organiser regions in endometrial hyperplasia and neoplasia. Pathol Res Pract 186:254, 1990
50. Niwa K, Yokoyama Y, Tanaka T et al: Silver-stained nucleolar organizer regions in the normal, hyperplastic and neoplastic endometrium. Virchows Arch A 419:493, 1991
51. Prasad C, Ireland K: Nucleolar organizer regions in neoplastic and non-neoplastic endometrium, abstracted. Mod Pathol 5:67A, 1992
52. Hachisuga T, Kaku T, Enjoji M: Carcinoma of the lower uterine segment. Clinicopathologic analysis of 12 cases. Int J Gynecol Pathol 8:26, 1989
53. Abeler VM, Kjorstad KE: Endometrial adenocarcinoma in Norway. Cancer 67:3093, 1991
54. Salm R: Mucin production of normal and abnormal endometrium. Arch Pathol 73:30, 1962
55. Fox H, Brander WL: A sertoliform endometrioid adenocarcinoma of the endometrium. Histopathology 13:584, 1988
56. Gernow A, Ahrentsen OD: Adenoid cystic carcinoma of the endometrium. Histopathology 16:197, 1990
57. Chan JKC: Cribriform endometrioid adenocarcinoma, not adenoid cystic carcinoma, of the endometrium (letter). Histopathology 16:317, 1990
58. Yorishima M, Hiura M, Moriwaki S et al: Clear cell carcinoma of the endometrium with lipid-producing activity. Histologic and ultrastructural study suggesting a unique neoplasm. Int J Gynecol Pathol 8:286, 1989
59. Harris HR: Foam cells in the stroma of carcinoma of the body of the uterus and uterine cervical polypi. J Clin Pathol 11:19, 1959
60. Salm R: Macrophages in endometrial lesions. J Pathol 83:405, 1962
61. Isaacson PG, Pilot JR, Gooselaw JG: Foam cells in the stroma in carcinoma of the endometrium. Obstet Gynecol 23:9, 1964
62. Fechner RE, Bossart MI, Spjut HI: Ultrastructure of endometrial stromal foam cells. Am J Clin Pathol 72:628, 1979
63. Fechner RE: Ultrastructure of endometrial stromal foam cells (letter). Am J Clin Pathol 73:732, 1980
64. Dawagne MP, Silverberg SG: Foam cells in endometrial carcinoma—a clinicopathologic study. Gynecol Oncol 13:67–75, 1982
65. Nogales FF, Gomez-Morales M, Raymundo C, Aguilar D: Benign heterologous tissue components associated with endometrial carcinoma. Int J Gynecol Pathol 1:286, 1982
66. Hendrickson MR, Ross J, Eifel P et al: Uterine papillary serous carcinoma. A highly malignant form of endometrial adenocarcinoma. Am J Surg Pathol 6:93, 1982
67. Chen JL, Trost DC, Wilkinson EJ: Endometrial papillary adenocarcinomas: two clinicopathological types. Int J Gynecol Pathol 4:279, 1985
68. Sutton GP, Brill L, Michael H et al: Malignant papillary lesions of the endometrium. Gynecol Oncol 27:294, 1987
69. Burke TW, Heller PB, Woodward JE et al: Treatment failure in endometrial carcinoma. Obstet Gynecol 75:96, 1990
70. O'Hanlan KA, Levine PA, Harbatkin D et al: Virulence of papillary endometrial carcinoma. Gynecol Oncol 37:112, 1990
71. Ward BG, Wright RG, Free K: Papillary carcinomas of the endometrium. Gynecol Oncol 39:347, 1990
72. Christopherson WM, Alberhasky RC, Connelly PJ: Carcinoma of the endometrium. I. A clinicopathologic study of clear-cell carcinoma and secretory carcinoma. Cancer 49:1511, 1982
73. Tobon H, Watkins GJ: Secretory adenocarcinoma of the endometrium. Int J Gynecol Pathol 4:328, 1985
74. Kusuyama Y, Yoshida M, Imai H et al: Secretory carcinoma of the endometrium. Acta Cytol 33:127, 1989
75. Kurman RJ, Scully RE: Clear cell carcinoma of the endometrium An analysis of 21 cases. Cancer 37:872, 1976
76. Silverberg SG, Makowski EL: Endometrial carcinoma in young women taking oral contraceptive agents. Obstet Gynecol 46:503, 1975
77. Silverberg SG, Makowski EL, Roche WD: Endometrial carcinoma in women under 40 years of age. Comparison of cases in oral

contraceptive users and non-users. Cancer 39:592, 1977

78. Hendrickson MR, Kempson RL: Ciliated carcinoma—a variant of endometrial adenocarcinoma: a report of 10 cases. Int J Gynecol Pathol 2:1, 1983

79. Haibach H, Oxenhandler RW, Luger AM: Ciliated adenocarcinoma of the endometrium. Acta Obstet Gynecol Scand 64:457, 1985

80. Silverberg SG, Mullen D, Faraci JA et al: Endometrial carcinoma: clinical–pathologic comparison of cases in postmenopausal women receiving and not receiving exogenous estrogens. Cancer 45:3018, 1980

81. Gould PR, Li L, Henderson DW et al: Cilia and ciliogenesis in endometrial adenocarcinomas. Arch Pathol Lab Med 110:326, 1986

82. Ng ABP: Mixed carcinoma of the endometrium. Am J Obstet Gynecol 102:506, 1968

83. Ng ABP, Reagan JW, Storaasli JP, Wentz WB: Mixed adenosquamous carcinoma of the endometrium. Am J Clin Pathol 59:765, 1973

84. Silverberg SG, Bolin MG, DeGiorgi LS: Adenoacanthoma and mixed adenosquamous carcinoma of the endometrium. A clinicopathologic study. Cancer 30:1307, 1972

85. Haqqani MT, Fox H: Adenosquamous carcinoma of the endometrium. J Clin Pathol 29:959, 1976

86. Alberhasky RC, Connelly PJ, Christopherson WM: Carcinoma of the endometrium. IV. Mixed adenosquamous carcinoma. A clinico-pathological study of 68 cases with long-term follow-up. Am J Clin Pathol 77:655, 1982

87. Demopoulos RI, Dubin N, Noumoff J et al: Prognostic significance of squamous differentiation in stage I endometrial adenocarcinoma. Obstet Gynecol 68:245, 1986

88. Salazar OM, DePapp EW, Bonfiglio TA et al: Adenosquamous carcinoma of the endometrium. Cancer 40:119, 1977

89. Zaino RJ, Kurman RJ: Squamous differentiation in carcinoma of the endometrium: a critical appraisal of adenoacanthoma and adenosquamous carcinoma. Semin Diagn Pathol 5:154, 1988

90. Zaino RJ, Kurman R, Herbold D et al: The significance of squamous differentiation in endometrial carcinoma. Data from a gynecologic oncology group study. Cancer 68:2293, 1991

91. Abeler VM, Kjorstad KE: Endometrial adenocarcinoma with squamous cell differentiation. Cancer 69:488, 1992

92. Sidaway MK, Silverberg SG: Endometrial carcinoma. Pathologic factors of therapeutic and prognostic significance. Pathol Annu 27:153, 1992

93. Hirose T, Sano T, Abe J et al: Spindle cell carcinoma of the uterus. Acta Pathol Jpn 37:997, 1987

94. Christopherson WM, Alberhasky RC, Connelly PJ: Glassy cell carcinoma of the endometrium. Hum Pathol 13:418, 1982

95. Arends JW, Willebrand D, DeKoning HJ et al: Adenocarcinoma of the endometrium with glassy-cell features—immunohistochemical observations. Histopathology 8:873, 1984

96. Dawson EC, Belinson JL, Lee K: Glassy cell carcinoma of the endometrium responsive to megestrol acetate. Gynecol Oncol 33:121, 1989

97. Hachisuga T, Sugimori H, Kaku T et al: Glassy cell carcinoma of the endometrium. Gynecol Oncol 36:134, 1990

98. Chen KTK, Kostich ND, Rosai J: Peritoneal foreign body granulomas to keratin in uterine adenoacanthoma. Arch Pathol Lab Med 108:359, 1978

99. Kim K, Scully RE: Peritoneal keratin granulomas with carcinomas of endometrium and ovary and atypical polypoid adenomyoma of endometrium. Am J Surg Pathol 14:925, 1990

100. Savage J, Subby W, Okagaki T: Adenocarcinoma of the endometrium with trophoblastic differentiation and metastases as choriocarcinoma: a case report. Gynecol Oncol 26:257, 1987

101. Pesce C, Merino MJ, Chambers JT, Nogales P: Endometrial carcinoma with trophoblastic differentiation. An aggressive form of uterine cancer. Cancer 68:1799, 1991

102. Tsoutsoplides GC: Ectopic production of human chorionic gonadotropin by a highly anaplastic adenocarcinoma of the endometrium. Am J Obstet Gynecol 136:694, 1980

103. Jones MA, Young RH, Scully RE: Endometrial adenocarcinoma with a component of giant cell carcinoma. Int J Gynecol Pathol 10:260, 1991

104. Silverberg SG: Case 6, Evening Gynecologic Pathology Specialty Conference, 78th Annual Meeting of the International Academy of Pathology, March 1988

105. Lauchlan SC: Tubal (serous) carcinoma of the endometrium. Arch Pathol Lab Med 105:615, 1981

106. Jeffrey JF, Krepart GV, Lotocki RJ: Papillary serous adenocarcinoma of the endometrium. Obstet Gynecol 67:670, 1986

107. Kuebler DL, Nikrui N, Bell DA: Cytologic features of endometrial papillary serous carcinoma. Acta Cytol 33:120, 1989

108. Abeler VM, Kjorstad KE: Serous papillary carcinoma of the endometrium: a histopathological study of 22 cases. Gynecol Oncol 39:266, 1990

109. Burrell MO, Franklin EW, Powell JL: Endometrial cancer: evaluation of spread and follow-up in one hundred eighty-nine patients with stage I or stage II disease. Am J Obstet Gynecol 144:181, 1982

110. Walker AN, Mills SE: Serous papillary carcinoma of the endometrium. A clinicopathological study of 11 cases. Diagn Gynecol Obstet 4:261, 1982

111. Chen SS, Lee L: Retroperitoneal lymph node metastases in stage I carcinoma of the endometrium: Correlation with risk factors. Gynecol Oncol 16:319, 1983

112. Sato N, Mori T, Orenstein JM, Silverberg SG: Ultrastructure of papillary serous carcinoma of the endometrium. Int J Gynecol Pathol 2:337, 1984

113. Fitzgerald D, Rosenthal S: Uterine papillary serous carcinoma. Complete response to combination chemotherapy. Cancer 56:1023, 1985

114. Chambers JT, Merino M, Kohorn EI et al: Uterine papillary serous carcinoma. Obstet Gynecol 69:109, 1987

115. Christman JE, Kapp DS, Hendrickson MR et al: Therapeutic approaches to uterine papillary serous carcinoma: A preliminary report. Gynecol Oncol 26:228, 1987

116. Fukuma K, Miyamura S, Thoya T et al: Uterine papillary serous carcinoma with high levels of serum carcinoembryonic antigen. Response to combination chemotherapy. Cancer 59:403, 1987

117. Ramirez-Gonzalez CE, Adamsons K, Mangual-Vazquez TY, Wallach RC: Papillary adenocarcinoma in the endometrium. Obstet Gynecol 70:212, 1987

118. Bitterman P, Potkul RK, Lewandowski GS, Kurman RJ: Papillary serous carcinoma of the endometrium and ovary: a comparative study of 40 cases, abstracted. Lab Invest 58:10A, 1988

119. Gallion HH, Van Nagell JR, Jr, Powell DF et al: Stage I serous papillary carcinoma of the endometrium. Cancer 63:2224, 1989

120. Rosenberg P, Risberg B, Askmalm L, Simonsen E: The prognosis in early endometrial carcinoma. The importance of uterine papillary serous carcinoma (UPSC), age, FIGO grade and nuclear grade. Acta Obstet Gynecol Scand 68:157, 1989

121. Tseng PC, Sprance HE, Carcangiu ML et al: CA 125, NB/70K, and lipid-associated sialic acid in monitoring uterine papillary serous carcinoma. Obstet Gynecol 74:384, 1989

122. Sasano H, Comerford J, Wilkinson DS et al: Serous papillary adenocarcinoma of the endometrium. Analysis of proto-oncogene amplification, flow cytometry, estrogen and progesterone receptors, and immunohistochemistry. Cancer 65:1545, 1990

123. Silva EG, Jenkins R: Serous carcinoma in endometrial polyps. Mod Pathol 3:120, 1990

124. Wilson TO, Podratz KC, Gaffey TA et al: Evaluation of unfavorable histologic subtypes in endometrial adenocarcinoma. Am J Obstet Gynecol 162:418, 1990

125. Frank AH, Tseng PC, Haffty BG et al: Adjuvant whole-abdominal radiation therapy in uterine papillary serous carcinoma. Cancer 68:1516, 1991

126. Kern SB: Prevalence of psammoma bodies in Papanicolaou-stained smears. Acta Cytol 35:81, 1991

127. Kubo K, Lee G, Yamauchi K, Kitagawa T: Alpha-fetoprotein-producing adenocarcinoma originating from a uterine body. Acta Pathol Jpn 41:399, 1991

128. Lee KR, Belinson JL: Relationship to non-invasive endometrial carcinoma. Relation-

ship to uterine papillary serous carcinoma. Am J Surg Pathol 15:965, 1991

129. Parkash V, Carcangiu ML: Uterine papillary serous carcinoma after radiation therapy for carcinoma of the cervix. Cancer 69:496, 1992

130. Swanson PE, Wick MR, Mills SE: Serous papillary endometrial carcinoma. An immunohistochemical comparison with endometrioid carcinoma, abstracted. Mod Pathol 4:62A, 1991

131. Sherman ME, Bitterman P, Rosenshein NB et al: Uterine serous carcinoma. A morphologically diverse neoplasm with unifying clinicopathologic features. Am J Surg Pathol 16:600, 1992

131a. Lee KR, Belinson JL: Papillary serous adenocarcinoma of the endometrium: a clinicopathologic study of 19 cases. Gynecol Oncol 46:51, 1992

131b. Rosenberg P, Wingren S, Simonsen E et al: Flow cytometric measurements of DNA index and S-phase on paraffin-embedded early stage endometrial cancer. An important prognostic factor. Gynecol Oncol 35:50, 1989

132. Silverberg SG, De Giorgi LS: Clear cell carcinoma of the endometrium. Clinical, pathologic, and ultrastructural findings. Cancer 31:1127, 1973

133. Iglesias J, Marquez M, Ausin J et al: Mesonephric adenocarcinoma of the endometrium. Report of three patients. Int J Gynecol Obstet 12:129, 1974

134. Rorat E, Ferenczy A, Richart RM: The ultrastructure of clear cell adenocarcinoma of endometrium. Cancer 33:880, 1974

135. Eastwood J: Mesonephroid (clear cell) carcinoma of the ovary and endometrium. A comparative prospective clinico-pathological study and review of the literature. Cancer 41:1911, 1978

136. Crum CP, Fechner RE: Clear cell adenocarcinoma of the endometrium. A clinicopathologic study of 11 cases. Am J Diagn Gynecol Obstet 1:261, 1979

137. Photopulos GJ, Carney CN, Edelman DA et al: Clear cell carcinoma of the endometrium. Cancer 43:1448, 1979

138. Wolinska WH, Melamed MR, de las Heras P, Delgado E: Clear cell endometrial adenocarcinoma in a young woman: report of a case detected by cytology. Gynecol Oncol 8:118, 1979

139. Giri PGS, Schneider V, Belgrad R: Clear cell carcinoma of the endometrium: an uncommon entity with a favorable prognosis. Int J Radiat Oncol Biol Phys 7:1383, 1981

140. Webb GA, Lagios MD: Clear cell carcinoma of the endometrium. Am J Obstet Gynecol 156:1486, 1987

141. Abeler VM, Kjorstad KE: Clear cell carcinoma of the endometrium: a histopathological and clinical study of 97 cases. Gynecol Oncol 40:207, 1991

142. Kanbour-Shakir A, Tobon H: Primary clear cell carcinoma of the endometrium: a clinicopathologic study of 20 cases. Int J Gynecol Pathol 10:67, 1991

143. Tiltman AJ: Mucinous carcinoma of the endometrium. Obstet Gynecol 55:244, 1980

144. Czernobilsky B, Katz Z, Lancet M, Gaton E: Endocervical-type epithelium in endometrial carcinoma. A report of 10 cases with emphasis on histochemical methods for differential diagnosis. Am J Surg Pathol 4:481, 1980

145. Ross JC, Eifel PJ, Cox RS et al: Primary mucinous adenocarcinoma of the endometrium. A clinicopathologic and histochemical study. Am J Surg Pathol 7:715, 1983

146. Melhem MF, Tobon H: Mucinous adenocarcinoma of the endometrium: a clinicopathological review of 18 cases. Int J Gynecol Pathol 6:347, 1987

147. Sorvari TE: A histochemical study of epithelial mucosubstances in endometrial and cervical adenocarcinomas. Acta Pathol Microbiol Scand Suppl 207:1, 1969

148. Young RH, Scully RE: Uterine carcinomas simulating microglandular hyperplasia: a report of six cases. Am J Surg Pathol 16:1092, 1992

149. Dabbs DJ, Geisinger KR, Norris HT: Intermediate filaments in endometrial and endocervical carcinomas. The diagnostic utility of vimentin patterns. Am J Surg Pathol 10:568, 1986

150. Azumi N, Jones M, Joyce J et al: Endometrial and endocervical adenocarcinomas: immunohistochemical studies and differentiating markers, abstracted. Mod Pathol 4:54A, 1991

151. Dallenbach-Hellweg G, Lang-Averous G,

Hahn U: The value of immunohisto-chemistry in the differential diagnosis of endometrial carcinomas, suppl. APMIS 23:91, 1991

152. Abeler V, Kjorstad KE: Endometrial squamous cell carcinoma: report of three cases and review of the literature. Gynecol Oncol 36:321, 1990

153. Lauritzen AF, Rye B, Vest S: Primary squamous-cell carcinoma of the endometrium. Acta Obstet Gynecol Scand 66:181, 1987

154. Cortes J, Rossello JJ, Llompart M: Primary squamous carcinoma of the endometrium. Case report. Eur J Gynaecol Oncol 9:246, 1988

155. Jeffers MD, McDonald GSA, McGuinness EP: Primary squamous cell carcinoma of the endometrium. Histopathology 19:177, 1991

156. Gedikoglu G, Demirel D, Gunhan O, Finci R: Endometrial squamous cell carcinoma. Acta Obstet Gynecol Scand 70:619, 1991

157. Orhon E, Ulgenalp I, Baser I et al: Primary squamous cell carcinoma of the endometrium. Eur J Cancer 27:946, 1991

158. Sluijmer AV, Ubachs JMH, Stoot JEGM et al: Clinical and pathological aspects of benign and malignant squamous epithelium of the corpus uteri: a report of two cases. Eur J Obstet Gynecol Reprod Biol 39:71, 1991

159. Adelson MD, Strumpf KB: Squamous cell carcinoma of the endometrium presenting as peritonitis with small bowel obstruction. Gynecol Oncol 45:214, 1992

160. Voet RL, Waisman J, Ballon SC: Intraepithelial epidermoid carcinoma of the cervix, endometrium, and a fallopian tube. Gynecol Oncol 8:349, 1979

161. Wilkinson M, Andrasako KP, Stafl A: Endometrial involvement by cervical intraepithelial neoplasia. Obstet Gynecol 55:378, 1980

162. Ryder DE: Verrucous carcinoma of the endometrium — a unique neoplasm with a long survival. Obstet Gynecol 59:78S, 1982

163. Hussain SF: Verrucous carcinoma of the endometrium. APMIS 96:1075, 1988

164. Abeler VM, Kjorstad KE, Nesland JM: Undifferentiated carcinoma of the endome-trium. A histopathologic and clinical study of 31 cases. Cancer 68:98, 1991

165. Bannatyne P, Russell P, Wills EJ: Argyrophilia and endometrial carcinoma. Int J Gynecol Pathol 2:235, 1983

166. Inoue M, DeLellis RA, Scully RE: Immunohistochemical demonstration of chromogranin in endometrial carcinomas with argyrophil cells. Hum Pathol 17:841, 1986

167. Inoue M, Ueda G, Yamasaki M et al: Immunohistochemical demonstration of peptide hormones in endometrial carcinoma. Cancer 54:2127, 1984

168. Ueda G, Yamasaki M, Inoue M, Kurachi K: A clinicopathologic study of endometrial carcinomas with argyrophil cells. Gynecol Oncol 7:223, 1979

169. Aguirre P, Scully RE, Wolfe HJ, DeLellis RA: Endometrial carcinoma with argyrophil cells: a histochemical and immunohistochemical analysis. Hum Pathol 15:210, 1984

170. Sivridis E, Buckley CH, Fox H: Argyrophil cells in normal, hyperplastic, and neoplastic endometrium. J Clin Pathol 37:378, 1984

171. Sato Y, Psaki M, Ueda G, Tanizawa O: Clinical significance of argyrophilia in endometrial carcinomas. Gynecol Oncol 25:53, 1986

172. Ueda G, Nishino T, Saito J et al: Detection of chromogranin in argyrophil cells of endometrial carcinoma. Gynecol Oncol 27:159, 1987

173. Berger G, Fetissof F, Vitrey D et al: Endometrial carcinoma of the intestinal type. A first case report. Appl Pathol 2:63, 1984

174. Cancer Committee Report to the General Assembly of FIGO: Classification and staging of malignant tumor in the female pelvis. Int J Gynecol Obstet 9:172, 1971

175. Lotocki RJ, Copeland M, DePetrillo AD, Muirhead W: Stage I endometrial adenocarcinoma: treatment results in 835 patients. Am J Obstet Gynecol 146:141, 1983

176. Figge DC, Otto PM, Tamimi HK, Greer BE: Treatment variables in the management of endometrial cancer. Am J Obstet Gynecol 146:495, 1983

177. Sutton GP, Geisler HE, Stehman FB et al: Features associated with survival and dis-

ease-free survival in early endometrial cancer. Am J Obstet Gynecol 160:1385, 1989

178. Morrow CP, Bundy BN, Kurman RK, et al: Relationship between surgical-pathological risk factors and outcome in clinical stage I and II carcinoma of the endometrium: a Gynecologic Oncology Group study. Gynecol Oncol 40:55, 1991

179. Hendrickson M, Ross J, Eifel PJ et al: Adenocarcinoma of the endometrium: analysis of 256 cases with carcinoma limited to the uterine corpus. Pathology review and analysis of prognostic variables. Gynecol Oncol 13:373, 1982

180. Christopherson WM, Connelly PJ, Alberhasky RC: Carcinoma of the endometrium. V. An analysis of prognosticators in patients with favorable subtypes and stage I disease. Cancer 51:1705, 1983

181. Mittal KR, Schwartz PE, Barwick KW: Architectural (FIGO) grading, nuclear grading and other prognostic indicators in stage I endometrial adenocarcinoma with identification of high-risk and low-risk groups. Cancer 61:538, 1988

182. Announcements. FIGO Stages: 1988 revision. Gynecol Oncol 35:125, 1989

183. Nielsen AL, Thomsen HK, Nyholm HCJ: Evaluation of the reproducibility of the revised 1988 International Federation of Gynecology and Obstetrics grading system of endometrial cancers with special emphasis on nuclear grading. Cancer 68:2303, 1991

184. Zaino R, Silverberg S, Norris H, Bundy B: The prognostic utility of nuclear grading versus architectural grading in endometrial adenocarcinoma, abstracted. Mod Pathol 5:70A, 1992

185. Ambros RA, Kurman RJ: Combined assessment of vascular and myometrial invasion as a model to predict prognosis in stage I endometrioid adenocarcinoma of the uterine corpus. Cancer 69:1424, 1992

185a. Tornos C, Silva EG, El-Naggar A, Burke TW: Aggressive stage I grade 1 endometrial carcinoma. Cancer 70: 790, 1992

186. Henson DE: The histological grading of neoplasms. Arch Pathol Lab Med 112:1091, 1988

187. Creasman WT, Morrow CP, Bundy BN et al: Surgical pathologic spread patterns of endometrial cancer. A gynecologic oncology group study. Cancer 60:2035, 1987

188. Piver MS, Lele S, Barlow JJ, Blumenson L: Paraaortic lymph node evaluation in stage I endometrial carcinoma. Obstet Gynecol 59:97, 1982

189. Gal D, Recio FO, Zamurovic D, Tancer ML: Lymphvascular space involvement—a prognostic indicator in endometrial adenocarcinoma. Gynecol Oncol 42:142, 1991

190. Grigsby PW, Perez CA, Kuten A et al: Clinical stage I endometrial cancer: Prognostic factors for local control and distant metastasis and implications of the new FIGO surgical staging system. Int J Radiat Oncol Biol Phys 22:905, 1992

190a. Gal D, Recio F, Zamurovic D: The new International Federation of Gynecology and Obstetrics surgical staging and survival rates in early endometrial carcinoma. Cancer 69:200, 1992

191. Templeton AC: Reporting of myometrial invasion by endometrial cancer. Histopathology 6:733–737, 1982

192. Lutz MH, Underwood PB, Jr, Kreutner A, Miller MC: Endometrial carcinoma: a new method of classification of therapeutic and prognostic significance. Gynecol Oncol 6:83, 1978

193. Doering DL, Barnhill DR, Weiser EB et al: Intraoperative evaluation of depth of myometrial invasion in stage I endometrial adenocarcinoma. Obstet Gynecol 74:930, 1989

194. Malviya VK, Deppe G, Malone JM, et al: Reliability of frozen section examination in identifying poor prognostic indicators in stage I endometrial adenocarcinoma. Gynecol Oncol 34:29, 1989

195. Fanning J, Tsukuda Y, Piver MS: Intraoperative frozen section diagnosis of depth of myometrial invasion in endometrial adenocarcinoma. Gynecol Oncol 37:47, 1990

196. Goff BA, Rice LW: Assessment of depth of myometrial invasion in endometrial adenocarcinoma. Gynecol Oncol 38:46, 1990

197. Noumoff JS, Menzin A, Mikuta J et al: The ability to evaluate prognostic variables on frozen section in hysterectomies performed for endometrial carcinoma. Gynecol Oncol 42:202, 1991

197a. Shim JU, Rose PG, Reale FR et al: Accuracy of frozen-section diagnosis at surgery in clinical stage I and II endometrial carcinoma. Am J Obstet Gynecol 166:1335, 1992

198. Mittal KR, Barwick KW: Diffusely infiltrating adenocarcinoma of the endometrium: a subtype with a poor prognosis. Am J Surg Pathol 12:754, 1988

199. Hernandez E, Woodruff JD: Endometrial adenocarcinoma arising in adenomyosis. Am J Obstet Gynecol 138:827, 1980

200. Hall JB, Young RH, Nelson JH, Jr: The prognostic significance of adenomyosis in endometrial carcinoma. Gynecol Oncol 17:32, 1984

201. Woodruff JD, Erozan YS, Genadry R: Adenocarcinoma arising in adenomyosis detected by atypical cytology. Obstet Gynecol 67:145, 1986

202. Kay S, Frable WJ, Goplerud DR: Endometrial carcinoma arising in a large polypoid adenomyoma of the uterus. Int J Gynecol Pathol 7:391, 1988

203. Mittal KR, Barwick KW: Effect of adenomyosis on prognosis in stage I endometrial adenocarcinoma, abstracted. Lab Invest 56:53A, 1987

204. Jacques SM, Lawrence WD: Endometrial adenocarcinoma with variable-level myometrial involvement limited to adenomyosis: a clinicopathologic study of 23 cases. Gynecol Oncol 37:401, 1990

205. Hanson MB, Van Nagell JR, Jr, Powell DE et al: The prognostic significance of lymphvascular space invasion in stage I endometrial cancer. Cancer 55:1753, 1985

206. Geisinger KR, Homesley HD, Morgan TM et al: Endometrial adenocarcinoma. A multiparameter clinicopathologic analysis including the DNA profile and the sex steroid hormone receptors. Cancer 58:1518, 1986

207. Sivridis E, Buckley CH, Fox H: The prognostic significance of lymphatic vascular space invasion in endometrial adenocarcinoma. Br J Obstet Gynaecol 94:991, 1987

208. Ambros RA, Kurman RJ: Identification of patients with stage I uterine endometrioid adenocarcinoma at high risk of recurrence by DNA ploidy, myometrial invasion, and vascular invasion. Gynecol Oncol 45:235, 1992

209. Spiegel GW: Free mucin (FM) in the myometrium associated with endometrial adenocarcinoma (ECA), abstracted. Mod Pathol 5:68A, 1992

210. Morrow CP, DiSaia PJ, Townsend DE: Current management of endometrial carcinoma. Obstet Gynecol 42:399, 1973

211. Homesley HD, Boronow RC, Lewis JL, Jr: Stage II endometrial adenocarcinoma. Memorial Hospital for Cancer, 1949–1965. Obstet Gynecol 49:604, 1977

212. Bruckman JE, Goodman RL, Murthy RL, Marck A: Combined irradiation and surgery in the treatment of stage II carcinoma of the endometrium. Cancer 42:1146, 1978

213. Surwit EA, Fowler WC Jr, Rogoff EE et al: Stage II carcinoma of the endometrium. Int J Radiat Oncol Biol Phys 5:323, 1979

214. Tak WK: Carcinoma of the endometrium with cervical involvement (stage II). Cancer 43:2504, 1979

215. Cox JD, Komaki R, Wilson JF, Greenberg M: Locally advanced adenocarcinoma of the endometrium: results of irradiation with and without subsequent hysterectomy. Cancer 45:715, 1980

216. Kinsella TJ, Bloomer WD, Lavin PT, Knapp RC: Stage II endometrial carcinoma: 10-year follow-up of combined radiation and surgical treatment. Gynecol Oncol 10:290, 1980

217. Berman ML, Afridi MA, Kanbour AI, Ball HG: Risk factors and prognosis in stage II endometrial cancer. Gynecol Oncol 14:49, 1982

218. Kadar NRD, Kohorn EI, LiVolsi VA, Kapp DS: Histologic variants of cervical involvement by endometrial carcinoma. Obstet Gynecol 59:85, 1982

219. Onsrud M, Aalders J, Abeler V, Taylor P: Endometrial carcinoma with cervical involvement (stage II): Prognostic factors and value of combined radiological-surgical treatment. Gynecol Oncol 13:76, 1982

220. Bigelow B, Vekshtein V, Demopoulos RI: Endometrial carcinoma, stage II: Route and extent of spread to the cervix. Obstet Gynecol 62:363, 1983

221. Wallin TE, Malkasian GD, Gaffey TA et al: Stage II cancer of the endometrium: A pathologic and clinical study. Gynecol Oncol 18:1, 1984

222. Grigsby PW, Perez CA, Camel HM et al: Stage II carcinoma of the endometrium: Results of therapy and prognostic factors. Int J Radiat Oncol Biol Phys 11:1915, 1985

223. Frauenhoffer EE, Zaino R, Wolff TV, Whitney CE: Value of endocervical curettage in the staging of endometrial carcinoma. Int J Gynecol Pathol 6:195, 1987

224. Larson DM, Copeland LJ, Gallagher HS et al: Nature of cervical involvement in endometrial carcinoma. Cancer 59:959, 1987

225. Larson DM, Copeland LJ, Gallagher HS et al: Prognostic factors in stage II endometrial carcinoma. Cancer 60: 1358, 1987

226. DiSaia PJ, Creasman WT (eds): Clinical Gynecologic Oncology. 3rd Ed. CV Mosby, St Louis, 1989, p. 107.

227. Weiner J, Bigelow B, Demopoulos RI et al: The value of endocervical sampling in the staging of endometrial carcinoma. Diagn Gynecol Obstet 2:265, 1989

228. Andersen ES: Stage II endometrial carcinoma: prognostic factors and the results of treatment. Gynecol Oncol 38:220, 1990

229. Lanciano RM, Curran WJ, Jr, Greven KM et al: Influence of grade, histologic subtype, and timing of radiotherapy on outcome among patients with stage II carcinoma of the endometrium. Gynecol Oncol 39:368, 1990

230. Caron C, Tetu B, Laberge G et al: Endocervical involvement by endometrial carcinoma on fractional curettage: A clinicopathological study of 37 cases. Mod Pathol 4:655, 1991

231. Fanning J, Alvarez PM, Tsukada Y, Piver MS: Prognostic significance of the extent of cervical involvement by endometrial cancer. Gynecol Oncol 40:46, 1991

232. Reisinger SA, Staros EB, Mohiuddin M: Survival and failure analysis in stage II endometrial cancer using the revised 1988 FIGO staging system. Int J Radiat Oncol Biol Phys 21:1027, 1991

233. Lurain JR, Rice BL, Rademaker AW et al: Prognostic factors associated with recurrence in clinical stage I adenocarcinoma of the endometrium. Obstet Gynecol 78:63, 1991

234. Fanning J, Alvarez PM, Tsukada Y, Piver MS: Cervical implantation metastasis by endometrial adenocarcinoma. Cancer 68:1335, 1991

235. Manetta A, Delgado G, Petrilli E et al: The significance of paraaortic node status in carcinoma of the cervix and endometrium. Gynecol Oncol 23:284, 1986

236. Boronow RC, Morrow CP, Creasman WT et al: Surgical staging in endometrial cancer: clinical–pathological findings of a prospective study. Obstet Gynecol 63:825, 1984

237. Schink JC, Lurain JR, Wallemark CB, Chmiel JS: Tumor size in endometrial cancer: a prognostic factor for lymph node metastasis. Obstet Gynecol 70:216, 1987

238. Schink JC, Rademaker AW, Miller DS, Lurain JR: Tumor size in endometrial cancer. Cancer 67:2791, 1991

239. Eifel P, Hendrickson M, Ross J et al: Simultaneous presentation of carcinoma involving ovary and the uterine corpus. Cancer 50:163, 1982

240. Zaino RJ, Unger ER, Whitney C: Synchronous carcinomas of the uterine corpus and ovary. Gynecol Oncol 19:329, 1984

241. Ulbright TM, Roth LM: Metastatic and independent cancers of the endometrium and ovary: a clinicopathologic study of 34 cases. Hum Pathol 16:28, 1985

242. Jambhekar NA, Sampat MB: Simultaneous endometrioid carcinoma of the uterine corpus and ovary: a clinicopathologic study of 15 cases. J Surg Oncol 37:20, 1988

243. Piura B, Glezerman M: Synchronous carcinomas of endometrium and ovary. Gynecol Oncol 33:261, 1989

244. Prat J, Matias-Guiu X, Barreto J: Simultaneous carcinoma involving the endometrium and ovary. A clinicopathologic, immunohistochemical, and DNA flow cytometric study of 18 cases. Cancer 68:2455, 1991

245. Young RH, Scully RE: Metastatic tumors in the ovary: a problem-oriented approach and review of the recent literature. Semin Diagn Pathol 8:250, 1991

246. Creasman WT, DiSaia PJ, Blessing J et al: Prognostic significance of peritoneal cytology in patienrs with endometrial cancer and preliminary data concerning therapy with intraperitoneal radiopharmaceuticals. Am J Obstet Gynecol 141:921, 1981

247. Harouny VR, Sutton GP, Clark SA et al: The importance of peritoneal cytology in endometrial carcinoma. Obstet Gynecol 72:394, 1988

248. Turner DA, Gershenson DM, Atkinson N et al: The prognostic significance of peritoneal cytology for stage I endometrial cancer. Obstet Gynecol 74:775, 1989

249. Szpak GA, Creasman WT, Vollmer RT, Johnston WW: Prognostic value of cytologic examination of peritoneal washings in patients with endometrial carcinoma. Acta Cytol 25:640, 1981

250. Yazigi R, Piver MS, Blumenson L: Malignant peritoneal cytology as prognostic indicator in stage I endometrial cancer. Obstet Gynecol 62:359, 1983

250a. Kennedy AW, Peterson GL, Becker SN et al: Experience with pelvic washings in stage I and II endometrial carcinoma. Gynecol Oncol 28:50, 1987

250b. Imachi M, Tsukamoto N, Matsuyama T, Nakano H: Peritoneal cytology in patients with endometrial carcinoma. Gynecol Oncol 30:76, 1988

250c. Mazurka JL, Krepart GV, Lotocki RJ: Prognostic significance of positive peritoneal cytology in endometrial carcinoma. Gynecol Oncol 158:303, 1988

251. Hirai Y, Fujimoto I, Yamauchi K et al: Peritoneal fluid cytology and prognosis in patients with endometrial carcinoma. Obstet Gynecol 73:335, 1989

252. Grimshaw RN, Tupper WC, Fraser RC et al: Prognostic value of peritoneal cytology in endometrial carcinoma. Gynecol Oncol 36:97, 1990

252a. Kadar N, Homesley HD, Malfetano JH: Positive peritoneal cytology is an adverse factor in endometrial carcinoma only if there is other evidence of extrauterine disease. Gynecol Oncol 46:145, 1992.

252b. Lurain JR: The significance of positive peritoneal cytology in endometrial cancer. Gynecol Oncol 46:143, 1992

253. Naus GJ, DeVere White R, Richart RM, Deitch AD: Predictive value of flow cytometic DNA content analysis of paraffin-embedded tissue in endometrial carcinoma, abstracted. Lab Invest 52:48A, 1985

254. Geisinger KR, Kute TE, Marshall RB et al: Analysis of the relationships of the ploidy and cell cycle kinetics to differentiation of the female sex steroid hormone receptors in adenocarcinoma of the endometrium. Am J Clin Pathol 85:536, 1986

255. Iverson OE: Flow cytometric deoxyribonucleic acid index: a prognostic factor in endometrial carcinoma. Am J Obstet Gynecol 155:770, 1986

256. Lindahl B, Alm P, Killander D et al: Flow cytometric DNA analysis of normal and cancerous human endometrium and cytological–histopathological correlations. Anticancer Res 7:781, 1987

257. Lindahl B, Alm P, Ferno M et al: Prognostic value of flow cytometrical DNA measurements in stage I–II endometrial carcinoma: correlations with steroid receptor concentration, tumor myometrial invasion, and degree of differentiation. Anticancer Res 7:791, 1987

258. Quillamor RM, Furlong JW, Hoschner JA, Wynn RM: Relative prognostic significance of DNA flow cytometry and histologic grading in endometrial carcinoma. Gynecol Obstet Invest 26:332, 1988

259. Wagenius G, Strang P, Boman K et al: Residual myometrial invasion after intracavitary irradiation of endometrial adenocarcinoma stages I and II. In Vivo 2:243, 1988

260. Stendahl U, Wagenius G, Strang P, Tribukait B: Flow cytometry in invasive endometrial carcinoma. Correlations between DNA content, S phase rate, and clinical parameters. In Vivo 2:123, 1988

261. Iverson OE, Utaaker E, Skaarland E: DNA ploidy and steroid receptors as predictors of disease course in patients with endometrial carcinoma. Acta Obstet Gynecol Scand 67:531, 1988

262. Britton LC, Wilson TO, Gaffey TA et al: Flow cytometric DNA analysis of stage I endometrial carcinoma. Gynecol Oncol 34:317, 1989

263. Britton LC, Wilson TO, Gaffey TA et al: DNA ploidy in endometrial carcinoma: major objective prognostic factor. Mayo Clin Proc 65:643, 1990

264. Newbury R, Schuerch C, Goodspeed N et al: DNA content as a prognostic factor in endometrial carcinoma. Obstet Gynecol 76:251, 1990

265. Symonds DA: Prognostic value of patho-

logic features and DNA analysis in endometrial carcinoma. Gynecol Oncol 39:272, 1990

266. Stendahl U, Strang P, Wagenius G et al: Prognostic significance of proliferation in endometrial adenocarcinomas: a multivariate analysis of clinical and flow cytometric variables. Int J Gynecol Pathol 10:271, 1991

267. Jacobsen M, Hoyer M, Bentzen SM, Nielsen K: DNA flow cytometry in uterine endometrial carcinoma, suppl. APMIS 23:107, 1991

268. Konski AA, Myles JL, Sawyer T et al: Flow cytometric DNA content analysis of paraffin block embedded endometrial carcinomas. Int J Radiat Oncol Biol Phys 21:1033, 1991

269. Wagenius G, Strang P, Bergstrom R et al: Prognostic indices in endometrial adenocarcinoma stages I and II. A study based on clinical, histopathological and flow cytometric variables. Anticancer Res 11:2137, 1991

270. Sorbe B, Risberg B, Frankendal B: DNA ploidy, morphometry, and nuclear grade as prognostic factors in endometrial carcinoma. Gynecol Oncol 38:22, 1990

270a. Dyas CH, Simmons TK, Ellis CN et al: Effect of deoxyribonucleic acid ploidy status on survival of patients with carcinoma of the endometrium. Surg Gynecol Obstet 174:133, 1992

271. Kauppila A, Janne O, Kujansuu E, Vihko R: Treatment of advanced endometrial adenocarcinoma with a combined cytotoxic therapy. Cancer 46:2162, 1980

272. Ehrlich CE, Young PCM, Cleary RE: Cytoplasmic progesterone and estradiol receptors in normal, hyperplasia, and carcinomatous endometria: therapeutic implications. Am J Obstet Gynecol 141:539, 1981

273. Kauppila A, Kujansuu E, Vihko R: Cytosol estrogen and progestin receptors in endometrial carcinoma of patients treated with surgery, radiotherapy, and progestin. Cancer 50:2157, 1982

274. Martin JD, Hahnel R, McCartney AJ, Woodings TL: The effect of estrogen receptor status on survival in patients with endometrial cancer. Am J Obstet Gynecol 147:322, 1983

275. Creasman WT, Soper JT, McCarty KS, Jr et al: Influence of cytoplasmic steroid receptor content on prognosis of early stage endometrial carcinoma. Am J Obstet Gynecol 151:922, 1985

276. Quinn MA, Cauchi M, Fortune DW: Endometrial carcinoma: steroid receptors and response to medroxyprogesterone acetate. Gynecol Oncol 21:314, 1985

277. Quinn MA, Pearce P, Fortune DW et al: Correlation between cytoplasmic steroid receptors and tumour differentiation and invasion in endometrial carcinoma. Br J Obstet Gynaecol 92:399, 1985

278. Geisinger KR, Marshall RB, Kute TE, Homesley HD: Correlation of female sex steroid hormone receptors with histologic and ultrastructural differentiation in adenocarcinoma of the endometrium. Cancer 58:1506, 1986

279. Budwit-Novotny DA, McCarty KS, Cox EB et al: Immunohistochemical analyses of estrogen receptor in endometrial adenocarcinoma using a monoclonal antibody. Cancer Res 46:5419, 1986

280. Kauppila AJI, Isotalo HE, Kivinen ST, Vihko RK: Prediction of clinical outcome with estrogen and progestin receptor concentrations and their relationships to clinical and histopathological variables in endometrial cancer. Cancer Res 46:5380, 1986

281. Liao BS, Twiggs LB, Leung BS et al: Cytoplasmic estrogen and progesterone receptors as prognostic parameters in primary endometrial carcinoma. Obstet Gynecol 67:463, 1986

282. Pertschuk LP, Beddoe AM, Gorelic LS, Shain SA: Immunocytochemical assay of estrogen receptors in endometrial carcinoma with monoclonal antibodies. Cancer 57:1000, 1986

283. Mutch DG, Soper JT, Budwit-Novotny DA et al: Endometrial adenocarcinoma estrogen receptor content: association of clinicopathologic features with immunohistochemical analysis compared with standard biochemical methods. Am J Obstet Gynecol 157:924, 1987

284. Thornton JG, Wells M: Oestrogen receptor

in glands and stroma of normal and neoplastic human endometrium: a combined biochemical, immunohistochemical, and morphometric study. J Clin Pathol 40:1437, 1987

285. Utaaker E, Iversen OE, Skaarland E: The distribution and prognostic implications of steroid receptors in endometrial carcinomas. Gynecol Oncol 28:89, 1987

286. Chambers JT, MacLusky N, Eisenfield A et al: Estrogen and progestin receptor levels as prognosticators for survival in endometrial cancer. Gynecol Oncol 31:65, 1988

287. Ehrlich CE, Young PCM, Stehman FB et al: Steroid receptors and clinical outcome in patients with adenocarcinoma of the endometrium. Am J Obstet Gynecol 158:796, 1988

288. Palmer DC, Muir IM, Alexander AI et al: The prognostic importance of steroid receptors in endometrial carcinoma. Obstet Gynecol 72:388, 1988

289. Borazjani G, Twiggs LB, Leung BS et al: Prognostic significance of steroid receptors measured in primary metastatic and recurrent endometrial carcinoma. Am J Obstet Gynecol 161:1253, 1989

290. Soper J, Segreti E, Novotny D et al: Endometrial cancer: correlations of ER and PgR–ICA with progression-free interval, abstracted. Mod Pathol 2:90A, 1989

291. Brustein S, Fruchter R, Greene GL, Pertschuk LP: Immunocytochemical assay of progesterone receptors in paraffin-embedded specimens of endometrial carcinoma and hyperplasia. A preliminary evaluation. Mod Pathol 2:449, 1989

292. De Cicco Nardone F, Benedetto MT, Rossiello F et al: Hormone receptor status in human endometrial carcinoma. Cancer 64:2572, 1989

293. Ingram SS, Rosenman J, Heath R et al: The predictive value of progesterone receptor levels in endometrial cancer. Int J Radiat Oncol Biol Phys 17:21, 1989

294. Segreti EM, Novotny DB, Soper JT et al: Endometrial cancer: histologic correlates of immunohistochemical localization of progesterone receptor and estrogen receptor. Obstet Gynecol 73:780, 1989

295. Carcangiu ML, Chambers JT, Voynick IM et al: Immunohistochemical evaluation of estrogen and progesterone receptor content in 183 patients with endometrial carcinoma. Part I: Clinical and histologic correlations. Am J Clin Pathol 94:247, 1990

296. Chambers JT, Carcangiu ML, Voynick IM, Schwartz PE: Immunohistochemical evaluation of estrogen and progesterone receptor content in 183 patients with endometrial carcinoma. Part II. Correlation between biochemical and immunohistochemical methods and survival. Am J Clin Pathol 94:255, 1990

297. Kleine W, Maier T, Geyer H, Pfleiderer A: Estrogen and progesterone receptors in endometrial cancer and their prognostic relevance. Gynecol Oncol 38:59,1990

298. Pickartz H, Beckmann R, Fleige B et al: Steroid receptors and proliferative activity in non-neoplastic and neoplastic endometria. Virchows Arch A 417:163, 1990

299. Soper JT, Segreti EM, Novotny DB et al: Estrogen and progesterone receptor content of endometrial carcinomas: comparison of total tissue versus cancer component analysis. Gynecol Oncol 36:363, 1990

300. Huang SJ, Cheng L, Lewin KJ, Fu YS: Immunohistochemical estrogen receptor assessment in hyperplastic, neoplastic, and physiologic endometria. Pathol Res Pract 187:487, 1991

301. Richardson GS, MacLaughlin DT: The status of receptors in the management of endometrial cancer. Clin Obstet Gynecol 29:628, 1986

302. Soper JT, Christensen CW: Steroid receptors and endometrial cancer. Clin Obstet Gynaecol 13:825, 1986

303. Chambers JT: Sex steroid receptors in endometrial cancer. Yale J Biol Med 61:339, 1988

304. Bauknecht T, Janz J, Kohler M et al: Human ovarian carcinomas: correlation of malignancy and survival with the expression of epidermal growth factor receptors (EGF-R) and EGF-like factors (EGF-F). Med Oncol Tumor Pharmacother 6:121, 1989

305. Berchuk A, Soisson AP, Olt GJ et al: Epidermal growth factor receptor expression

in normal and malignant endometrium. Am J Obstet Gynecol 161:1247, 1989

306. Garuti G, Genazzani AR: Human *neu* oncogene is expressed in endometrial but not in ovarian adenocarcinomas. [Letter.] Cancer 67:1713, 1991

307. Borst MP, Baker VV, Dixon D et al: Oncogene alterations in endometrial carcinoma. Gynecol Oncol 38:364, 1990

308. Brumm C, Riviere A, Wilckens C, Loning T: Immunohistochemical investigation and Northern Blot analysis of c-*erb*B-2 expression in normal, premalignant and malignant tissues of the corpus and cervix uteri. Virchows Arch A 417:477, 1990

309. Berchuk A, Rodriguez G, Kinney RB et al: Overexpression of HER-2/*neu* in endometrial cancer is associated with advanced stage disease. Am J Obstet Gynecol 164:15, 1991

310. Bigsby RM, Aixin L, Bomalaski J et al: Immunohistochemical study of HER-2/*neu*, epidermal growth factor receptor, and steroid receptor expression in normal and malignant endometrium. Obstet Gynecol 79:95, 1992

311. Agnantis NJ, Spandidos DA, Mahera H et al: Immunohistochemical study of *ras* oncogene expression in endometrial and cervical human lesions. Eur J Gynaecol Oncol 9:360, 1988

312. Long CA, O'Brien TJ, Sanders M et al: *ras* Oncogene is expressed in adenocarcinoma of the endometrium. Am J Obstet Gynecol 159:1512, 1988

313. Enomoto T, Inoue M, Perantoni AO et al: K-*ras* activation in neoplasms of the human female reproductive tract. Cancer Res 50:6139, 1990

314. Enomoto T, Inoue M, Perantoni AO et al: K-*ras* activation in premalignant and malignant epithelial lesions of the human uterus. Cancer Res 51:5308, 1991

314a. Mizuuchi H, Nasim S, Kudo R et al: Clinical implications of K-*ras* mutations in malignant epithelial tumors of the endometrium. Cancer Res 52:2777, 1992

315. Kacinski BM, Carter D, Mittal K et al: High level expression of *fms* proto-oncogene mRNA is observed in clinically aggressive human endometrial adenocarcinomas. Int J Radiat Oncol Biol Phys 15:823, 1988

316. Azuma C, Safi F, Kimura T et al: Steroid hormones induce macrophage colony-stimulating factor (MCSF) and MCSF receptor mRNAs in the human endometrium. J Mol Endocrinol 5:103, 1990

317. Bur ME, Perlman C, Edelmann L et al: p53 expression in neoplasms of the uterine corpus. Am J Clin Pathol 98:81, 1992

318. Kohler MF, Berchuk A, Davidoff AM et al: Overexpression and mutation of p53 in endometrial carcinomas. Cancer Res 52:1622, 1992

319. Silverberg SG, Mullen D, Faraci JA et al: Endometrial carcinoma: clinical–pathological comparison of cases in postmenopausal women receiving and not receiving exogenous estrogens. Cancer 45:3018, 1980

320. Bokhman JV: Two pathogenetic types of endometrial cancer. Gynecol Oncol 15:10, 1983

6

Pure Mesenchymal Tumors

Philip B. Clement

This chapter discusses the pathology of pure mesenchymal tumors of the uterus, (our classification of which is reproduced in Table 6-1), with an emphasis on malignant forms; the latter account for approximately 3 percent of uterine cancers. Benign tumors are also considered, but primarily with regard to their differential with sarcomas, as their typical gross and microscopic features are well known. The procedure for mitosis counting in mesenchymal tumors is discussed in the appendix to this chapter (p. 317).

SMOOTH MUSCLE TUMORS

LEIOMYOMA VARIANTS

Although most uterine leiomyomas are obviously benign and most uterine leiomyosarcomas obviously malignant on histologic examination, a number of variants of clinically benign leiomyomas may be misinterpreted as leiomyosarcoma or some other uterine neoplasm. Similar variants may be occasionally encountered as a pure or predominant component of intravenous leiomyomatosis (p. 288). Unless otherwise noted, these tumors have a clinical presentation similar to that of typical leiomyomas. Although their gross appearance may resemble that of typical leiomyoma, leiomyoma variants may have macroscopic features characteristic of that variant; in other

cases, their gross features may incorrectly suggest the diagnosis of leiomyosarcoma.

Leiomyomas that are unusually cellular but otherwise typical (devoid of nuclear atypia, a mitotic rate of 4 or fewer mitotic figures per 10 high-power field [MF/10 HPF] are referred to as *cellular leiomyomas*[1–7] (Fig. 6-1). On gross examination, they may resemble typical leiomyomas but sometimes have a more fleshy, tan-brown sectioned surface. Hemorrhage, necrosis, slightly infiltrative borders, or combinations thereof, are present in a minority of cases[3, 4, 7] (as in Fig. 6-2). Such tumors should be particularly thoroughly sampled to exclude a diagnosis of leiomyosarcoma or smooth muscle tumor of uncertain malignant potential. The frequent dense cellularity of cellular leiomyomas may result in a close resemblance to an endometrial stromal nodule on low-power examination, or less commonly, if its borders are infiltrative, a low-grade endometrial stromal sarcoma. The presence of a fascicular growth pattern, thick-walled blood vessels, fusiform nuclei, and focal merging with the adjacent myometrium indicates a smooth muscle origin. It is worth noting that although smooth muscle tumors typically have large, thick-walled vessels, in contrast to the typical small vessels of stromal tumors, vessels of the latter type may be seen in some leiomyomas; with possible rare exceptions, however, they are not as diffusely distributed as in stromal tumors. Because of the frequent immunoreactivity of endo-

Table 6-1. Classification of Pure Mesenchymal Tumors of the Uterus

Smooth muscle tumors
  Leiomyoma
    Variants
      Cellular
      With bizarre nuclei
      Mitotically active
      Apoplectic
      Myxoid
      Hydropic
      With benign heterologous elements
      Schwannoma-like
      Epithelioid
      Others
  Leiomyosarcoma
    Variants
      Myxoid
      Epithelioid
  Smooth muscle tumors of uncertain malignant
    potential
  Smooth muscle tumors with unusual growth
    patterns
      Diffuse leiomyomatosis
      Leiomyoma with vascular invasion
      Intravenous leiomyomatosis
      Benign metastasizing leiomyoma
      Peritoneal leiomyoma
      Diffuse peritoneal leiomyomatosis
Endometrial stromal tumors
  Stromal nodule
  Low-grade endometrial stromal sarcoma
  High-grade endometrial stromal sarcoma and
    other high-grade endometrial sarcomas
Mixed endometrial stromal and smooth muscle
  tumors
Rare sarcomas
  Homologous
    Angiosarcoma and related tumors
    Malignant fibrous histiocytoma (and variants)
  Heterologous
    Rhabdomyosarcoma, pleomorphic and
      embryonal (sarcoma botryoides)
    Chondrosarcoma
    Osteosarcoma
    Liposarcoma
  Of uncertain histogenesis
    Alveolar soft part sarcoma
    Malignant rhabdoid tumor
Rare benign mesenchymal tumors

metrial stromal cells for smooth muscle markers,[8, 9] immunohistochemical stains for intermediate filaments have limited value in the differential diagnosis.

Occasional leiomyomas contain cells with bizarrely shaped, multilobated or multinucleated, hyperchromatic nuclei; the chromatin sometimes has a smudged ap-

pearance. These tumors are variously referred to as "symplastic," "atypical," or "bizarre" leiomyoma, or *leiomyoma with bizarre nuclei,* a term we prefer (Figs. 6-2 and 6-3).[1, 2, 5–7, 10, 11] The gross features are identical to those described for cellular leiomyomas (Fig. 6-2). The bizarre nuclei may contain cytoplasmic pseudoinclusions.[4, 7] A diagnostic impression of leiomyosarcoma can be enhanced in such cases when degenerating or karyorrhectic nuclei are mistaken for atypical mitotic figures (Fig. 6-3). Foci of hemorrhage or necrosis, or both, are seen in a few cases.[7] The cells with bizarre nuclei are often scattered singly or in small groups in an otherwise typical leiomyoma, and this finding, together with a paucity of unequivocal mitotic figures, premenopausal age, and an occasional association with exogenous progestins,[11] usually facilitate the correct diagnosis. When the cells with bizarre nuclei are more diffusely distributed, appreciation that the nuclear atypia is not accompanied by significant mitotic activity and awareness of this entity should establish the correct diagnosis.

Although mitotic activity, with rare exceptions, is one of the cardinal histologic features of leiomyosarcoma, it has been recently shown that otherwise typical or cellular leiomyomas with up to 15 MF/10 HPF have a benign course, even after myomectomy, provided that they are benign by other criteria (Fig. 6-4). The terms "*mitotically active leiomyoma*" (MAL)[12–14] or "*leiomyoma with increased mitotic figures*"[2] have been suggested for such tumors. At least 60 percent of MALs were submucosal in one study.[14] In two series, a diagnosis of MAL was allowable only in the absence of nuclear pleomorphism,[13, 14] whereas in a third series, mild or even moderate nuclear pleomorphism did not exclude the diagnosis.[12] In as many as 15 percent of MALs, there is microscopic vascular invasion within the confines of the tumor.[14] In contrast to leiomyosarcomas,

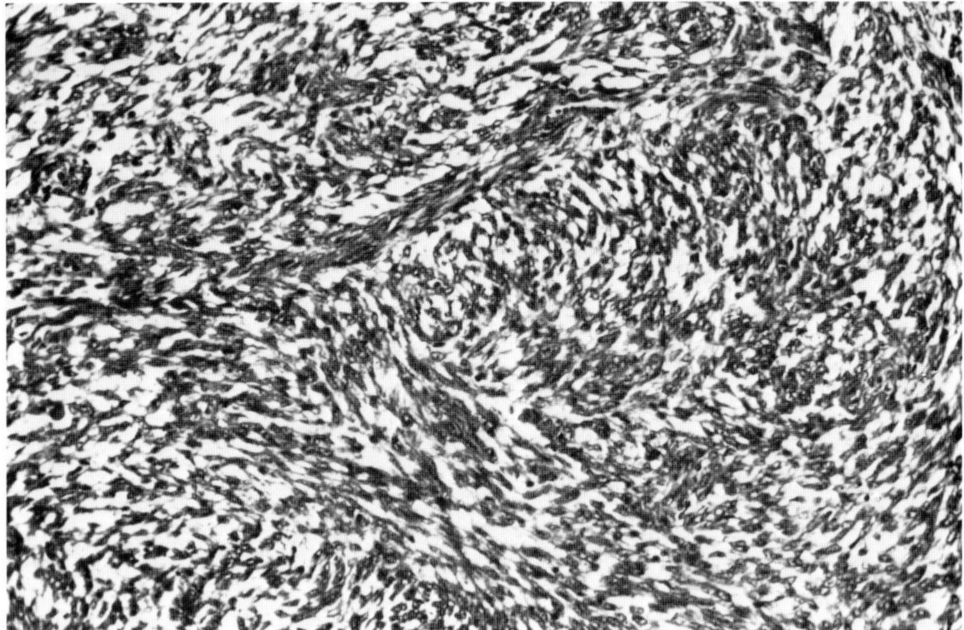

Fig. 6-1. Cellular leiomyoma. Note fascicular growth pattern of spindle cells.

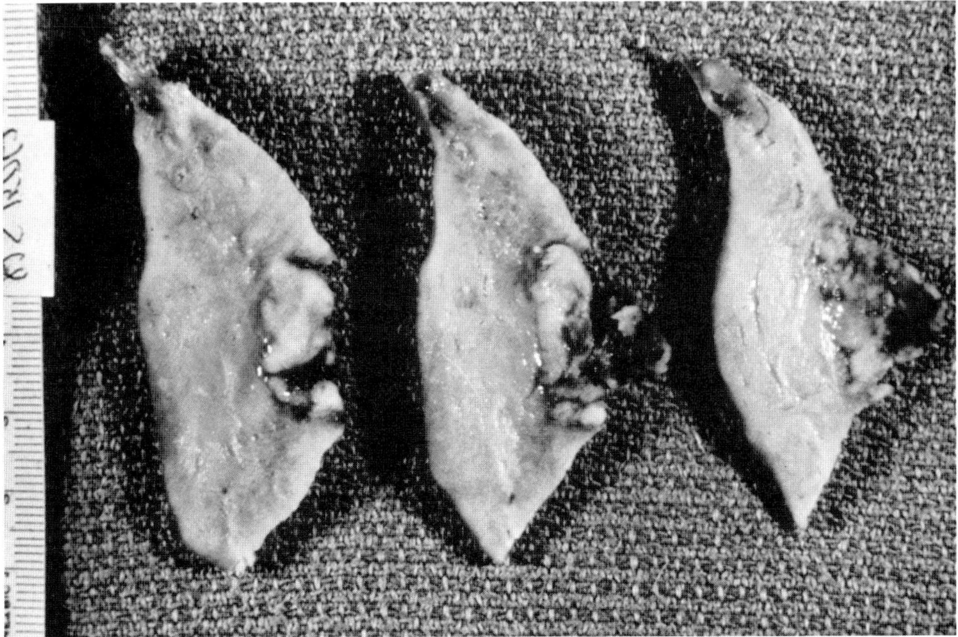

Fig. 6-2. Leiomyoma with bizarre nuclei, sectioned surface. The tumor is fleshy with foci of hemorrhage and is less well circumscribed than a typical leiomyoma.

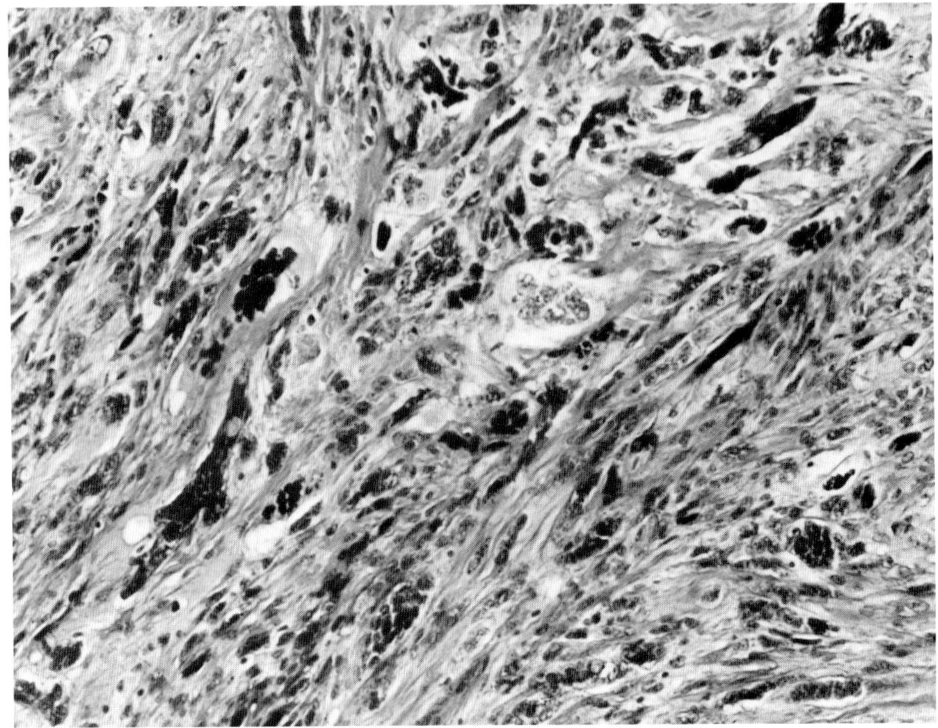

Fig. 6-3. Leiomyoma with bizarre nuclei.

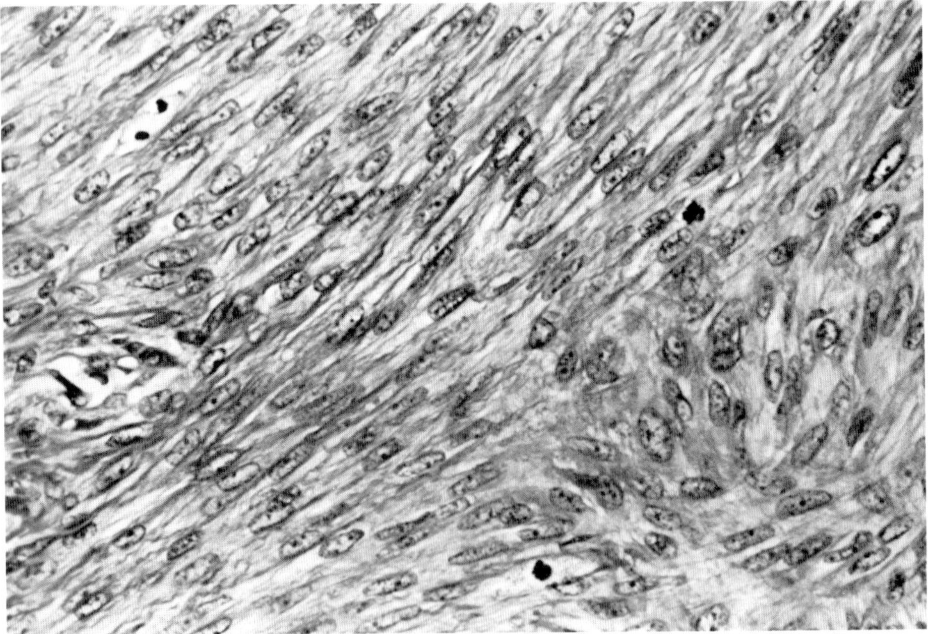

Fig. 6-4. Mitotically active leiomyoma.

most MALs lack worrisome gross features, but the presence of the latter does not exclude the diagnosis. In one series, for example, 37 percent of the tumors contained soft, fleshy, or cystic areas and 19 percent had visible areas of hemorrhage.[13] In additional contrast to leiomyosarcomas, MALs almost invariably occur in women of reproductive age and are typically associated with the secretory phase of the menstrual cycle, pregnancy, or the use of exogenous hormones.[13–16] These observations suggest that the mitotic activity in at least some MALs is due to an exogenous or endogenous progestational effect.

Leiomyomas from pregnant patients or those on progestins may be misinterpreted as leiomyosarcoma. There may be a history of rapid growth of the leiomyoma (which may also occur with clomiphene or tamoxifen therapy),[1, 17] leading to clinical suspicion of a sarcoma. Parenthetically, we have seen cases of leiomyoma in the absence of either clinical setting in which there is a clinical history of "rapid growth." On pathologic examination, the pregnancy or progestin-related changes include hemorrhage, edema, myxoid change, focal hypercellularity, nuclear pleomorphism, and increased mitotic activity.[18] So-called red degeneration of uterine leiomyomas, although observed in nonpregnant patients, is characteristic of pregnancy; it was encountered in one-third of leiomyomas from pregnant women in one study[20] (Fig. 6-5). The cause of the lesion is unclear, but it appears to be the result of variable degrees of infarction, hemorrhage with subsequent hemolysis, and hyalinization within a leiomyoma.[18]

Recently, the designations *"apoplectic leiomyoma"*[19] and *"hemorrhagic cellular leiomyoma"*[20] have been used to refer to a particular constellation of changes occurring within leiomyomas in women taking oral contraceptives or who are pregnant. Patients may present during pregnancy or the puerperium with acute abdominal signs secondary to rupture of the tumor into the

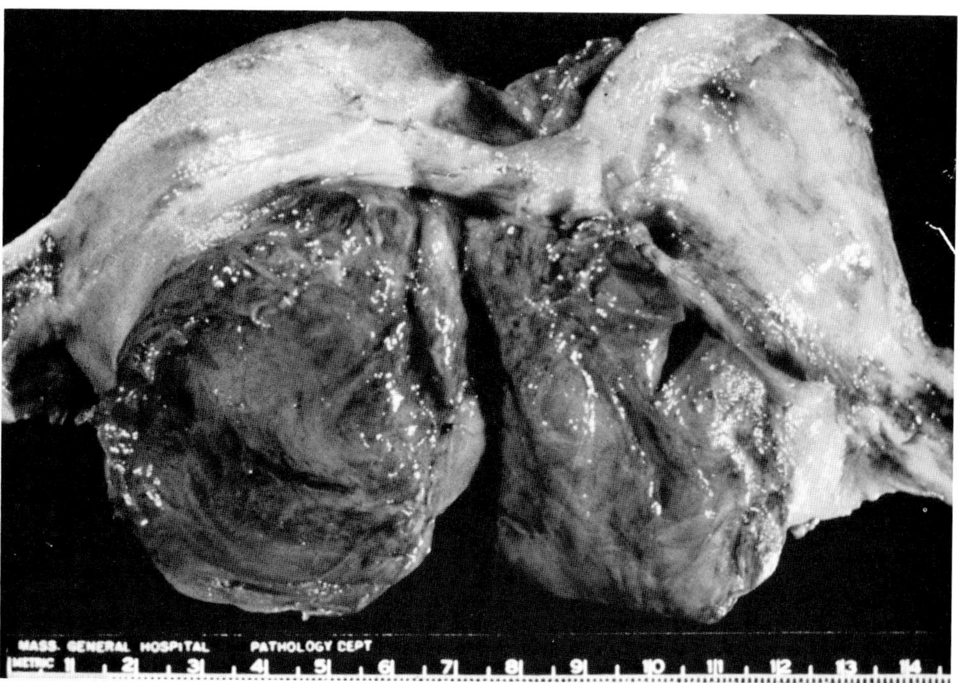

Fig. 6-5. Leiomyoma removed from pregnant patient showing "red degeneration."

peritoneal cavity. On gross examination, hemorrhage within one or more leiomyomas, which may be accompanied by cystic change, is the cardinal feature. Microscopic examination indicates a densely cellular proliferation of smooth muscle cells surrounding stellate zones of recent hemorrhage (Fig. 6-6). The cells lack malignant nuclear features, but as many as 8 MF/10 HPF have been encountered in some cases.[20] Vascular alterations, including intimal myxoid change and fibrosis, medial hypertrophy, fibrinoid necrosis, and thrombosis, may be encountered within the leiomyomas or the surrounding myometrium. Because of these pregnancy-related changes and the rarity of leiomyosarcomas in the reproductive age group, a diagnosis of uterine leiomyosarcoma should be rendered with caution in a pregnant patient or one on hormonal medication.

Some of the findings described in apoplectic leiomyomas may also be encountered in *leiomyomas treated with go-nadotropin-releasing hormone agonists* (GnRH-a) that reduce the size of leiomyomas prior to their removal. Although one recent study[21] found no significant difference between those leiomyomas treated with GnRH-a and controls, another study[22] found that the treated tumors had irregular borders, areas of markedly increased cellularity, hyalinization, infarct-like necrosis, and vascular changes (Fig. 6-7). The last alteration consisted of mural thickening secondary to smooth muscle proliferation, myxoid change, and fibrinoid degeneration.[22] None of the tumors had more than 3 mitotic figures per 50 HPF.[22]

Myxoid leiomyomas are uncommon in our experience, and many tumors referred to as such are more appropriately diagnosed as "hydropic leiomyomas." Myxoid and hydropic degeneration may be difficult to distinguish from each other with routine stains. Hendrickson and Kempson[23] refer to myxoid change as the presence of "scattered nuclei embedded in an amorphous,

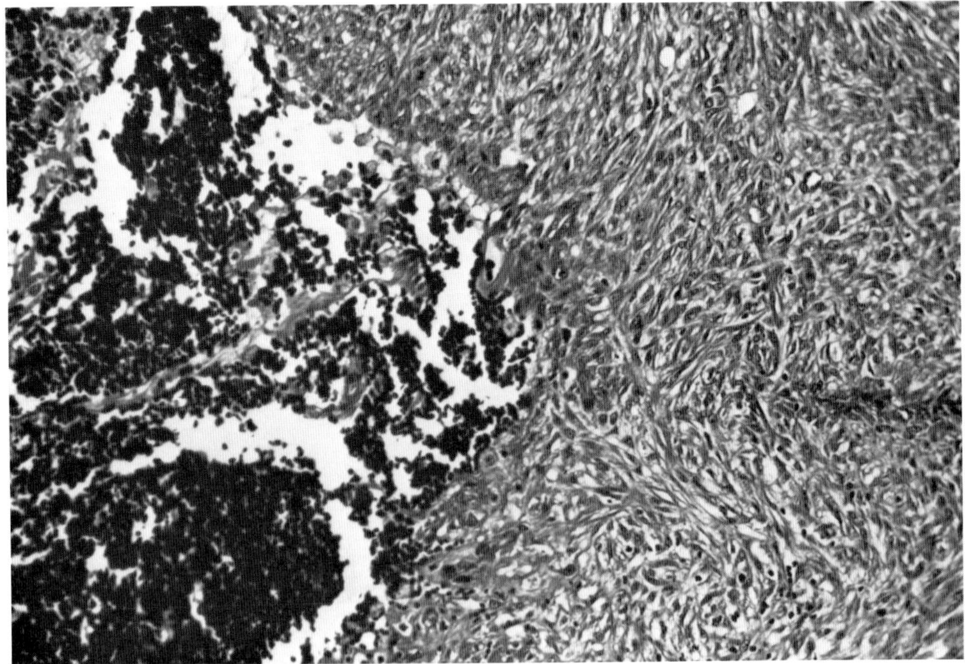

Fig. 6-6. "Apoplectic" leiomyoma in pregnant patient. Note focal area of recent hemorrhage surrounded by cellular smooth muscle.

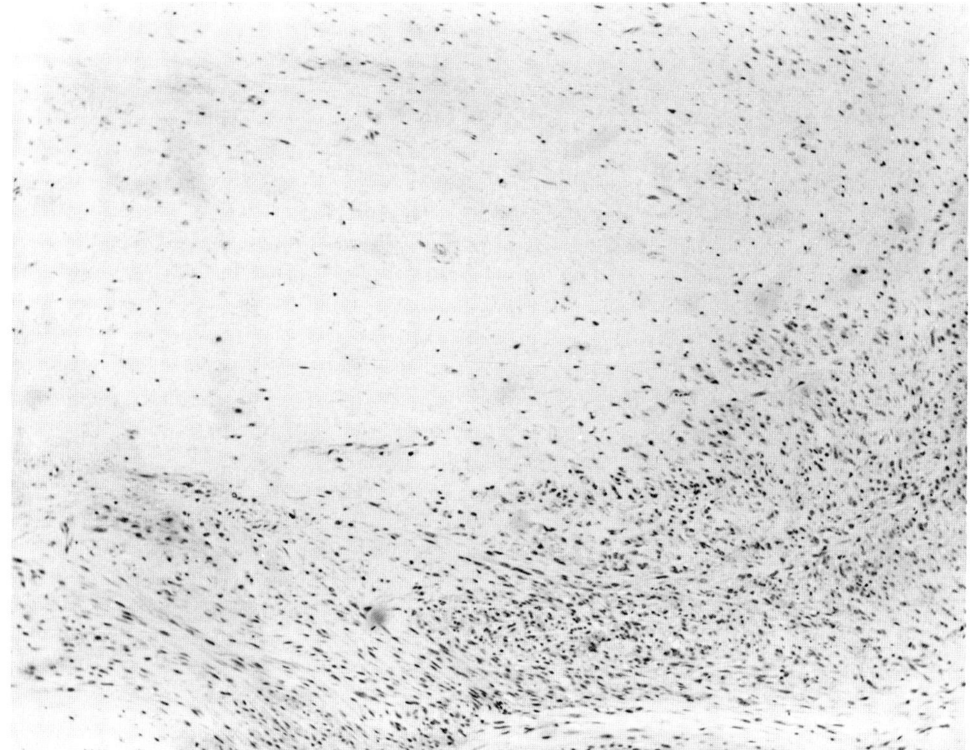

Fig. 6-7. Leiomyoma removed from patient treated with gonadotropin-releasing-hormone agonist. Large area of necrosis is surrounded by cellular smooth muscle.

pale-staining, slightly blue, fibrillar matrix" and mucoid degeneration as "pools of blue mucinous matrix separating muscle fibers." There appears to be little value in distinguishing between "myxoid" and "mucoid" degeneration, as these investigators acknowledge. We reserve the term *"myxoid leiomyoma"* for leiomyomas characterized by abundant acellular material rich in acid mucins, as confirmed by alcian blue or colloidal iron stains (Fig. 6-8). Applying this criterion, myxoid degeneration is much less common than hydropic degeneration in our experience, and is frequently a feature of uterine leiomyomas encountered during pregnancy.[18] Myxoid leiomyomas are usually grossly well circumscribed and resemble extrauterine myxomas, being composed of homogeneous, soft, gray, jellylike material.[24] On microscopic examination, the neoplastic cells are often stellate in shape and

widely separated by the extracellular material. Diffuse myxoid change may result in a microscopic appearance indistinguishable from a myxoma (p. 317),[24] and distinction of the two lesions may require immunohistochemical or ultrastructural confirmation[24] of smooth muscle differentiation within the tumor. Myxoid leiomyomas must also be distinguished from myxoid leiomyosarcomas (p. 279).

We have recently reported a series of uterine leiomyomas with prominent degrees of hydropic change, *"hydropic leiomyomas,"* that created problems in differential diagnosis.[25] Hydropic degeneration is typically accompanied by variable amounts of hyalinization ("hyaline degeneration") within the leiomyoma. Marked degrees of hydropic degeneration may result in cystic degeneration; occasional large myometrial cysts represent leiomy-

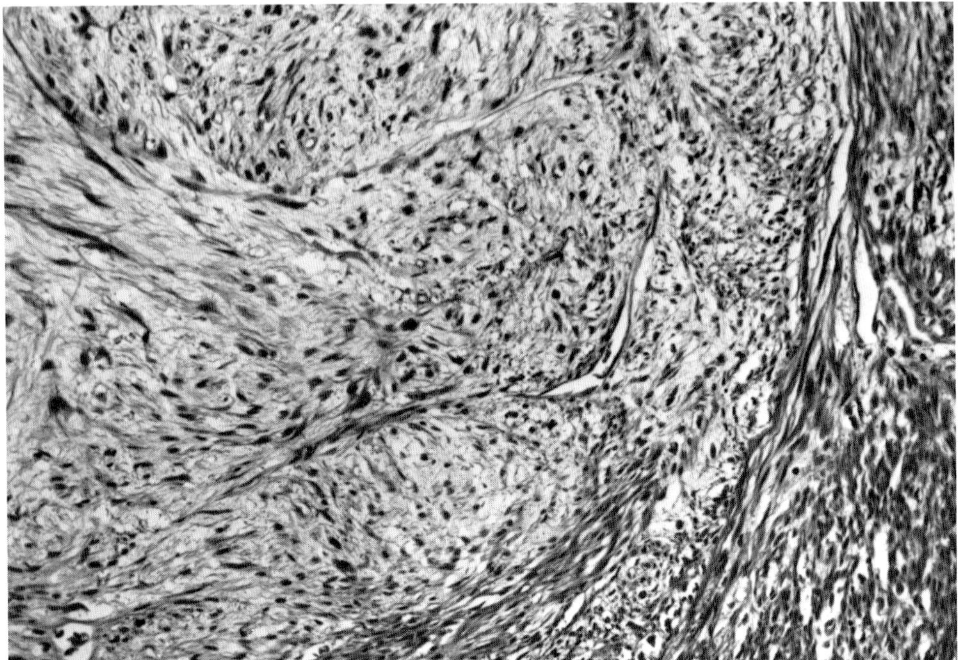

Fig. 6-8. Leiomyoma with myxoid degeneration. Pale intercellular material was strongly alcianophilic.

omas with total or subtotal cystic degeneration.[26] In some hydropic leiomyomas, sparsely cellular hydropic connective tissue subdivides part or all of the leiomyoma into numerous, small, typically nonhydropic leiomyomatous nodules (Figs. 6-9 and 6-10), resulting in a false impression that the nodules are lying within vascular spaces. In such cases, there has been confusion on both gross and microscopic examination with intravenous leiomyomatosis (p. 288). In contrast to the latter, immunohistochemical stains for factor VIII-related antigen and *Ulex europaeus* confirm an absence of endothelial cells surrounding the nodules and lining the pseudovascular spaces (Fig. 6-10B). Additional diagnostic problems have resulted in hydropic leiomyomas when hydropic changes have extended beyond the confines of the leiomyoma, in some cases suggesting invasion; myxoid leiomyosarcoma was an initial diagnostic consideration in some of these cases.

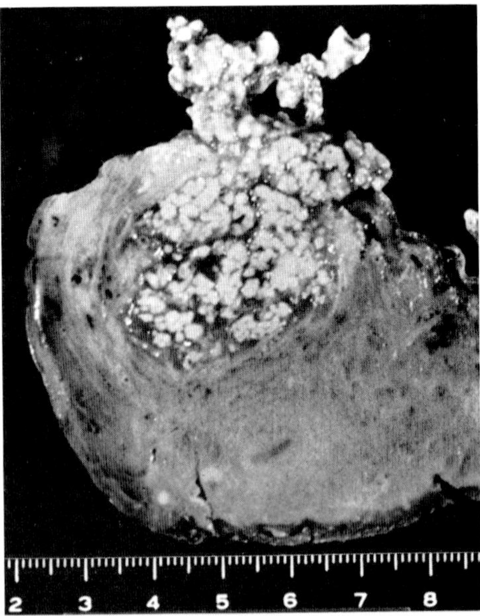

Fig. 6-9. Leiomyoma with perinodular hydropic degeneration. A leiomyoma is subdivided into numerous small nonhydropic nodules that are separated by hydropic connective tissue. (From Clement et al.,[25] with permission.)

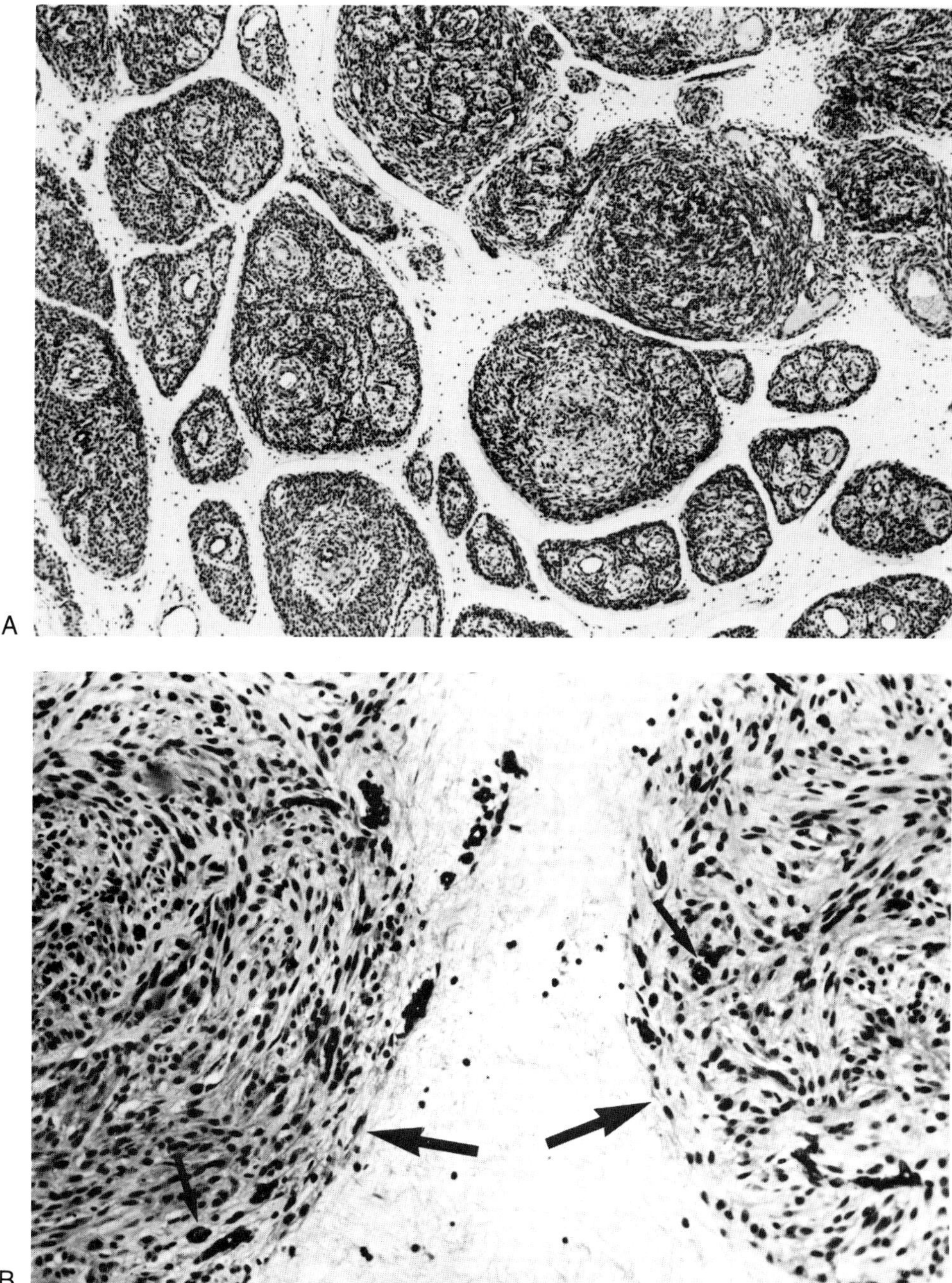

Fig. 6-10. Leiomyoma with perinodular hydropic degeneration. (A) Nodules of cellular smooth muscle (some of which contain thick-walled blood vessels) are separated by pale hydropic connective tissue. The appearance mimics that of intravenous leiomyomatosis (compare with Figs. 6-29 and 6-30). (B) Same case stained for *Ulex europaeus*. In contrast to intravenous leiomyomatosis, there is an absence of endothelial cells ensheathing the nodules of smooth muscle (large arrows). Note immunoreactivity of endothelial cells lining the blood vessels with the nodules (small arrows).

Finally, marked degrees of hydropic change may result in extensive or subtotal obliteration of the usual architecture of the leiomyoma, often accompanied by numerous thick-walled blood vessels, that tends to obscure its smooth muscle nature.[25] Awareness of these changes combined with mucin stains and with immunohistochemical stains for endothelial antigens facilitates the diagnosis.

Occasional otherwise typical leiomyomas contain mature heterologous elements. The most common of these are *lipoleiomyomas*[27–32]; some of the reported examples have contained cells with bizarre nuclei.[31, 32] The differential diagnosis of these lesions includes the much rarer pure lipomas (p. 317) and liposarcomas of the uterus (p. 312). Even rarer are *leiomyomas with osseus*[33] or *chondroid metaplasia or skeletal muscle differentiation.*[34] Mazur and Kraus[24] have described a *leiomyoma with tubules,* in which the latter were lined by uniform cuboidal cells that had the ultrastructural features of mesothelial cells.[24] The features of this tumor overlap with those of adenomatoid tumors (see Ch. 8). *Schwannoma-like leiomyomas* characterized by palisading nuclei and Antoni A and B type patterns within the tumors appear on ultrastructural examination to be true leiomyomas devoid of schwannian differentiation.[1, 2, 10, 24, 35]

Some leiomyomas contain prominent numbers of inflammatory and other cells of hematopoietic type. *"Pyomyomas"* are a result of bacterial infection within a leiomyoma.[36, 37] Pathologic examination reveals a leiomyoma with abscess cavities and large numbers of neutrophils; bacteria may be demonstrable. Rarely leiomyomas contain *massive lymphoid infiltrates* (see Ch. 4) or are the site of extramedullary hematopoiesis.[38] Typical leiomyomas may contain numerous histiocytes demonstrable with immunohistochemical stains,[39] and leiomyomas or lipoleiomyomas may contain striking collections of mast cells[27, 40] (see Ch. 4) or eosinophils, or both.[27]

LEIOMYOSARCOMA

Clinical Features. Leiomyosarcomas account for approximately 45 percent of uterine sarcomas.[1–7, 10, 12, 41, 42] The tumors may be found from the third to ninth decades, but the vast majority of affected patients are over the age of 40. In some series, there is an increased incidence in blacks.[5] Patients usually present with abnormal vaginal bleeding pain, or both, and usually have an enlarged uterus on pelvic examination. Although rapid enlargement of a myometrial tumor suggests leiomyosarcoma, a similar finding occurs in leiomyomas in women taking exogenous hormones and occasionally in patients with apparently typical leiomyomas with no obvious predisposing cause. In rare patients, the presenting manifestations of the tumor have been related to tumor rupture (and hemoperitoneum),[43, 44] extrauterine extension (present in one-third to one-half of cases), or metastases.[1] One uterine leiomyosarcoma was associated with fever, eosinophilia, and alkaline phosphatase production.[45] Cytologic evaluation and examination of curettings are unrewarding in patients with leiomyosarcoma, except in those with tumors that are submucosal or protrude into the endometrial cavity.[1] Occasional patients with high-stage disease have had an elevated serum level of CA-125 at presentation; this marker may also be useful in detecting recurrent tumor.[46] Rare patients with leiomyosarcomas have had prior pelvic irradiation.[5]

Gross Features. Leiomyosarcomas are typically large solitary masses with a mean (or median) diameter in several large series of 10 cm[3–7]; in one series,[10] however, 25 percent of tumors were less than 5 cm in diameter. Approximately two-thirds of leiomyosarcomas are intramural, one-fifth submucosal, and one-tenth subserosal. They are almost always less circumscribed than leiomyomas and cannot be shelled out from the adjacent myometrium. The cut surface is typically bulging, soft, fleshy, and focally necrotic and hemorrhagic without the whorled appearance characteristic of a leiomyoma (Fig. 6-11). Gross evidence of vascular invasion is rare. Five percent of these tumors originate in the cervix, where they usually form an intramural or an intraluminal mass.[47] Although leiomyosarcomas are frequently associated with benign leiomyomas in the same uterus,[6, 10] convincing examples of leiomyosarcomas arising in a leiomyoma or leiomyoma variant are very rare[3, 6, 10, 48] (Fig. 6-12).

Microscopic Features. Most leiomyosarcomas of the uterus are obviously malignant on microscopic examination, the cardinal histologic features being hypercellularity of at least moderate degree, usually moderate to marked degrees of nuclear pleomorphism, and a high mitotic rate (at least 5 but usually more than 15 MF/10 HPF)[1–7, 10, 12, 41, 42] (Figs. 6-13 and 6-14). Very rare leiomyosarcomas have high mitotic rates with only minimal nuclear atypia.[10] Additional supportive but nondiagnostic features that are commonly present include an infiltrating border, necrosis, and atypical mitotic figures[2, 12]; in rare cases, massive necrosis has been attributed to preoperative therapy with a GnRH-a.[49] Giant cells with bizarre nuclear features and intranuclear cytoplasmic inclusions, similar to those occurring in leiomyomas with bizarre nuclei, may be encountered.[7] Vascular invasion is present in 10 to 20 percent of tumors.[3, 7]

Most leiomyosarcomas are sufficiently well differentiated, at least focally, to permit recognition of their smooth muscle nature. Immunohistochemical stains for smooth muscle markers[50–52] and ultrastructural examination[53, 54] may facilitate the diagnosis, but these procedures are rarely necessary. In this context, it should be remembered that leiomyosarcomas can be

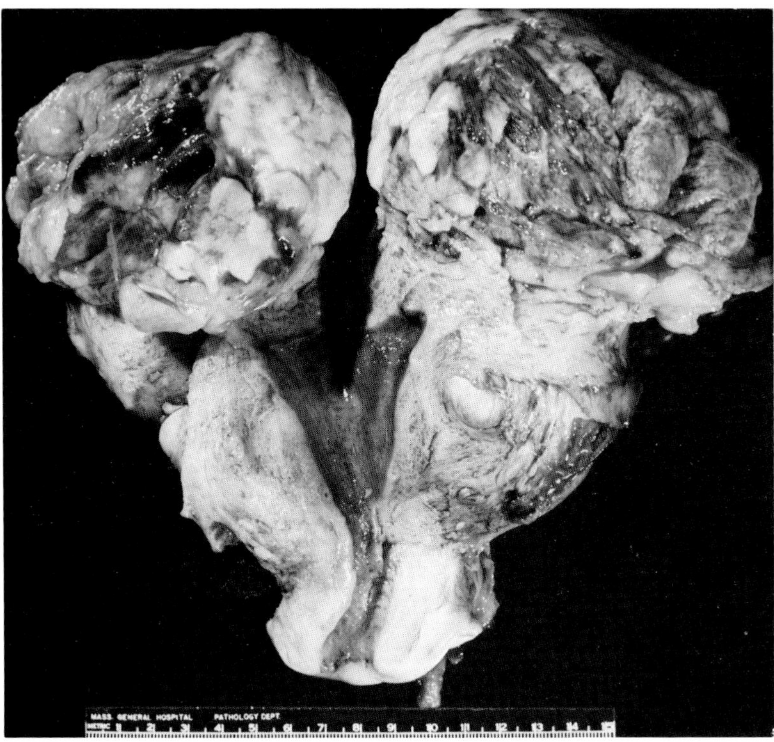

Fig. 6-11. Leiomyosarcoma. Large, poorly circumscribed mural mass has a fleshy, focally hemorrhagic and necrotic sectioned surface.

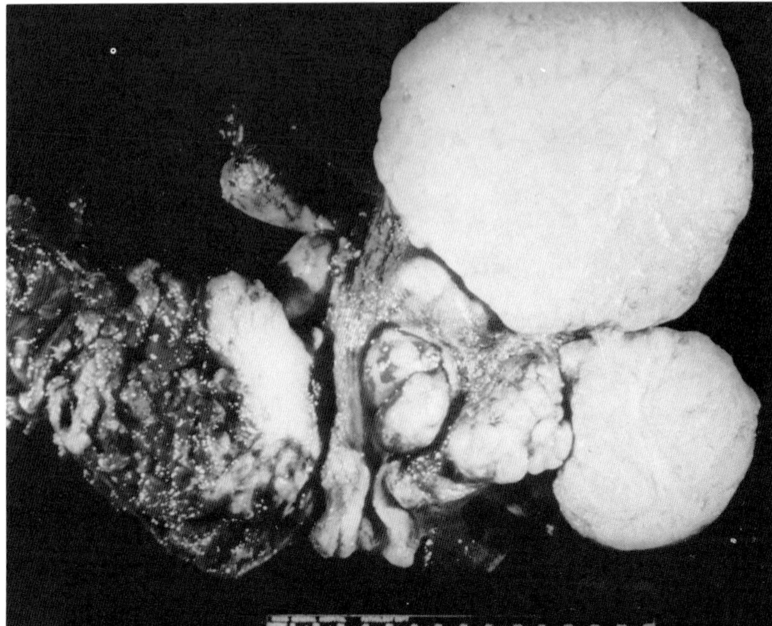

Fig. 6-12. Leiomyosarcoma arising from a leiomyoma. Mass on the left consisted predominantly of leiomyosarcoma (fleshy hemorhagic areas) admixed with a benign leiomyoma (pale area). Multiple typical leiomyomas are also present in the myometrium.

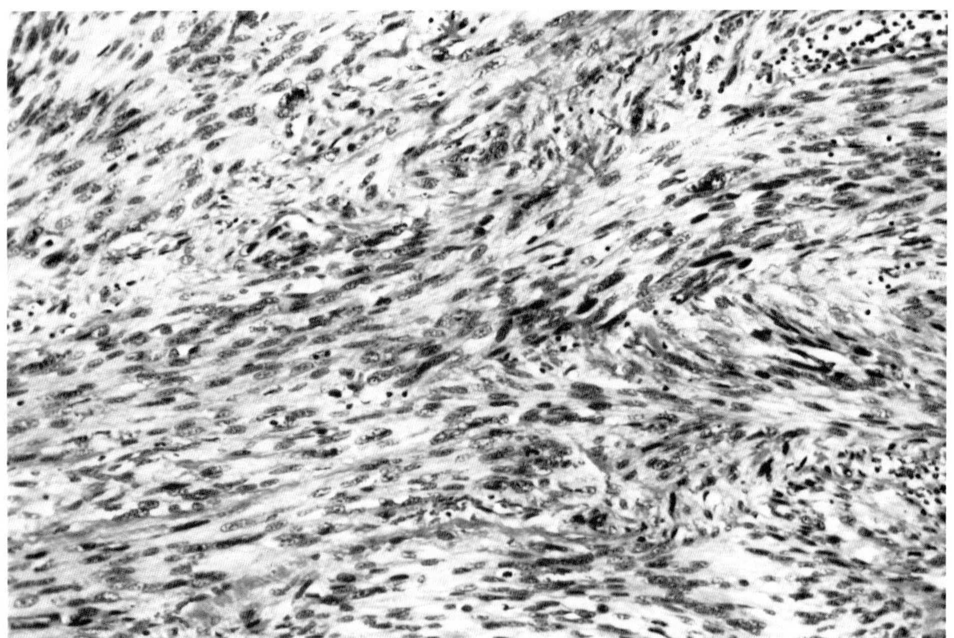

Fig. 6-13. Leiomyosarcoma. Note fascicular growth pattern, hypercellularity, and nuclear pleomorphism.

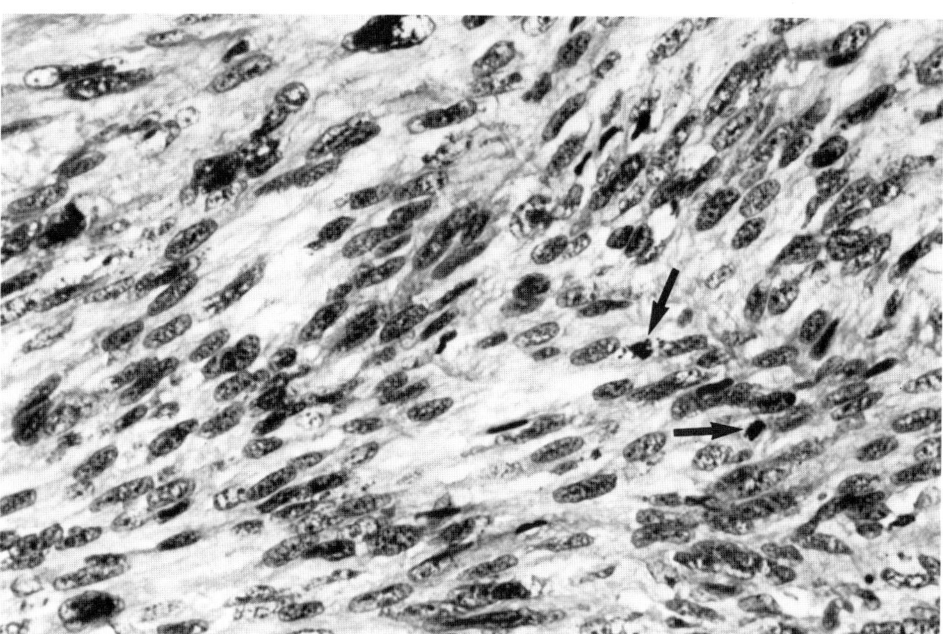

Fig. 6-14. Leiomyosarcoma. Higher-power view of Figure 6-13. Note mitotic figures (arrows).

immunoreactive for cytokeratin and epithelial membrane antigen,[55] and that the neoplastic cells of endometrial stromal sarcomas and the sarcomatous component of malignant müllerian mixed tumors (MMMTs) (see Ch. 7) are commonly immunoreactive for smooth muscle antigens.

Rare leiomyosarcomas have contained a prominent component of osteoclast-type giant cells within the primary and metastatic tumor[10, 51, 56–59] (Fig. 6-15). In some cases, the giant cell component of the tumor has resembled benign giant cell tumor of bone,[56] whereas in others, the mononuclear cells separating the osteoclastic giant cells have been cytologically malignant.[57] In one case, an otherwise typical leiomyosarcoma and a malignant osteoclastic giant cell tumor appeared as two adjacent tumors with different gross, histologic, ultrastructural, and immunohistochemical features[59] Immunohistochemical studies have suggested a macrophage origin for the osteoclastic giant cells, which are likely reactive in nature.[58]

Devaney and Tavassoli[51] recently described two cases of what they refer to as xanthomatous leiomyosarcoma. On gross examination, these tumors were focally or diffusely yellow and, on microscopic examination, were characterized by large cells with abundant cytoplasm containing lipid vacuoles and multiple or multilobated nuclei sometimes disposed in a wreathlike arrangement. The xanthomatous cells grew in solid sheets or were intimately admixed with the spindled smooth muscle cells. Mitotic figures were numerous ($>$10 MF/10 HPF) in both the xanthomatous and spindle cell areas.

Behavior, Prognostic Features, and Treatment. Leiomyosarcomas are aggressive tumors, with survival rates of only 15 to 25 percent in most series.[3–7, 10, 41] The median survival has been variable, ranging from only 13 months in one study[6] to 43 months in a more recent series.[10] In the latter series, 55 percent of patients who died from tumor had both local recurrence and distant metastases, 39 percent had distant

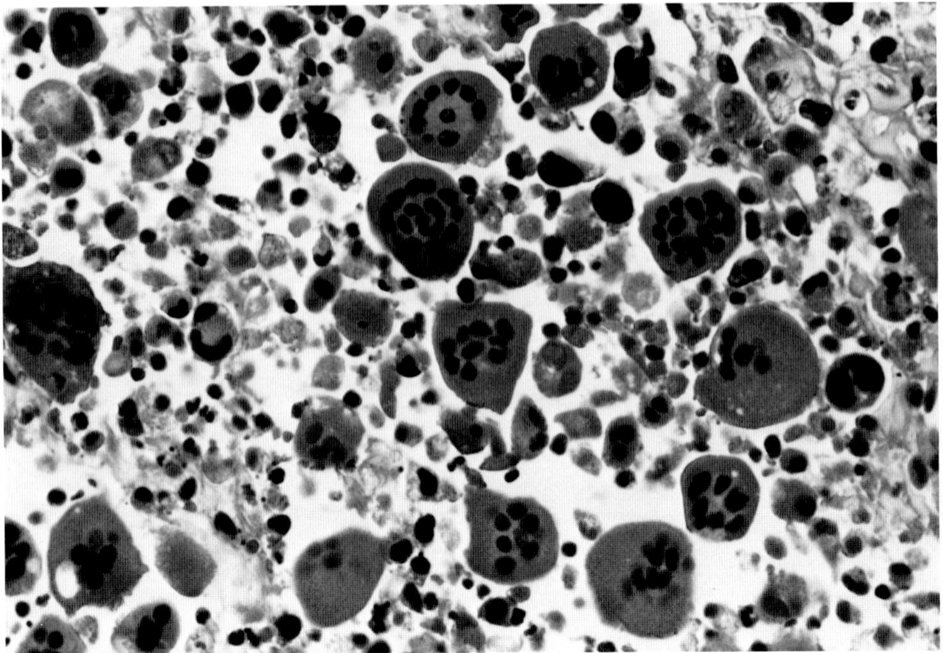

Fig. 6-15. Leiomyosarcoma with prominent numbers of osteoclast-type giant cells.

metastases only, and 6 percent had local recurrence only.[10] Rare patients die from tumor 10 or more years after hysterectomy[7] In one series, autopsies of patients dying with leiomyosarcoma documented pelvic and intra-abdominal visceral involvement (all cases), metastases to lungs and pleura (80 percent of cases), abdominopelvic lymph nodes (47 percent), kidneys (33 percent), and liver (20 percent).[3]

There has been no consistency among various studies with respect to showing a correlation between survival and age (or menopausal status) of the patient, clinical stage, tumor size, pushing versus infiltrative borders, the presence or absence of necrosis, mitotic rate, degree of nuclear pleomorphism, and vascular invasion.[10, 41, 42] One recent study, however, concluded that tumor size was a major prognostic parameter: five of eight patients with tumors less than 5 cm in diameter survived, whereas all the patients with tumors larger than 5 cm in diameter died from tumor.[10] Another recent study has suggested that DNA ploidy pat-

tern of LMSs may have prognostic significance.[60] Curative treatment for leiomyosarcomas requires complete surgical extirpation of the tumor. Pelvic irradiation may decrease the risk of local recurrence, but in most studies has not affected survival.[42] Similarly, adjuvant chemotherapy does not appear to improve survival rates.[41]

Differential Diagnosis. The differential diagnosis of leiomyosarcomas is usually with one or other of the leiomyoma variants discussed earlier. Although the latter may have one or even two worrisome microscopic features, none are characterized by the triad of hypercellularity, marked nuclear atypia, and high mitotic rate that characterize most leiomyosarcomas. Uterine smooth muscle tumors characterized by unusual growth patterns but a cytologically benign appearance (p. 287) are readily distinguishable from leiomyosarcoma. Although low-grade endometrial stromal sarcomas occasionally exhibit focal smooth muscle differentiation and are frequently immunoreactive for smooth muscle antigens, their characteristic population of mitotically inactive, small, uniform, endometrial stromal-type cells, their distinctive vascular pattern, their typical involvement of the endometrium, and their characteristic permeative invasion of the myometrium and myometrial vascular spaces readily facilitate their differentiation from leiomyosarcoma. Leiomyosarcomas should also be distinguished from other high-grade pure homologous sarcomas of the uterus, most of which have been variously referred to as "high-grade endometrial stromal sarcoma," "poorly differentiated endometrial sarcoma," or "high-grade undifferentiated uterine sarcoma" (p. 307). Unlike leiomyosarcoma, these tumors typically involve the endometrium and lack overt smooth muscle differentiation. The differential diagnosis of leiomyosarcomas with osteoclastic giant cells is with pure giant cell tumors of the uterus (p. 311), whereas the differential diagnosis of leiomyosarcomas with xanthomatous cell is with malignant fibrous histiocytomas and liposarcomas of the uterus (pp. 311–312).

Myxoid Leiomyosarcoma

Myxoid leiomyosarcoma[61–66] is a rare variant of uterine LMS that may create diagnostic problems because its myxoid appearance may obscure its smooth muscle nature, and because its mitotic inactivity may lead to a misdiagnosis of a benign tumor. The presenting clinical features resemble those of patients with typical uterine leiomyosarcoma. On gross examination, the tumors are usually found within the myometrium; three tumors located predominantly within the broad ligament were considered to have arisen within the outer myometrium.[61, 65] The tumors have ranged from 5 to 16 cm in diameter and typically exhibit a strikingly gelatinous cut surface and an apparently well-circumscribed border (Fig. 6-16). On microscopic examination, however, the tumors typically infiltrate the myometrium in irregular tongues, and in some cases, myometrial veins (Fig. 6-17). Most or all of the tumor is characterized by an abundant paucicellular myxoid matrix (Fig. 6-7) that is weakly basophilic

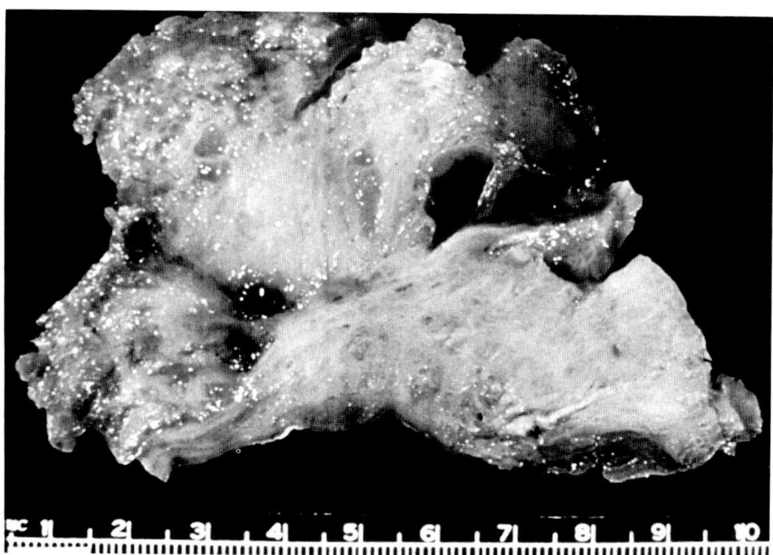

Fig. 6-16. Myxoid leiomyosarcoma. Gelatinous tumor has a deceptively well-circumscribed border with the surrounding myometrium. (From Clement et al.,[249] with permission.)

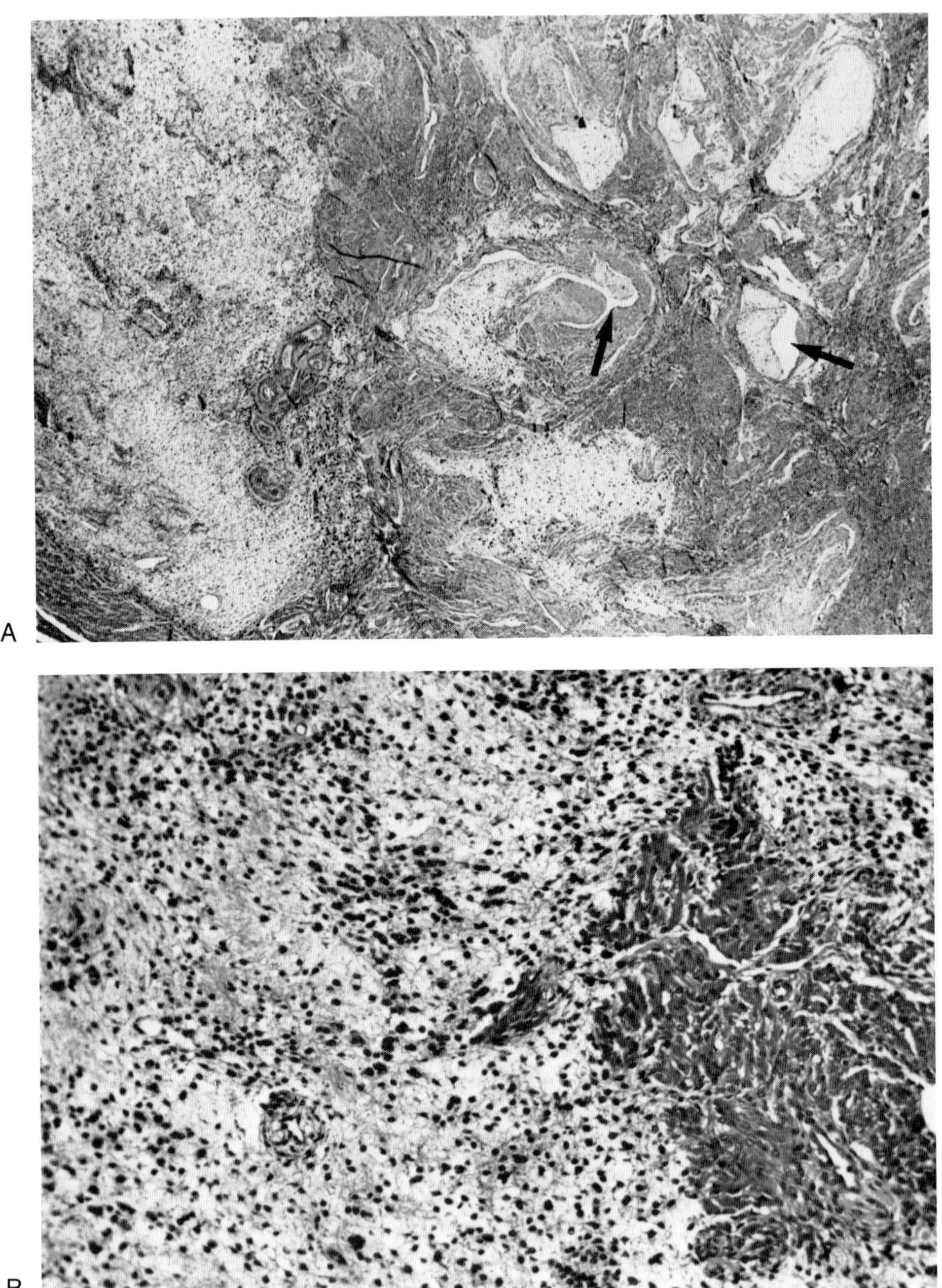

Fig. 6-17. Myxoid leiomyosarcoma. **(A)** The tumor infiltrates the myometrium in irregular tongues. Note invasion of myometrial veins (arrows). **(B)** The tumor is composed of small cells with scant cytoplasm within a myxoid matrix. Note infiltrative border with myometrial smooth muscle. (From Clement et al.,[249] with permission.)

or eosinophilic, weakly positive with the periodic acid-Schiff (PAS) and mucicarmine methods, and strongly positive with alcian blue and colloidal iron staining. Most of the material that stains with colloidal iron is not removed by hyaluronidase pretreatment. The majority of the tumor cells have scant cytoplasm with oval, spindle, or stellate nuclei with inapparent nucleoli and a low mitotic rate (0 to 2 MF/10 HPF) (Fig. 6-17B). Focally, the tumor cells may exhibit mild to moderate degrees of nuclear pleomorphism and occasional multinucleated cells may be present. The tumor cells may be uniformly distributed throughout the myxoid stroma, arranged in thin fascicles, or surround cavities filled with myxoid material. Nonmyxoid areas, present to a variable degree, usually exhibit architectural and cytologic features that help establish the smooth muscle nature of the neoplastic cells; greater degrees of nuclear pleomorphism and mitotic activity may also be present in such areas. Electron microscopic examination of several cases has shown evidence of smooth muscle differentiation.[61, 66]

Recurrent tumor, distant metastases, or both have appeared at posthysterectomy intervals of 6 months to 10 years in almost all reported cases with follow-up data. Most of these patients died from tumor or were alive with tumor at last follow-up. The morphologic features, including the mitotic rate, of the recurrent tumor are generally similar to those of the primary tumor. In occasional cases, however, there is more obvious smooth muscle differentiation or a higher mitotic rate. Rarely, a myxoid appearance may be present within metastatic or recurrent leiomyosarcoma that was absent within the primary tumor.[65]

Myxoid leiomyosarcoma should be differentiated from myxoid leiomyomas as well as the myxoid variant of intravenous leiomyomatosis. The myxoid leiomyoma and the extravascular tumor of myxoid IVL are well circumscribed on histologic examination in comparison to the markedly infiltrative borders of myxoid leiomyosarcoma. It may be difficult, however, to distinguish between these lesions in a curettage specimen; a hysterectomy may be necessary in order to determine the margin of a myxoid lesion.

Epithelioid Smooth Muscle Tumors

Rare smooth muscle tumors, composed predominantly or entirely of polygonal cells, have been referred to as leiomyoblastoma, epithelioid smooth muscle tumors, or clear cell smooth muscle tumors.[10, 67–81] We agree with others[10, 70, 79] who discourage the use of the term "leiomyoblastoma" for these tumors, a designation that incorrectly implies a highly malignant tumor composed of primitive cells. Epithelioid smooth muscle tumors with a pure or predominant plexiform pattern have been designated plexiform tumors[69, 72, 73] or, when small (less than 1 cm), "plexiform tumorlets."[75, 76] Occasional otherwise typical leiomyomas contain minor scattered foci of epithelioid cells. Rare examples of intravenous leiomyomatosis are composed predominantly or exclusively of epithelioid cells (p. 288).

The clinical presentation of epithelioid smooth muscle tumors does not differ significantly from that of typical leiomyomas[70]; plexiform tumorlets are usually incidental findings.[75] On gross examination, many epithelioid leiomyomas resemble typical leiomyomas, but some are fleshy (lacking a whorled cut surface) (Fig. 6-18), are poorly circumscribed, and contain foci of hemorrhage and necrosis, resulting in an appearance that may suggest leiomyosarcoma. Some epithelioid leiomyosarcomas have had obviously malignant features on gross examination.[77] Plexiform tumorlets are typically microscopic (Fig. 6-19), although they are rarely recognized grossly as small leiomyomas, and are frequently multiple (as many as 14).[75] Although more common in the myometrium, plexiform tu-

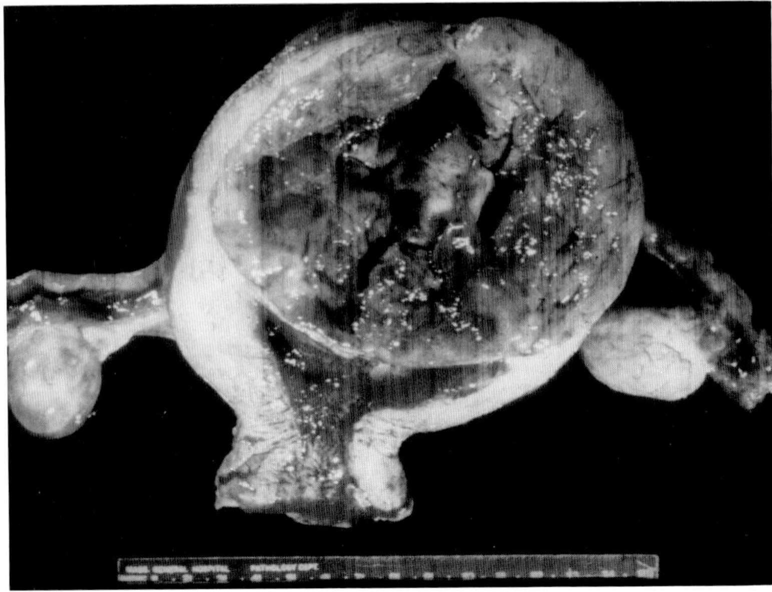

Fig. 6-18. Epithelioid leiomyoma. Sectioned surface is fleshy and lacks the typical whorled appearance of the usual leiomyoma.

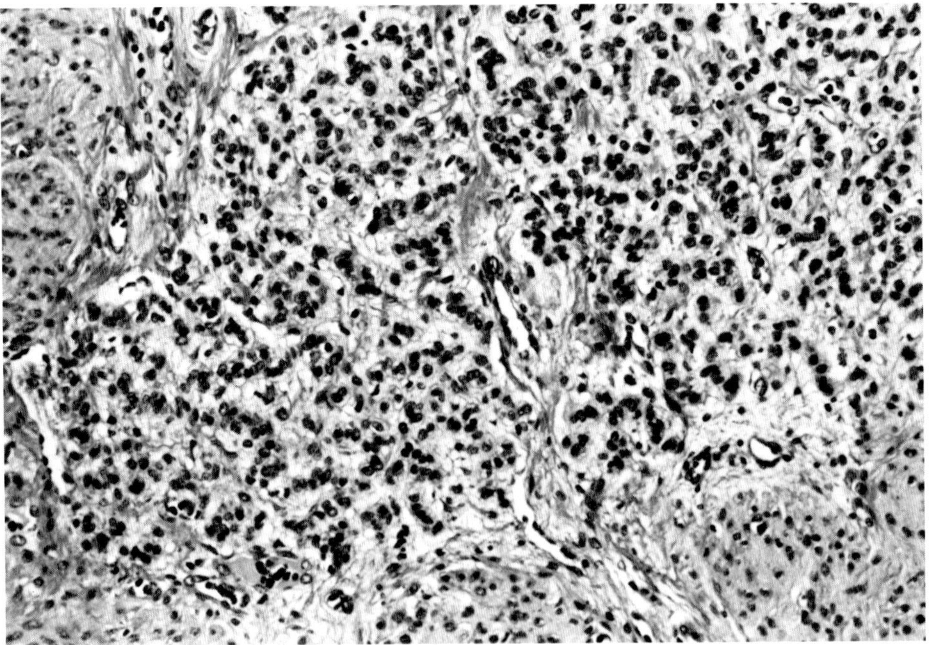

Fig. 6-19. Plexiform tumorlet within myometrium. Numerous similar microscopic lesions were present throughout the myometrium.

morlets may occasionally involve, or be confined to, the endometrium.[75] Occasional epithelioid smooth muscle tumors have arisen within the cervix.[78]

The neoplastic cells grow in sheets, nests, or long cords that are sometimes disposed in a focal plexiform pattern (Figs. 6-19 to 6-23). Stromal hyalinization may be slight and focal, or marked and diffuse, particularly in association with a plexiform pattern (Fig. 6-20). The cells are predominantly or exclusively round or polygonal. In one-half of cases, foci of spindle-shaped cells characteristic of typical smooth muscle tumors are present, and as noted above, the epithelioid cells may be scattered as small nests or cords throughout an otherwise typical leiomyoma (Fig. 6-22), or leiomyosarcoma,[81] an appearance that should not be mistaken for metastatic carcinoma. The cytoplasm is usually eosinophilic (Fig. 6-23) but may be clear (Figs. 6-21 and 6-22); in about 25 percent of cases, the entire tumor is composed of clear cells

(clear cell leiomyoma) (Fig. 6-21). Cytoplasmic glycogen is present in one-half of cases and small amounts of lipid less often, although both substances have been surprisingly absent in some clear cell tumors.[67] Rarely, the cells may have very scant cytoplasm.[81] The round or angular nucleus is typically central, but it may be eccentric, occasionally resulting in a signet-ring appearance. Nuclear pleomorphism is usually minimal, but occasionally moderate to marked (Fig. 6-24), and rarely, the nuclei are bizarre[32, 78] in one such case, adipocytes with bizarre nuclei were also present.[32] The mitotic rate is generally less than 3 MF/10 HPF, but several clinically malignant tumors (i.e., epithelioid leiomyosarcomas) have had more than 5 MF/10 HPF[70, 77] (Fig. 6-23). Most of the tumors extend into the adjacent myometrium; vascular invasion within the tumors was found in 15 percent of cases in one study.[70] Immunohistochemical[76, 78, 80] and ultrastructural[69, 71–73, 76, 78–80] examination has confirmed the smooth

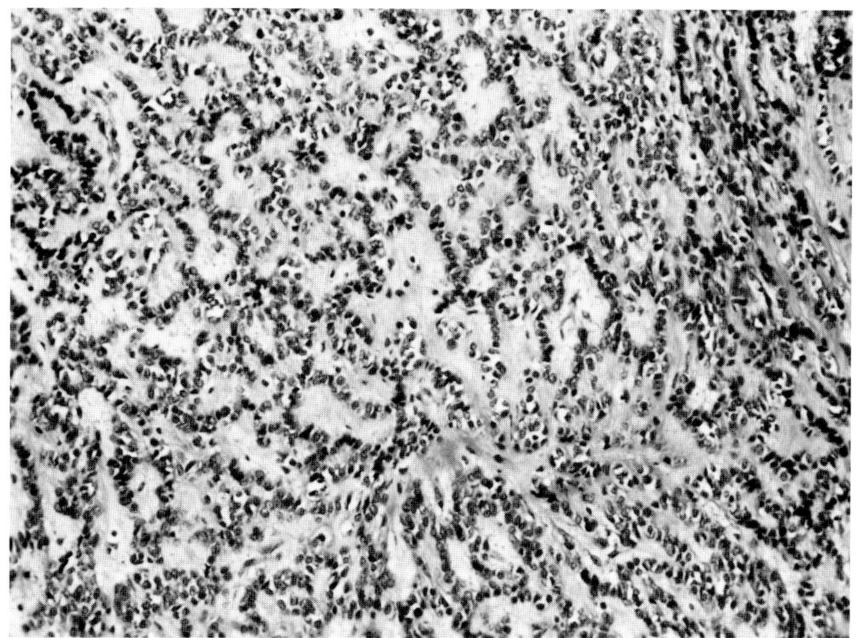

Fig. 6-20. Epithelioid leiomyoma with plexiform pattern. Tumor was a 10-cm mass that projected into the endometrial cavity.

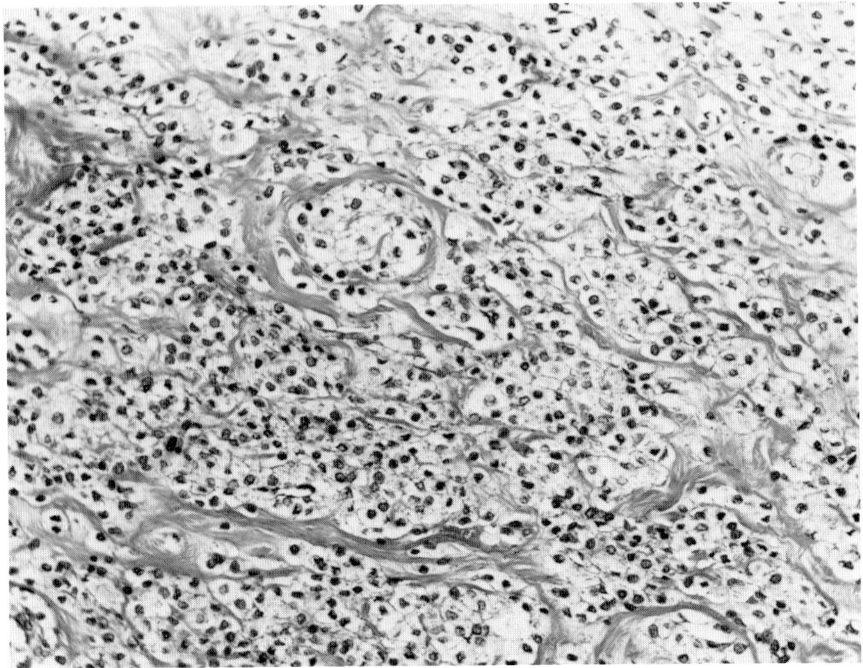

Fig. 6-21. Epithelioid leiomyoma, clear cell type.

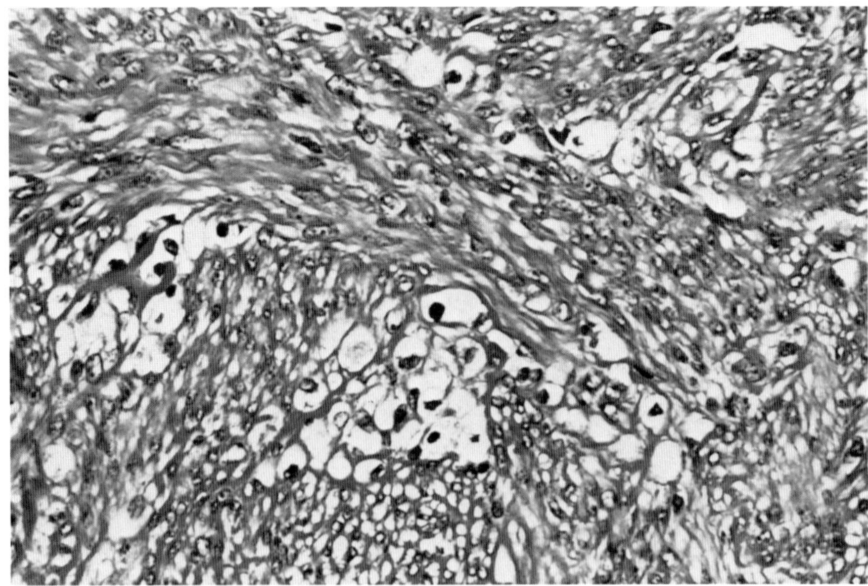

Fig. 6-22. Otherwise typical leiomyoma with scattered nests of epithelioid clear cells.

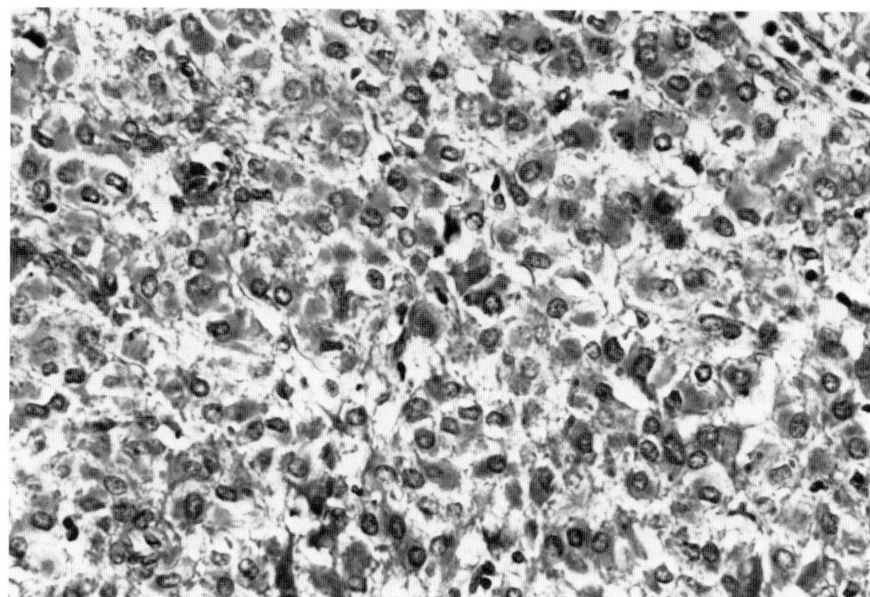

Fig. 6-23. Epithelioid leiomyoma, eosinophilic cell type.

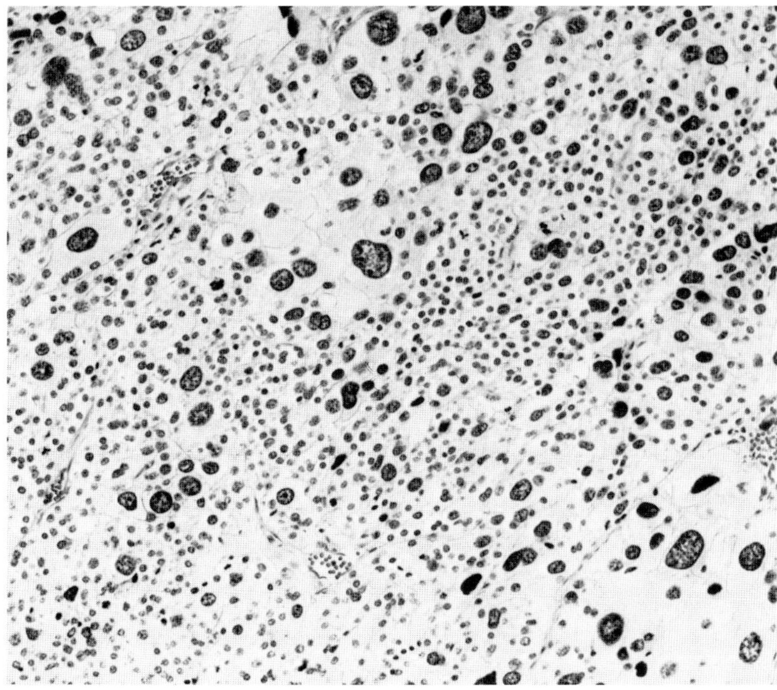

Fig. 6-24. Epithelioid leiomyosarcoma. Tumor cells have abundant clear cytoplasm and marked nuclear pleomorphism. Mitotic figures are not clearly seen at this magnification but were numerous.

muscle nature of the tumors. The clarity of the cytoplasm in clear cell leiomyomas has been attributed to large numbers of distended mitochondria in some studies[71, 80] or to cytolysosomes in others.[79]

Three of 6 tumors in one series[68] and 3 of 26 in another[70] recurred or metastasized; recurrent tumor may appear 5 or more years after hysterectomy.[70] In the second series, the malignant tumors exhibited one or more of the following features: a component of eosinophilic cells, an infiltrating margin, necrosis, a diameter greater than 6 cm, and the absence of a hyaline stroma.[70] Neither the mitotic rate nor the presence or absence of vascular invasion appeared to be prognostically useful. Because reliable microscopic criteria for predicting their behavior have not been established, only epithelioid smooth muscle tumors that are small (less than 5 cm) and mitotically inactive (not exceeding 1 MF/10 HPF) and that lack significant atypicality and necrosis should be considered benign.[70] Tumors with five or more MF/10 HPF should be considered epithelioid leiomyosarcoma.[70] Tumors that are neither clearly benign nor leiomyosarcoma should be considered of uncertain malignant potential.

The differential diagnosis of epithelioid smooth muscle tumors includes primary endometrial carcinomas (see Ch. 5) and metastatic carcinomas (see Ch. 8), especially those composed of eosinophilic or clear cells. Most such carcinomas, however, will exhibit, at least focally, overt glandular or squamous differentiation. Clear cell carcinomas of the endometrium, for example, usually have tubulocystic and papillary, in addition to diffuse, growth patterns. Tumor confined to the myometrium obviously favors an epithelioid smooth muscle tumor over a primary endometrial carcinoma; carcinomas metastatic to the uterus, however, may involve only the myometrium. Dense, pericellular reticulin patterns are more in keeping with an epithelioid smooth muscle tumor than a carcinoma. In rare cases, immunohistochemical or ultrastructural studies may be needed to facilitate the diagnosis. Clear and eosinophilic cells, as well as plexiform patterns, may be encountered in uterine tumors resembling ovarian sex-cord tumors (see Ch. 7). Primary cervical or metastatic malignant melanomas, especially amelanotic examples, are also in the differential diagnosis because of their frequent content of epithelioid and spindle cells with eosinophilic cytoplasm. Immunoreactivity for S-100 and HMB 45, and lack of reactivity for smooth muscle markers, obviously favor a diagnosis of melanoma.

SMOOTH MUSCLE TUMORS OF UNCERTAIN MALIGNANT POTENTIAL

Uterine smooth muscle tumors that are unclassifiable by current criteria as unequivocally benign or malignant have been referred to as "smooth muscle tumors of uncertain malignant potential" (STUMP).[82] These tumors have not been studied in sufficient numbers to allow prediction of their behavior based on their morphological features. Although there is as yet no uniform microscopic definition of STUMP, the criteria used by Kempson and Hendrickson[2] include the presence of (1) cytologic atypia and 2 to 4 MF/10 HPF; (2) more than 15 MF/10 HPF in the absence of hypercellularity and cytologic atypia; and (3) mitotic counts less than those above in the presence of abnormal mitotic figures or necrotic tumor cells. However, it should be noted that benign leiomyomas may undergo infarction and necrosis, and necrosis may occur in leiomyomas secondary to hormonal therapy and pregnancy. O'Connor and Norris[13] render a diagnosis of STUMP in the presence of 5 to 9 MF/10 HPF and mild (grade 1/3) nuclear atypia. Because some STUMP may ultimately prove to be low-grade leiomyosarcomas, hysterectomy and long-term follow-up are indicated.[1]

Smooth Muscle Tumors With Unusual Growth Patterns

It has already been noted that occasional leiomyoma variants may have infiltrative borders with the surrounding myometrium, a finding that has no prognostic significance. In addition, rare cytologically benign smooth muscle tumors of the uterus may have worrisome growth patterns that may simulate those of a malignant tumor, including leiomyosarcoma. The usual lack of nuclear pleomorphism and absence of significant mitotic activity in these disorders, however, exclude the diagnosis of sarcoma.

Diffuse Leiomyomatosis

Diffuse leiomyomatosis of the uterus is a rare benign disorder characterized by symmetric uterine enlargement due to the presence of countless, confluent, leiomyomatous nodules within the myometrium[83] (Figs. 6-25 and 6-26). The clinical presentation is similar to that of patients with typical uterine leiomyomas. In one case, however, there was a history of rapid uterine enlargement associated with clomiphene therapy.[84] Microscopic examination reveals that the nodules, including many not appreciable grossly, consist of cytologically benign, typically cellular, mitotically inactive smooth muscle (Fig. 6-26). A focal proliferation of perivascular smooth muscle cells has been encountered within the nodules and occasionally, the intervening myometrium.[83] Superimposed apoplectic changes (p. 269) were seen in the clomiphene-treated patient cited above who was also treated with norethindrone preoperatively.[84] The differential diagnosis includes rare cases of uterine involvement by lymphangioleiomyomatosis (LAL).[85] In one such case, the myometrium was involved

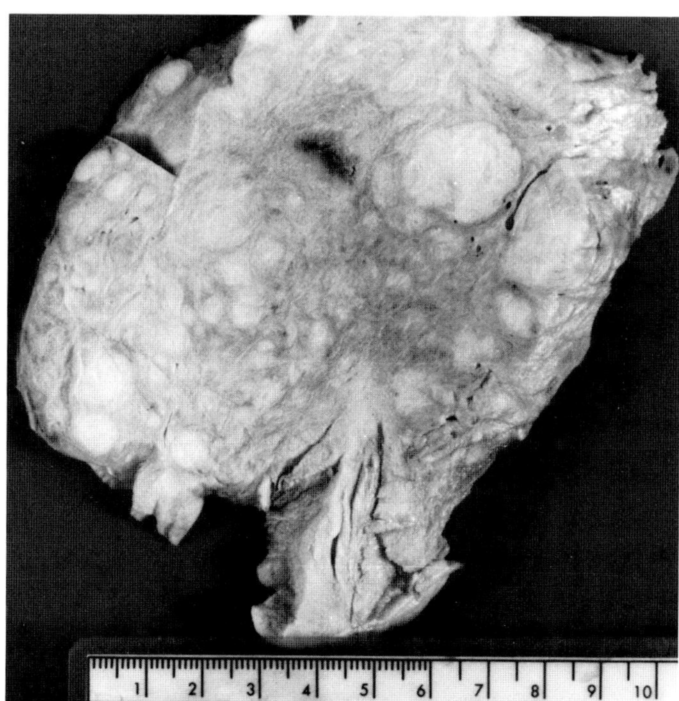

Fig. 6-25. Diffuse leiomyomatosis. The myometrium is replaced by numerous confluent nodules. (From Clement and Young,[83] with permission.)

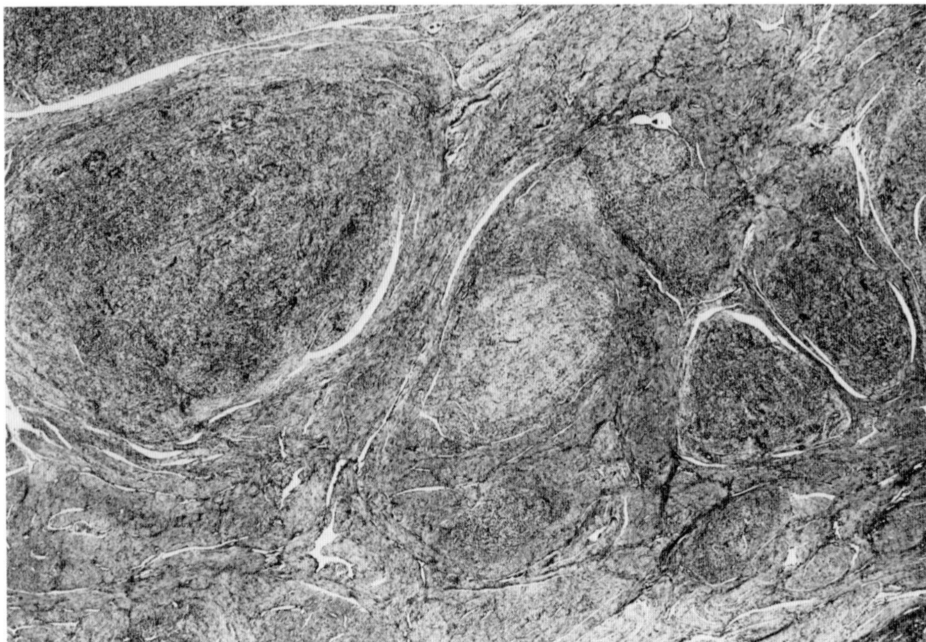

Fig. 6-26. Diffuse leiomyomatosis. Confluent nodules of cellular smooth muscle are present within the myometrium. (From Clement and Young,[83] with permission.)

by numerous microscopic foci of LAL that consisted of irregular nodules of smooth muscle that protuded into lymphatics.[85]

Leiomyoma With Vascular Invasion

The term *leiomyoma with vascular invasion* has been applied to rare otherwise typical leiomyomas or leiomyoma variants with microscopic intravascular growth confined to the tumor.[1, 2] In most patients, it appears that this intravascular growth is clinically inconsequential, although no large series of these tumors with long-term follow-up has been reported. Some cases may represent a precursor to intravenous leiomyomatosis or account for cases of benign metastasizing leiomyoma.

Intravenous Leiomyomatosis

Intravenous leiomyomatosis is an uncommon uterine tumor characterized by the presence of intravenous proliferations of benign-appearing smooth muscle in the absence of, or outside the confines of, a leiomyoma.[86–92] The clinial presentation is usually similar to that of typical uterine leiomyomas, although rare patients have presented with manifestations relating to cardiac involvement.[88] Extrauterine extension, particularly within the veins of the broad ligament, and less often in ovarian and vaginal veins, has been reported in 80 percent of cases, and in 40 percent of such cases, the tumor has reached the right side of the heart, sometimes with fatal results.[88] Extrauterine extension may be diagnosed intraoperatively or on gross examination of the hysterectomy specimen, but in other cases is evident only after the patient has presented with recurrent tumor in the pelvis or heart, in some cases many years after hysterectomy. Rare cases have been associated with solitary metastases (lungs, pelvic lymph nodes),[89, 92] as in benign metastasizing leiomyoma (see below).

The uterus is usually enlarged and bosselated with thickening of the myometrium by

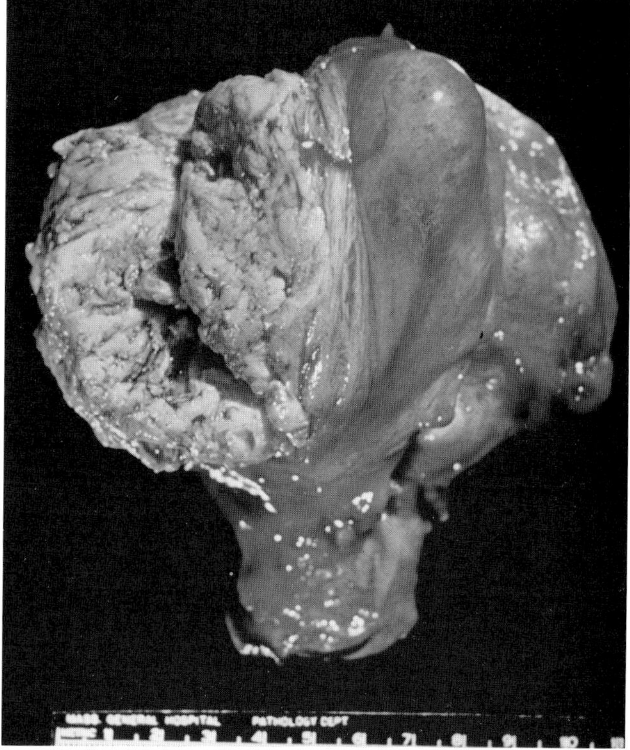

Fig. 6-27. Intravenous leiomyomatosis. The subserosal mass is composed of closely packed, coiled masses. (From Clement,[88] with permission.)

multinodular, rubbery, gray-white masses (Fig. 6-27). Although not always appreciated on initial examination of the hysterectomy specimen, the diagnostic gross feature is the presence of one or more wormlike extensions of tumor within myometrial or parametrial vessels (Fig. 6-28). Leiomyomas are also usually present, but occasionally all discernible tumor is intravascular without a discrete mass. Microscopic examination reveals endothelium-coated plugs of cytologically be-

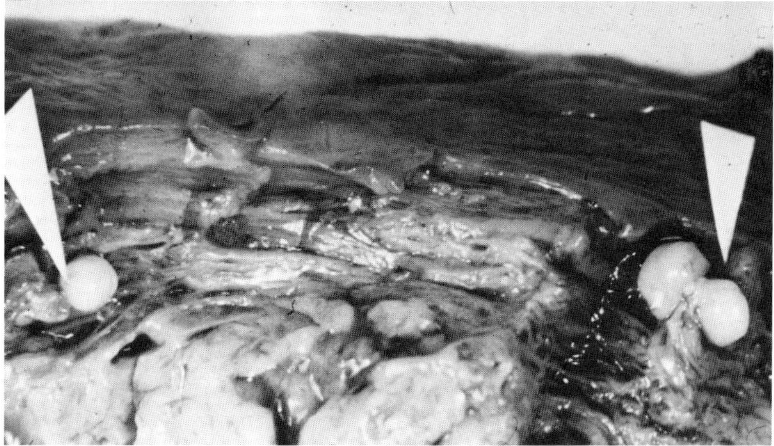

Fig. 6-28. Intravenous leiomyomatosis. Wormlike plugs of tumor protrude from the sectioned surfaces of myometrial vessels.

nign smooth muscle within myometrial vessels outside one or more leiomyomas (Figs. 6-29 and 6-30). When the vessels contain thrombi or communicate with large veins, they can be identified as veins, but other involved vessels may be lymphatics. In areas in which the intravenous tumor is attached to a vessel wall, it may merge with and appear to arise from a subendothelial smooth muscle proliferation, or it may be continuous with an extravascular leiomyoma. The intravascular growth usually resembles a typical leiomyoma, but rarely has the appearance of a leiomyoma variant, including cellular leiomyoma, leiomyoma with bizarre nuclei (Fig. 6-31), lipoleiomyoma, myxoid leiomyoma, and epithelioid leiomyoma (Fig. 6-32).[88–90] The intravascular tumor is characterized by a clefted or lobulated contour, extensive hydropic change or hyalinization, and a content of numerous thick-walled vessels (Figs. 6-29 and 6-30). Mitotic figures are usually rare, but in the cellular variants as many as 4

MF/10 HPF have been encountered.[89, 92] The extravascular tumor may be less well circumscribed than a typical leiomyoma and often exhibits hydropic degeneration.

The intravascular tumor of intravenous leiomyomatosis should be disintinguished from typical leiomyomas that are partially surrounded by compressed vascular spaces as well as from typical leiomyomas with artifactual retraction from the surrounding myometrium.[88] Stains for endothelial antigens (*Ulex europaeus*, factor VIII-related antigen) may be useful in problematic cases.[88, 89] The differential diagnosis also includes leiomyoma with vascular invasion, leiomyomas with perinodular hydropic change (p. 271), and, particularly with the cellular variant, low-grade endometrial stromal sarcoma. In contrast to intravenous leiomyomatosis, the latter tumor typically lacks thick-walled vessels and lobulation and hydropic degeneration in its intravascular extensions, and usually involves the endometrium as well as the myometrium.

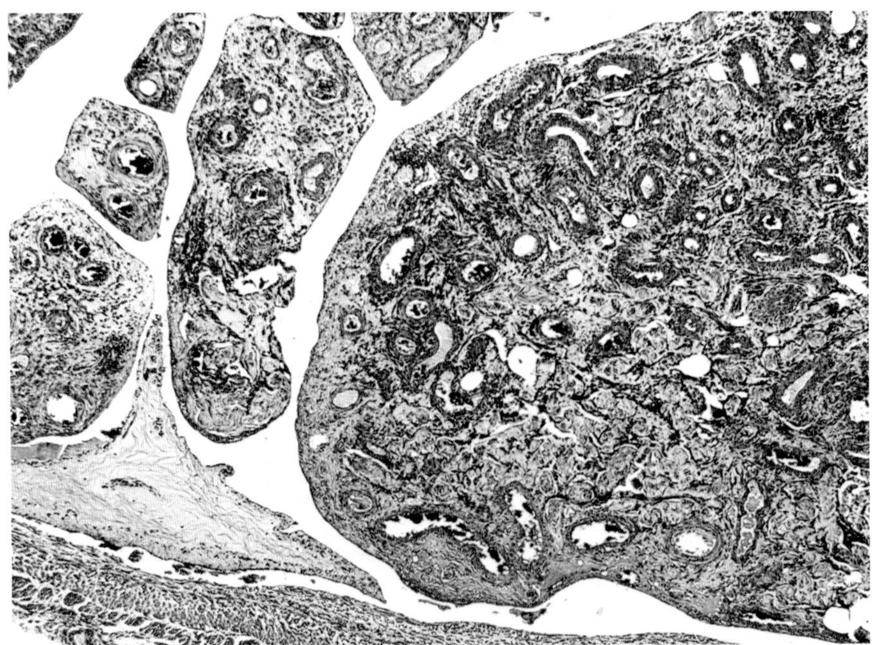

Fig. 6-29. Intravenous leiomyomatosis. Intravascular tumor is lobulated. Note numerous thick-walled blood vessels within the intravascular tumor.

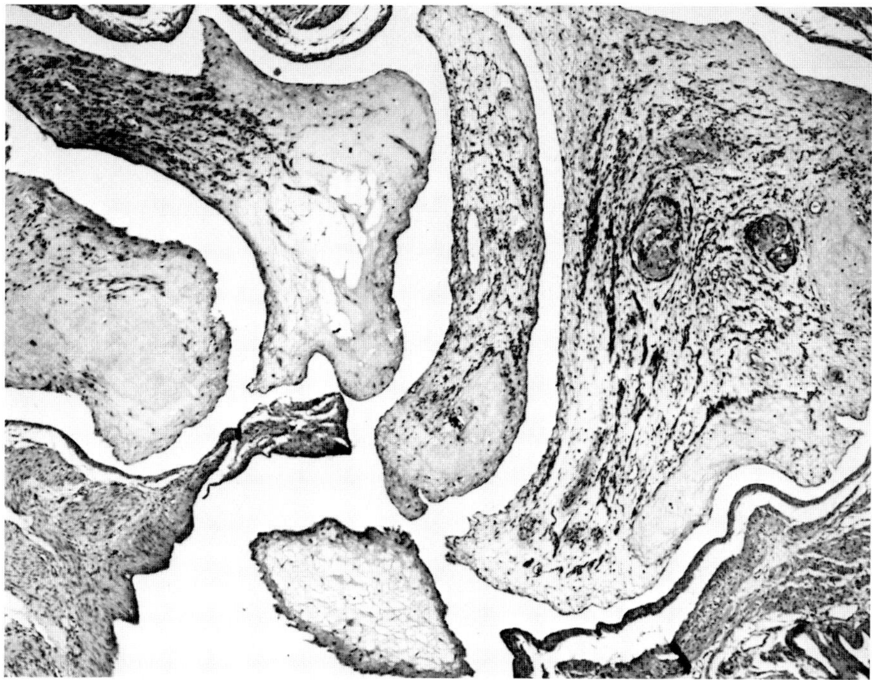

Fig. 6-30. Intravenous leiomyomatosis. Intravascular tumor is markedly hydropic.

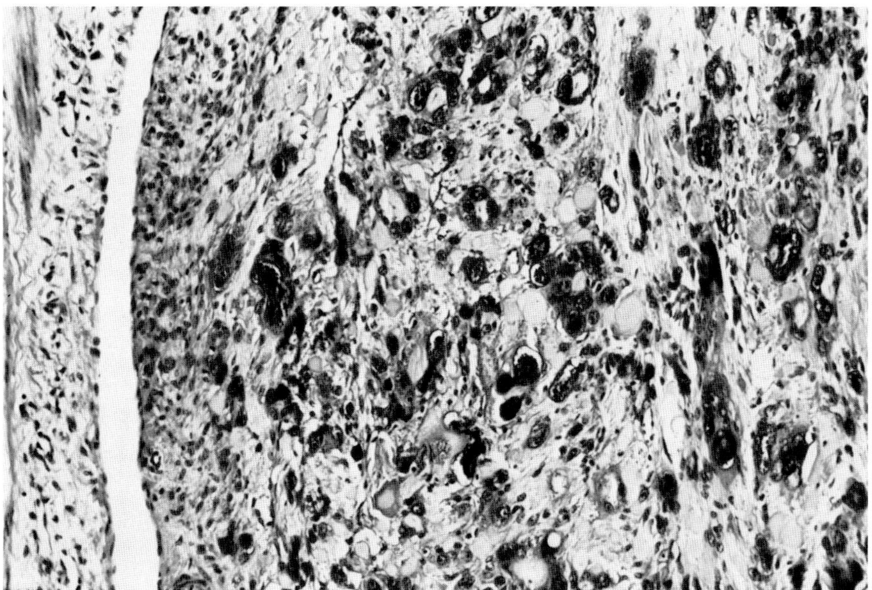

Fig. 6-31. Intravenous leiomyomatosis with bizarre nuclei. Intravascular plug of tumor is composed of cells with bizarre nuclei (vein lumen is a slitlike space at the extreme left).

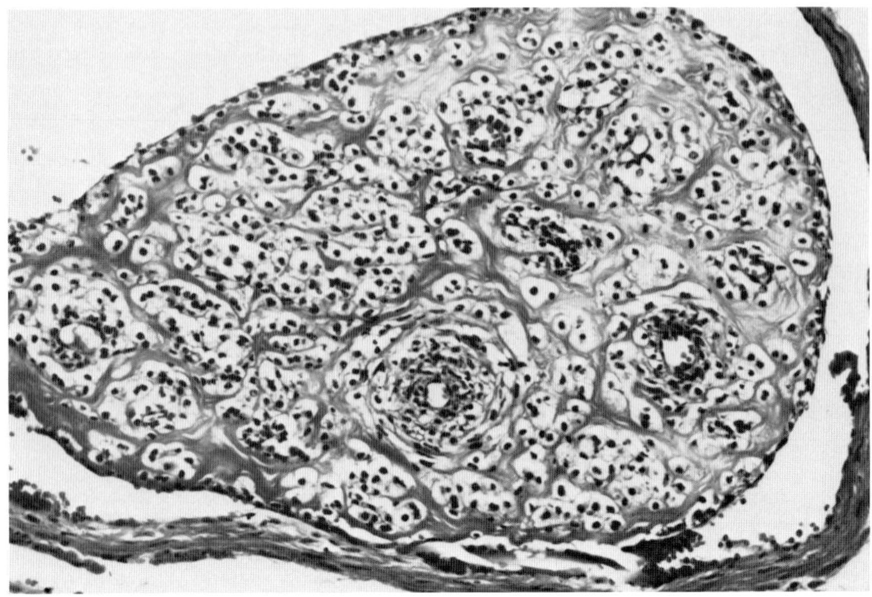

Fig. 6-32. Intravenous leiomyomatosis, epithelioid cell type. Intravascular tumor is composed of epithelioid cells with clear cytoplasm. (From Clement,[88] with permission.)

The primary treatment of intravenous leiomyomatosis is hysterectomy and excision of any extrauterine tumor to the extent that is technically feasible. Because of the presence of estrogen receptors within the neoplastic tissue in some cases, tamoxifen has been suggested as a potentially useful drug in controlling unresectable tumor.[91, 93] Periodic postoperative ultrasonic or magnetic resonance imaging (MRI) studies may be useful in detecting and monitoring the growth of residual intravascular tumor.[88, 94, 95]

Benign Metastasizing Leiomyoma

Benign metastasizing leiomyoma is an exceedingly rare disorder characterized by the presence of single or multiple pulmonary nodules composed of benign-appearing mitotically inactive smooth muscle in women who have had typical uterine leiomyomas.[96–107] Spread to the retroperitoneal and mediastinal lymph nodes[96, 97, 102, 105, 107] and other sites, such as bone[4, 104] and soft tissue,[104, 106] has been reported less often, with or without associated pulmonary involvement. The pulmonary tumors, which range up to 10 cm in diameter, are circumscribed, and may be solid or contain cysts filled with fluid. The uterus, which has been removed many years previously in most of the cases, contains typical leiomyomas, which are usually multiple. The diagnosis of benign metastasizing leiomyoma should only be rendered in cases in which the uterine leiomyomas have been thoroughly sampled to exclude leiomyosarcoma or intravenous leiomyomatosis. The possibility of an extrauterine leiomyosarcoma (gastrointestinal tract, retroperitoneum) should also be investigated.[2] On microscopic examination the pulmonary metastases are typically circumscribed; entrapment of bronchioalveolar epithelium can result in the formation of

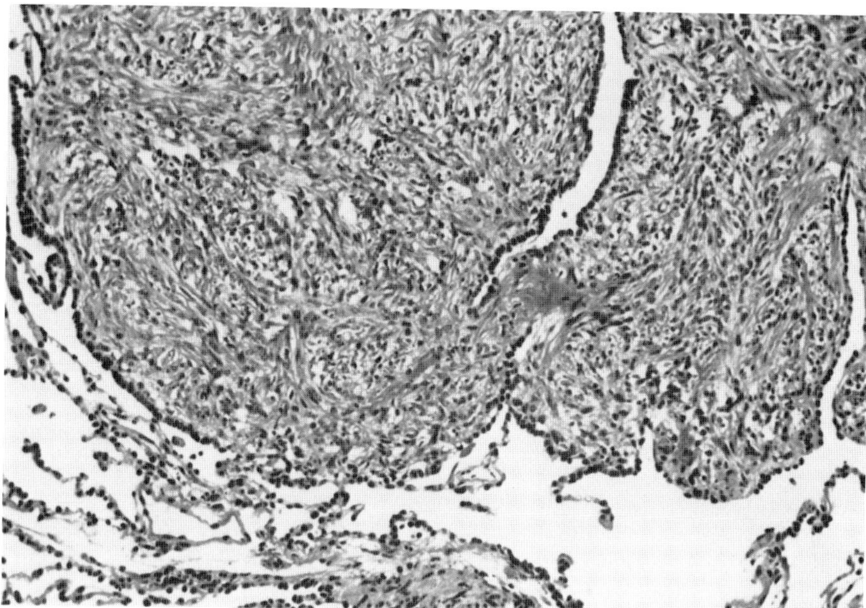

Fig. 6-33. Benign metastasizing leiomyoma. Nodule of benign-appearing smooth muscle is present within the lung. Entrapped slit-shaped glands lined by bronchioalveolar epithelium are present within the nodule.

glandlike spaces, which may be cystic and contain mucin (Fig. 6-33).

The metastasizing leiomyoma should be differentiated from the lesions of pulmonary lymphangiomyomatosis.[85, 103] In pulmonary lymphangiomyomatosis, which is sometimes associated with tuberous sclerosis, proliferating smooth muscle infiltrates the pleura, septa and bronchial and alveolar walls accompanied by honeycombing and bulla formation. Pulmonary vessels, particularly lymphatics, and lymph nodes are also involved in the myoproliferative process. As noted previously, uterine involvement is rare, but uterine leiomyomas, which are probably coincidental, may be present.[85]

The extreme rarity of primary pulmonary smooth muscle tumors, the association with uterine leiomyomas and the occasional additional involvement of pelvic and abdominal lymph nodes indicate that the pulmonary nodules encountered in this disorder are metastatic. Additional evidence includes the presence of estrogen receptors in the metastatic tumor in some cases,[101] an occasional reduction in their size during pregnancy[96, 98] and a cessation in their growth after oophorectomy[103] or the menopause, indicating hormone dependence in at least some cases.

Peritoneal Leiomyomas

The term peritoneal (parasitic) leiomyoma has been applied to otherwise unremarkable, usually solitary (one or occasionally a few), leiomyomas or leiomyoma variants attached to the pelvic peritoneum in women who usually have uterine leiomyomas. The peritoneal tumors in such cases are presumed to originate from subserosal pedunculated uterine leiomyomas that become attached to, and vascularized by, the pelvic peritoneum, eventually losing their attachment to the uterus.

Diffuse Peritoneal Leiomyomatosis

Parasitic leiomyomas contrast with a disorder that is characterized by numerous leiomyomatous nodules involving the peritoneum (including in some cases the uterine serosa), and which is referred to as *"diffuse peritoneal leiomyomatosis"* (DPL). Although this disorder is considered primarily a peritoneal, rather than a uterine, lesion, it is appropriately discussed here as it falls into the realm of the gynecologist and gynecologic pathologist.

In DPL (also known as leiomyomatosis peritonealis disseminata), the multiple peritoneal nodules are composed predominantly or exclusively of benign-appearing smooth muscle cells. Approximately 60 examples of this disorder have been reported.[18, 108] The age range has been 22 to 54 years, with a mean of 37 years, with the exception of one case in a 69-year-old woman involving a lesion that was an incidental finding at autopsy.[109] Forty percent of the reported cases have occurred in black women. The patients fall into three groups: pregnant or puerperal women (43 percent), oral contraceptive users (27 percent), and women in neither of those categories (30 percent).[18] A single case has been associated with a granulosa cell tumor.[110] In pregnant women, the disorder is usually an incidental finding during the course of a laparoscopy or laparotomy for cesarean section or postpartum tubal ligation. Symptoms in nonpregnant women and in some symptomatic pregnant women are usually related to the coexistence of uterine leiomyomas; in other cases, a diagnostic laparotomy was prompted by palpation of pelvic nodules.

Several to innumerable, firm, discrete, solid, round nodules are scattered over the parietal pelvic peritoneum and omentum, producing a matted nodularity or an ill-defined sheetlike thickening that can simulate metastatic tumor (Fig. 6-34). The nodules range in size from microscopic to 10 cm in diameter,[111] although most are less than 0.5 cm. Similar nodules also frequently involve the serosa of the uterus, ovary, bowel, and mesentery; less commonly, the upper ab-

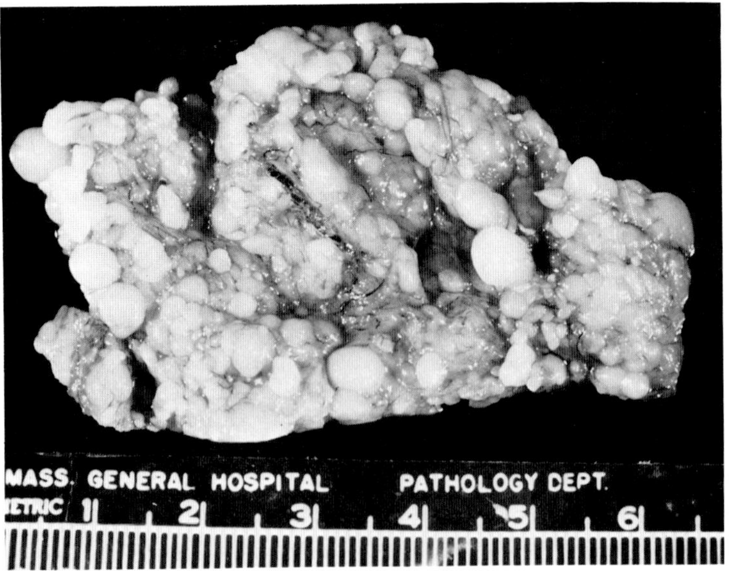

Fig. 6-34. Diffuse peritoneal leiomyomatosis involving the omentum. (From Clement et al.,[18] with permission.)

dominal peritoneum[112] is affected. One case of simultaneous pelvic lymph node involvement has also been reported.[113]

On microscopic examination, the nodules have the appearance of typical leiomyomas, usually with no significant nuclear pleomorphism or mitotic activity (Figs. 6-35 and 6-36). Occasionally, they are more cellular and may contain up to 3 MF/10 HPF.[108] Decidual cells and cells intermediate in appearance between muscle and decidual cells have been found to be admixed with the smooth muscle cells in many of the pregnant patients.[108] Foci of endometriosis or endosalpingiosis have likewise been identified in continuity with the nodules in 10 percent of cases.[18] The smooth muscle cells have been immunoreactive for both estrogen receptors (ER) and progesterone receptors (PR) in some cases.[114] Ultrastructural studies have confirmed the presence of smooth muscle cells, sometimes admixed with myofibroblasts, fibroblasts, and, in pregnant patients, decidual cells.[18]

With the exception of two cases (see below), there have been no reports of progressive disease on follow-up examination, despite incomplete excision. In several pregnant patients who had a second-look procedure when they were no longer pregnant, the nodules had completely or partially regressed. After frozen section confirmation of the diagnosis, conservative therapy is indicated, although the disorder may recur in subsequent pregnancies.[108, 115] One otherwise typical case of peritoneal leiomyomatosis in a pregnant woman was associated with uterine leiomyomas and multiple pulmonary nodules of benign-appearing smooth muscle, with the latter likely representing spread from the patient's uterine leiomyomas (benign metastasizing leiomyoma).[116]

There have been two cases of peritoneal leiomyomatosis with malignant transforma-

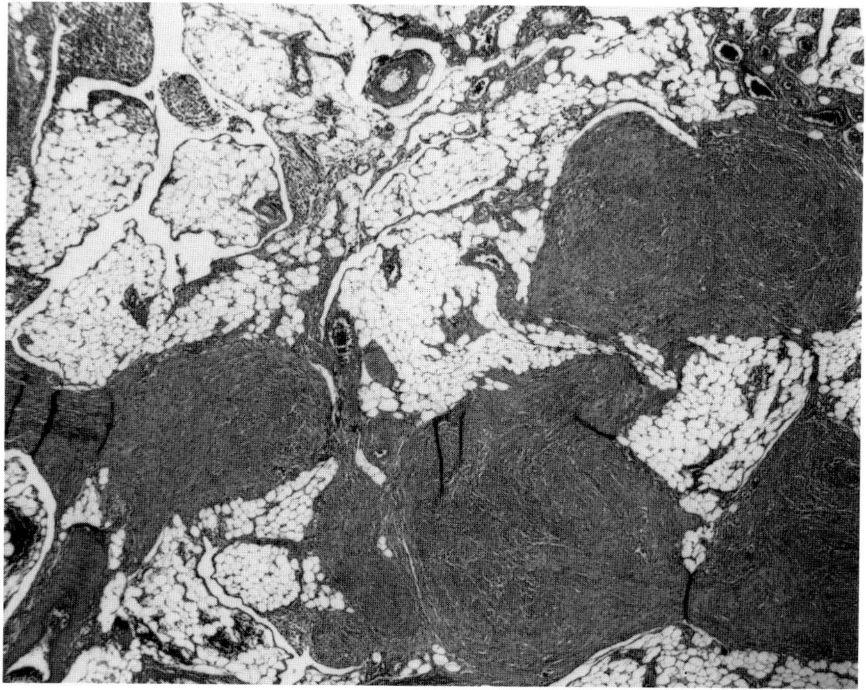

Fig. 6-35. Diffuse peritoneal leiomyomatosis involving the omentum. Multiple focally confluent nodules of smooth muscle partially replace the omental fat.

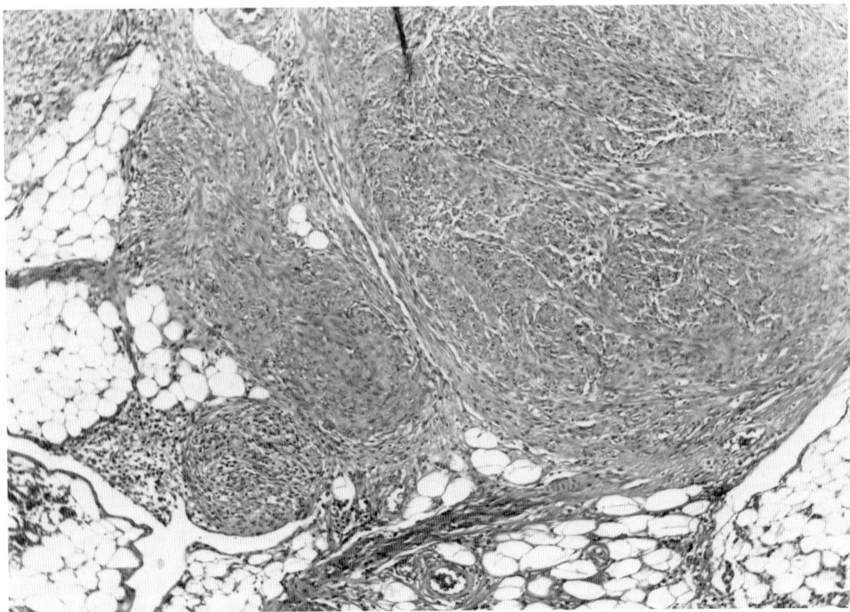

Fig. 6-36. Diffuse peritoneal leiomyomatosis involving the omentum. The nodules are composed of benign smooth muscle.

tion.[117, 118] In one case, peritoneal leiomyomatosis identified at the time of cesarean section in a 27-year-old woman was followed 6 months later by rapid growth of pelvic tumor and widespread bony metastases; the patient died as a result of tumor progression within 2 years.[117] The recurrent tumor within the pelvis and bone had the appearance of leiomyosarcoma. In the other case, typical peritoneal leiomyomatosis was diagnosed in a 25-year-old woman who was found 1 year later to have multiple masses ranging up to 10 cm in diameter throughout the peritoneal cavity.[118] Biopsies of these nodules revealed poorly differentiated leiomyosarcoma. The patient refused treatment and died 22 months after the initial diagnosis of peritoneal leiomyomatosis.

DPL is considered the result of metaplastic transformation of submesothelial mesenchymal cells into smooth muscle cells. The submesothelial location of the nodules and the occasional juxtaposition to other metaplastic lesions (ectopic decidua, endometriosis, endosalpingiosis) support this interpretation. The association with pregnancy or hormone administration in 70 percent of cases, the reduction in size of the tumors after pregnancy, surgical castration, or in one case, GnRH-a,[119] and the production in guinea pigs of similar uterine and submesothelial nodules by the administration of estrogen alone or in combination with progesterone, suggest a hormonal background for this disorder.[120–122] The submesothelial mesenchymal cells in patients with DPL may possess an unusual sensitivity to steroid hormones.[108] The high levels of estrogen and progesterone binding demonstrated biochemically within the nodules in one case[123] and the immunoreactivity of the lesional cells for ER and PR noted in several other cases (as noted above)[114] are consistent with this hypothesis. In the only other case in which hormone receptor assays were performed biochemically, however, the levels of estrogen and progesterone receptors were considerably lower than those of the normal myometrium and uterine leiomyomas.[112]

ENDOMETRIAL STROMAL TUMORS

Endometrial stromal tumors, which account for 10 to 15 percent of nonepithelial uterine cancers, are composed exclusively or almost exclusively of neoplastic cells that resemble the endometrial stromal cells of a proliferative endometrium.[124–167a] Rare stromal tumors with circumscribed borders are designated stromal nodules, and are clinically benign.[132] Those with infiltrating borders, designated *endometrial stromal sarcomas* (ESSs), have been subdivided on the basis of mitotic activity and nuclear pleomorphism into low-grade ESS (endolymphatic stromal myosis; endometrial stromatosis) and high-grade ESS.[125] Recently, however, some investigators have suggested that the terms poorly differentiated endometrial sarcoma[133] or "high-grade undifferentiated uterine sarcoma"[2] are more appropriate for the high-grade tumors, as most lack overt endometrial stromal differentiation; some of these tumors may not be of endometrial stromal origin. These observations notwithstanding, pure high-grade homologous endometrial sarcomas (whatever their histogenesis) and similar tumors arising in the endocervix ("endocervical stromal sarcomas") are most conveniently discussed in this section.

Clinical Features. ESSs usually occur in middle-aged women, with mean (or median) ages ranging among series from 42 to 58 years.[124, 125, 128, 132, 135, 137, 148] In contrast to patients with MMMTs and endometrial carcinomas, 75 percent of cases occur in patients under 50 years of age[139]; occasional cases occur in adolescents and children.[4, 125] In one study, patients with high-grade tumors (poorly differentiated

endometrial sarcomas) were significantly older than patients with low-grade ESSs, with median ages of 61 and 39 years, respectively.[133] There is no association with risk factors that are known to exist for endometrial carcinoma, although rare tumors have arisen in patients with prolonged estrogenic stimulation[168, 169] or a history of pelvic irradiation.[125]

The most frequent symptom is abnormal vaginal bleeding that is usually more severe than in patients with leiomyomas, and less commonly, pelvic or abdominal pain; occasional patients are asymptomatic.[132, 135, 137] Pelvic examination typically reveals an enlarged uterus with an irregular contour and, occasionally, tumor protruding through the external os. Since most tumors involve the endometrium, the diagnosis can often be made on a curettage specimen. Rare presentations of low-grade ESS have included recurrent cervical "polyps" over a 3-year period,[130] hematuria secondary to involvement of the urinary bladder,[149] presentation as a primary ovarian tumor due to metastases to one or both ovaries,[160] and those relating to pulmonary metastases appearing before recognition of the primary tumor.[1, 146] A few patients with ESS have had a synchronous endometrial adenocarcinoma.[135, 145]

At the time of hysterectomy, approximately one-sixth to one-third of patients with low-grade ESS have evidence of extrauterine extension of tumor.[124, 128, 133, 155] In some cases, the latter takes the form of wormlike plugs of tumor within the vessels of the broad ligament, the adnexae, the vagina, or extragenital pelvic organs.[124, 128, 133]

Gross Appearance. Stromal nodules are well-circumscribed, nonencapsulated, usually solitary, round to oval tumors (Fig. 6-37) that are located in the myometrium (60 percent), myometrium and endometrium (33 percent), or, rarely, the endometrium alone (7 percent).[132] Approximately 20 percent protrude into the endometrial

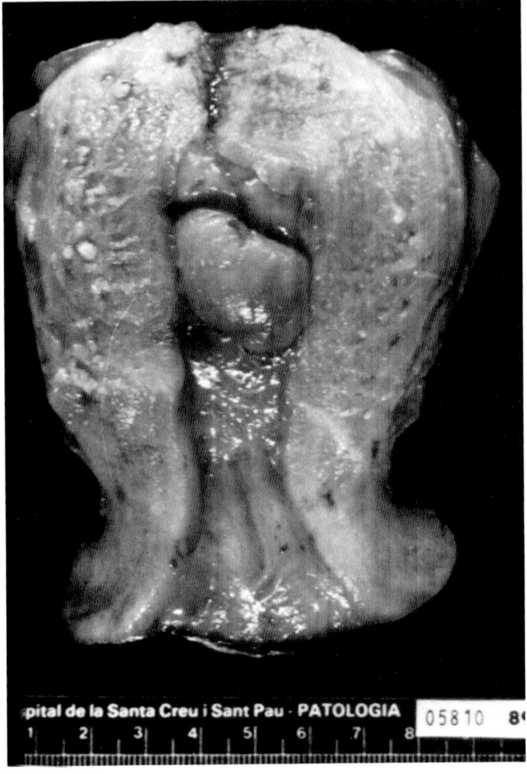

Fig. 6-37. Endometrial stromal nodule forming polypoid mucosal mass. (From Lloreta and Prat,[167a] with permission.)

cavity (Fig. 6-37). The median diameter in one series was 4.0 cm (range 0.8 to 15 cm).[132]

Low-grade ESSs form single or multiple, predominantly (or occasionally exclusively) intramural masses that frequently protrude into the endometrial cavity[125, 128] (Figs. 6-38 to 6-40). Nodular or diffuse permeation of the myometrium is common (Figs. 6-38 to 6-40), with extension to the serosa in approximately one-half of cases. Occasional cases are deceptively well circumscribed on gross examination and may resemble a leiomyoma.[2, 137] Six percent of low-grade ESSs involved the cervix in one large series; one-half of these were considered cervical primaries.[155] The neoplastic tissue of stromal nodules and low-grade ESSs is typically soft, fleshy and tan to yellow to orange, with a bulging cut surface. Areas of myxoid or cystic degeneration, necrosis, and hemorrhage may be seen, but

these features are more common in the high-grade tumors. In ESSs, wormlike plugs of tumor within myometrial and extrauterine pelvic vessels may be recognized on gross examination of the hysterectomy specimen (Figs. 6-40 and 6-41).

The gross appearance of the high-grade endometrial sarcomas may resemble that of low-grade ESSs, but more commonly they resemble MMMTs, forming one or more fungating, polypoid or plaquelike, fleshy, gray-white to gray-yellow endometrial masses, often with prominent hemorrhage and necrosis.[129, 133] Myometrial invasion is common, but the diffuse permeation of the myometrium and myometrial and extrauterine vascular spaces that characterize the low-grade tumors is usually not seen. Endocervical stromal sarcomas are typically polypoid or diffusely infiltrative tumors but rarely appear as an indurated ulcer.[47]

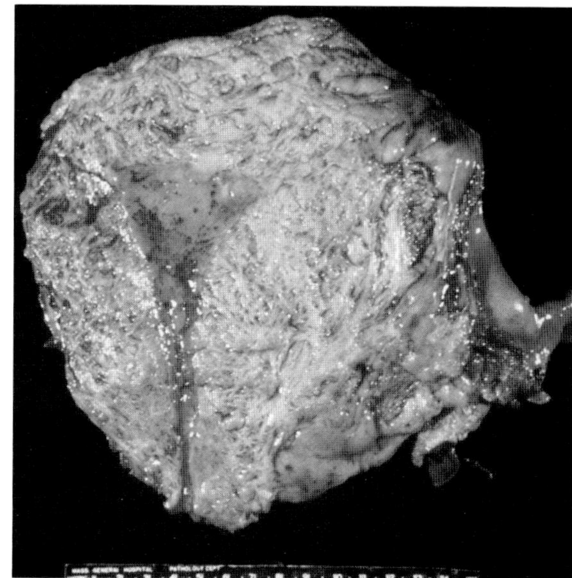

Fig. 6-38. Low-grade endometrial stromal sarcoma involving the uterus (the cervix has been amputated). Note permeation of myometrium and parametrial tissues by tumor.

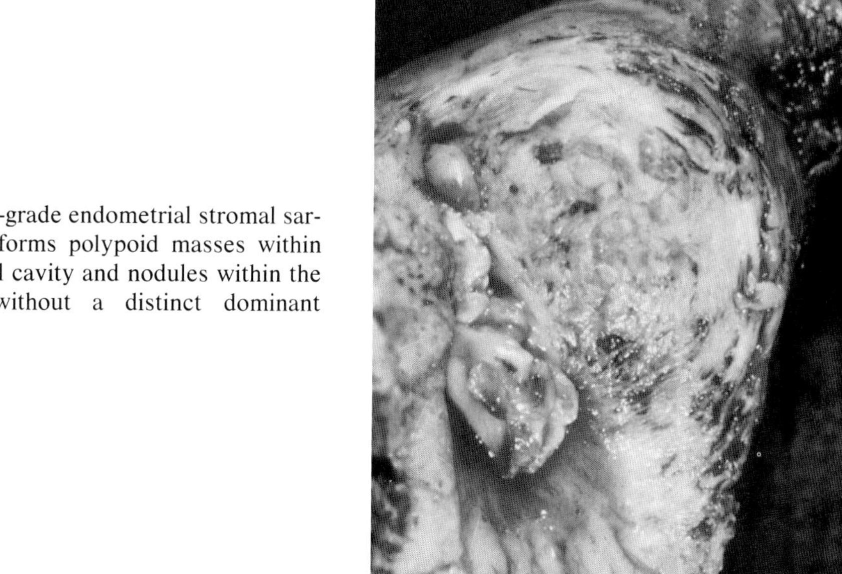

Fig. 6-39. Low-grade endometrial stromal sarcoma. Tumor forms polypoid masses within the endometrial cavity and nodules within the myometrium without a distinct dominant mass.

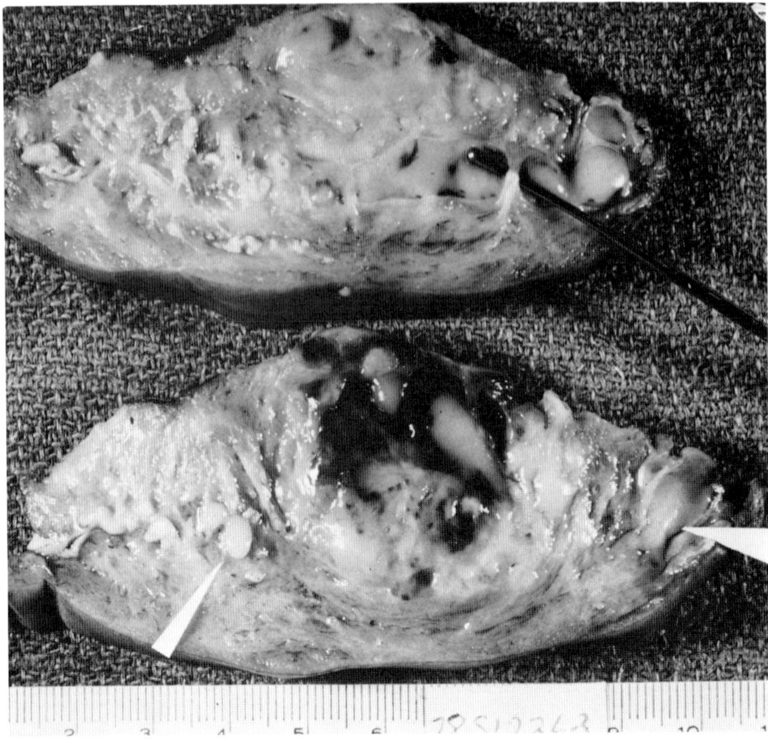

Fig. 6-40. Low-grade endometrial stromal sarcoma. Fleshy, focally hemorrhagic mass deeply infiltrates the myometrium and myometrial vessels (the latter indicated by arrows and probe).

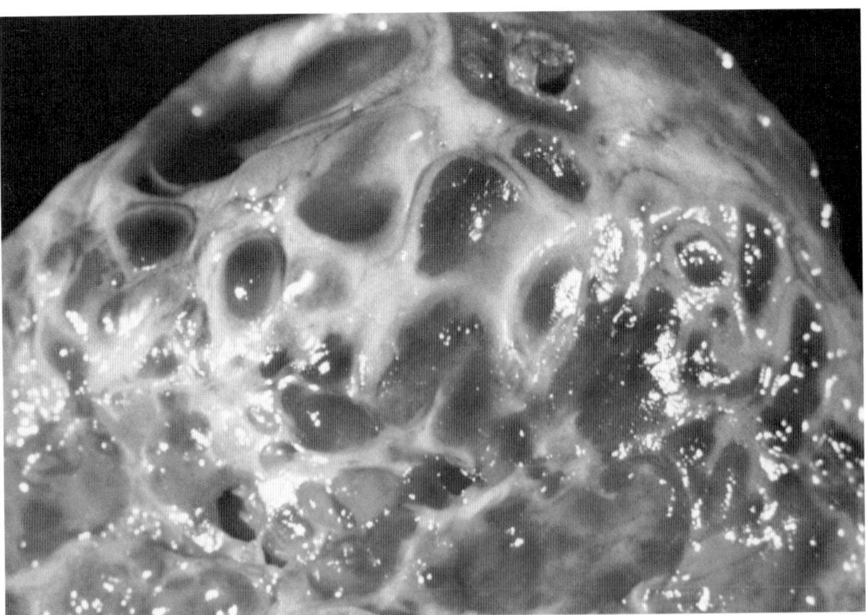

Fig. 6-41. Ovarian involvement by low-grade endometrial stromal sarcoma of uterus. Sectioned surface of the ovary is replaced with multiple nodules, most of which represent plugs of tumor within vessels.

Microscopic Features of Stromal Nodules and Low-Grade ESSs. Stromal nodules have well-circumscribed borders (Fig. 6-42), although rare fingerlike projections measuring up to 3 mm in size do not exclude the diagnosis; myometrial and vascular invasion is absent.[132, 137, 155] By contrast, low-grade ESSs, in addition to involving the endometrium in most cases, permeate the myometrium in irregular tongues, and myometrial as well as extrauterine veins and lymphatics frequently contain extensions of the tumor (Fig. 6-43). A distinction between an endometrial stromal nodule and a low-grade ESS can rarely be made on a curettage specimen, since the appearance of the interface of the tumor with the myometrium is the essential criterion in the differential diagnosis.

Aside from the differences noted above, stromal nodules and low-grade ESSs have an identical histologic appearance. Both are cellular tumors characterized by uniform, oval to spindle-shaped cells of endometrial stromal type; significant degrees of nuclear pleomorphism and tumor giant cells are absent (Figs. 6-44 and 6-45). A network of small arteries resembling the spiral arteries of the late secretory endometrium is typically present, and the neoplastic cells are focally disposed in a whorled pattern around the vessels (Fig. 6-45). The cytoplasm of the cells contains stainable lipid in one-half of cases, and cells with foamy cytoplasm (tumor cells, foamy histiocytes, or both) are prominent in some cases.[125, 128, 132, 137, 155] A partial decidual alteration of the tumor cells may reflect an endogenous or exogenous progestational effect.[126] Foci of smooth muscle differentiation or cells with differentiation that is ambiguous between stromal and smooth muscle cells are occasionally seen in both tumors.[133, 137, 155, 167a] A stromal nodule with skeletal muscle differentiation has been recently reported.[167a] The mitotic rate of stromal nodules and low-grade ESSs is usually very low. More than 90 percent of the stromal nodules in the series reported by Tavassoli and Norris had 3 or fewer MF/10 HPF, and almost one-half of cases had no discernible mitotic activity; rare cases have

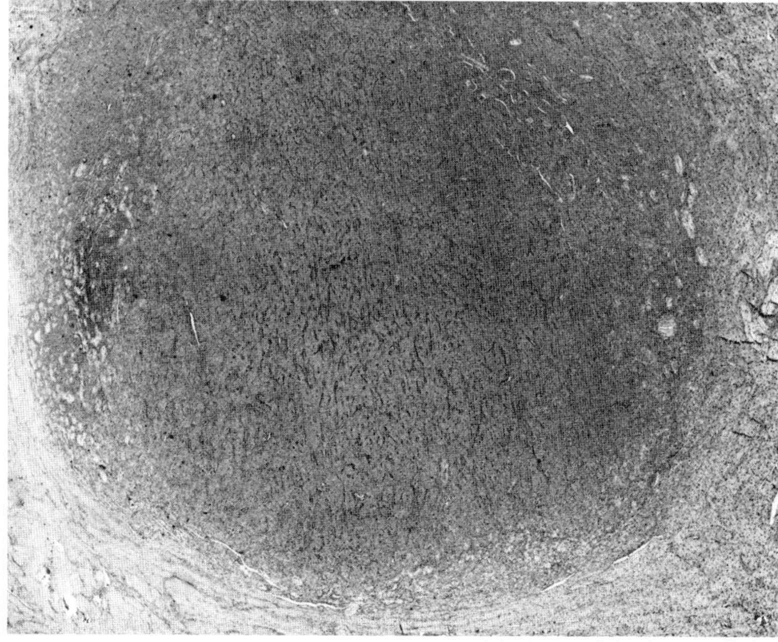

Fig. 6-42. Scanning view of endometrial stromal nodule within the myometrium. Note its well-circumscribed border.

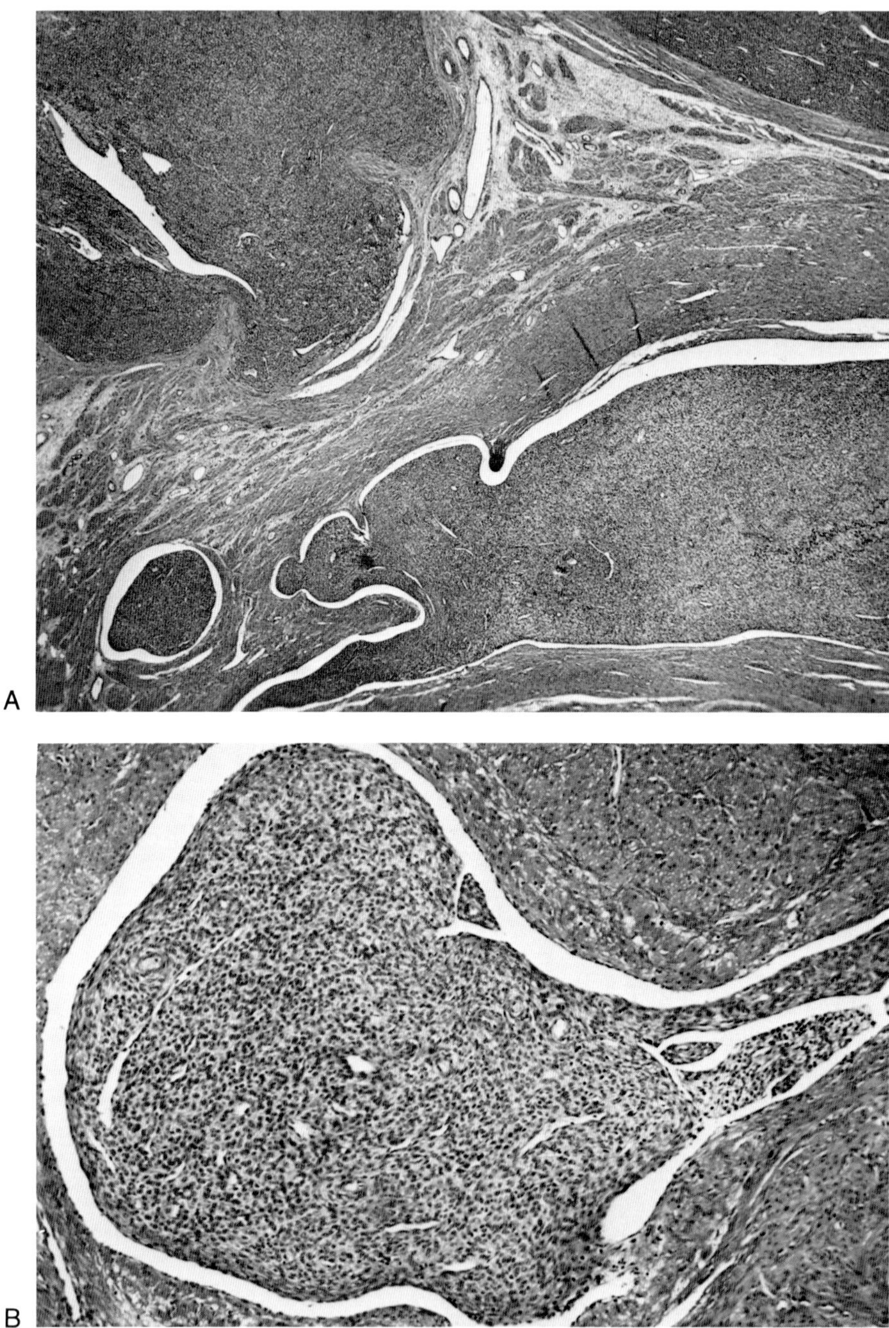

Fig. 6-43. Low-grade endometrial stromal sarcoma invading myometrium **(A)** and myometrial vessels **(A & B).**

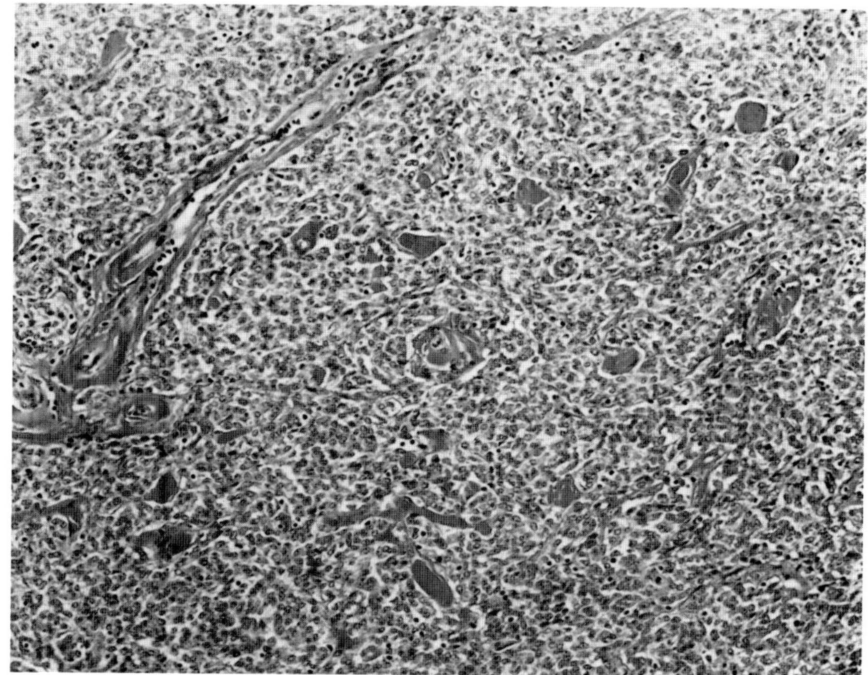

Fig. 6-44. Low-grade endometrial stromal sarcoma. Note focal plaquelike hyalinization.

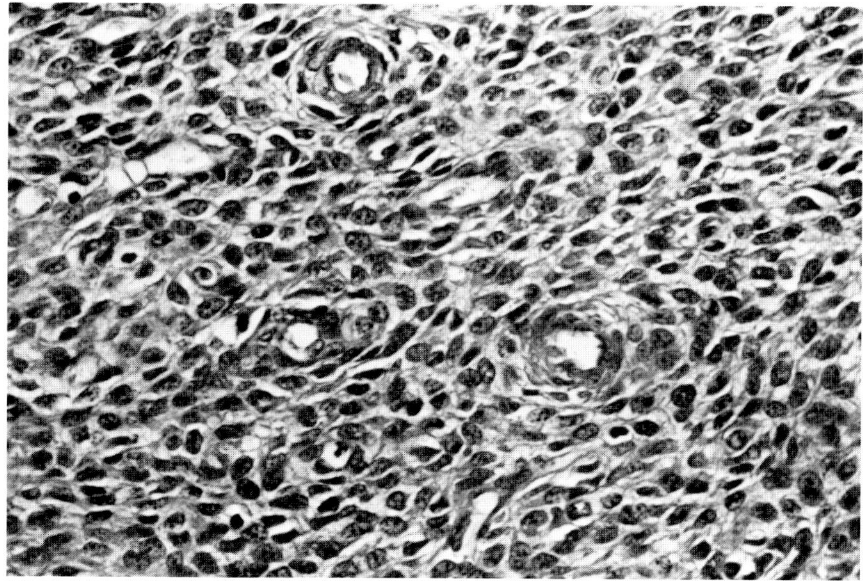

Fig. 6-45. Low-grade endometrial stromal sarcoma. Note uniform population of endometrial stromal-type cells and network of small blood vessels.

higher mitotic rates (as high as 15 MF/10 HPF).[132] Similarly, low-grade ESSs usually have 3 or fewer MF/10 HPF; higher mitotic rates can be encountered occasionally, however, and do not exclude the diagnosis.[133, 155]

Collagen in the form of hyalinized, occasionally calcified, plaques or perivascular hyalinization is a common finding (Fig. 6-44) and may be prominent, even obscuring the basic pattern of the tumor.[125, 128, 132, 133, 137] In some cases, hyalinization within the centers of one or more nodules of tumor may radiate to their periphery, resulting in a stellate pattern of collagen deposition. Rare ESSs have contained microscopic foci of osteoid or mature bone.[124] Reticulin stains usually reveal a dense network of fibrils surrounding individual cells or small groups of cells.[124, 125] Necrosis is typically absent or inconspicuous, in contrast to the high-grade tumors.

Although glandular differentiation has not been specifically noted in most published series of endometrial stromal tumors, rare, focally distributed, benign endometrioid glands,[124, 125, 132] or occasionally, glands lined by clear cells,[1] have been described in occasional stromal nodules and low-grade ESS. The presence of the glands has typically not created problems in diagnosis, nor has had any demonstrable effect on the behavior of the tumor. In contrast, we have encountered several low-grade ESSs with prominent numbers of benign, atypical, or carcinomatous endometrioid glands within the primary or recurrent tumor[165] (Figs. 6-46 to 6-48). Lesions referred to as "atypical endometriosis"[166] may represent extrauterine examples of ESSs with prominent glandular differentiation (Fig. 6-46).

Glandular differentiation should be distinguished from the more common type of differentiation within stromal nodules[132]

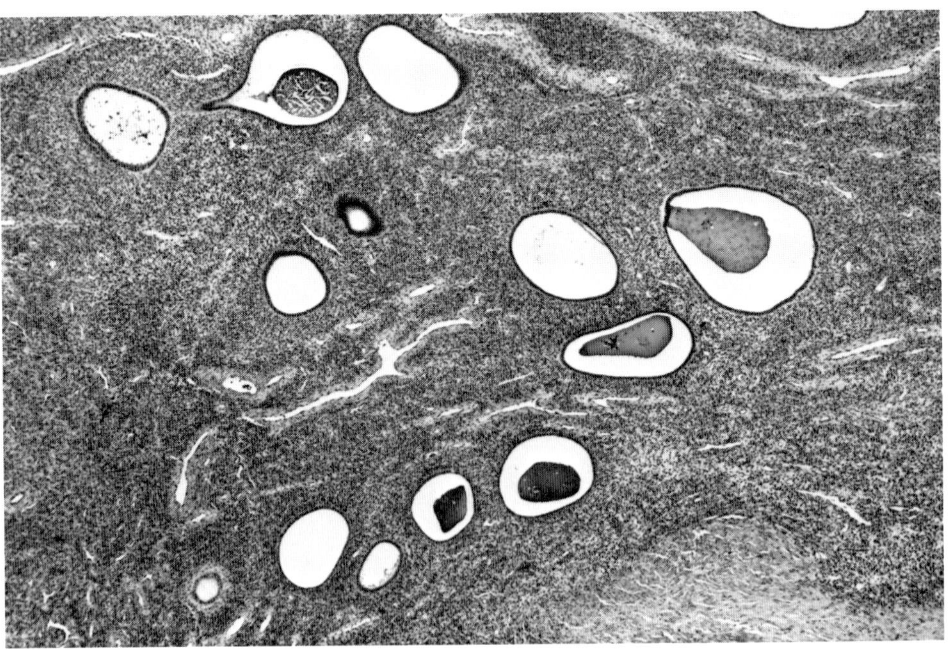

Fig. 6-46. Low-grade endometrial stromal sarcoma, pelvic recurrence. There is prominent glandular differentiation within the tumor, resulting in an appearance in this field that is similar to endometriosis. More typical stromal sarcoma was present in other fields.

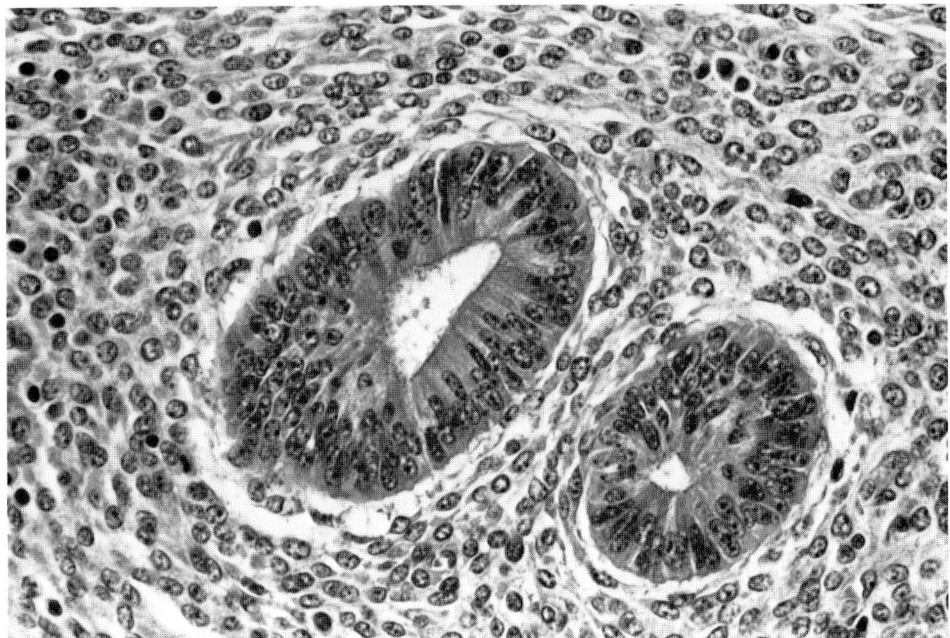

Fig. 6-47. Low-grade endometrial stromal sarcoma with endometrioid glandular differentiation. Tumor illustrated in this field was deep in the myometrium and focally simulated adenomyosis.

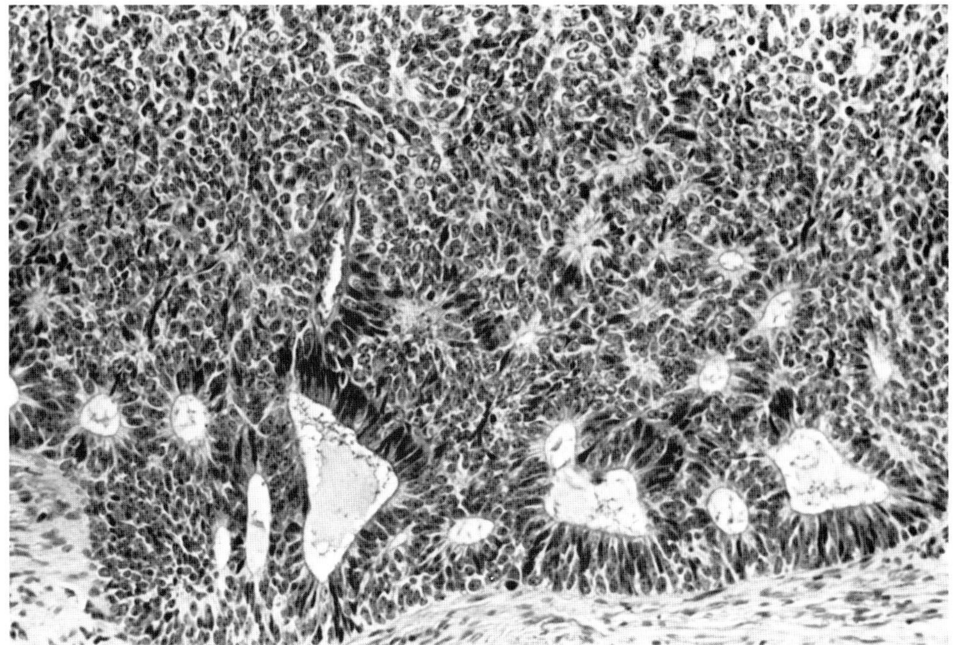

Fig. 6-48. Low-grade endometrial stromal sarcoma with atypical endometrioid glandular differentiation. Stromal cells (top) merge with atypical columnar cells that line confluent glands.

and ESSs that has been referred to as "epithelial-like"[1, 125, 137, 164] or, as we prefer, "sex-cord-like."[127, 137] When these sex-cord-like elements (SCLEs) form the predominant or exclusive component of a uterine tumor, the designation uterine tumor resembling ovarian sex cord tumor has been used[127] (see Ch. 7). SCLEs take the form of aggregated cells, sometimes with an epithelioid appearance and variable amounts of eosinophilic cytoplasm, arranged in small nests, cords, trabeculae (Fig. 6-49), and solid or hollow tubules.[125, 127, 128, 132, 134, 137, 141, 155, 164] The last three are often arranged in plexiform patterns (Fig. 6-49), and in some cases ramifying slitlike spaces impart a retiform pattern. Nests of cells with abundant lipid-rich cytoplasm have also been described in some cases. The SCLEs are typically surrounded but not penetrated by reticulin.[127, 137]

Rare uterine tumors exhibit histologic evidence of prominent endometrial stromal and smooth muscle differentiation in different areas of the same tumor (stromomyoma)[170]; in other cases, the differentiation is ambiguous.[2] That such tumors exist is not surprising, given the metaplastic potential of the endometrial stromal cell, the minor foci of smooth muscle differentiation observed in occasional stromal nodules and ESSs (see above), the overlapping immunoprofiles of uterine smooth muscle tumors and endometrial stromal tumors (see below), and the lack of a sharp distinction between the ultrastructural features of stromal and smooth muscle cells.[2] The behavior of such tumors is uncertain as no clinicopathologic study of a large series of cases has been performed. Kempson and Hendrickson, however, have found that infiltrating uterine tumors with combined stromal-smooth muscle or ambiguous differentiation behave like ESSs and suggest that such tumors be treated as if they were purely stromal.[2, 155]

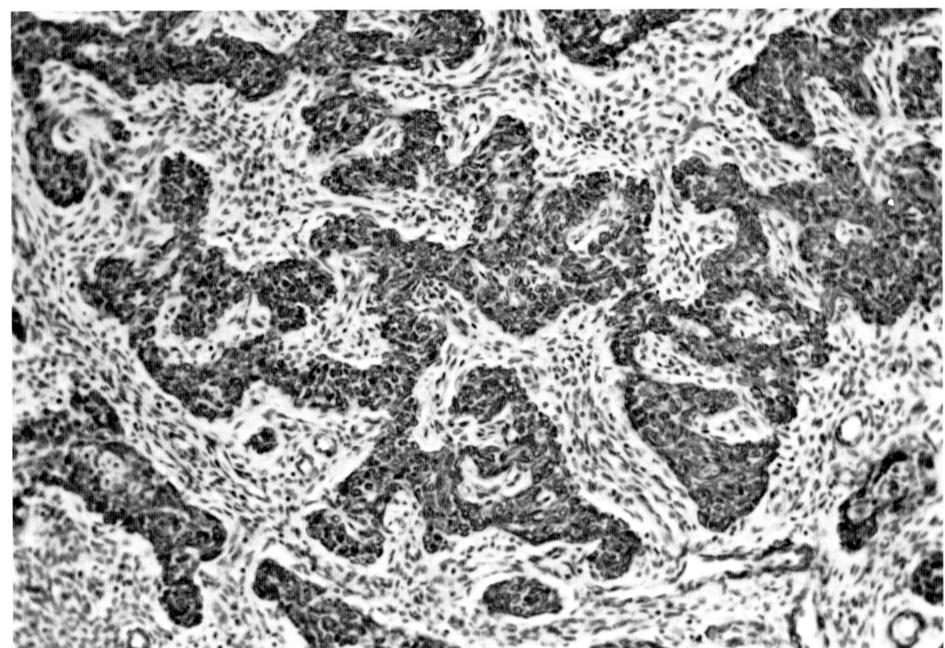

Fig. 6-49. Low-grade endometrial stromal sarcoma with sex-cord-like elements. Tumor cells form trabeculae that are arranged in a plexiform pattern. Cells within the trabeculae were immunoreactive for desmin and smooth muscle actin.

Microscopic Features of High-Grade Endometrial and Endocervical Sarcomas. Most of the tumors previously interpreted as high-grade ESS appear to represent a heterogeneous group that are composed of spindle to polygonal cells with marked degrees of nuclear pleomorphism (Fig. 6-50), including multinucleated giant cells, and mitotic rates greater than 10 MF/10 HPFs, often exceeding 20 or 30 MF/10 HPF.[2, 129, 133] In additional contrast to low-grade ESS, atypical mitotic figures are also commonly encountered.[147, 155] The distinctive vascular pattern, the focal hyalinization, and the SCLEs of the low-grade tumors are typically absent. Although rare high-grade endometrial sarcomas have had foci suggestive of heterologous differentiation,[133] similar tumors with overt heterologous differentiation are most appropriately classified as pure heterologous sarcomas (p. 312). In contrast to low-grade ESSs, there is usually destructive invasion of the myometrium, and although vascular invasion is common in the high-grade tumors, it lacks the characteristic permeative pattern seen in low-grade ESS. Necrosis is often prominent.[129, 147]

As the cells of the high-grade tumors bear little or no resemblance to endometrial stromal cells, they are of uncertain and possibly variable origin. As has already been noted, "poorly differentiated endometrial sarcoma[133] or "high-grade undifferentiated uterine sarcoma"[2] have been recently proposed as appropriate designations for these tumors. It has been suggested that some of them may be monophasic variants of MMMTs in which the carcinomatous component has been obliterated by the sarcomatous component.[133] Indeed, additional histologic sampling of an apparently pure high-grade endometrial sarcoma may reveal rare foci of carcinoma that were missed on initial sampling, warranting a final diagnosis of MMMT. Rare examples of high-grade endometrial sarcomas may have arisen from a low-grade ESS, possibly represent-

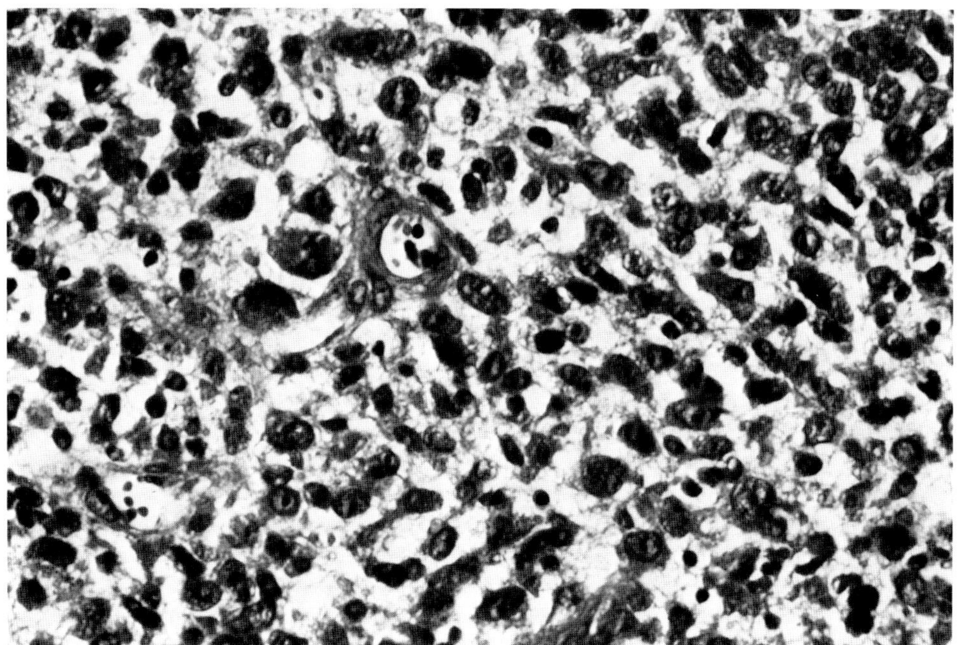

Fig. 6-50. High-grade undifferentiated endometrial sarcoma. Note marked nuclear pleomorphism and lack of endometrial stromal differentiation.

mend diagnostic imaging of the uterus. If the lesion appears to be well circumscribed with these techniques, local excision may be technically feasible.

In contrast, low-grade ESS are tumors of low malignant potential; pelvic or abdominal recurrences develop in from one-third to one-half of patients.[125, 126, 128, 133, 137, 139, 155, 158, 159] In rare cases, the recurrent tumor has been within the inferior vena cava or heart, as in some patients with intravenous leiomyomatosis (p. 288).[144, 150] The tumors typically have an indolent growth with a tendency to late recurrence; the interval before recurrence in one large series varied from 3 months to 23 years, with a median interval of 3 years.[139] In the Stanford study,[155] the median time between hysterectomy and relapse correlated with the surgical stage: 5.4 years for patients with stage I tumors compared with 9 months in patients with stage III to IV disease. Patients with multiple recurrences occurring over three decades following hysterectomy have been reported.[151] Blood-borne metastases are unusual, and as with recurrences may not appear until many years or even decades after hysterectomy. Pulmonary metastases occurred in 10 percent of stage I patients in the Stanford study, with a median time to discovery of 9.6 years after hysterectomy.[146, 155] Bone and other sites are involved less commonly.

Recurrent or metastatic low-grade ESS is sometimes misdiagnosed by the pathologist because of the often long postoperative intervals and because the secondary tumor may sometimes have an unusual gross or histologic appearance. Ovarian involvement, for example, may sometimes be misinterpreted as a primary ovarian endometrioid stromal sarcoma or other tumors, such as a sex-cord-stromal tumor.[160] We have also seen occasional cases in which SLCEs that were minor in amount in the primary tumor were prominent within re-

current tumor, creating problems in interpretation. Cystic pulmonary metastases have been misinterpreted as cystic hamartomas,[140, 146] and pulmonary involvement in other cases has been misdiagnosed as oat cell carcinoma.[155] The possibility of metastatic ESS should always be considered when dealing with a benign-appearing, monomorphous spindle cell pulmonary neoplasm in a female patient.[146, 155]

In many cases recurrent or even metastatic ESS may remain localized for long periods and be amenable to successful treatment by resection, radiation therapy, progestin therapy, or combinations thereof.[126, 128, 135–137, 139, 142, 154, 155, 157, 159] Approximately 90 percent of patients in two studies[139, 155] and 100 percent of patients in another study[125] survived 10 years. Some patients, however, may die from tumor progression after 10 years, and tumor-related deaths have occurred as late as 30 years after presentation.[155]

The only significant predictor of recurrence (and survival) in low-grade ESS is the surgical stage. In the Stanford study,[155] tumor recurred in 36 percent of patients with stage I disease compared to 76 percent of patients with stage III to IV disease. The corresponding survival rates were 92 percent (stage I) and 66 percent (stage III to IV). Other studies, however, have found 100 percent survival rates even in stage III patients;[139] this high survival rate is at least partially attributable to successful progestagen therapy. In the Stanford series, tumor size, mitotic rate and nuclear atypia were not predictive of recurrence in patients with stage I tumors.[155] Although there was a significantly increased recurrence rate in tumors with SCLEs, the overall survival rate was not affected. Adjuvant pelvic irradiation did not result in any statistically significant decrease in the relapse rate for stage I tumors.[155] Conservation of adnexae may be associated with an increased recurrence rate, because adnexal extensions of tumor are not always visible at operation,[126, 158] and because of the possible stimulatory effects of estrogen from the retained ovary.[154] In one study,[125] recurrences in patients with stage I tumors were confined to those who had had a subtotal hysterectomy.

These observations suggest that the appropriate initial management for patients with ESS is total abdominal hysterectomy including bilateral salpingo-oophorectomy and wide parametrial excision. Tumor samples should be analyzed for hormone receptors and patients with stage I tumors that contain receptors should be treated with progestagens. Postoperative radiation may be justifiable in patients with stage I tumors that are receptor poor. Higher-stage tumors should be excised to the extent technically feasible and the patients given postoperative hormonal therapy or radiation therapy, or both.

In contrast to the foregoing, high-grade endometrial sarcomas are aggressive tumors, with death from abdominopelvic recurrence and lymphatic and hematogenous metastases within 3 years after hysterectomy in most of the cases.[2, 4, 125, 129, 133] Tumors limited to the endometrium may have a more favorable prognosis.[133] Preoperative or postoperative radiation may decrease the frequency of pelvic recurrence.[1, 158] Higher survival rates have been reported in some series in which tumors were considered high-grade based solely on a high mitotic rate; at least some of these tumors would be considered low-grade ESS by current criteria.[125, 158] Endocervical stromal sarcomas also behave aggressively. Seven of 13 patients with follow-up died of recurrent or metastatic tumor within 2 years of treatment; an eighth patient was alive with pulmonary metastases 14 months after hysterectomy.[172] Five patients without recurrence in the series of Abell and Ramirez were described as having "better differentiated lesions."[47]

RARE SARCOMAS

HOMOLOGOUS SARCOMAS

Rare examples of *malignant vascular tumors* have been reported under the designations malignant hemangioendothelioma,[174] angiosarcoma[175–178] and hemangiopericytoma.[179, 180] In our opinion, many, if not most of the uterine tumors designated hemangiopericytoma, based on the published illustrations, likely represent endometrial stromal sarcomas. The former term should be reserved for those tumors with the characteristic branching, staghorn-shaped vessels with open lumina that characterize hemangiopericytomas in extrauterine sites. Twelve uterine examples of pure angiosarcoma (or malignant hemangioendothelioma) have been reported in females 17 to 36 years of age.[174–178] The tumors morphologically resembled angiosarcomas in other sites, and the majority of them pursued a malignant course.

Nine uterine *malignant fibrous histiocytomas* (or variants thereof, including fibroxanthosarcoma and malignant giant cell tumor) have been reported.[181–187] Similar tumors have also occurred as a component of a müllerian mixed tumor[188] (see Ch. 7) or, as previously noted, admixed with uterine leiomyosarcoma. The differential diagnosis also includes endometrial carcinomas with a prominent component of giant cell carcinoma or osteoclastic giant cells (see Ch. 5). Patients with malignant fibrous histiocytomas or variants have ranged in age from 43 to 75, and typically presented with abnormal vaginal bleeding and a large pelvic mass; two patients had lung metastases at presentation.[182, 184] Large, fleshy polypoid masses with prominent hemorrhage and necrosis typically involved the endometrium and myometrium; in one case, the tumor arose in the cervix. On microscopic examination, the cellular tumors consisted of varying combinations of pleomorphic epithelioid and spindled mononuclear cells, benign-appearing multinucleated cells resembling osteoclasts or Touton giant cells, malignant giant cells with multiple bizarre nuclei, and foamy histiocytes. Six of the nine patients died from tumor or were alive with metastatic tumor at the time of reporting.

HETEROLOGOUS SARCOMAS

Heterologous Sarcomas Other Than Sarcoma Botryoides

Aside from embryonal rhabdomyosarcoma (sarcoma botryoides) of the cervix (see below), uterine sarcomas containing heterologous elements in the absence of epithelial elements are rare, and include *pleomorphic rhabdomyosarcoma,*[189–193] *chondrosarcoma,*[194, 195] *osteosarcoma,*[190, 196–202] and *liposarcoma.*[190, 203, 204] These tumors typically occur in elderly women who present with abnormal vaginal bleeding and an enlarged uterus. Large polypoid masses usually fill the endometrial cavity, often prolapsing through the external os, and frequently invade the myometrium; occasional tumors are confined to the myometrium[194, 200] or cervix.[196, 199, 203] The sectioned surfaces of uterine chondrosarcomas, osteosarcomas, and liposarcomas may grossly resemble their extrauterine counterparts. Occasional tumors have had an associated leiomyosarcomatous component.[190, 194, 196, 204] Pleomorphic rhabdomyosarcomas are usually more diffusely cellular than embryonal rhabdomyosarcomas, lacking edematous zones and a cambium layer, and contain large numbers of pleomorphic cells with abundant eosinophilic cytoplasm, including numerous diagnostic rhabdomyoblasts. The behavior of pure heterologous sarcomas is similar to or possibly even more aggressive than that of other high-grade uterine sarcomas; the vast majority of tumors follow a malignant clinical course with local recurrence and hematogenous dissemination.

The differential diagnosis of heterologous sarcomas is usually with müllerian mixed tumors with heterologous elements (see Ch. 7), which in contrast to pure heterologous sarcomas, contain a carcinomatous component (MMMTs) or a benign glandular component (müllerian adenosarcomas). The glandular elements of the mixed tumors may be sparsely distributed; before a diagnosis of pure heterologous sarcoma is rendered, the tumor should be thoroughly examined histologically to exclude an integral epithelial component. Pure heterologous sarcomas are readily distinguished from other uterine tumors that may contain benign heterologous elements such as leiomyomas (p. 274) and endometrial adenocarcinomas (see Ch. 5). Pleomorphic rhabdomyosarcomas should be distinguished not only from embryonal rhabdomyosarcomas, but also from rhabdomyomas and malignant rhabdoid tumors (see below).

Sarcoma Botryoides

The vast majority of sarcoma botryoides (embryonal rhabdomyosarcoma) of the uterus have arisen within the cervix[189, 205–212]; occasional cases have been confined to the corpus or have involved both corpus and cervix.[189, 206] Although these tumors have been encountered in patients over a wide age range, including infants and postmenopausal women, most cases occur in young women, with a mean age of 18 years in the largest series of cervical tumors.[208] This age predilection contrasts with the almost exclusive occurrence of sarcoma botryoides of the vagina in infants. The patients usually present with vaginal bleeding, tissue protruding from the introitus, or both. On gross examination, the cervical tumors are usually 3 to 4 cm in diameter, polypoid, sometimes pedunculated, smooth, glistening or myxoid, and fo-

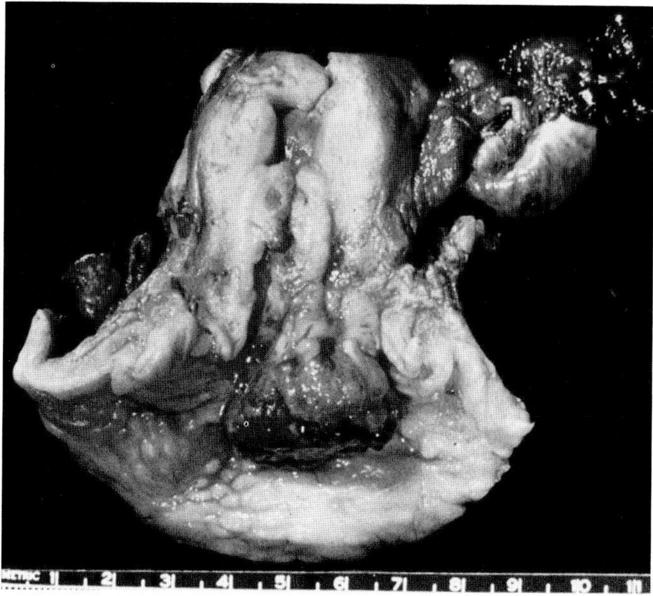

Fig. 6-52. Embryonal rhabdomyosarcoma of uterine cervix. Endocervical polypoid mass protrudes through the external os. (From Clement,[250] with permission.)

cally hemorrhagic (Fig. 6-52). A botryoid appearance characteristic of vaginal tumors is uncommon, and in some cases the tumor may resemble a benign endocervical polyp.

On microscopic examination, the uterine tumors resemble their vaginal counterparts, with a cambium layer lying subjacent to the surface epithelium (Fig. 6-53) and in some cases surrounding an occasional, entrapped endocervical (or endometrial) gland. The cambium layer is composed of plump, mitotically active spindle cells with scanty cytoplasm and hyperchromatic nuclei. In the deeper edematous zones of the tumor, rhabdomyoblasts appearing as strap-shaped cells with abundant eosinophilic cytoplasm, with or without cytoplasmic cross striations, are a cardinal feature (Fig. 6-54). These cells, however, may be sparsely distributed, and a diligent search may be required to find them. The strap cells are typically immunoreactive for myoglobin, desmin, or both. The atypicality of the neoplastic cells varies from mild to severe; in one study, the mitotic rate in the most cellular areas of the tumor ranged from 2 to 12 MF/10 HPF.[208] In the same study, 45 per-

cent of tumors contained minor foci of hyaline cartilage. In the cervix, tumor cells may invade the overlying squamous epithelium, but this is a less common feature than in vaginal tumors. Invasion of the cervical wall or myometrium may occur but is uncommon.

In contrast to patients with sarcoma botryoides of the vagina, the majority of patients with uterine tumors have a favorable prognosis. In a recent review, 80 percent of patients with cervical tumors were alive with no evidence of disease (mean follow-up period, 68 months); the corresponding figure for stage I tumors (representing 75 percent of patients) was 88 percent.[207] Of the 13 cases reported by Daya and Scully,[208] the only patient who died of tumor had deep invasion. Although most patients reported in the literature have had a radical operation, sometimes followed by chemotherapy, an apparent cure has been achieved in some patients with polypectomy or cervicectomy, with or without chemotherapy.[208, 212] Occasional tumors, however, may be aggressive, such as one recently reported by Perrone et al.[211] that

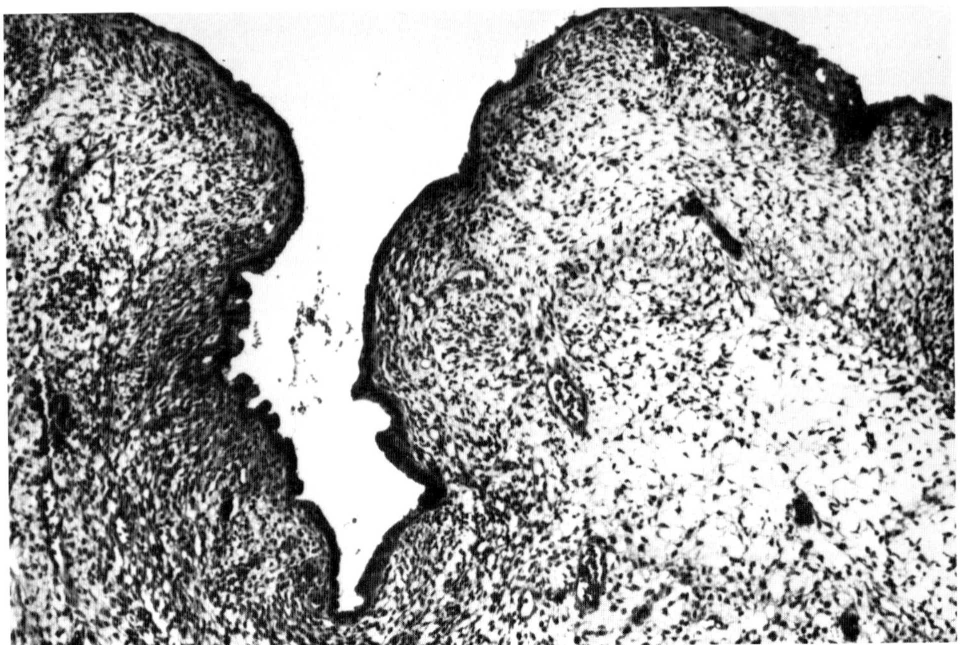

Fig. 6-53. Embryonal rhabdomyosarcoma of uterine cervix. Subepithelial cambium layer is present. Deeper zones of the tumor are edematous.

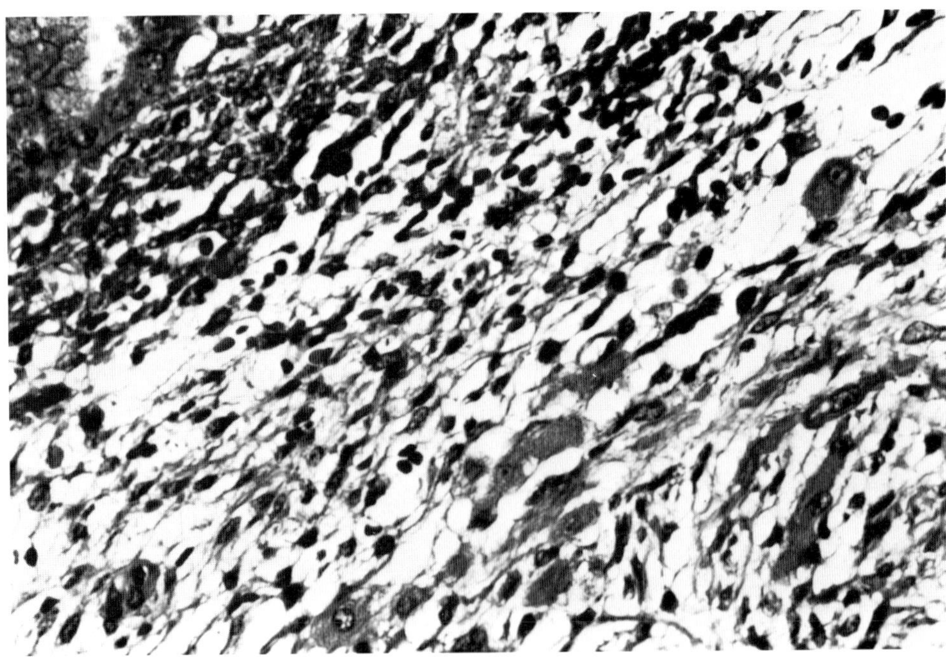

Fig. 6-54. Embryonal rhabdomyosarcoma of uterine cervix. High-power view of tumor illustrated in Figure 6-53. Small cells with scant cytoplasm are admixed with rhabdomyoblasts.

resulted in the death of a young woman 21 months after presentation. That tumor, however, was deeply invasive, invaded the deep cervical lymphatics, and contained a focal component that resembled alveolar rhabdomyosarcoma. We have seen a similar case (Fig. 6-55). As a sarcoma botryoides containing a component of alveolar rhabdomyosarcoma may be unusually aggressive, the presence of the latter should be specifically noted in the pathology report.

The differential diagnosis of sarcoma botryoides of the uterus includes pleomorphic rhabdomyosarcoma, benign polyps, rhabdomyomas, poorly differentiated endometrial and endocervical stromal sarcomas, and müllerian adenosarcomas. Benign endocervical or endometrial polyps, especially if large, are uncommon in the first two decades. Before a diagnosis of benign polyp is rendered in this setting, the lesion should be thoroughly examined histologically for evidence of a cambium layer, stromal mitotic figures, and rhabdomyoblasts. The distinction of sarcoma botryoides from fibroepithelial polyps with stromal atypia is discussed in Chapter 1. In the female genital tract, rhabdomyomas are most common in the vulvovaginal region of middle-aged women, but two cases presenting as polypoid endocervical lesions have been reported.[213] One patient was of unknown age and the other was 40 years old. Both lesions were of fetal myxoid histologic type with rhabdomyoblasts scattered throughout a myxoid and edematous stroma. In contrast to embryonal rhabdomyosarcoma, a cambium layer, densely cellular areas of small cells, mitotic figures, and invasion of the overlying epithelium or the cervical wall were absent. In another case, a cervical polypoid mass in a 15-year-old girl was reported as a possible intermediate form between a fetal myxoid rhabdomyoma and an embryonal rhabdomyosarcoma.[214]

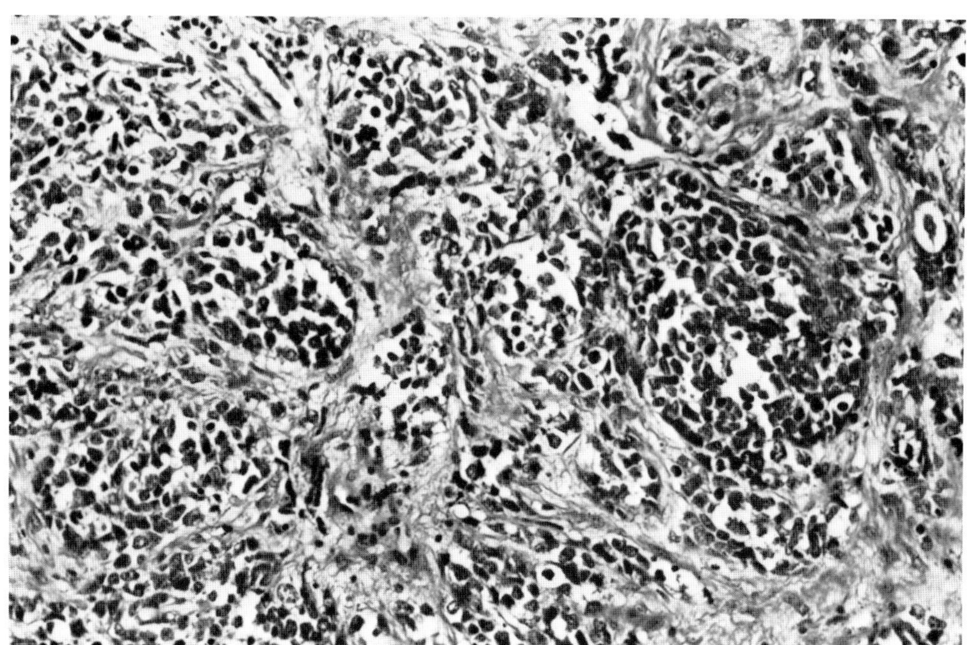

Fig. 6-55. Focus resembling alveolar rhabdomyosarcoma in an otherwise typical embryonal rhabdomyosarcoma of the cervix.

Poorly differentiated endometrial and endocervical stromal sarcomas, in contrast to sarcoma botryoides, typically occur in an older age group and lack a cambium layer and diagnostic rhabdomyoblasts. The presence of nodules of mature cartilage favors a diagnosis of sarcoma botryoides. Adenosarcomas merit consideration in the differential diagnosis because they may also occur as a polypoid lesion within the cervix or endometrium of a young woman; in addition, heterologous elements, including rhabdomyoblasts and cartilage, may be present on histologic examination. In contrast to sarcoma botryoides with occasional entrapped glands, the glands of adenosarcomas are usually more numerous and more uniformly distributed, are often lined by a variety of müllerian epithelia that exhibit mitotic activity, and may contain intraluminal stromal papillae.

SARCOMAS OF UNCERTAIN HISTOGENESIS

Alveolar Soft Part Sarcoma

Ten *alveolar soft part sarcomas* (ASPS) have been recently documented within the uterus, seven in the cervix and three in the corpus.[215-223] All the tumors were encountered in women of reproductive age (14 to 43 years; mean, 35 years) who typically presented with abnormal vaginal bleeding, a cervical mass that was sometimes polypoid, or both. The smallest tumor was an incidental finding within a hysterectomy specimen.[216] Gross examination has revealed a well-circumscribed solid mass, 0.4 to 7 cm in diameter, usually within the superficial cervical stroma or myometrium; one tumor was deep in the myometrium. Microscopic examination has shown the characteristic features of ASPS (Fig. 6-56),

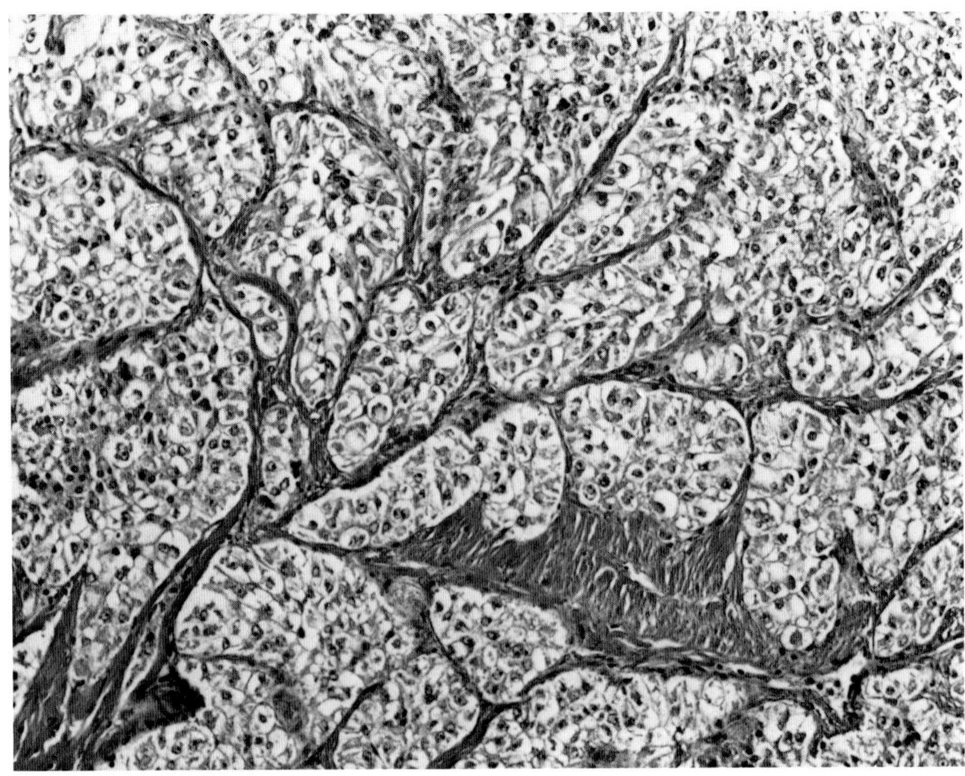

Fig. 6-56. Alveolar soft part sarcoma of the myometrium.

recognition of which should enable distinction from other tumors. In problem cases, a PAS stain should be obtained in an attempt to highlight the distinctive intracytoplasmic needle-shaped crystals. Metastasis has been documented in only one patient who had a microscopic focus of tumor within an obturator lymph node.[215] Postoperative follow-up information, available in nine cases, has been uneventful, although in most cases the follow-up period was brief.

Malignant Rhabdoid Tumor

Three uterine tumors resembling *malignant rhabdoid tumors* have been described.[224–227] Two of the cases, encountered in women 39 and 46 years of age, were considered to have the typical microscopic, immunohistochemical, and ultrastructural features of malignant rhabdoid tumors as encountered in extrauterine sites.[224, 226] One of them was a polypoid endometrial mass that was 8.5 cm at its widest and invaded over one-half of the myometrial thickness. The patient died of widespread tumor 17 months after hysterectomy.[226] The other typical rhabdoid tumor was a myometrial mass 9 cm in diameter.[224] A vaginal recurrence appeared 4 months after hysterectomy[224] and the patient died of tumor dissemination less than 1 year after diagnosis.[227] In the third case, the uterus of a 66-year-old woman contained a fungating mass that filled the endometrial cavity, invaded the wall of the uterus, and involved adnexal structures and pelvic lymph nodes.[225] In contrast to the other cases, the tumor was interpreted as arising from the endometrial stroma and therefore was considered an endometrial stromal sarcoma with rhabdoid differentiation.

RARE BENIGN MESENCHYMAL TUMORS

Aside from leiomyomas and adenomatoid tumors (see Ch. 8), benign mesenchymal tumors in the uterus are rare, and include pure lipomas,[23, 24, 228, 229] vascular tumors (hemangiomas and lymphangiomas of both typical and cavernous type; hemangiomyomas)[230–235] a fibro-osteochondroma,[236] and myxomas.[237, 238] It is noteworthy that the myxomas were encountered in two patients with the complex of myxomas (usually of the heart, skin, and breast) and primary pigmented nodular adrenocortical disease (Carney's complex).[237, 238] The myometrial tumors, which were 1.5 cm and 2.0 cm in maximum dimension, were well circumscribed, and on microscopic examination resembled typical myxomas (Fig. 6-57).

APPENDIX: MITOSIS COUNTING IN MESENCHYMAL TUMORS OF THE UTERUS

The mitotic activity of uterine smooth muscle tumors, and to a lesser extent, tumors in the adenofibroma-adenosarcoma spectrum (see Ch. 7), is the single most important guide to their behavior, albeit not the only one. Although the interobserver reproducibility of mitotic counts has been questioned,[239] it has been shown that interpathologist assessment of mitotic activity is remarkably consistent provided that the pathologist is experienced in this procedure and that certain guidelines are followed.[1, 2, 240–244]

The tumor must be promptly and thoroughly fixed. A number of studies have shown that the mitotic counts of a tumor decline if fixation is delayed and that this decline is proportional not only to the delay but also to the mitotic rate of the tumor.[240, 245–247] Tumors with the highest mitotic rates are associated with the greatest decline in mitotic counts.[246] Although it has been suggested that this apparent decline in mitotic counts is due to mitotic figures (MF) going to completion in unfixed tissue, it has been shown more recently that this phenomenon is at least partially attributable to reduced identifiability of mitotic figures re-

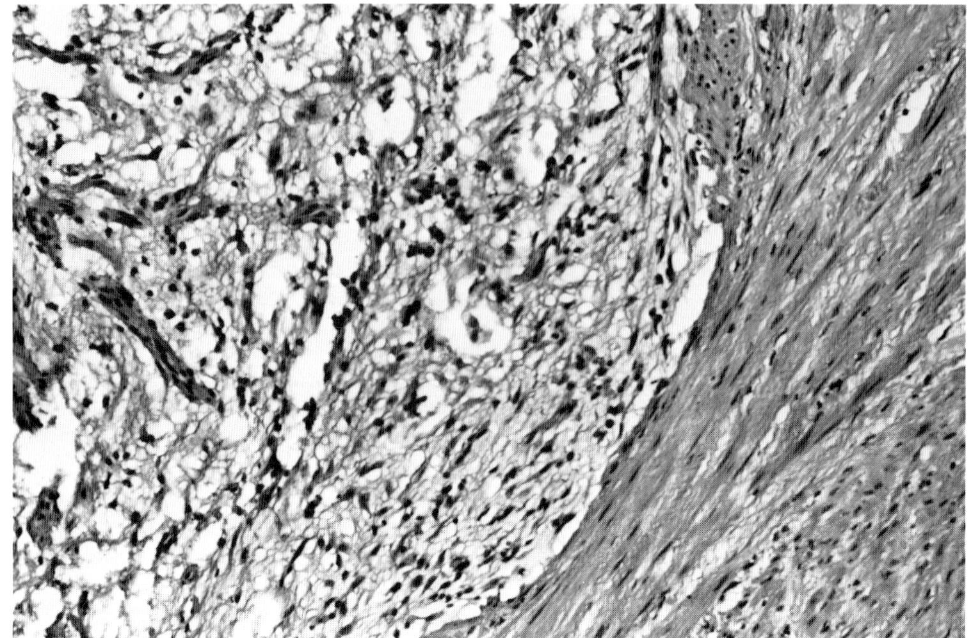

Fig. 6-57. Myometrial myxoma from patient with primary pigmented nodular adrenocortical disease. (Case courtesy of Dr. J. A. Carney, Mayo Clinic.)

lated to delayed fixation.[244, 246] Donhuijsen et al.[246] found that despite a decline in mitotic counts with delayed fixation, flow cytometric data did not change substantially, and that there was only a slight increase in G2 + M − phase fraction associated with delayed fixation. These observations indicate that a tumor on which mitotic counts are to be performed should be fixed as soon as possible after its removal; large tumors should be thoroughly sectioned before immersion in formalin to permit adequate penetration of the fixative.[1]

The tumor must be thoroughly and judiciously sampled. The need for appropriate sampling is underscored by one study in which all five leiomyosarcomas that were initially misdiagnosed as benign were inadequately sampled.[7] Most observers suggest that adequate sampling of a worrisome smooth muscle tumor requires at least one block per centimeter in diameter of tumor or at least 10 blocks, whichever is greater.[1, 241, 242] The border of the tumor

with the surrounding myometrium and areas of the tumor that are suspicious on gross examination (fleshy, hemorrhagic, or necrotic foci) should be well sampled. Tumors with unusual histologic features or with marked variability in cellularity and mitotic rates from one area to another or tumors with borderline counts may require additional sampling.

The histologic slides must be of good technical quality. The slides should be thinly cut, not exceeding 4 to 5 μm in thickness and not overstained with hematoxylin.[241, 242] Norris[242] has found that in some cases it is necessary to perform mitotic counts on slides stained with the mucicarmine method when excessive nuclear staining persists in sections stained with hematoxylin and eosin (H&E)

The mitotic counts are performed in the most mitotically active areas of the tumor. Only unequivocal MFs are counted, and care must be taken not to mistake bizarre, pyknotic, or karyorrhectic nuclei, leukocytes, mast cells, or precipitated hematoxylin for MF.[241, 242] The presence of atypical mitotic figures should be noted. Suspicious MFs should not be counted, and in cases with numerous suspicious MFs, the blocks should be recut and the slides restained.[242] If the problem persists, a mitotic count may still not be performable. In other cases, mitotic counts will be unreliable because of extensive necrosis[10] or because of large numbers of cells with bizarre, hyperchromatic or karyorhectic nuclei.

At least 50 consecutive HPF should be counted by recording the number of MF in each of five different sets of 10 consecutive HPF. The final mitotic count for the tumor (expressed as the number of mitotic figures per 10 HPF) has been determined from either (1) the set of 10 HPF that yielded the highest count, or (2) the average count obtained from all five sets.[14] The first method appears to be the one currently used by most investigators. We are aware of only one published study that compared the mitotic counts obtained by both methods. In that study (of mitotically active leiomyomas), Prayson and Hart found that counts ranged from 5 to 15 MF/10 HPF using the first method and from 4.2 to 10.2 MF/10 HPF with the second method.[14]

Finally, if the mitosis counts are part of a study that is to be published, the area of the HPF should be measured and expressed in mm^2. It has been shown that there can be a wide variation in the area of a standard $450\times$ HPF because of the differences in relative magnification provided by various eyepieces.[248] Recording the area of the HPF thereby facilitates the comparison of data between different studies.

Mitosis counting is a time-consuming and tedious procedure that must be performed compulsively and at an unhurried pace. Performed in this manner and with adherence to the guidelines discussed above, it can be the source of diagnostically valuable information.

REFERENCES

1. Zaloudek CJ, Norris HJ: Mesenchymal tumors of the uterus. p. 1. In Fenoglio CM, Wolff M (eds): Progress in Surgical Pathology. Vol. III. Masson USA, New York, 1981
2. Kempson RL, Hendrickson MR: Pure mesenchymal neoplasms of the uterine corpus: selected problems. Semin Diagn Pathol 5:172, 1988
3. Taylor HB, Norris HJ: Mesenchymal tumors of the uterus. IV. Diagnosis and prognosis of leiomyosarcoma. Arch Pathol Lab Med 82:40, 1966
4. Kempson RL, Bari W: Uterine sarcomas. Classification, diagnosis, and prognosis. Hum Pathol 1:331, 1970
5. Christopherson WM, Williamson EO, Gray LA: Leiomyosarcoma of the uterus. Cancer 29:1512, 1972
6. Hart WR, Billman JK: A reassessment of uterine neoplasms originally diagnosed as leiomyosarcomas. Cancer 41:1902, 1978
7. Burns B, Curry RH, Bell MEA: Morphologic features of prognostic significance in uterine smooth muscle tumors: a review of eighty-four cases. Am J Obstet Gynecol 135:109, 1979
8. Farhood AI, Abrams J: Immunohistochemistry of endometrial stromal sarcoma. Hum Pathol 22:224, 1991
9. Franquemont DW, Frierson HF, Mills SE: An immunohistochemical study of normal endometrial stroma and endometrial stromal neoplasms. Evidence for smooth muscle differentiation. Am J Surg Pathol 15:861, 1991
10. Evans HL: Smooth muscle neoplasms of the uterus other than ordinary leiomyoma. A study of 46 cases, with emphasis on diagnostic criteria and prognostic factors. Cancer 62:2239, 1988.
11. Fechner RE: Atypical leiomyomas and synthetic progestin therapy. Am J Clin Pathol 49:697, 1968
12. Perrone T, Dehner LP: Prognostically favorable "mitotically active" smooth-muscle tumors of the uterus. A clinicopathologic study of 10 cases. Am J Surg Pathol 12:1, 1988

13. O'Connor DM, Norris HJ: Mitotically active leiomyomas of the uterus. Hum Pathol 21:223, 1990

14. Prayson RA, Hart WR: Mitotically active leiomyomas of the uterus. Am J Clin Pathol 97:14, 1992

15. Tiltman AJ: The effect of progestins on the mitotic activity of uterine fibromyomas. Int J Gynecol Pathol 4:89, 1985

16. Kawaguchi K, Fujii S, Konishi I et al: Mitotic activity in uterine leiomyomas during the menstrual cycle. Am J Obstet Gynecol 160:637, 1989

17. Dilts PV Jr, Hopkins MP, Chang AE, Cody RL: Rapid growth of leiomyoma in patient receiving tamoxifen. Am J Obstet Gynecol 166:167, 1992

18. Clement PB, Young RH, Scully RE: Non-trophoblastic pathology of the female genital tract and peritoneum associated with pregnancy. Semin Diagn Pathol 6:372, 1989

19. Myles JL, Hart WR: Apoplectic leiomyomas of the uterus. A clinicopathologic study of five distinctive hemorrhagic leiomyomas associated with oral contraceptive usage. Am J Surg Pathol 9:798, 1985

20. Norris HJ, Hilliard GD, Irey NS: Hemorrhagic cellular leiomyomas ("apoplectic leiomyoma") of the uterus associated with pregnancy and oral contraceptives. Int J Gynecol Pathol 7:212, 1988

21. Smiddy M, Silverberg SG: Pathologic features of uterine leiomyomas following treatment with leuprolide acetate, abstracted. Am J Clin Pathol 97:448, 1992

22. August C, Kepic T, Meier L, Valle J: Histologic findings in uterine leiomyomata of women treated with gonadotropin-releasing hormone agonists, abstracted. Am J Clin Pathol 97:448, 1992

23. Hendrickson MR, Kempson RL: Surgical pathology of the uterine corpus. p. 473. In Bennington JL (ed): Major Problems in Pathology, Vol 12. WB Saunders, Philadelphia, 1980

24. Mazur MT, Kraus FT: Histogenesis of morphologic variations in tumors of the uterine wall. Am J Surg Pathol 4:59, 1980

25. Clement PB, Young RH, Scully RE: Diffuse, perinodular, and other patterns of hydropic degeneration within and adjacent to uterine leiomyomas: problems in differential diagnosis. Am J Surg Pathol 16:26, 1992

26. Lee SS, Herlitzka AJ: Giant myometrial cyst: report of a case. Iowa Med 77:24, 1987

27. Jacobs DS, Cohen H, Johnson JS: Lipoleiomyomas of the uterus. Am J Clin Pathol 44:45, 1965

28. Willen R, Gad A, Willen H: Lipomatous lesions of the uterus. Virchows Arch [A] 377:351, 1978

29. Pounder DJ: Fatty tumours of the uterus. J Clin Pathol 35:1380, 1982

30. Sieinski W: Lipomatous neometaplasia of the uterus. Report of 11 cases with discussion of histogenesis and pathogenesis. Int J Gynecol Pathol 8:357, 1989

31. Lin M, Hunai J: Atypical lipoleiomyoma of the uterus. Acta Pathol Jpn 41:164, 1991

32. Brooks JJ, Wells GB, Yeh I, LiVolsi VA: Bizarre epithelioid lipoleiomyoma of the uterus. Int J Gynecol Pathol 11:144, 1992

33. Novak ER, Woodruff JD: Novak's Gynecologic and Obstetric Pathology with Clinical and Endocrine Relations. 8th Ed. WB Saunders, Philadelphia, 1979

34. Martin-Reay DG, Christ ML, LaPata RE: Uterine leiomyoma with skeletal muscle differentiation. Am J Clin Pathol 96:344, 1991

35. Gisser SD, Young I: Neurilemoma-like uterine myomas: an ultrastructural reaffirmation of their non-Schwannian nature. Am J Obstet Gynecol 129:389, 1977

36. Case Records of the Massachusetts General Hospital: Case 23–1985. N Engl J Med 312:1505, 1985

37. Prichard JG, Lowenstein MH, Silverman IJ, Brennan JC: *Streptococcus milleri* pyomyoma simulating infective endocarditis. Obstet Gynecol 68:46S, 1986

38. Schmid C, Beham A, Kratochvil P: Haematopoesis in a degenerating leiomyoma. Arch Gynecol Obstet 248:81, 1991

39. Adany R, Fodor F, Molnar P: Increased density of histiocytes in uterine leiomyomas. Int J Gynecol Pathol 9:137, 1990

40. Crow J, Wilkins M, Howe S et al: Mast cells in the female genital tract. Int J Gynecol Pathol 10:230, 1991

41. Barter JF, Smith EB, Szpak CA et al:

Leiomyosarcoma of the uterus: Clinicopathologic study of 21 cases. Gynecol Oncol 21:220, 1985.

42. Larson B, Silfversward C, Nilsson B, Pettersson F: Prognostic factors in uterine leiomyosarcoma. A clinical and histopathological study of 143 cases. The Radiumhemmet series 1936–1981. Acta Oncol 29:185, 1990

43. Lazaro NA, Batts JA Jr, Rishi A et al: Rupture of leiomyosarcoma uteri with hemoperitoenum clinically simulating ruptured ectopic pregnancy. J Reprod Med 24:174, 1980

44. Marua R, Olesnicky G: Uterine leiomyosarcoma presenting with haemoperitoneum. Med J Aust 148:655, 1988

45. Bodon GR, Mijangos JA: Alkaline phosphatase-producing leiomyosarcoma of the uterus. Am J Surg 124:673, 1972

46. Patsner B, Mann WJ: Use of serum CA-125 in monitoring patients with uterine sarcoma. Cancer 62:1355, 1988

47. Abell MR, Ramirez JA: Sarcomas and carcinosarcomas of the uterine cervix. Cancer 31:1176, 1973

48. Scurry J, Hack M: Leiomyosarcoma arising in a lipoleiomyoma. Gynecol Oncol 39:381, 1990

49. Hitti IF, Glasberg SS, McKenzie C, Meltzer BA: Uterine leiomyosarcoma with massive necrosis diagnosed during gonadotropin-releasing hormone analog therapy for presumed uterine fibroid. Fertil Steril 56:778, 1991

50. Azumi H, Ben-Ezra J, Battifora H: Immunophenotypic diagnosis of leiomyosarcomas and rhabdomyosarcomas with monoclonal antibodies to muscle-specific actin and desmin in formalin-fixed tissue. Mod Pathol 1:469, 1988

51. Devaney K, Tavassoli FA: Immunohistochemistry as a diagnostic aid in the interpretation of unusual mesenchymal tumors of the uterus. Mod Pathol 4:225, 1991

52. Marshall RJ, Braye SG: Alpha-1-antitrypsin, alpha-1-antichymotrypsin, actin, and myosin in uterine sarcomas. Int J Gyncol Pathol 4:346, 1985

53. Ferenczy A, Richart RM, Okagaki T: A comparative ultrastructural study of leiomyosarcoma, cellular leiomyoma, and leiomyoma of the uterus. Cancer 28:1004, 1971

54. Mackay B, Ro J, Floyd C, Ordonez NG: Ultrastructural observations on smooth muscle tumors. Ultrastruct Pathol 11:593, 1987

55. Miettinen M: Immunoreactivity for cytokeratin and epithelial membrane antigen in leiomyosarcoma. Arch Pathol Lab Med 112:637, 1988

56. Darby AJ, Papadaki L, Beilby JOW: An unusual leiomyosarcoma of the uterus containing osteoclast-like giant cells. Cancer 36:495, 1975

57. Pilon V, Parikh N, Maccera J: Malignant osteoclast-like giant cell tumor associated with a uterine leiomyosarcoma. Gynecol Oncol 23:381, 1986

58. Marshall RJ, Braye SG, Jones DB: Leiomyosarcoma of the uterus with giant cells resembling osteoclasts. Int J Gynecol Pathol 5:260, 1986

59. Sienski W: Malignant giant cell tumor associated with leiomyosarcoma of the uterus. Cancer 65:1838, 1990

60. Tsushima K, Stanhope CR, Gaffey TA, Lieber MM: Uterine leiomyosarcomas and benign smooth muscle tumors: usefulness of nuclear DNA patterns studied by flow cytometry. Mayo Clin Proc 63:248, 1988

61. King ME, Dickersin GR, Scully RE: Myxoid leiomyosarcoma of the uterus. A report of six cases. Am J Surg Pathol 6:589, 1982

62. Chen KTK: Myxoid leiomyosarcoma of the uterus. Int J Gynecol Pathol 3:389, 1984

63. Pounder DJ, Iyer PV: Uterine leiomyosarcoma with myxoid stroma. Arch Pathol Lab Med 109:762, 1985

64. Salm R, Evans DJ: Myxoid leiomyosarcoma. Histopathology 9:159, 1985

65. Peacock G, Archer S: Myxoid leiomyosarcoma of the uterus: case report and review of the literature. Am J Obstet Gynecol 160:1515, 1989

66. Shroff CP, Deodhar KP, Bhagwat AG: Myxoid leiomyosarcoma of the uterus—a case report with light microscopic and ultrastructural appraisal. Tumori 70:561, 1984

67. Rywlin AM, Recher L, Benson J: Clear cell leiomyoma of the uterus: report of 2

cases of a previously undescribed entity. Cancer 17:100, 1964

68. Lavin L, Hajdu SI, Foote FW, Jr: Gastric and extragastric leiomyoblastomas. Clinicopathologic study of 44 cases. Cancer 29:305, 1972

69. Goodhue WW, Susin M, Kramer EE: Smooth muscle origin of uterine plexiform tumors. Ultrastructural and histochemical evidence. Arch Pathol Lab Med 97:263, 1974

70. Kurman RJ, Norris HJ: Mesenchymal tumors of the uterus. VI. Epithelioid smooth muscle tumors including leiomyoblastoma and clear-cell leiomyoma. A clinical and pathological analysis of 26 cases. Cancer 37:1853, 1976

71. Chang V, Aikawa M, Druet R: Uterine leiomyoblastoma. Ultrastructural and cytologic studies. Cancer 39:1563, 1977

72. Fisher ER, Paulson JD, Gregorio RM: The myofibroblastic nature of the uterine plexiform tumor. Arch Pathol Lab Med 102:477, 1978

73. Nunez-Alonso C, Battifora HA: Plexiform tumors of the uterus: Ultrastructural study. Cancer 44:1707, 1979

74. Haberstroh WD, Reamer JF, Slate WG: Epithelioid leiomyoma of the uterus. Obstet Gynecol 57:86S, 1981

75. Kaminski PF, Tavassoli FA: Plexiform tumorlet: a clinical and pathologic study of 15 cases with ultrastructural observations. Int J Gynecol Pathol 3:124, 1984

76. Balaton AJ, Vuong PN, Vaury P, Baviera EE: Plexiform tumorlet of the uterus: immunohistochemical evidence for smooth muscle origin. Histopathology 10:749, 1986

77. Buscema J, Carpenter SE, Rosenshein NB, Woodruff JD: Epithelioid leiomyosarcoma of the uterus. Cancer 57:1192, 1986

78. Ito H, Sasaki H, Miyagawa K, Tahara E: Bizarre leiomyoblastoma of the cervix uteri. Immunohistochemical and ultrastructural study. Acta Pathol Jpn 36:1737, 1986

79. Mazur MT, Priest JE: Clear cell leiomyoma (leiomyoblastoma) of the uterus: Ultrastructural observations. Ultrastruct Pathol 10:249, 1986

80. Hyde KE, Geisinger KR, Marshall RB, Jones TL: The clear-cell variant of uterine epithelioid leiomyoma. An immunohistochemical and ultrastructural study. Arch Pathol Lab Med 113:551, 1989

81. Seidman JD, Yetter RA, Papadimitriou JC: Epithelioid component of uterine leiomyosarcoma simulating metastatic carcinoma. Arch Pathol Lab Med 116:287, 1992

82. Kempson RL: Sarcomas and related neoplasms. p. 298. In Norris HJ, Hertig AT (eds): The uterus. International Academy of Pathology Monograph. Williams & Wilkins, Baltimore, 1973

83. Clement PB, Young RH: Diffuse leiomyomatosis of the uterus: a report of four cases. Int J Gynecol Pathol 6:322, 1987

84. Lai FM, Wong FWS, Allen PW: Diffuse leiomyomatosis with hemorrhage. Arch Pathol Lab Med 115:834, 1991

85. Lack EE, Dolan MF, Finisio J et al: Pulmonary and extrapulmonary lymphangioleiomyomatosis. Am J Surg Pathol 10:650, 1986

86. Norris HJ, Parmley T: Mesenchymal tumors of the uterus. V. Intravenous leiomyomatosis. A clinical and pathological study of 14 cases. Cancer 36:2164, 1975

87. Nogales FF, Navarro N, de Victoria JMM et al: Uterine intravascular leiomyomatosis: An update and report of seven cases. Int J Gynecol Pathol 6:331, 1987

88. Clement PB: Intravenous leiomyomatosis. Pathol Ann 23(2):153, 1988

89. Clement PE, Young RH, Scully RE: Intravenous leiomyomatosis of the uterus. A clinicopathological analysis of 16 cases with unusual histologic features. Am J Surg Pathol 12:932, 1988

90. Brescia RJ, Tazelaar HD, Hobbs J, Miller AW: Intravascular lipoleiomyomatosis: A report of two cases. Hum Pathol 20:252, 1989

91. Suginami H, Kaura R, Ochi H, Matsuura S: Intravenous leiomyomatosis with cardiac extension: successful surgical management and histopathologic study. Obstet Gynecol 76:527, 1990

92. Slavin J, Mulvany N: Intravenous leiomyomatosis—a review, abstracted. Pathology 24:7, 1992

93. Tierney WM, Ehrlich CE, Bailey JC et al:

Intravenous leiomyomatosis of the uterus with extension into the heart. Am J Med 69:471, 1980

94. Rotter AJ, Lundell CJ: MR of intravenous leiomyomatosis of the uterus extending into the inferior vena cava. J Comput Assist Tomogr 15:690, 1991

95. Kawakami S, Sagoh T, Kumada H et al: Intravenous leiomyomatosis of uterus: MR appearance. J Comput Assist Tomogr 15:68, 1991

96. Boyce CR, Buddhdev HN: Pregnancy complicated by metastasizing leiomyoma of uterus. Obstet Gynecol 42:252, 1973

97. Abell MR, Littler ER: Benign metastasizing uterine leiomyoma. Cancer 36:2206, 1975

98. Horstmann JP, Pietra GG, Harman JA et al: Spontaneous regression of pulmonary leiomyomas during pregnancy. Cancer 39:314, 1977

99. Tench WD, Dail D, Gmelich JT, Matani N: Benign metastasizing leiomyomas: a review of 21 cases, abstracted. Lab Invest 38:37, 1978

100. Wolff M, Silva F, Kaye G: Pulmonary metastases (with admixed epithelial elements) from smooth muscle neoplasms. Am J Surg Pathol 3:325, 1979

101. Cramer SF, Meyer JS, Kraner JF et al: Metastasizing leiomyoma of the uterus. Cancer 45:932, 1980

102. Deppe G, Clachko M, Deligdisch L, Cohen CJ: Uterine fibroleiomyomata with aortic node metastases. Int J Gynaecol Obstet 18:1, 1980

103. Banner AS, Carrington CB, Emory WB et al: Efficacy of oophorectomy in lymphangioleiomyomatosis and benign metastasizing leiomyoma. N Engl J Med 305:204, 1981

104. Gatti J, Morvan GG, Henin D et al: Leiomyomatosis metastasizing to the spine. J Bone Joint Surg 65A:1163, 1983

105. Rigaud C, Bogomoletz WV: Leiomyomatosis in pelvic lymph node (letter). Arch Pathol Lab Med 107:153, 1983

106. Evans AJ, Wiltshaw E, Kochanowski SJ et al: Metastasizing leiomyoma of the uterus and hormonal manipulations. Br J Obstet Gynaecol 93:646, 1986

107. Barter JF, Szpak C, Creasman W.T: Uterine leiomyomas with retroperitoneal lymph node involvement. South Med J 80. 1320, 1987

108. Tavassoli FA, Norris HJ: Peritoneal leiomyomatosis (leiomyomatosis peritonealis disseminata): a clinicopathologic study of 20 cases with ultrastructural observations. Int J Gynecol Pathol 1:59, 1982

109. Erbstroesser E, Lessel W: Leiomyomatosis peritonealis disseminata. Zentralbl Chir 107:223, 1982

110. Willson JR, Peale AR: Multiple peritoneal leiomyomas associated with a granulosa-cell tumor of the ovary. Am J Obstet Gynecol 64:204, 1952

111. Taubert H, Wissner SE, Haskins AL. Leiomyomatosis peritonealis disseminata. An unusual complication of genital leiomyomata. Obstet Gynecol 25:561, 1965

112. Walley VM: Leiomyomatosis peritonealis disseminata (letter). Int J Gynecol Pathol 2:222, 1983

113. Hsu YK, Rosenshein NB, Parmley TH et al: Leiomyomatosis in pelvic lymph nodes. Obstet Gynecol 57:91S, 1981

114. Due W, Pickartz H: Immunohistochemical detection of estrogen and progesterone receptors in disseminated peritoneal leiomyomatosis. Int J Gynecol Pathol 8:46, 1989

115. Lim OW, Segal A, Ziel HK: Leiomyomatosis peritonealis disseminata associated with pregnancy. Obstet Gynecol 55:122, 1980

116. Barnes HM, Richardson PJ: Benign metastasizing leiomyoma. J Obstet Gynaecol Br Commonw 80:569, 1973

117. Rubin SC, Wheeler JE, Mikuta JJ: Malignant leiomyomatosis peritonealis disseminata. Obstet Gynecol 68:126, 1986

118. Akkersdijk GJM, Flu PK, Giard RWM et al: Malignant leiomyomatosis peritonealis disseminata. Am J Obstet Gynecol 163:591, 1990

119. Clavero PA, Nogales FF, Ruis-Avila I et al: Regression of peritoneal leiomyomatosis after treatment with gonadotropin releasing hormone analogue. Int J Gynecol Cancer 2:52, 1992

120. Fujii S, Nakashima N, Okamura H et al: Progesterone-induced smooth muscle-like

cells in the subperitoneal nodules produced by estrogen. Experimental approach to leiomyomatosis peritonealis disseminata. Am J Obstet Gynecol 139:164, 1981

121. Lipschutz A, Vargas L, Jr: Structure and origin of uterine and extragenital fibroids induced experimentally in the guinea pig by prolonged administration of estrogen. Cancer Res 1:236, 1941

122. Lipschutz A: Experimental fibroids and the antifibromatogenic action of steroid hormones JAMA 120:171, 1942

123. Sutherland JA, Wilson EA, Edger DE, Powell D: Ultrastructure and steroid-binding studies in leiomyomatosis peritonealis disseminata. Am J Obstet Gynecol 136:992, 1980

124. Jensen PA, Dockerty MB, Symmonds RE, Wilson RB: Endometrioid sarcoma ("stromal endometriosis"). Report of 15 cases including 5 with metastases. Am J Obstet Gynecol 95:79, 1966

125. Norris HJ, Taylor HB: Mesenchymal tumors of the uterus. I. A clinical and pathologic study of 53 endometrial stromal tumors. Cancer 19:755, 1966

126. Baggish MS, Woodruff JD: Uterine stromatosis. Clinicopathologic features and hormone dependency. Obstet Gynecol 40:487, 1972

127. Clement PB, Scully RE: Uterine tumors resembling ovarian sex-cord tumors. Am J Clin Pathol 66:512, 1976

128. Hart WR, Yoonessi M: Endometrial stromatosis of the uterus. Obstet Gynecol 49:393, 1977

129. Yoonessi M, Hart WR: Endometrial stromal sarcomas. Cancer 40:898, 1977

130. Mazur MT, Askin FB: Endolymphatic stromal myosis. Unique presentation and ultrastructural study. Cancer 42:2661, 1978

131. Smith ML, Faaborg LL, Newland JR: Dedifferentiation of endolymphatic stromal myosis to poorly differentiated uterine stromal sarcoma. Gynecol Oncol 9: 108, 1980

132. Tavassoli FA, Norris HJ: Mesenchymal tumours of the uterus. VII. A clinicopathological study of 60 endometrial stromal nodules. Histopathology 5:1, 1981

133. Evans HL: Endometrial stromal sarcoma and poorly differentiated endometrial sarcoma. Cancer 50:2170, 1982

134. Paulsen SM, Nielsen VT, Hansen P, Ferenczy A: Endolymphatic stromal myosis with focal tubular-glandular differentiation (biphasic endometrial stromal sarcoma). Ultrastruct Pathol 3:31, 1982

135. Thatcher SS, Woodruff JD: Uterine stromatosis: a report of 33 cases. Obstet Gynecol 59:428, 1982

136. Baker VV, Walton LA, Fowler WC, Jr, Currie JL: Steroid receptors in endolymphatic stromal myosis. Obstet Gynecol 63:72S, 1984

137. Fekete PS, Vellios F: The clinical and histologic spectrum of endometrial stromal neoplasms: a report of 41 cases. Int J Gynecol Pathol 3:198, 1984

138. Lantta M, Kahanpaa K, Karkkainen J et al: Estradiol and progesterone receptors in two cases of endometrial stromal sarcoma. Gynecol Oncol 18:233, 1984

139. Piver MS, Rutledge FN, Copeland L et al: Uterine endolymphatic stromal myosis: A collaborative study. Obstet Gynecol 64:173, 1984

140. Case Records of the Massachusetts General Hospital. Case 32-1985. N Engl J Med 313:374, 1985

141. Yu TJ, Iwasaki I, Teratani T et al: Circumscribed endometrial stromatosis of the uterus with marked epitheliogenesis. Gynecol Oncol 24:367, 1986

142. Katz L, Merino MJ, Sakamoto H, Schwartz PE: Endometrial stromal sarcoma: a clinicopathologic study of 11 cases with determination of estrogen and progestin receptor levels in three tumors. Gynecol Oncol 26:87, 1987

143. Lifschitz-Mercer B, Czernobilsky B, Dgani R et al: Immunocytochemical study of an endometrial diffuse clear cell stromal sarcoma and other endometrial stromal sarcomas. Cancer 59:1494, 1987

144. Whitlach SP, Meyer RL: Recurrent endometrial stromal sarcoma resembling intravenous leiomyomatosis. Gynecol Oncol 28:121, 1987

145. Ohta H, Nozawa S, Hosoda Y: Endolymphatic stromal myosis coexisting with adenocarcinoma of the uterus. Ultrastruct Pathol 12:659, 1988

146. Abrams J, Talcott J, Corson JM: Pulmonary metastases in patients with low-grade endometrial stromal sarcoma. Am J Surg Pathol 13:133, 1989

147. August CZ, Bauer KD, Lurain J, Murad T: Neoplasms of endometrial stroma: histopathologic and flow cytometric analysis with clinical correlation. Hum Pathol 20:232, 1989

148. De Fusco PA, Gaffey TA, Malkasian GD, Jr et al: Endometrial stromal sarcoma: review of Mayo Clinic experience 1945–1980. Gynecol Oncol 35:8, 1989

149. Dgani R, Shoham Z, Czernobilsky B et al: Endolymphatic stromal myosis (endometrial low-grade stromal sarcoma) presenting with hematuria: A diagnostic challenge. Gynecol Oncol 35:262, 1989

150. Montag TW, Manart FD: Endolymphatic stroma myosis: surgical and hormonal therapy for extensive venous recurrence. Gynecol Oncol 33:255, 1989

151. Styron SL, Burke TW, Linville WK: Low-grade endometrial stromal sarcoma recurring over three decades. Gynecol Oncol 35:275, 1989

152. Taina E, Maenpaa J, Erkkola R et al: Endometrial stromal sarcoma: a report of nine cases. Gyneco Oncol 32:156, 1989

153. Tosi P, Sforza V, Santopietro R: Estrogen receptor content, immunohistochemically determined by monoclonal antibodies, in endometrial stromal sarcoma. Obstet Gynecol 73:75, 1989

154. Berchuk A, Rubin SC, Hoskins WJ et al: Treatment of endometrial stromal tumors. Gynecol Oncol 36:60, 1990

155. Chang KL, Crabtree GS, Lim-Tan SK et al: Primary uterine endometrial stromal neoplasms. A clinicopathologic study of 117 cases. Am J Surg Pathol 14:415, 1990

156. Chumas JC, Pastner B, Mann WJ: High-grade pelvic sarcoma after radiation therapy for low-grade endometrial stromal sarcoma. Gynecol Oncol 36:428, 1990

157. Dunton CJ, Kelsten ML, Brooks SE et al: Low-grade stromal sarcoma: DNA flow cytometric analysis and estrogen progesterone receptor data. Gynecol Oncol 37:268, 1990

158. Larson B, Silfversward C, Nilsson B, Pettersson F: Endometrial stromal sarcoma of the uterus. A clinical and histopathologic study. The radiumhemmet series 1936–1981. Eur J Obstet Gynecol Reprod Biol 35:239, 1990

159. Mansi JL, Ramachandra S, Wiltshaw E, Fisher C: Endometrial stromal sarcomas. Gynecol Oncol 36:113, 1990

160. Young RH, Scully RE: Sarcomas metastatic to the ovary: a report of 21 cases. Int J Gynecol Pathol 9:231, 1990

161. Binder SW, Nieberg RK, Cheng L, Al-Jitawi S: Histologic and immunohistochemical analysis of nine endometrial stromal tumors: an unexpected high frequency of keratin protein positivity. Int J Gynecol Pathol 10:191, 1991

162. El-Naggar A, Abdul-Karim FW, Silva EG et al: Uterine stromal neoplasms: a clinicopathologic and DNA flow cytometric correlation. Hum Pathol 22:897, 1991

163. Hitchock CL, Norris HJ: Flow cytometric analysis of endometrial stromal sarcoma. Am J Clin Pathol 97:267, 1992

164. Lillemoe TJ, Perrone T, Norris HJ, Dehner LP: Myogenous phenotype of epithelial-like areas in endometrial stromal sarcomas. Arch Pathol Lab Med 115:215, 1991

165. Clement PB, Scully RE: Endometrial stromal sarcomas of the uterus with extensive endometrioid glandular differentiation. A report of three cases that caused problems in differential diagnosis. Int J Gynecol Pathol 11:163, 1992

166. Kempson RL, Hendrickson MR: Pure mesenchymal neoplasms of the uterine corpus. p. 426. In Fox H (ed): Haines and Taylor's Obstetrical and Gynaecological Pathology. Churchill Livingstone, New York, 1987

167. Sabini G, Chumas JC, Mann WJ: Steroid hormone receptors in endometrial stromal sarcoma. A biochemical and immunohistochemical study. Am J Clin Pathol 97:381, 1992

167a. Lloreta J, Prat J: Endometrial stromal nodule with smooth and skeletal muscle components simulating stromal sarcoma. Int J Gynecol Pathol 11:293, 1992

168. Press MF, Scully RE: Endometrial "sarcomas" complicating ovarian thecoma, polycystic ovarian disease and estrogen therapy. Gynecol Oncol 21:135, 1985

169. Altaras MM, Jaffe R, Cohen I et al: Role of prolonged excessive estrogen stimulation in the pathogenesis of endometrial sarcomas: Two cases and a review of the literature. Gynecol Oncol 38:273, 1990

170. Roth LM, Senteny GE: Stromomyoma of the uterus. Ultrastruct Pathol 9:137, 1985

171. Jaffe R, Altaras M, Bernheim J, Aderet NB: Endocervical stromal sarcoma—a case report. Gynecol Oncol 22:105, 1985

172. Abdul-Karim FW, Bazi TM, Sorensen K, Nasr MF: Sarcoma of the uterine cervix: clinicopathologic findings in three cases. Gynecol Oncol 26:103, 1987

173. Clement PB, Scully RE: Mullerian adenosarcoma of the uterus. A clinicopathological analysis of 100 cases with a review of the literature. Hum Pathol 21:363, 1990

174. Ehrmann RL, Griffiths CT: Malignant hemangioendothelioma of the uterus, Gynecol Oncol 8:376, 1979

175. Ongkasuwan C, Taylor JE, Tang C, Prempree T: Angiosarcoma of the uterus and ovary: clinicopathologic report. Cancer 49:1469, 1982

176. Witkin GB, Askin F, Geratz D, Reddick RL: Angiosarcoma of the uterus: a light microscopic, immunohistochemical, and ultrastructural study. Int J Gynecol Pathol 6:176, 1987

177. Milne DS, Hinshaw K, Malcolm AJ, Hilton P: Primary angiosarcoma of the uterus: a case report. Histopathology 16:203, 1990

178. Quinonez GE, Paraskevas MP, Diocee MS, Lorimer SM: Angiosarcoma of the uterus: a case report. Am J Obstet Gynecol 164:90, 1991

179. Sooriyaarachchi GS, Ramirez G, Roley EL: Hemangiopericytoma of the uterus: report of a case with a comprehensive review of the literature. J Surg Oncol 10:399, 1978

180. Buscema J, Klein V, Rotmensch J et al: Uterine hemangiopericytoma. Obstet Gynecol 69:104, 1987

181. Bonfiglio TA, Patten SF, Jr, Woodworth FE: Fibroxanthosarcoma of the uterine cervix: cytopathologic and histopathologic manifestations. Acta Cytol 20:501, 1976

182. Kindblom L, Seidal T: Malignant giant cell tumor of the uterus. Acta Pathol Microbiol Immunol Scand A 89:179, 1981

183. Takaki Y, Kishikawa M, Sekine I et al: Primary malignant fibrous histiocytoma of the endometrium. Acta Pathol Jpn 33:823, 1983

184. Chou S, Fortune D, Beischer NA et al: Primary malignant fibrous histiocytoma of the uterus—ultrastructural and immunocytochemical studies of two cases. Pathology 17:36, 1985

185. Fujii S, Kanzaki H, Konishi I et al: Malignant fibrous histiocytoma of the uterus. Gynecol Oncol 26:319, 1987

186. Torrisi A, Georgino F, Onnis GL, Minucci D: Cytological patterns of primary malignant uterine fibrous histiocytoma. Eur J Gynaecol Oncol 11:343, 1990

187. Magni E, Lauritzen AF, Wilken-Jensen C, Horn T: Malignant giant cell tumour of the uterus, Suppl. APMIS 23:113, 1991

188. Auerbach HE, LiVolsi VA, Merino MJ: Malignant mixed mullerian tumors of the uterus. An immunohistochemical study. Int J Gynecol Pathol 7:123, 1988

189. Hart WR, Craig JR: Rhabdomyosarcomas of the uterus. Am J Clin Pathol 70:217, 1978

190. Vakiani M, Mawad J, Talerman A: Heterologous sarcomas of the uterus. Int J Gynecol Pathol 1:211, 1982

191. Siegal GP, Taylor LL III, Nelson KG et al: Characterization of a pure heterologous sarcoma of the uterus: rhabdomyosarcoma of the corpus. Int J Gynecol Pathol 2:303, 1983

192. Jaworski RC Rencoret RH, Moir DH: Pleomorphic rhabdomyosarcoma of the uterus. Case report with a review of the literature. Br J Obstet Gynaecol 91:1269, 1984

193. Podczaski E, Sees J, Kaminski P et al: Rhabdomyosarcoma of the uterus in a postmenopausal patient. Gynecol Oncol 37:439, 1990

194. Clement PB: Chondrosarcoma of the uterus: report of a case and review of the literature. Hum Pathol 9:726, 1978

195. Kofinas AD, Suarez J, Calame RJ, Chipeco Z: Chondrosarcoma of the uterus. Gynecol Oncol 19:231, 1984

196. Crum CP, Rogers BH, Andersen W: Osteosarcoma of the uterus: case report of review of the literature. Gynecol Oncol 9:256, 1980

197. Jotkowitz MW, Valentine R: A rare pelvic mass: osteosarcoma of the body of the uterus. Aust NZ J Obstet Gynaecol 25:132, 1985

198. Piscioli F, Govoni E, Polla E et al: Primary osteosarcoma of the uterine corpus. Report of a case and critical review of the literature. Int J Gynaecol Obstet 23:377, 1985

199. Bloch T, Roth LM, Stehman FB et al: Osteosarcoma of the uterine cervix associated with hyperplastic and atypical mesonephric rests. Cancer 62:1594, 1988

200. Basolo F, Pingitore R, Gadducci A: Osteosarcoma of the myometrium synchronous with bilateral papillary cystadenocarcinoma of the ovary and papillary adenocarcinoma of the cervix. Tumori 74:227, 1988

201. Caputo MG, Reuter KL, Reale F: Primary osteosarcoma of the uterus. Br J Radiol 63:578, 1990

202. De Young B, Bitterman P, Lack EE: Primary osteosarcoma of the uterus: Report of a case with immunohistochemical study. Mod Pathol 5:212, 1992

203. Veliath AJ, Hannah P, Ratnakar C et al: Primary liposarcoma of the cervix: a case report. Int J Gynaecol Obstet 16:75, 1978

204. Bapat K, Brustein S: Uterine sarcoma with liposarcomatous differentiation: Report of a case and review of the literature. Int J Gynecol Obstet 28:71, 1989

205. Copeland LJ, Gershenson DM, Saul PB et al: Sarcoma botryoides of the female genital tract. Obstet Gynecol 66:262, 1985

206. Montag TW, d'Ablaing G, Schlaerth JB et al: Embryonal rhabdomyosarcoma of the uterine corpus and cervix. Gynecol Oncol 25:171, 1986

207. Brand E, Berek JS, Nieberg RK, Hacker NF: Rhabdomyosarcoma of the uterine cervix. Sarcoma botryoides. Cancer 60:1552, 1987

208. Daya DA, Scully RE: Sarcoma botryoides of the uterine cervix in young women: a clinicopathological study of 13 cases. Gynecol Oncol 29:290, 1988

209. Hays DM, Shimada H, Raney RB, Jr et al: Clinical staging and treatment results in rhabdomyosarcoma of the female genital tract among children and adolescents. Cancer 61:1893, 1988

210. Loughlin KR, Retik AB, Weinstein HJ et al: Genitourinary rhabdomyosarcoma in children. Cancer 63:1600, 1989

211. Perrone T, Carson LF, Dehner LP: Rhabdomyosarcoma with heterologous cartilage of the uterine cervix: A clinicopathologic and immunohistochemical study of an aggressive neoplasm in a young female. Med Pediatr Oncol 18:72, 1990

212. Gordon AH, Montag TW: Sarcoma botryoides of the cervix: excision followed by adjuvant chemotherapy for preservation of reproductive function. Gynecol Oncol 36:119, 1990

213. Di Sant' Agnese PA, Knowles DM II: Extracardiac rhabdomyoma: a clinicopathologic study and review of the literature. Cancer 46:780, 1980

214. Wertheim RA, Krebs H, Frable WJ: Intermediate form of cervical fetal rhabdomyoma? A case report. Diagn Gynecol Obstet 4:57, 1982

215. Flint A, Gikas PW, Roberts JA: Alveolar soft part sarcoma of the uterine cervix. Gynecol Oncol 22:263, 1985

216. Gray GF, Glick AD, Kurtin PJ, Jones HW III: Alveolar soft part sarcoma of the uterus. Hum Pathol 17:297, 1986

217. Kopolovic J, Weiss DB, Dolberg L et al: Alveolar soft-part sarcoma of the female genital tract. Case report with ultrastructural findings. Arch Gynecol 240:125, 1987

218. Foschini MP, Ceccarelli C, Eusebi V et al: Alveolar soft part sarcoma: immunological evidence of rhabdomyoblastic differentiation. Histopathology 13:101, 1988

219. Foschini MP, Eusebi V, Tison V: Alveolar soft part sarcoma of the cervix uteri. A case report. Pathol Res Pract 184:354, 1989

220. Abeler V, Nesland JM: Alveolar soft-part sarcoma in the uterine cervix. Arch Pathol Lab Med 113:1179, 1989

221. Sahin AA, Silva EG, Ordonez NG: Alveolar soft part sarcoma of the uterine cervix. Mod Pathol 2:676, 1989

222. Nolan NPM, Gaffney EF: Alveolar soft part sarcoma of the uterus. Histopathology 16:97, 1990

223. Guillon L, Lamoureux E, Masse S, Costa J: Alveolar soft-part sarcoma of the uterine corpus: histological, immunocytochemical

and ultrastructural study of a case. Virchows Arch [A] 418:467, 1991

224. Cho KR, Rosenshein NB, Epstein JI: Malignant rhabdoid tumor of the uterus. Int J Gynecol Pathol 8:381, 1989

225. Fitko R, Brainer J, Schink JC, August CZ: Endometrial stromal sarcoma with rhabdoid differentiation (letter). Int J Gynecol Pathol 9:379, 1990

226. Cattani MG, Viale G, Santini D, Martinelli: GN: Malignant rhabdoid tumour of the uterus: an immunohistochemical and ultrastructural study: Virchows Archiv 420A:459, 1992

227. Cho KR, Epstein JI: Authors' response (letter). Int J Gynecol Pathol 9:381, 1990

228. Salm R: The histogenesis of uterine lipomas. Beitr Pathol Bd 149:284, 1973

229. Dharkar DD, Kraft JR, Gangadharam D: Uterine lipomas. Arch Pathol Lab Med 105:43, 1981

230. Gusdon JP: Hemangioma of the cervix. Four new cases and a review. Am J Obstet Gyencol 91:204, 1965

231. Ahern JK, Allen NH: Cervical hemangioma: a case report and review of the literature. J Reprod Med 21:228, 1978

232. Salm R: Cavernous lymphangioma of the uterus. Am J Obstet Gynecol 80:365, 1960

233. Chestnut DH, Szpak CA, Fortier KJ, Hammond CB: Uterine hemangioma associated with infertility. South Med J 81:926, 1988

234. Bowers VM, King JD: Benign hemangiomyoma of the uterus. Obstet Gynecol 49:38S, 1977

235. Jameson CF: Angiomyoma of the uterus in a patient with tuberous sclerosis. Histopathology 16:202, 1990

236. Fukuoka M, Fujii S, Konishi I et al: Fibro-osteochondroma of the uterus. Obstet Gynecol 70:517, 1987

237. Carney JA, Young WF, Jr: Primary pigmented nodular adrenocortical disease and its associations. Endocrinologist 2:6, 1992

238. Barlow JF, Abu-Gazeleh S, Tam GE et al: Myxoid tumor of the uterus and right atrial myxomas. South Dakota J Med 36:9, 1983

239. Silverberg SG: Reproducibility of the mitosis count in the histologic diagnosis of smooth muscle tumors of the uterus. Hum Pathol 7:451, 1976

240. Scully RE: Mitosis counting I (editorial.) Hum Pathol 7:481, 1976

241. Kempson RL: Mitosis counting. II (editorial). Hum Pathol 7:482, 1976

242. Norris HJ: Mitosis counting. III (editorial). Hum Pathol 7:483, 1976

243. Donhuijsen K: Mitotis counts: reproducibility of significance in grading malignancy. Hum Pathol 17:1122, 1986

244. Baak JPA: Mitosis counting in tumors. (Editorial.) Hum Pathol 21:683, 1990

245. Franzini DA, Silva EG, Maizel A: Variability of mitotic count dependent on fixation time, abstracted. Lab Invest 44:20A, 1981

246. Donhuijsen K, Schmidt U, Hirche H et al: Changes in mitotic rate and cell cycle fractions caused by delayed fixation. Hum Pathol 21:709, 1990

247. Cross SS, Start RD, Smith JHF: Does delay in fixation affect the number of mitotic figures in processed tissue? J Clin Pathol 43:597, 1990

248. Ellis PSJ, Whitehead R: Mitosis counting—a need for reappraisal. Hum Pathol 12:3, 1981

249. Clement PB, Prat J, Young RH: Diagnostic problems in gynecological tumor pathology. Mod Pathol 3:234, 1990.

250. Clement PB: Miscellaneous primary and metastatic tumors of the uterine cervix. Semin Diagn Pathol 7:228, 1990.

7

Tumors With Mixed Epithelial and Mesenchymal Elements

Philip B. Clement and Robert E. Scully

A variety of uterine tumors are characterized by a focal or diffuse admixture of epithelial and mesenchymal elements. Our classification of these tumors is listed in Table 7-1. Endometrial stromal tumors with epithelial elements are discussed in Chapter 6.

MALIGNANT MÜLLERIAN MIXED TUMOR (CARCINOSARCOMA)

CLINICAL FEATURES

Although *carcinosarcoma* is now the recommended term for these tumors in the International Society of Gynecological Pathologists/World Health Organization (ISGP/WHO) classification, the succinct acronym for *malignant müllerian mixed tumor* (MMMT) is used here. In the older literature, the term *carcinosarcoma* has been used as a synonym for all MMMTs by some investigators but only for the homologous form by others. Whatever term is used should be modified by the term *homologous* or *heterologous*, to avoid confusion.

Although MMMTs are the most common form of uterine "sarcoma", they account for only 1 to 2 percent of all uterine cancers in the western world[1-55]; some studies, however, indicate a recent increase in their frequency.[22] Patients with MMMTs are almost exclusively postmenopausal, with a median age at diagnosis ranging from 62 to 68 years.[1-25] Approximately a dozen cases, however, have been reported in females under 40 years of age, including very rare examples in children.[22, 33-38] There appears to be a higher frequency in black patients.[24, 39] Infertility, hypertension, obesity, and diabetes are present in some patients,[1, 3, 4, 6, 7, 11, 14, 18, 22] but the association with these disorders is not as strong as it is with endometrial carcinoma.

In some series of MMMTs, particularly those in the older literature, as many as 37 percent of patients have had a history of pelvic radiation,[1, 4, 5, 7, 9, 11, 14, 15, 22–24, 40, 41] with an estimated average of 10 percent. Similarly, analyses of uterine tumors arising after pelvic radiation have shown a disproportionate number of MMMTs.[40] The mean interval between the radiation and the diagnosis of the tumor was 11, 16, and 24 years in three studies,[23, 40, 41] and the tumors have usually occurred in slightly younger patients than those without a history of radiation therapy. Occasional MMMTs have arisen in women after prolonged unopposed endogenous or exogenous estrogen exposure,[34, 35, 36] consistent with the presence of estrogen receptors in these neoplasms.[42–44] Patients with MMMTs appear to be at increased risk of a second primary malignant tumor, which was found in one-fourth of patients in two recent studies.[14, 16]

329

Table 7-1. Uterine Tumors With Mixed Epithelial and Mesenchymal Elements

Malignant müllerian mixed tumors (carcinosarcomas), homologous and heterologous
Müllerian adenofibroma
Müllerian adenosarcoma
Müllerian carcinofibroma and carcinomesenchymoma
Endometrial stromal tumors with focal epithelial differentiation
Uterine tumors resembling ovarian sex-cord tumors
Adenomyoma, including atypical polypoid adenomyoma

The most common symptom is abnormal vaginal bleeding; pelvic or abdominal pain is also frequent. As many as 50 percent of patients have clinical evidence of extrauterine disease at presentation (clinical stage III to IV)[14, 17, 18]; such patients may have clinical manifestations related to gastrointestinal or urinary tract involvement.[4, 5] In occasional patients, the tumor is discovered because of an abnormal Papanicolaou smear.[1] Pelvic examination usually discloses an enlarged and irregular uterus or an abdominal mass. In about one-half of cases, tumor protrudes through the external os. MMMTs that have extended beyond the uterus at the time of diagnosis may be associated with palpable parametrial or adnexal involvement.[4, 5] The diagnosis can frequently be made prior to hysterectomy by a dilatation and curettage (D&C), although in some curettage specimens only one neoplastic component is found[45] and the diagnosis is not made until the hysterectomy specimen has been examined. There should be a high index of suspicion for the diagnosis in a postmenopausal woman with a polypoid uterine mass in whom a D&C shows an anaplastic tumor. The majority of patients in one study had elevated serum levels of CA-125 at the time of presentation[46]; determinations of this antigen may be useful in monitoring the effects of therapy in these patients. Unique presentations of MMMTs have included an association with a viable gestation,[47] uterine rupture and hemoperitoneum,[48] hyper- catecholaminemia,[49] and elevated serum levels of alpha-fetoprotein (AFP).[50]

GROSS APPEARANCE

MMMTs are usually large, soft, broad-based, polypoid tumors that often fill the endometrial cavity (Fig. 7-1), frequently protruding through the external os. Rare tumors appear to be multicentric, with two or more separate exophytic masses.[6, 18] The surface of the tumor is characteristically smooth, in contrast to the more rough and irregular surface of a typical endometrial carcinoma. The cut surface is usually fleshy, often with areas of hemorrhage, necrosis, and cystic degeneration. Gritty or hard areas may be produced by the presence of bone or cartilage; the latter may have a translucent appearance. Myometrial invasion is usually evident. The cervix may be involved secondarily by downgrowth of tumor, and rare MMMTs are primary in the endocervix.[5, 6, 9, 28, 38, 45, 51–54]

MICROSCOPIC APPEARANCE

Microscopic examination characteristically reveals an intimate admixture of malignant epithelial (carcinomatous) and malignant mesenchymal (sarcomatous) components (Figs. 7-2 to 7-6), although in areas of an individual tumor, only one component may be present. Most MMMTs contain poorly differentiated epithelial and mesenchymal components, but a rare example is composed of well-differentiated carcinoma and well-differentiated sarcoma (Fig. 7-6). In such a case, a special notation attesting to the unusually high degree of differentiation should be provided.

The carcinoma in more than 90 percent of cases is an adenocarcinoma, typically high grade, that is usually endometrioid or serous (Fig. 7-2) and less often clear cell (Fig. 7-5), mucinous or nonspecific in appear-

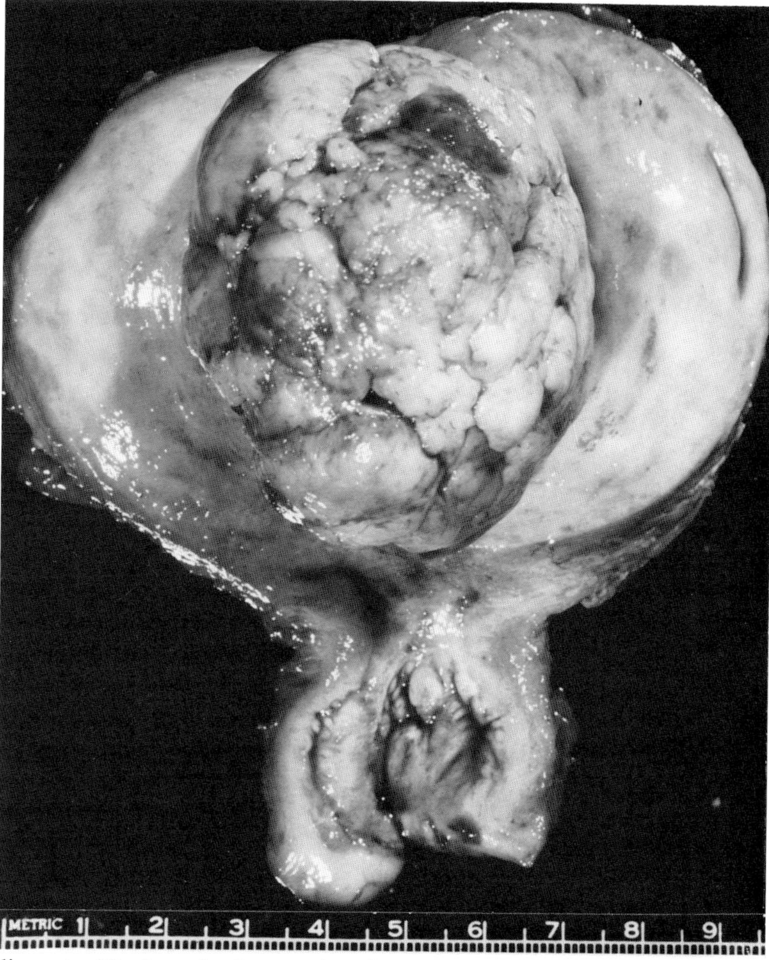

Fig. 7-1. Malignant müllerian mixed tumor (carcinosarcoma). A polypoid mass fills the endometrial cavity.

ance (Fig. 7-3), alone or in combination. In occasional MMMTs, rare glands may lack frankly malignant features, exhibiting a benign or dysplastic appearance. Squamous cell carcinoma alone is found in approximately 5 percent of cases, but more frequently it is admixed with an adenocarcinomatous component.[55] It has been suggested that MMMTs with squamous elements more commonly arise within the cervix.[51, 55] One MMMT contained foci of small cell neuroendocrine carcinoma,[56] and as noted below, a recent immunohistochemical study has found neuroendocrine

differentiation in 17 percent of otherwise typical MMMTs.[32]

The sarcomatous component of MMMTs may be homologous or heterologous. Homologous sarcoma typically has the appearance of a spindle cell sarcoma (Figs. 7-2 and 7-3), resembling high-grade endometrial stromal sarcoma, leiomyosarcoma, fibrosarcoma, malignant fibrous histiocytoma, undifferentiated sarcoma, or any combination thereof. Bizarre cells with eosinophilic cytoplasm but no cross-striations may be present, but they should not be considered rhabdomyoblasts on the basis of light mi-

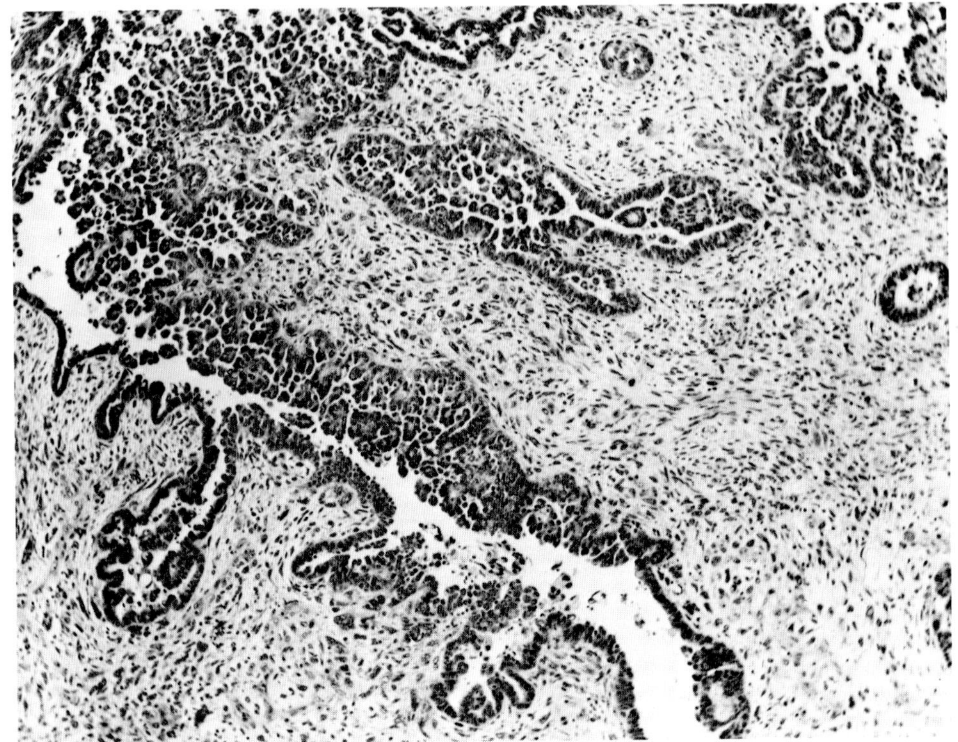

Fig. 7-2. Malignant müllerian mixed tumor (homologous) in which most of the carcinomatous component is papillary serous carcinoma.

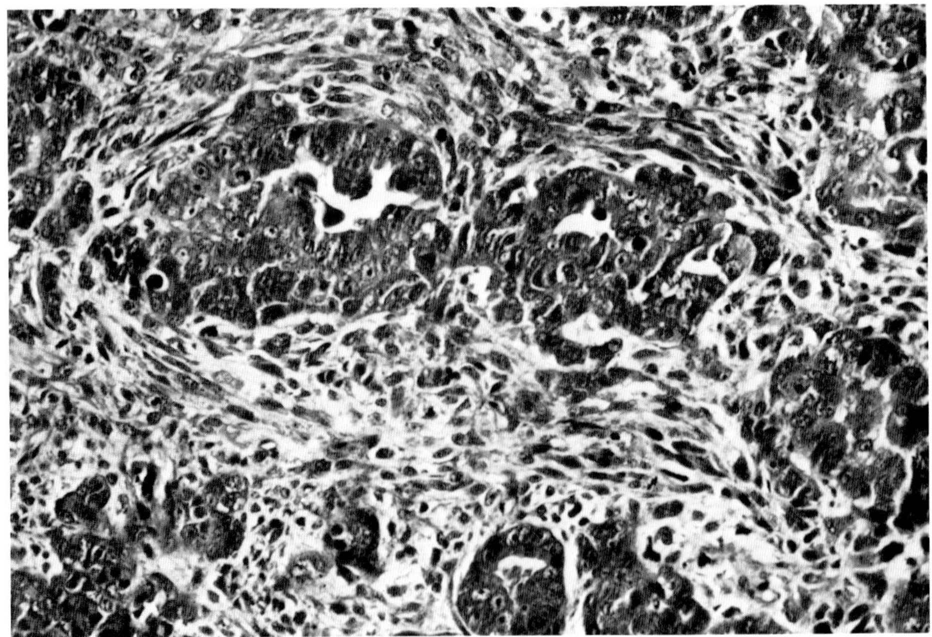

Fig. 7-3. Malignant müllerian mixed tumor, homologous. Poorly differentiated glands are surrounded by a high-grade spindle cell sarcoma.

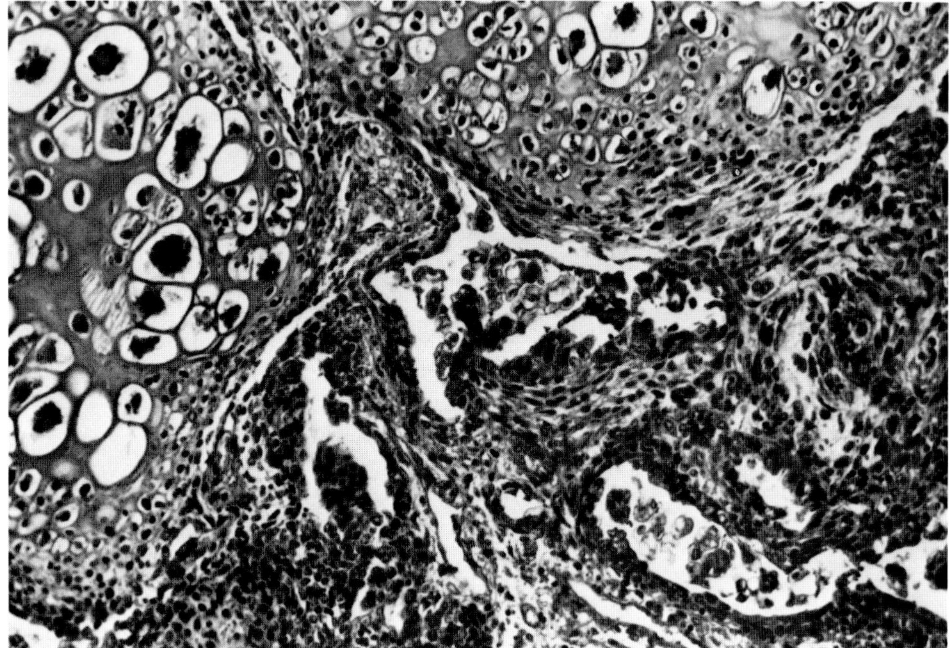

Fig. 7-4. Malignant müllerian mixed tumor, heterologous, composed of an admixture of adenocarcinoma and chondrosarcoma.

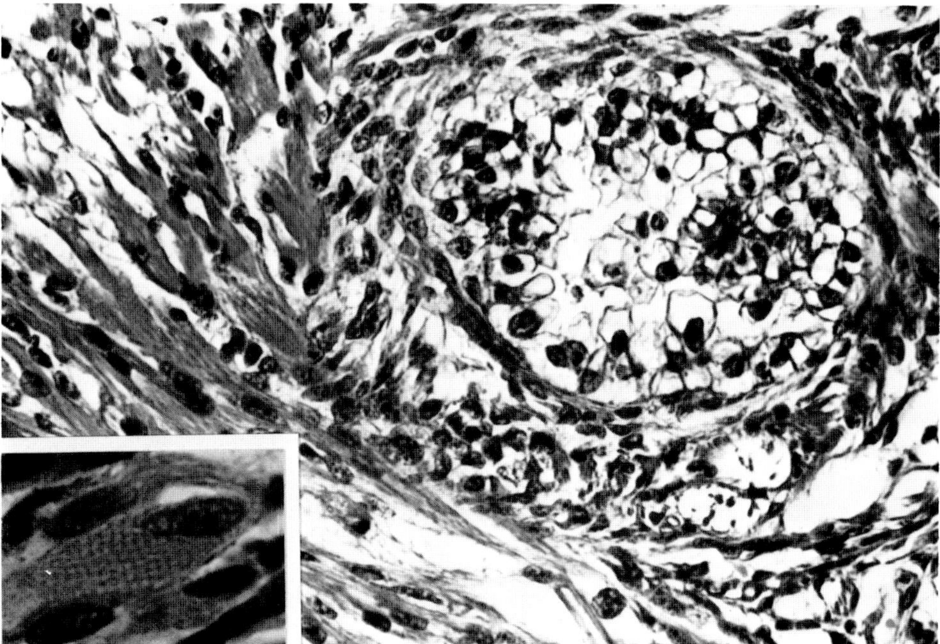

Fig. 7-5. Malignant müllerian mixed tumor, heterologous, composed of an admixture of clear cell carcinoma and strap-shaped sarcomatous cells with fibrillar cytoplasm that was eosinophilic. Cross-striations were identified within some of the stromal cells (inset), confirming rhabdomyoblastic differentiation.

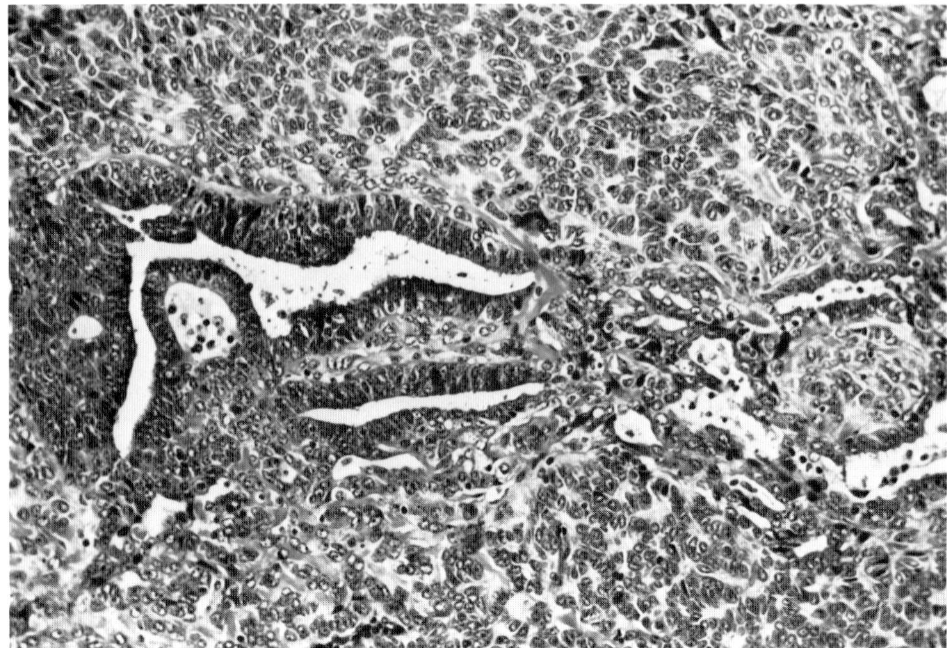

Fig. 7-6. Low-grade malignant müllerian mixed tumor. The tumor is composed of a low-grade endometrioid adenocarcinoma admixed with a low-grade sarcoma resembling endometrial stromal sarcoma.

croscopic examination of routinely stained sections alone. Edematous or myxoid areas are common. In the heterologous tumors, the heterologous foci typically merge with and appear to be derived from undifferentiated homologous sarcoma. Heterologous tumors contain one or more of the following elements, in descending order of frequency: rhabdomyoblasts (Fig. 7-5); mature-appearing cartilage or chondrosarcoma (Fig. 7-4); osteoid, bone, or osteosarcoma; and liposarcoma.

Homologous and heterologous MMMTs have occurred with approximately equal frequency in most studies. Heterologous tumors, have predominated, however, in some series of postradiation MMMTs,[41] as well as in other series in which an assiduous seach for heterologous elements has been performed.[12] It has been suggested that because these elements are often sparsely and irregularly distributed, heterologous tumors are probably underdiagnosed and truly homologous tumors may be rare.[12]

Eosinophilic hyaline droplets are commonly present in both uterine and ovarian MMMTs[57, 58] (Fig. 7-7). Dictor[58] has described the features of these droplets in detail based on their presence in 21 of 22 ovarian MMMTs. They are 1 to 50 μm in diameter and are usually arranged in grape-like clusters within the perinuclear cytoplasm; extracellular droplets, however, are also commonly present.[58] The droplets stain consistently with periodic acid-Schiff (PAS) after diastase digestion and are light blue to deep purple with phosphotungstic acid staining. In some tumors, they may be inconspicuous, whereas in others large numbers of closely packed droplets may be a striking finding. The droplets are most commonly within mesenchymal cells in edematous or myxomatous areas, but in approximately one-half of Dictor's cases,

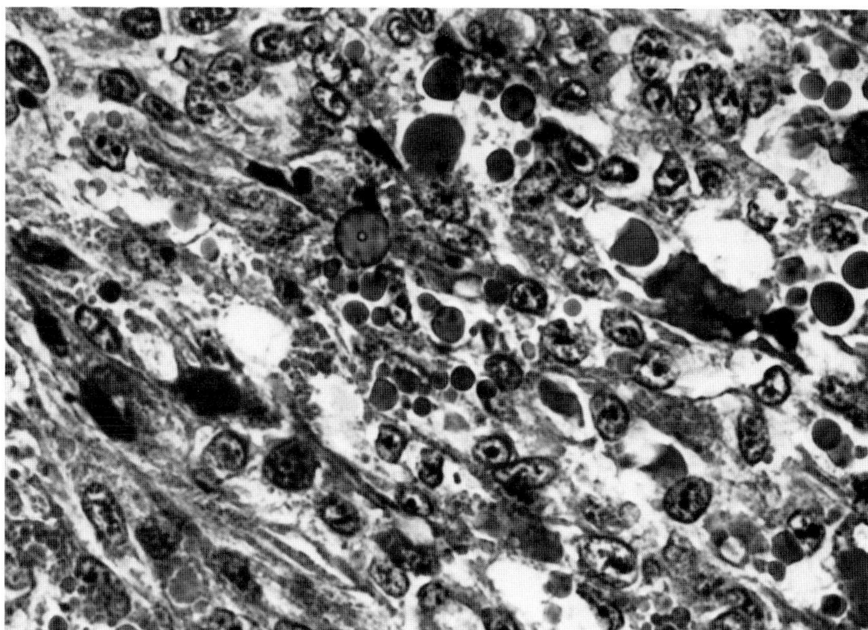

Fig. 7-7. Malignant müllerian mixed tumor. Numerous hyaline bodies are present within the sarcomatous component of the tumor.

they were also within carcinoma cells. On ultrastructural examination, they consist of granular material of medium electron density.[57]

The rarest type of differentiation in MMMTs is neural. Young et al. described an MMMT with focal glial differentiation[59] and found another possible example of such an occurrence in the older literature.[60] More recently, Gersell et al.[61] have reported an MMMT with extensive differentiation into glial and neuronal elements.

Eighty percent of MMMTs invade beyond the inner third of the myometrium, and 40 percent extend into the outer third.[62] Myometrial lymphatic and vascular invasion is present in almost all the cases. Rare MMMTs may be confined to an otherwise typical endometrial polyp.[22, 30, 63–65] The uninvolved endometrium may be the site of an atypical endometrial hyperplasia or contain pure endometrial carcinoma in as many as one-half of the cases.[3]

The histology of metastatic tumor has been specifically documented in several recent large studies, with conflicting results. In one study,[27] metastases in all cases consisted exclusively of carcinoma; in the second,[30] metastases in 75 percent of cases were purely carcinomatous, 15 percent were carcinosarcomatous, and 10 percent were purely sarcomatous; in the third study,[32] 62 percent of metastases were carcinosarcomatous, 18 percent purely carcinomatous, and 20 percent purely sarcomatous.

Immunohistochemical Findings

Recent immunohistochemical studies of MMMTs[66–77] have revealed simultaneous expression of epithelial markers (cytokeratin, EMA) and vimentin in both the epithelial and stromal components of MMMTs,[27, 30, 31, 69, 76, 77] indicating an overlap with the immunoprofile of endometrial adenocarcinomas.[77] Nonetheless, these markers may be useful in accentuating the biphasic pattern of MMMTs, inasmuch as the immunoreactivity for the epithelial markers and vimentin is more diffuse and intense in the carcinomatous and sarcomatous components, respectively[32] (Fig. 7-8). Immunoreactivity for a variety of muscle markers, including actin, desmin, myosin, and myoglobin, is almost invariably confined to the sarcomatous cells; cells with nonspecific features and rhabdomyoblasts (Fig. 7-9) may be immunoreactive with these markers.[27, 31, 32, 67] Myoglobin appears to be the most specific but least sensitive marker for rhabdomyoblasts.[32] Both the epithelial and stromal components are frequently immunoreactive for α_1-antitrypsin (AAT) and α_1-antichymotrypsin.[67]

Immunohistochemical stains may also be useful in unmasking neuroendocrine differentiation within MMMTs. In one study,[32] one-sixth of otherwise typical MMMTs showed evidence of such differentiation, as manifested by reactivity for chromogranin (CG), Leu-7, neuron-specific enolase (NSE), and synaptophysin (SP), alone or in combination; isolated staining for NSE or Leu-7 in the absence of other neuroendocrine markers was not considered diagnostic of neuroendocrine differentiation. In the same study, reactivity for CG, Leu-7, and SP was usually multifocal and confined to poorly differentiated, solid, carcinomatous areas.[32] A small cell carcinomatous component within one MMMT (p. 331) stained positively with the Grimelius method and for NSE.[56] The neuroectodermal differentiation in an MMMT noted above was reflected by immunoreactivity for glial fibrillary acidic protein (GFAP), S-100, and NSE.[61] Within this context, it is noteworthy that expression of GFAP has been demonstrated within otherwise nonspecific neoplastic spindle cells in 9 of 13 MMMTs in one study.[73, 74]

Hyaline droplets have been shown to be

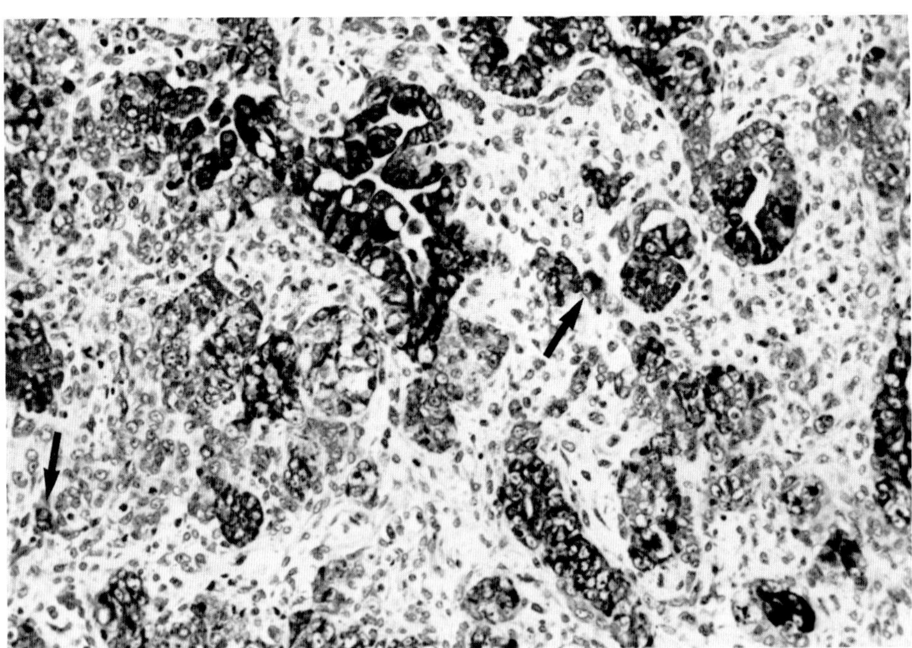

Fig. 7-8. Malignant müllerian mixed tumor, immunohistochemical stain for cytokeratin. Most of the immunoreactivity is within the adenocarcinomatous component. Occasional stromal cells, however, are also immunoreactive (arrows).

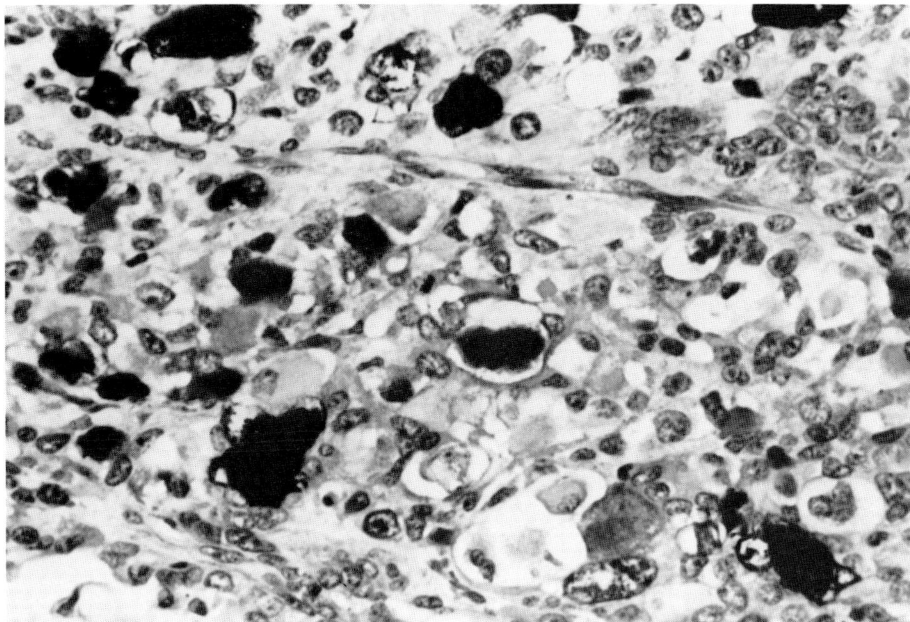

Fig. 7-9. Malignant müllerian mixed tumor, immunohistochemical stain for myoglobin. Polygonal cells with abundant eosinophilic cytoplasm suspicious for rhabdomyoblasts with routine stains (but that lacked obvious cross-striations) are focally immunoreactive for myoglobin confirming rhabdomyoblastic differentiation.

consistently positive for AAT, although it is unclear whether it is a secretory product of the tumor cells or is derived from the serum.[57, 72] In the case of the AFP-secreting MMMT cited above, the AFP was confined immunohistochemically to the epithelial component.[50] Chondrosarcomatous elements are typically immunoreactive for S-100 protein.

DIFFERENTIAL DIAGNOSIS

In a tumor that is an otherwise typical endometrial carcinoma, a question of MMMT may be raised by the presence of foci exhibiting possible sarcomatous differentiation. Similarly, as previously noted (see Ch. 5), the squamous elements in some endometrial carcinomas may be composed of malignant spindle cells potentially mimicking the sarcomatous component of a MMMT. Features that favor sarcoma (versus sarcomatoid carcinoma) in such cases include sharp demarcation from the obvious epithelial component, a dense pattern of reticulin fibers, the presence of heterologous elements, strong and diffuse vimentin immunoreactivity, and immunoreactivity for one or more of the muscle antigens noted above. Ultrastructural studies may also be useful in confirming sarcomatous differentiation.

Evans has designated endometrial sarcomas composed exclusively of highly mitotic, pleomorphic, polygonal, and spindle-shaped cells as *poorly differentiated endometrial sarcomas;* differentiation into tissue resembling endometrial stroma or into heterologous elements was absent in his cases.[78] The close resemblance of these neoplasms to the homologous sarcomatous component of MMMTs, in addition to their highly malignant behavior, suggests that they may be monophasic variants of homologous MMMTs, or MMMTs with sarcomatous overgrowth of the epithelial elements. The rare uterine tumors that resemble malignant fibrous histiocytomas may be in the same category[79–81] (see Ch. 6).

Benign heterologous mesenchymal elements are encountered rarely within otherwise typical endometrial adenocarcinomas[82] (see Ch. 5), within uterine leiomyomas (see Ch. 6), or in the absence of a neoplasm (see Ch. 4), and their presence should therefore not be considered diagnostic of an MMMT. Malignant heterologous mesenchymal elements can be found in the uterus in the absence of an epithelial element in cases of pure heterologous sarcomas (see Ch. 6), although the latter diagnosis should be rendered only after thorough sampling of the tumor has excluded a carcinomatous component. The differential diagnosis of MMMTs with neuroectodermal differentiation includes rare cases of primary endometrial glioma and primitive neuroectodermal tumor (see Ch. 8).

BEHAVIOR AND PROGNOSTIC FACTORS

MMMTs are highly malignant. Five-year survival rates from most studies in the last two decades have ranged between 15 and 40 percent (all stages).[1–29] The corresponding survival rate for patients with surgical stage I and II disease has ranged from 40 to 60 percent.[13, 24, 25, 30, 83] Median survival times have ranged from 7 months to 1.8 years.[2–5, 7]

The most important prognostic factor is the extent of tumor at the time of treatment. Most survivors have tumors confined to the endometrium and inner myometrium.[8, 11, 12, 16, 17, 22, 27, 30, 84] Tumors confined to an endometrial polyp are associated with a relatively favorable prognosis,[22, 30] and in one study, pedunculated MMMTs had a significantly better prognosis than those that were sessile.[29]

The much poorer survival associated with deeper invasion is related to the high frequency of lymphatic and hematogenous involvement. DiSaia et al. found pelvic and paraaortic lymph node metastases in 36 percent and 14 percent, respectively, of clinical stage I cases, but metastases occurred only in patients with neoplasms invading the outer half of the myometrium.[62] Similar figures were obtained in another study.[24] In a recent large series, lymph node metastases were also associated with invasion of the cervix or lower uterine segment.[30] Tumor size, histologic grading, mitotic activity, and the presence or absence of heterologous elements have not been consistently useful in determining the prognosis of patients with MMMTs. Vascular or lymphatic invasion has been an adverse prognostic indicator in some studies,[18, 24, 29–31] but not in others.[7, 22, 23, 25, 27] Two groups of investigators have recently found that a component of papillary serous carcinoma[23, 30] or clear cell carcinoma[30] was an adverse prognostic indicator.

A number of studies have shown that as many as 50 percent of clinical stage I tumors are associated with extrauterine spread at operation,[4, 15, 18, 24, 26] indicating that clinical staging in these patients is a poor discriminator of outcome and is misleading as a guideline for therapy.[15, 18] The presence of malignant cells in peritoneal washings at the time of hysterectomy is an adverse prognostic sign, even in patients with pathologic stage I disease.[85, 86]

Ninety percent of recurrences occur within 2 years.[83] Most patients die as a result of complications of tumor growth within the pelvis and abdomen, although most of such patients also have hematogenous spread, most commonly to the lungs, liver, bone, and brain.[1–7, 14, 15, 87–89]

MANAGEMENT

Patients with clinical stage I and II disease should undergo a staging laparotomy; if no extrauterine disease is found, a total abdominal hysterectomy with bilateral salpingo-oophorectomy is indicated.[15, 17, 87] Adjuvant preoperative or postoperative radiation has decreased the frequency of pelvic recurrence in some studies but has not increased survival.[2, 17, 19, 88, 90, 91] Several recent studies have indicated that combination chemotherapy may be effective for patients with tumor confined to the uterus and may prolong survival in patients with more advanced disease.[11, 91–94]

<h3 align="center">HISTOGENESIS</h3>

Traditionally, it has been hypothesized that MMMTs are derived from multipotential mullerian cells (possibly endometrial stromal cells) that are capable of simultaneous carcinomatous and sarcomatous differentiation. The presence of identical immunohistochemical markers in both components of MMMTs lends credence to this theory.[32] The same observations, however, have led some investigators to conclude that at least some, or possibly all, MMMTs are metaplastic carcinomas.[27, 30, 77] Other observations used to support this hypothesis include the frequent association of MMMTs with otherwise typical endometrial adenocarcinomas in the same hysterectomy specimen[3]; the finding that occasional, apparently pure, endometrial adenocarcinomas recur or metastasize as MMMT[95, 96]; a metastatic pattern of MMMTs similar to that of endometrial adenocarcinomas and dissimilar to other uterine sarcomas[27, 30]; and the observation that recurrent or metastatic tumor in patients with MMMT is often purely carcinomatous (p. 335).[27, 30] These observations notwithstanding, MMMTs have distinctive clinical and pathological features which warrant their separate classification. These highly aggressive tumors are fatal in the vast majority of patients, with a prognosis significantly worse than that of poorly differentiated endometrial adenocarcinomas or any prognostically unfavorable subtype

thereof.[97] Unlike metaplastic carcinomas in other sites, there is usually no merging of the two components of MMMTs at either the histologic or ultrastructural level,[69] and heterologous mesenchymal elements are common.

MÜLLERIAN ADENOFIBROMA AND ADENOSARCOMA

Because müllerian adenofibromas (papillary adenofibroma, cystadenofibroma) and adenosarcomas share many clinical and pathologic features, they will be considered together. They are much less common than MMMTs, although approximately 275 such tumors have been reported in the literature.[98–159] The term *adenofibroma*, or a variation thereof, has been applied to approximately 10 percent of these tumors, with the term *adenosarcoma* assigned to most of the remainder. In some studies, however, the two tumors have been referred to collectively as *"benign and low-grade variants of mixed mullerian tumors"*[119] or as uterine *"cystosarcoma phyllodes,"*[120] terms that reflect uncertainty regarding prognostic factors in patients with these tumors.

<h3 align="center">CLINICAL FEATURES</h3>

The tumors usually occur in postmenopausal women; the median age of patients with adenosarcoma in the largest series was 58 years.[151] In contrast to MMMTs, however, approximately 30 percent of adenosarcomas are found in patients under 50 years of age, and 11 cases have occurred in the second decade. The occasional association of adenosarcomas with hyperestrinism (exogenous estrogen, ovarian thecoma, Stein-Leventhal syndrome)[35, 151] or prior pelvic radiation[151] suggests their possible etiologic role in some cases. Tamoxifen therapy may have played a role in the development of an adenosarcoma from an adenomyoma in one recently described

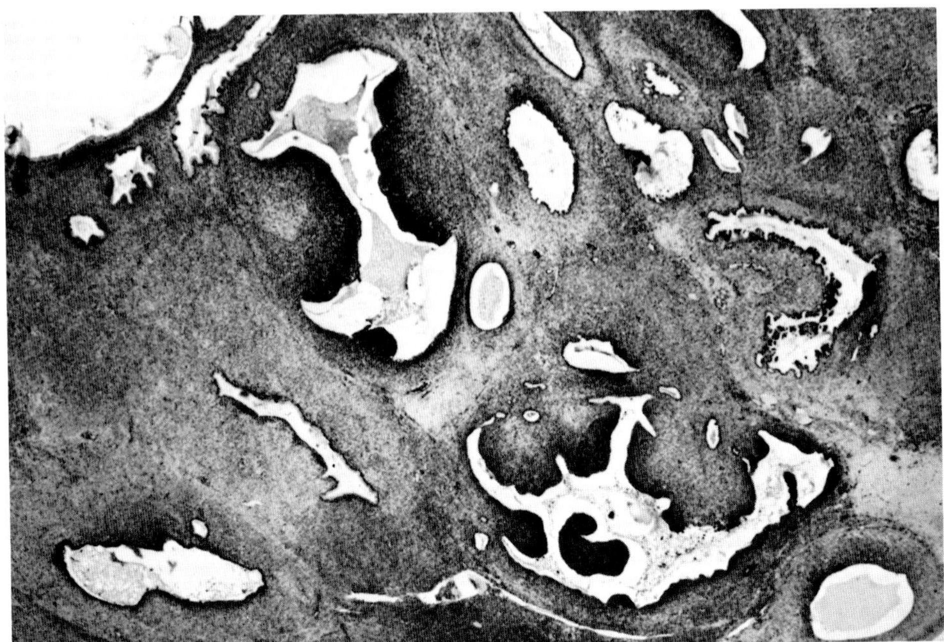

Fig. 7-11. Müllerian adenosarcoma. The sarcomatous stroma is condensed around the glands, many of which are cystic. The stroma forms intraglandular polypoid projections.

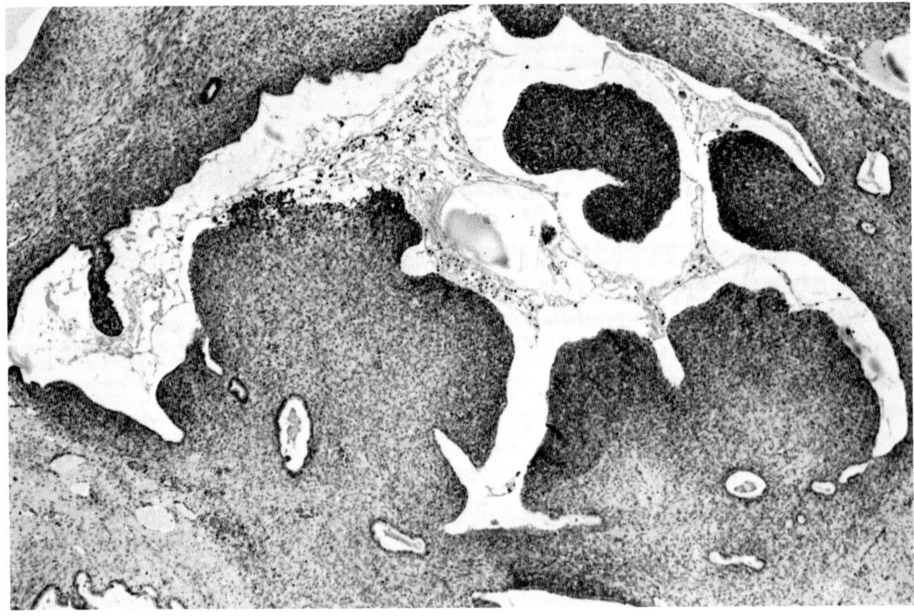

Fig. 7-12. Müllerian adenosarcoma, higher-power view of Figure 7-11.

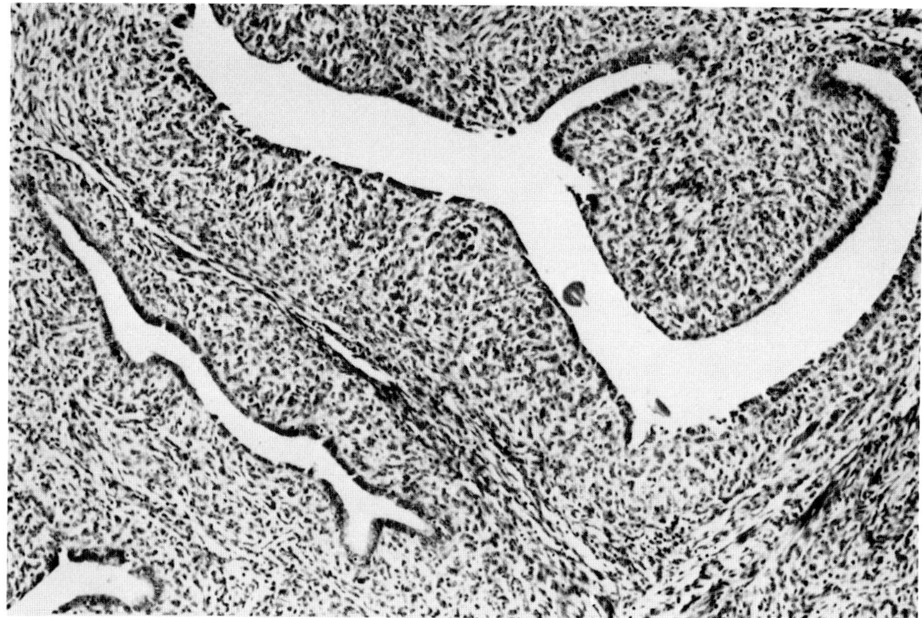

Fig. 7-13. Müllerian adenosarcoma. Slit-shaped endometrioid glands with a benign appearance are surrounded by a sarcoma resembling low-grade endometrial stromal sarcoma.

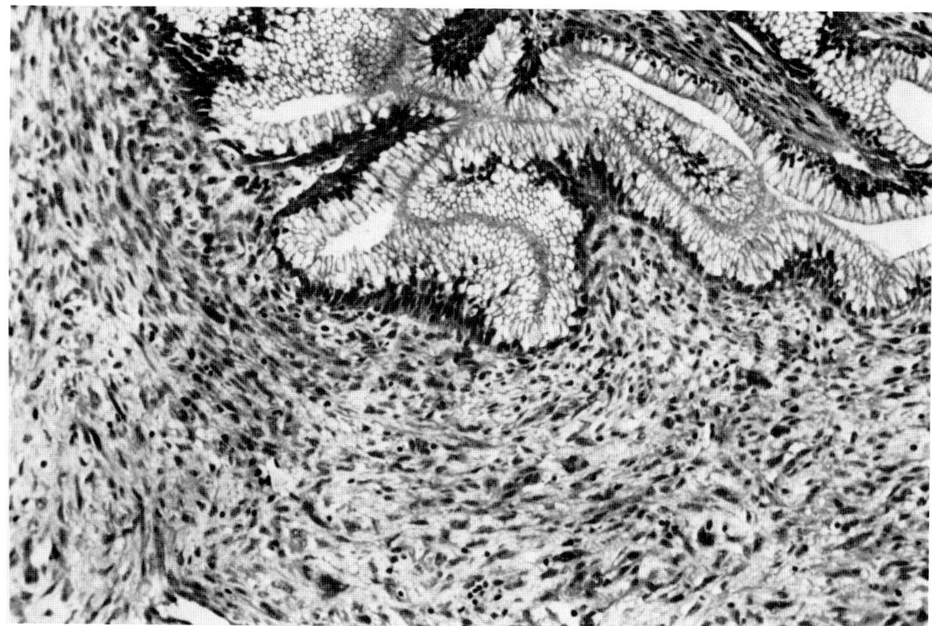

Fig. 7-14. Müllerian adenosarcoma. Benign-appearing mucinous glands are surrounded by a fibro-sarcomatous stroma.

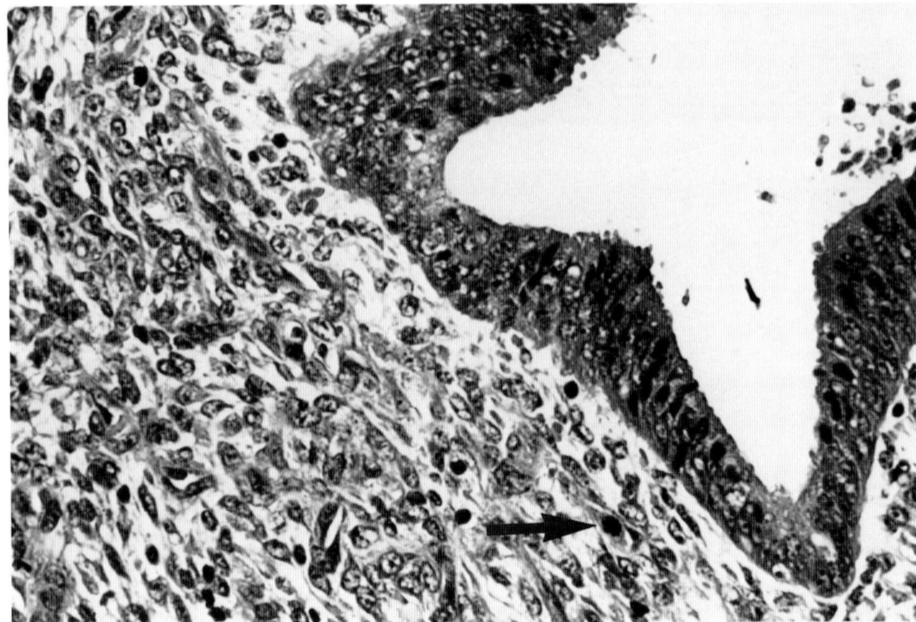

Fig. 7-15. Müllerian adenosarcoma. Atypical endometrioid gland is surrounded by a sarcomatous component resembling low-grade endometrial stromal sarcoma. Note mitotic figures in sarcomatous cells (arrow).

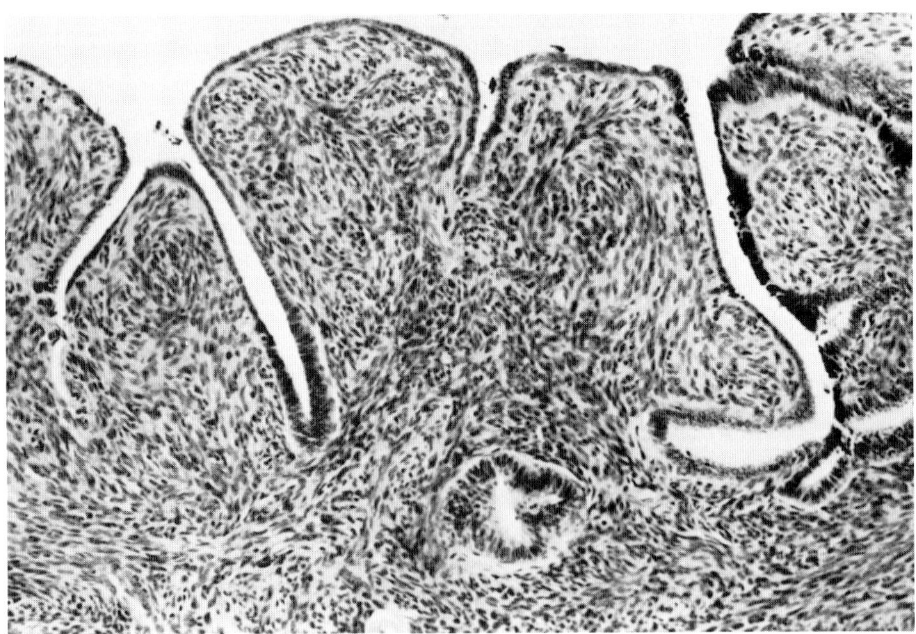

Fig. 7-16. Müllerian adenofibroma. Benign endometrioid epithelium lines stromal papillae (that were on the surface of the tumor) and occasional glands. The stroma is composed of benign fibroblasts devoid of mitotic activity (see Fig. 7-17).

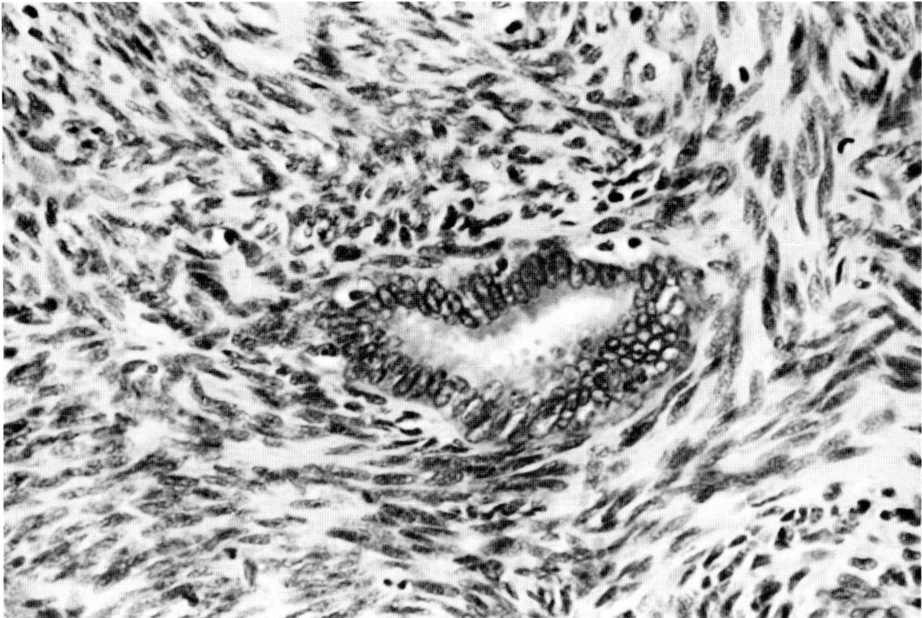

Fig. 7-17. Müllerian adenofibroma, higher-power view of tumor illustrated in Figure 7-16.

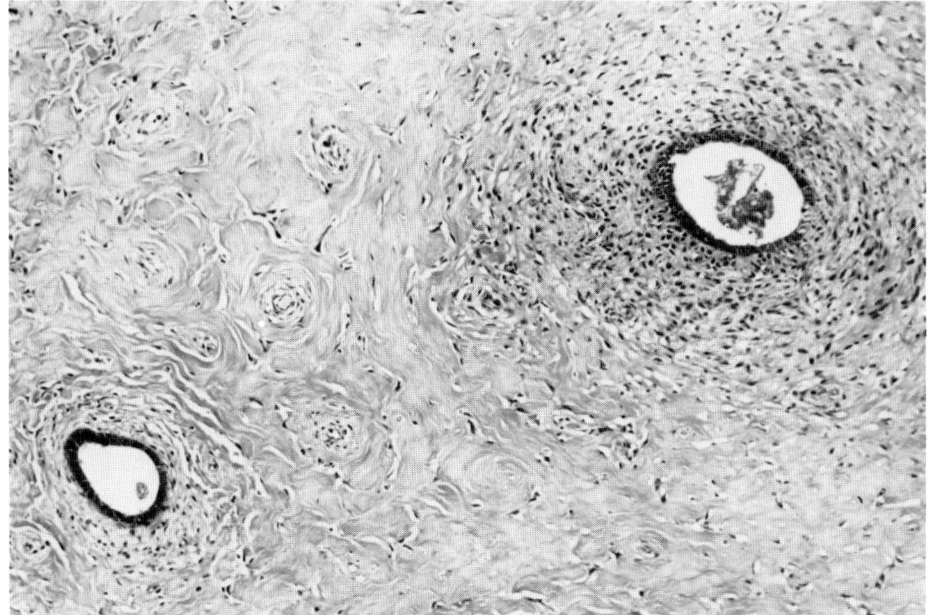

Fig. 7-18. Müllerian adenosarcoma with extensive hyalinization of stroma. The appearance in this field potentially mimics that of a benign endometrial polyp; stromal condensation, however, is still apparent around one of the glands. The stroma was more overtly sarcomatous in other areas. (From Clement and Scully,[151] with permission.)

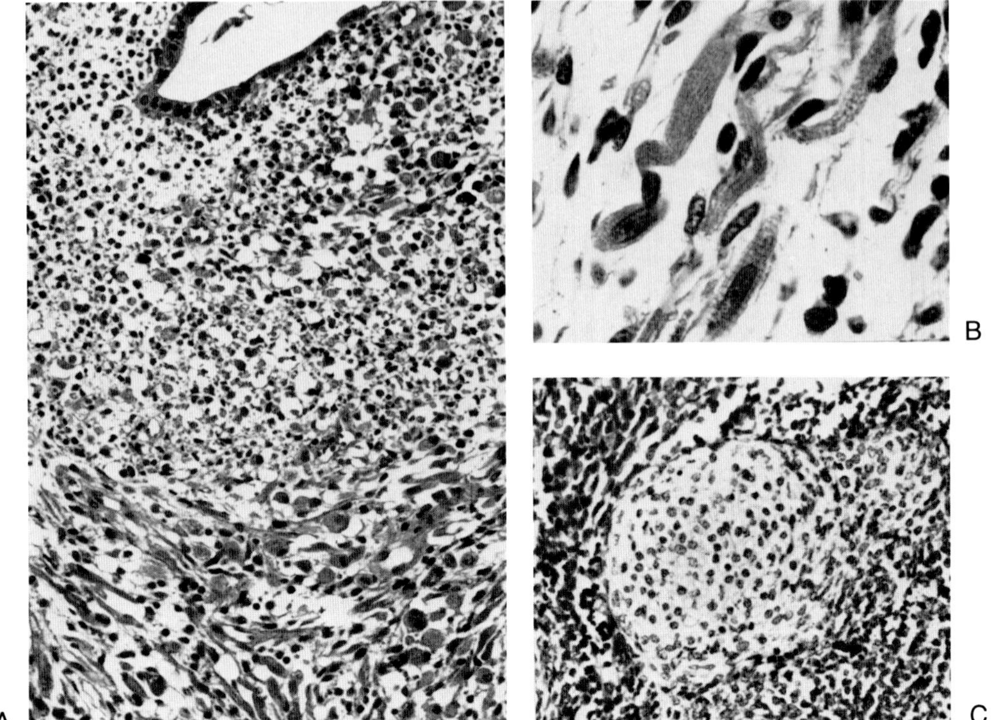

Fig. 7-19. Müllerian adenosarcoma with heterologous elements. The sarcomatous stroma is predominantly embryonal rhabdomyosarcoma **(A)**. Some of the rhabdomyoblasts exhibit cytoplasmic cross-striations **(B)**. The stroma also contains occasional nodules of fetal-type cartilage **(C)**. (From Clement and Scully,[151] with permission.)

dometrial stromal sarcoma (Figs. 7-13 and 7-15), fibrosarcoma (Fig. 7-14), or combinations thereof.[151] Minor foci of smooth muscle differentiation of typical or epithelioid type have been encountered in occasional cases.[125, 151] In one recently reported case, the stromal component of an adenosarcoma consisted exclusively of angiosarcoma.[155] The stromal cells exhibit nuclear atypia that is usually mild or moderate (Figs. 7-13 and 7-15), but occasionally marked (Fig. 7-14). Stromal mitotic figures (MF) are an almost constant finding (Fig. 7-15), and more than 80 percent of tumors exhibit a mitotic rate of 4 or more MF per 10 high-power fields (HPF).[151] The mitotic rates are highly variable from one tumor to another, however, with a range of 1 to 40 MF/10 HPF (mean 9) in the largest series in

the literature.[151] Characteristically, the stroma is more cellular around the glands, creating a cufflike appearance, and intraluminal polypoid or papillary stromal projections are common (Figs. 7-11 and 7-12). The stroma at a distance from the glands is often less cellular; in some tumors, the stroma is composed predominantly of sparsely cellular, myxoid, or hyalinized fibrous tissue, imparting a deceptively benign appearance to large areas of the tumor (Fig. 7-18). Approximately 20 percent of adenosarcomas contain heterologous elements, which have varied from minor foci of fat, cartilage, or rhabdomyoblasts to embryonal rhabdomyosarcoma occupying most or all of the stroma.[151, 157] Some of the cases with the latter type of stroma have also contained nodules of fetal-type carti-

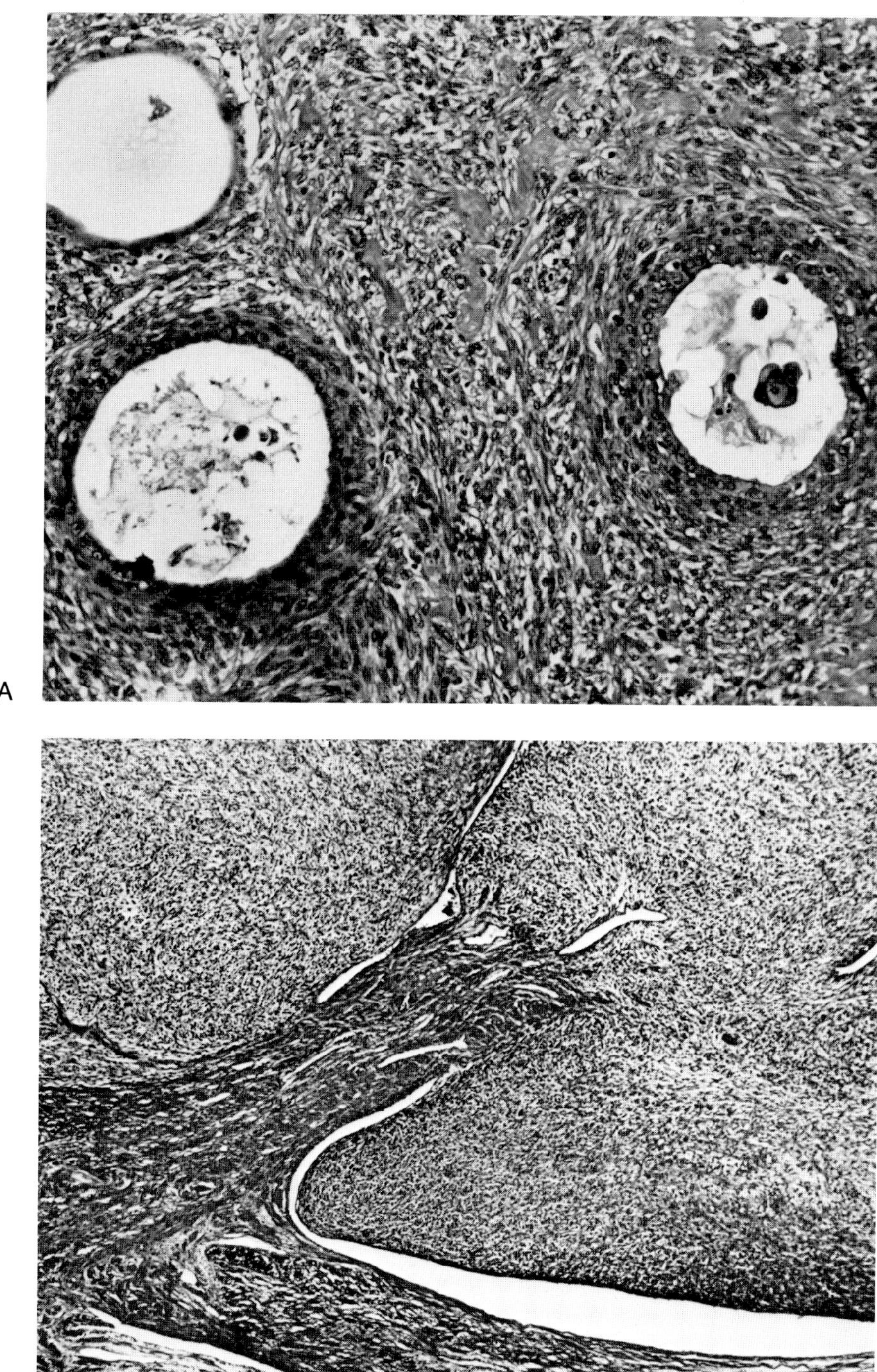

Fig. 7-20. Müllerian adenosarcoma with sarcomatous overgrowth. **(A)** The superficial part of the tumor consists of typical adenosarcoma composed of benign-appearing glands and a sarcomatous stromal component resembling low-grade endometrial stromal sarcoma (mitotic rate, 6 MF/10 HPF). **(B)** Deeper aspect of the same tumor consists of pure endometrial stromal sarcoma that had greater degrees of nuclear pleomorphism and a higher mitotic rate (35 MF/10 HPF) than the sarcomatous component of the typical adenosarcoma.

lage[151] (Fig. 7-19) similar to those occurring in some cases of embryonal rhabdomyosarcoma of the vagina and cervix. One adenosarcoma contained stromal elements suggestive of neuroepithelial differentiation.[110]

Adenofibromas are usually noninvasive, but three examples have invaded the endocervical wall or the myometrium; in one of them, myometrial vessels were invaded as well.[119, 152] Approximately one-sixth of adenosarcomas invade the myometrium, although in only 20 percent of such cases does the invasion extend beyond the inner one-half of the myometrium.[151] The invasive borders are usually well circumscribed, but occasional tumors invade in irregular tongues. Rare adenosarcomas invade myometrial vessels in a pattern similar to that of low-grade endometrial stromal sarcoma.[151]

Occasional adenosarcomas are focally overgrown by the stromal component (*müllerian adenosarcoma with sarcomatous overgrowth*) (MASO).[148, 157] In one series of 10 cases, a pure homologous sarcoma, typically of higher grade and with a higher mitotic rate than those of the associated adenosarcoma, focally replaced the tumor[148] (Fig. 7-20). In contrast to typical adenosarcomas, myometrial invasion was present in 6 of the 10 cases, reaching the serosa in 3 of them (Fig. 7-20). Pure sarcoma occupied at least 25 percent of the tumor volume in the reported cases. MASOs accounted for less than 10 percent of adenosarcomas in one series of consultation cases[148, 151] but accounted for 55 percent of adenosarcomas in another series based on a Gynecologic Oncology Group (GOG) study.[157] The MASOs in the GOG study were also associated with a much higher frequency of myometrial (and lymphatic) invasion than in cases of typical adenosarcoma.[157] In contrast to the other series of MASOs,[148] the pure sarcoma in almost 60 percent of MASOs in the GOG

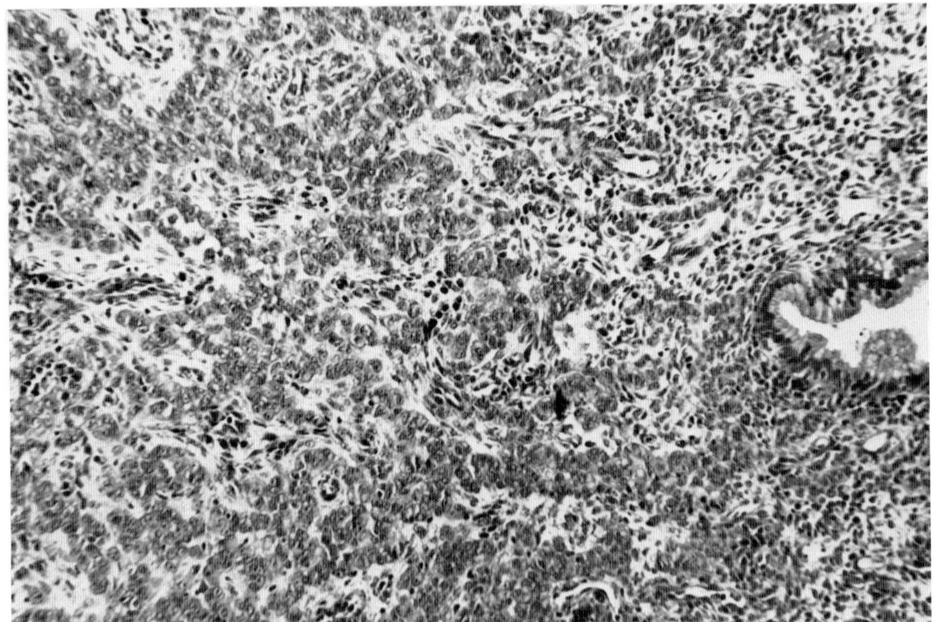

Fig. 7-21. Müllerian adenosarcoma with sex-cord–like elements. A neoplastic gland is present at the extreme right. Most of the stromal component of the tumor is composed of granulosa-like cords in a plexiform arrangement.

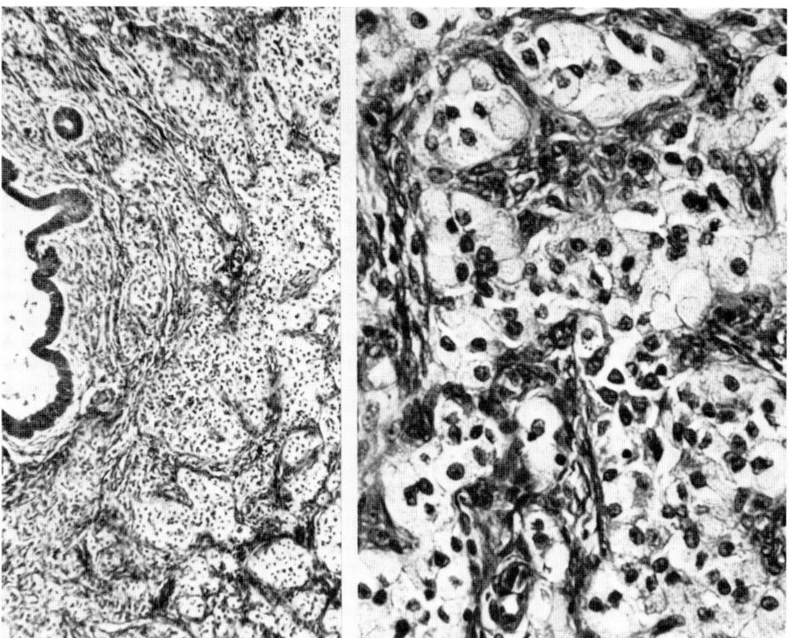

Fig. 7-22. Müllerian adenosarcoma with sex-cord–like elements. **(A)** Neoplastic glands are present at extreme left. The stroma of the tumor consists of irregular nests and trabeculae composed of cells with abundant pale cytoplasm. **(B)** Higher-power view of the stroma shows that the cells have abundant foamy cytoplasm and bland nuclear features.

study consisted of a prominent component of rhabdomyosarcoma.

A second type of stromal proliferation in adenosarcomas was documented in a series of eight adenosarcomas that contained foci of sex-cord–like elements (SCLEs) within their stromal component[149]; two other similar cases have been reported.[141, 156] The SCLEs, which accounted for 5 to 50 percent of the tumors, were composed of benign-appearing cells of epithelial type that were arranged in solid nests, trabeculae, and solid or hollow tubules (Fig. 7-21 and 7-22). The cells often contained abundant eosinophilic or foamy lipid-rich cytoplasm (Fig. 7-22). The SCLEs were similar to those encountered in some endometrial stromal tumors (see Ch. 6) and in the rare uterine tumors resembling ovarian sex cord tumors (see p. 353).

CRITERIA FOR DISTINGUISHING ADENOFIBROMAS AND ADENOSARCOMAS

The histologic dividing line between adenofibromas and adenosarcomas has not been clearly established. Zaloudek and Norris have stated that the stromal mitotic rate is the most reliable criterion in the differential diagnosis.[125] Because all the clinically malignant tumors in their series of cases had stromal mitotic counts of 4 or more MF/10 HPF, they concluded that only tumors with that degree of mitotic activity should be designated adenosarcomas. Four of the 10 clinically malignant adenosarcomas in their series, however, had mitotic rates of only 4 or 5/10 HPF; the difference between such counts and a "benign" count of 3 MF/10 HPF is within interobserver variation. Also, counting mitotic figures in these tumors may be difficult because of variations in cellularity; in some cases, for example, the mitotically active areas are confined to thin rims around the glands. Finally, Zaloudek and Norris reported a 5-year follow-up on only 4 of the 10 tumors they designated as adenofibromas, all of which were treated by hysterectomy. Even a 5-year follow-up is inadequate to evaluate the behavior of these tumors since adenosarcomas often recur betweeen 5 and 10 years postoperatively.

We have encountered in our series,[151] as well as in the literature,[130] a number of tumors with 2 or 3 MF/10 HPF and extrauterine disease at presentation or that recurred after hysterectomy. Thus it appears that almost any measurable degree of stromal mitotic activity in these tumors can be associated with a malignant behavior. We currently diagnose as adenosarcoma tumors with 2 or more MF/10 HPF, a mitotic rate that will detect almost all tumors with a malignant potential. Because rare essentially amitotic tumors with marked stromal cellularity, stromal atypia or both have recurred after hysterectomy, we also consider tumors with these features low-grade adenosarcomas. If these criteria are applied, adenofibromas account for only 5 percent of tumors in the adenofibroma-adenosarcoma group; the former diagnosis is rendered only after the tumor has been extensively sampled to exclude foci exhibiting mitotic activity, marked cellularity, or stromal cell atypia. This evaluation usually requires hysterectomy.

Differential Diagnosis

The differential diagnosis of adenofibroma and adenosarcoma includes benign endometrial polyps as well as other tumors characterized by a mixture of epithelial and mesenchymal elements. In endometrial polyps, the stroma may resemble that of the adjacent endometrium or may be less cellular and often sclerotic. If its stromal component is unusually cellular or mitotically active, if its glandular cells differ in appearance from those of the adjacent endometrium, or if periglandular cuffing or intraglandular stromal papillae are present, the diagnosis of adenosarcoma should be seriously considered. The atypical polypoid adenomyoma (p. 358) has a stromal component that consists predominantly of fascicles of benign, cellular smooth muscle, which may show mitotic activity, and a glandular component that is less cystic and generally more atypical than that of an adenosarcoma and usually contains prominent numbers of squamous morules. Occasional MMMTs have foci in which the glandular component lacks frankly malignant features, but most of the glands are frankly carcinomatous and focally confluent. Endometrial stromal sarcomas typically lack the integral glandular component of the adenosarcoma, although their periphery may contain occasional entrapped glands or, in a minority of cases there may be focal prominent glandular differentiation within the tumor (see Ch. 6). Unlike adenosarcomas, endometrial stromal sarcomas typically have highly infiltrative borders with extensive myometrial and vascular penetration. A final consideration in the differential diagnosis of adenosarcoma is the very rare uterine Wilms' tumor (see Ch. 8).

Behavior

Tumors fulfilling our criteria for adenofibroma are associated with a benign postoperative course, although they may recur after local excision.[119] Similarly, the follow-up was uneventful at the time of reporting in the three cases of invasive adenofibroma referred to above.[119, 152] In contrast to MMMTs, adenosarcomas typically have a low malignant potential, manifested primarily by vaginal (Fig. 7-23) or abdominopelvic

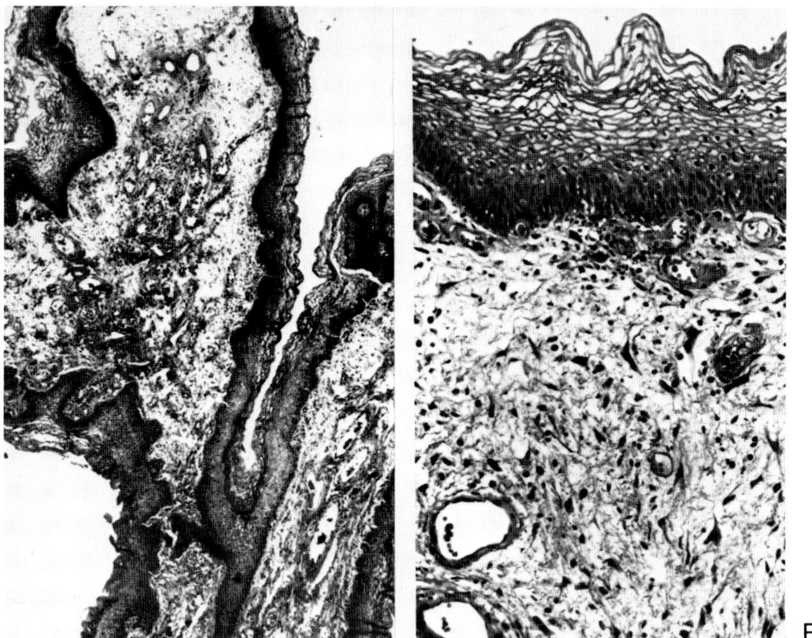

Fig. 7-23. Müllerian adenosarcoma, polypoid vaginal recurrence. The recurrent tumor mimics a fibroepithelial polyp at both low-power **(A)** and high-power **(B)** magnifications. No glandular component was identified. (From Clement and Scully,[151] with permission.)

recurrence (Fig. 7-24) in approximately one-fourth of cases; hematogenous spread occurs in less than 5 percent.[125, 151] Even in the clinically malignant cases, the recurrent tumor has often been indolent. In one-third of cases with recurrences in one large series, the recurrent tumor appeared 5 or more years after hysterectomy, and rare tumors recurred 10 or more years after hysterectomy.[151] Long-term clinical follow-up is therefore essential in these patients. The recurrent tumor has been a pure sarcoma in 70 percent of the cases (Figs. 7-23 and 7-24), an adenosarcoma in almost 30 percent (Fig. 7-24), and a carcinosarcoma in a single case.[151] Rarely recurrent tumor has contained heterologous elements or foci of carcinoma that were not present in the primary tumors.[151] Blood-borne metastases have been pure sarcomas. The mitotic rate and grade of the recurrent tumor may be lower than, similar to, or in one-half of cases, higher than those of the original adenosar-

coma. In some of the cases in which the initial recurrence was an adenosarcoma, subsequent recurrences have been pure sarcomas (Fig. 7-24).

The risk of recurrence in adenosarcomas correlates with the presence of myometrial invasion.[125, 151, 157] In the largest literature series, the risk of recurrence in the absence of invasion was 12.7 percent and the risk in the presence of invasion 46 percent.[151] Although such cases are rare, there is a suggestion that the risk of recurrence may be even higher in tumors with deep myometrial invasion.[125, 151] The only other feature that correlates with an increased risk of recurrence is sarcomatous overgrowth.[148, 157] In the aforementioned study of 10 cases of adenosarcomas with sarcomatous overgrowth, recurrent tumor, hematogenous metastases, and death from tumor occurred in 70 percent, 40 percent, and 60 percent of patients, respectively.[148] Corresponding figures for recurrence and death

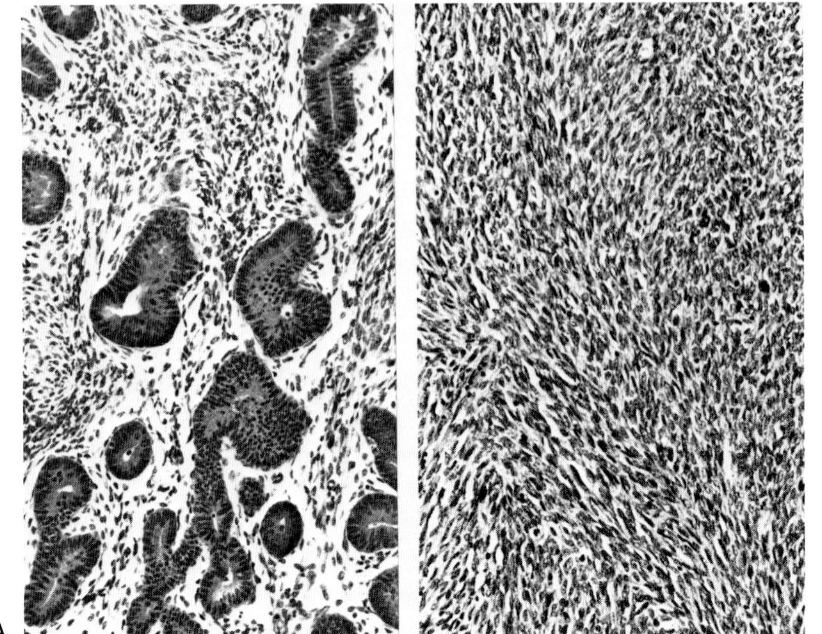

Fig. 7-24. Müllerian adenosarcoma, pelvic recurrence. The first recurrence **(A)**, 6 years after hysterectomy, consists of benign-appearing glands admixed with a low-grade sarcomatous stroma. The second recurrence 1 year later **(B)**, consists exclusively of a high-grade sarcoma. (From Clement and Scully,[151] with permission.)

from tumor in the GOG series of adenosarcomas with sarcomatous overgrowth were 44 percent and 31 percent.[157] Two of 17 tumors with sarcomatous overgrowth in that study were also associated with pelvic lymph node metastases. The areas of sarcomatous overgrowth accounted for at least 25 percent of the tumor volume in these series, but it was noted in another study that even smaller foci of pure high-grade sarcoma may indicate an increased likelihood of aggressive behavior.[151] Adenosarcomas with sarcomatous overgrowth therefore have a malignant potential similar to that of other high-grade uterine sarcoma, such as MMMT and leiomyosarcoma.

When tumors fulfilling the criteria presented above for adenofibroma are excluded, the stromal mitotic rate does not appear to be of prognostic importance. The presence of heterologous elements was not associated with an increased risk of recurrence in one large study of typical adenosarcomas.[151] Extensive rhabdomyosarcomatous differentiation was accompanied by a higher rate of recurrence in another study, but all such tumors also had sarcomatous overgrowth by the rhabdomyosarcoma.[157]

TREATMENT

In young patients with endometrial or endocervical adenofibromas, in whom the preservation of fertility is a consideration, local excision by curettage or polypectomy may be curative.[151] It is important, however, that the specimen be thoroughly examined to exclude adenosarcoma, and that the patient be followed closely for evidence of local recurrence. Adenofibromas in older patients are most easily managed by hysterectomy, unless such an operation is contraindicated.

The recommended therapy for adenosarcomas is almost always hysterectomy, usually accompanied by bilateral salpingooophorectomy. Although typical adenosarcomas are almost always stage I at presentation, the GOG study concluded that a staging procedure (including peritoneal washings) should be performed.[157] Staging would be particularly important if sarcomatous overgrowth is diagnosed or suspected in a curettage specimen. As adjuvant postoperative radiation or chemotherapy appears to have had no demonstrable value in reducing the likelihood of recurrent tumor,[151] such therapy should probably be reserved, if it is to be used at all, for patients with invasive tumors or tumors with sarcomatous overgrowth. Recurrent tumor was successfully treated by local excision in 50 percent of cases in one series,[151] although in another series, all but two patients with recurrent tumor died of tumor progression or were alive with tumor at the time of reporting.[125]

MÜLLERIAN CARCINOFIBROMA AND CARCINOMESENCHYMOMA

Very rare uterine tumors are characterized by a malignant epithelial component and a benign mesenchymal component. Several such tumors have been designated *carcinofibroma* because the mesenchymal element consisted of abundant fibromatous tissue.[160, 161] In such cases, however, it is difficult to prove that the fibrous component is neoplastic and not reactive. The term has also been applied,[119, 160, 161] inappropriately in our opinion, to otherwise typical tumors in the adenofibroma-adenosarcoma spectrum with foci of in situ or invasive adenocarcinoma.[99, 119]

A more convincing example of a tumor in this category has been labeled *carcino-*

mesenchymoma.[162] A well-circumscribed myometrial tumor in a 50-year-old woman was composed of adenocarcinoma, growing in glandular and papillary patterns, intimately admixed with a major component of benign smooth muscle, cartilage, and adipose tissue.[162]

UTERINE TUMORS RESEMBLING OVARIAN SEX-CORD TUMORS

We have applied the term *uterine tumor resembling ovarian sex-cord tumor* (*UTROSCT*) to a heterogeneous group of rare neoplasms characterized by pure or prominent microscopic patterns that resemble those of ovarian sex-cord tumors (granulosa cell and Sertoli cell tumors).[163–172] Several tumors reported as "granulosa cell tumors" of the uterus belong in this category.[173, 174] The histologic appearance of these neoplasms merges almost imperceptibly with that of endometrial stromal tumors exhibiting less than predominant epithelial differentiation (see Ch 6).

CLINICAL FEATURES

The patients are in the reproductive and postmenopausal age groups, with an age range of 16 to 73 years (mean, 47 years).[172] The presenting clinical manifestations are usually abnormal vaginal bleeding, uterine enlargement ascribed to "fibroids" or a pelvic mass, or both; occasional patients have had pelvic pain or discomfort or have been asymptomatic. Unique presentations have included uterine rupture, tumor prolapse through the external os, and masculinization.[172] In approximately 25 percent of cases, tumor tissue has been obtained by curettage, biopsy, or polypectomy prior to hysterectomy; rarely, no residual tumor has been found in the hysterectomy specimen in these cases.[172] At the time of hysterectomy, the tumors are almost invariably confined to the uterus (stage I). Extrauterine tumor, however, has been documented intraoperatively in four patients, involving bowel, ovary, omentum, and liver, alone or in combination.[172] One of these four patients had serosal involvement by the primary tumor, a finding that was present in three additional cases not associated with extrauterine spread.

GROSS APPEARANCE

On gross examination (Figs. 7-25 and 7-26), UTROSCTs are generally solid, round, well-circumscribed myometrial masses that range from 0.7 to 20 cm in diameter (mean, 5.7 cm); rare tumors have been predominantly cystic.[163, 172] Occasional tumors have had infiltrative margins or foci of vascular invasion that were macroscopically visible.[172] UTROSCTs are usually mural but are occasionally submucosal or subserosal; the submucosal and subserosal tumors may be polypoid and, in such cases, focal hemorrhage is sometimes encountered within them. Rare tumors have been located predominantly within the endometrium or endocervix. The cut surfaces are often yellow, but occasionally gray to tan, and are soft, fleshy, and homogeneous without the whorled pattern of a leiomyoma (Figs. 7-25 and 7-26).

MICROSCOPIC APPEARANCE

The cardinal feature of UTROSCTs on microscopic examination is a variety of epithelial and stromal patterns that create a resemblance to those of ovarian sex-cord tumors, especially granulosa cell and Sertoli cell tumors (Figs. 7-27 to 7-29). In the largest series of UTROSCTs (92 cases), the tumors were separated into two groups.[172] Group I (25 cases) was characterized by a predominant component of cells resembling endometrial stromal or smooth muscle cells and a minor component (10 to 50 percent) of sex-cord-like elements (SCLEs), whereas in group II tumors (67 cases), the latter component predominated. Almost 60

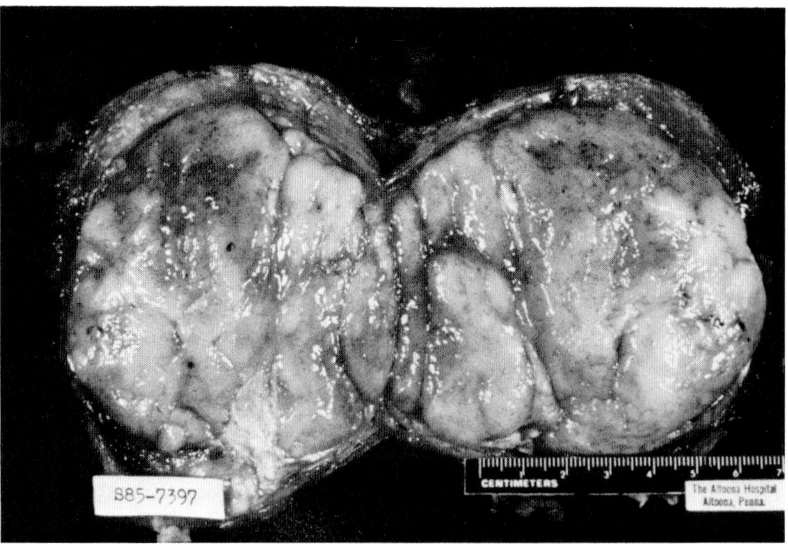

Fig. 7-25. Uterine tumor resembling ovarian sex-cord tumor. The well-circumscribed tumor is surrounded by myometrium and has a fleshy, lobulated cut surface, which was tan. (From Clement and Scully,[188] with permission.)

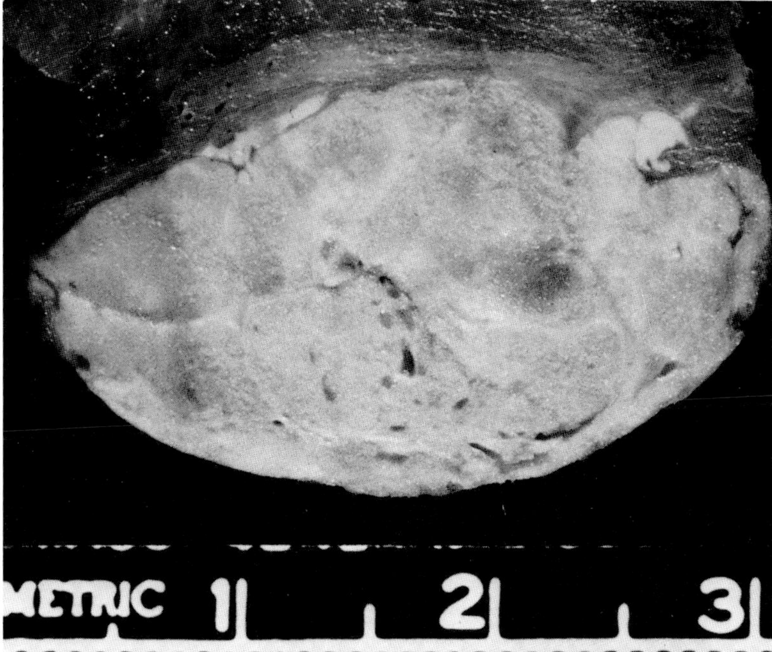

Fig. 7-26. Uterine tumor resembling ovarian sex-cord tumor. Well-circumscribed mural tumor exhibits a faintly lobulated, fleshy (yellow) cut surface (tumor was completely surrounded by myometrium, some of which has become detached). (From Clement and Scully,[163] with permission.)

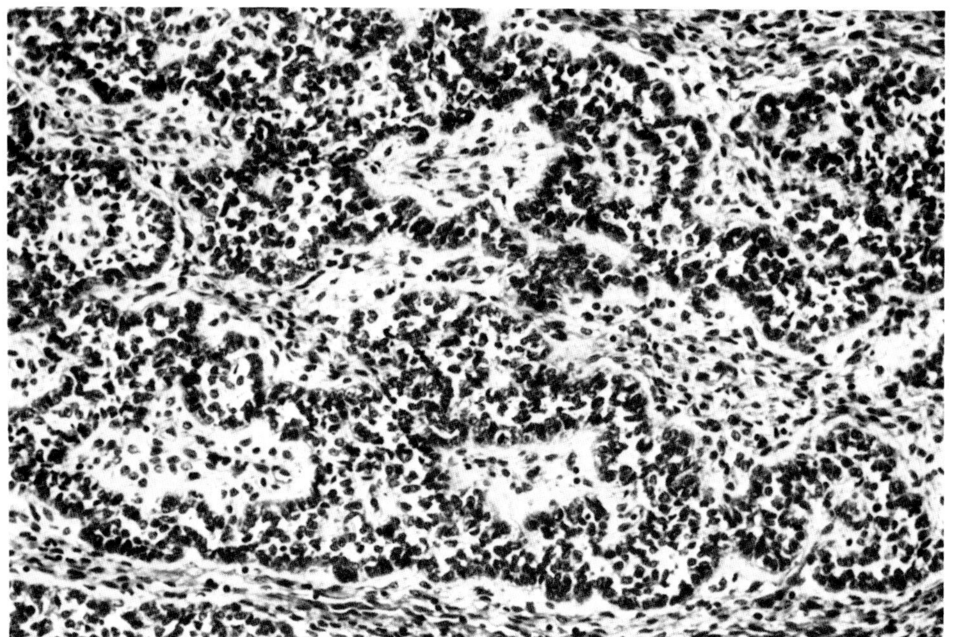

Fig. 7-27. Uterine tumor resembling ovarian sex-cord tumor. The tumor is composed of cellular trabeculae arranged in a plexiform pattern simulating a granulosa cell tumor.

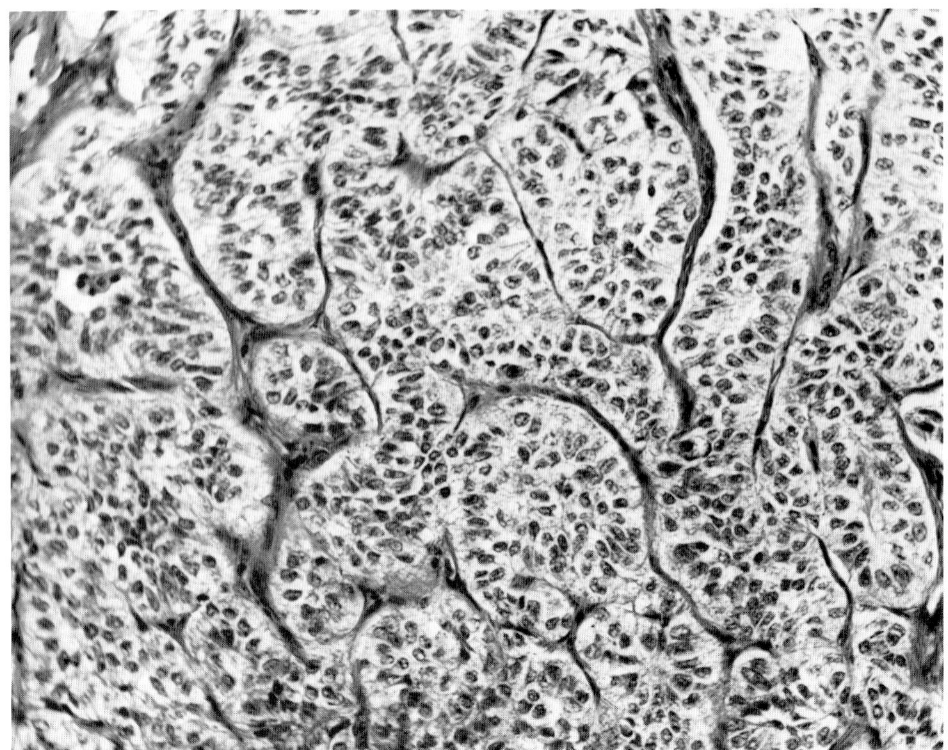

Fig. 7-28. Uterine tumor resembling ovarian sex-cord tumor. Microscopic appearance of the tumor illustrated in Figure 7-26. Solid sertoliform tubules are lined by cells with abundant vacuolated cytoplasm, which was rich in lipid.

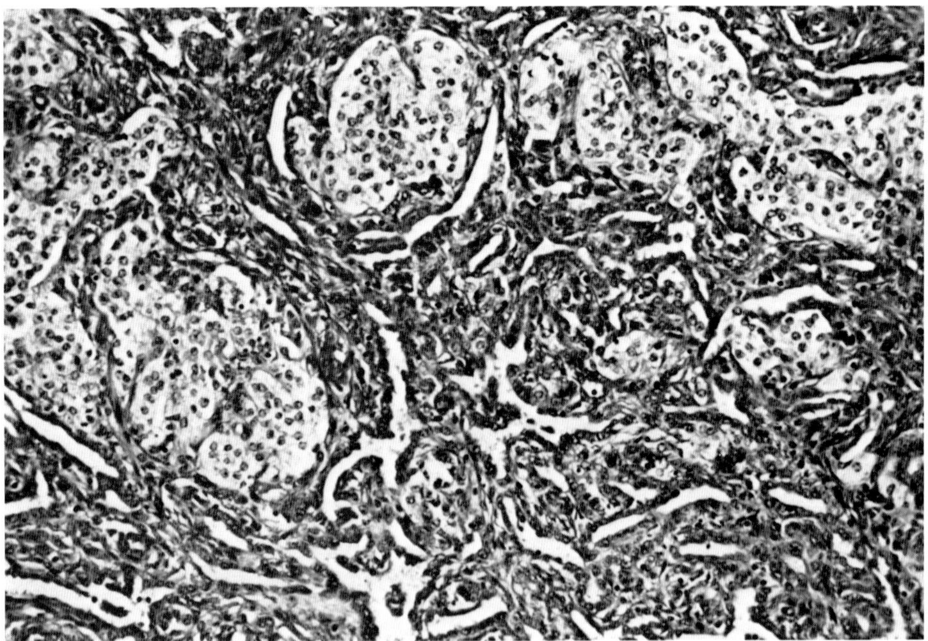

Fig. 7-29. Uterine tumor resembling ovarian sex-cord tumor. Tumor cells with scant cytoplasm line ramifying slitlike spaces imparting a retiform pattern. Admixed are solid nests of cells with abundant foamy cytoplasm.

percent of group I tumors and 10 percent of group II tumors had an infiltrating border similar to that of low-grade endometrial stromal sarcomas (ESSs), despite being grossly well demarcated.[172] The SCLEs typically consist of, alone or in combination, anastomosing cords one to two cells in width or broader trabeculae, small nests, and sertoliform tubular structures (Figs. 7-27 to 7-29). Call-Exner–like bodies were found in 8 percent of group I tumors and 17 percent of group II tumors. The epithelial-like cells within the SCLEs vary from small, round and regular with scanty cytoplasm to large with abundant eosinophilic, clear, or foamy cytoplasm that is often lipid rich (Fig. 7-26 to 7-29). The nuclei are generally small and regular with little pleomorphism and indistinct nucleoli. Nuclear grooves are rare or absent, and mitotic figures are typically scarce.

The stroma ranges from scanty to abundant and from moderately cellular to hypocellular and hyalinized. Twelve percent of group I tumors and 22 percent of the group II tumors in the series cited above were considered to have a stromal component of smooth muscle, characterized by bundles of cells with elongated nuclei, and occasionally cells with ample eosinophilic cytoplasm resembling the cells of typical and epithelioid smooth muscle tumors, respectively.[172] Leydig cell-like or theca cell-like differentiation has not been observed in UTROSCTs, although lipid-laden stromal cells of questionable origin have been present in some cases[167] (Fig. 7-29). Vascular invasion was observed in 32 percent of group I tumors and 19 percent of group II tumors.[172]

In one immunohistochemical study of UTROSCTs, most of the tumors were immunoreactive for both mesenchymal and epithelial markers.[171] The SCLEs were immunoreactive for vimentin in all cases, for cytokeratin in 55 percent of cases, for EMA in 10 percent of cases, and, surprisingly, for desmin in 43 percent of cases.[171] Other immunohistochemical studies of SCLEs in UTROSCTs (and ESSs) have also reported frequent immunoreactivity for smooth muscle antigens.[175–177] Ultrastructural study of one tumor revealed cells with features of both endometrial stromal and smooth muscle cells,[164] and in another case, cells with desmosomes, tonofilaments and microvilli lining glandular spaces.[167]

HISTOGENESIS

Because of the close resemblance of these tumors to ovarian sex-cord tumors, a possible origin from displaced ovarian tissue has been considered. However, the neoplastic cells lack the characteristic pale nuclei with grooves and typical Call-Exner body formation of ovarian granulosa cell tumors, and with one exception,[172] there has been no clinical evidence of endocrine function in the reported cases. In one case, however, structures resembling Charcot-Bottcher filament bundles, characteristic inclusions of testicular Sertoli cells, were enigmatically present.[169] The histologic heterogeneity of these tumors suggests the possibility of more than a single cell of origin. The similarity of the epithelial patterns to those seen focally in endometrial stromal tumors strongly supports a derivation from endometrial stromal cells in most cases. The plexiform pattern in some cases, which may be similar to that seen in epithelioid smooth muscle tumors and plexiform tumorlets, favors a smooth muscle origin in other cases.[178, 179] Some UTROSCTs may represent combined smooth muscle-endometrial stromal tumors (stromomyomas).[164, 175]

BEHAVIOR

Most UTROSCTs are clinically benign. In the study cited above, recurrent tumor developed in 10 patients (15 percent) at an average of 6 years after initial therapy (range 2 to 12 years).[172] Secondary recurrences were seen in two of these patients at intervals of 1 and 13 years after the first recurrence. Seven of the ten patients ultimately died of tumor. Recurrences were associated with one or more of the following features: serosal rupture, vessel invasion, stromal predominance, and cytologic atypia.

ATYPICAL POLYPOID ADENOMYOMA

Approximately 1 percent of benign polypoid tumors of the endometrium have a stroma composed of smooth muscle rather than the endometrial or fibrous stroma of the typical endometrial polyp. When these adenomyomas lack atypical architectural or cytologic features on microscopic examination ("typical" polypoid adenomyomas) (see Ch. 4), they pose no diagnostic problem. In 1981, however, Mazur focused attention on the presence of atypical features in some adenomyomas that occasionally led to confusion with a malignant tumor.[180] Approximately 40 of these atypical polypoid adenomyomas have now been reported.[180–185]

CLINICAL FEATURES

Atypical polypoid adenomyomas (APAs) characteristically occur in premenopausal women usually in their fourth or fifth decade (average age 39 years); in rare cases, the tumor is encountered after the menopause.[181] The APAs have been reported in patients with Turner's syndrome, at least two of whom had been on long-term estrogen therapy.[183] The presenting symptom is almost always abnormal vaginal bleeding. Pelvic examination is usually negative, although rare tumors have been visible as polypoid masses projecting through the external os.[183]

GROSS APPEARANCE

Most or all of the lesion is usually curetted out in fragments, and thus gross descriptions of intact tumors are few. The lesions typically involve the lower uterine segment, and less commonly the endocervix or upper corpus. APAs are usually solitary and less than 2 cm in diameter[181] (Fig. 7-30), although multiple tumors and examples up to 6 cm (Fig. 7-31) have been described.[183] The cut surfaces are yellow-tan to gray to white, solid, bulging, lobulated or bosselated, and firm to rubbery. The tumors may be pedunculated or sessile and are well demarcated from the underlying myometrium.

MICROSCOPIC APPEARANCE

On histologic examination, APAs are composed of endometrial glands admixed with smooth mucle (Figs. 7-32 to 7-35). The glands exhibit varying degrees of architectural and cytologic atypia with mitotic activity; in occasional cases, a cribriform pattern (Fig. 7-34) and severe cytologic atypia may be present focally.[181] In 90 percent of cases, squamous morules are present and may be extensive, obliterating glandular lumens (Figs. 7-34 and 7-35), and occasionally containing areas of central necrosis. The squamous foci uncommonly exhibit focal keratization; peritoneal keratin granulomas may be seen in such cases.[187] Mucinous metaplasia[183] and in pregnant patients, a focal Arias-Stella-like reaction,[181] have also been rarely encountered.

The cellular stromal component consists of interlacing bundles of smooth muscle cells that appear benign (Figs. 7-32 to 7-35) but exhibit mild to moderate atypia in a mi-

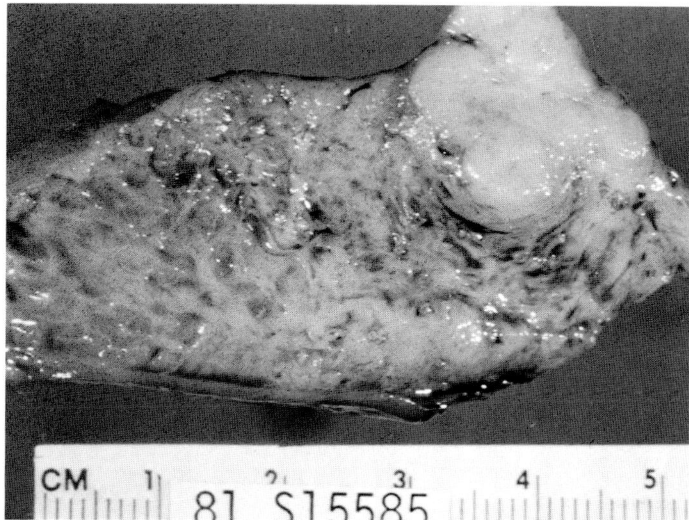

Fig. 7-30. Atypical polypoid adenomyoma. The lobulated mass is well demarcated from the subjacent myometrium.

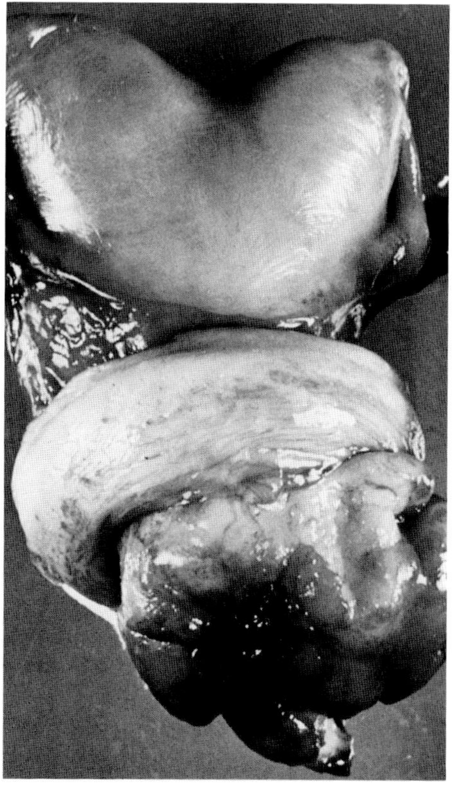

Fig. 7-31. Atypical polypoid adenomyoma. The tumor, which arose in a patient with Turner's syndrome, has prolapsed through the external os. Its base of attachment was in the lower uterine segment. (From Clement and Young,[183] with permission.)

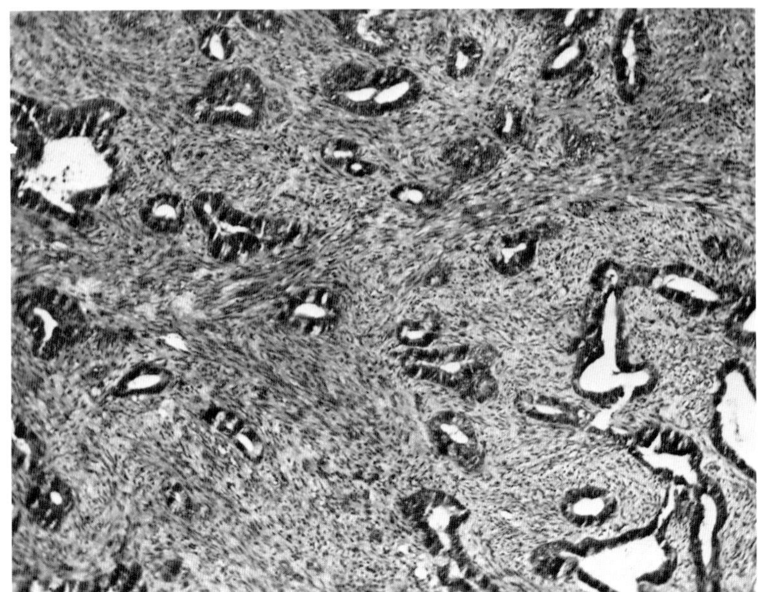

Fig. 7-32. Atypical polypoid adenomyoma. Endometrial-type glands are admixed with cellular smooth muscle.

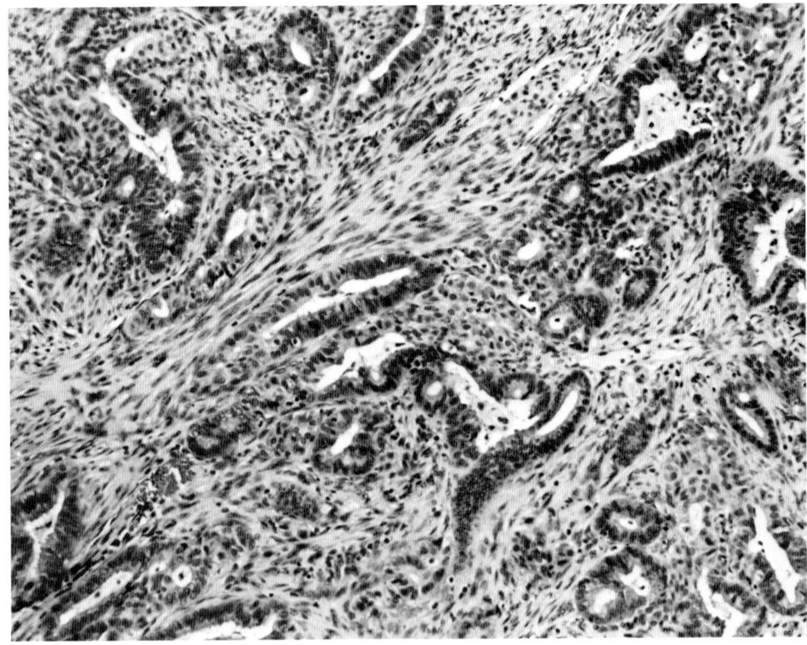

Fig. 7-33. Atypical polypoid adenomyoma. Focally crowded endometrial glands of irregular size and shape are disposed within cellular smooth muscle.

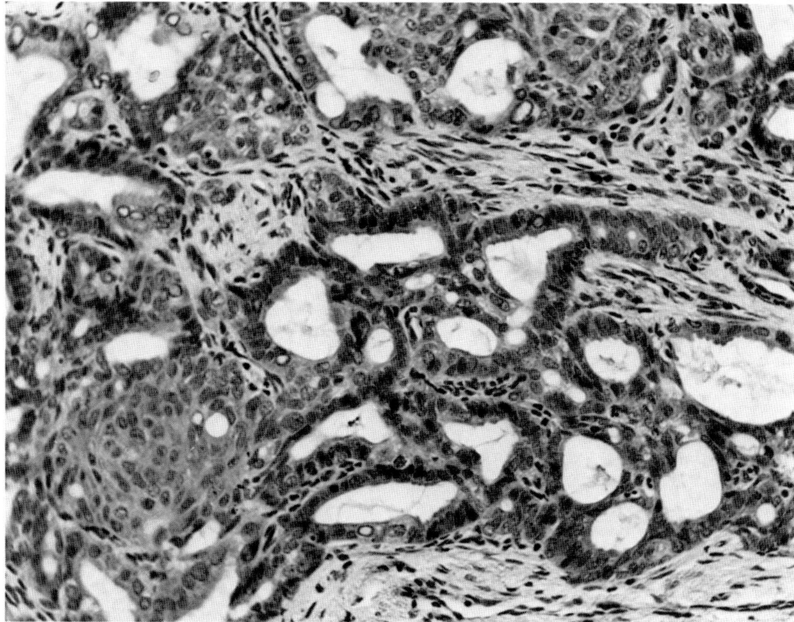

Fig. 7-34. Atypical polypoid adenomyoma. A focal cribriform pattern is seen within the glandular component. The atypical epithelial cells, however, lack frankly malignant features. Note squamous morules.

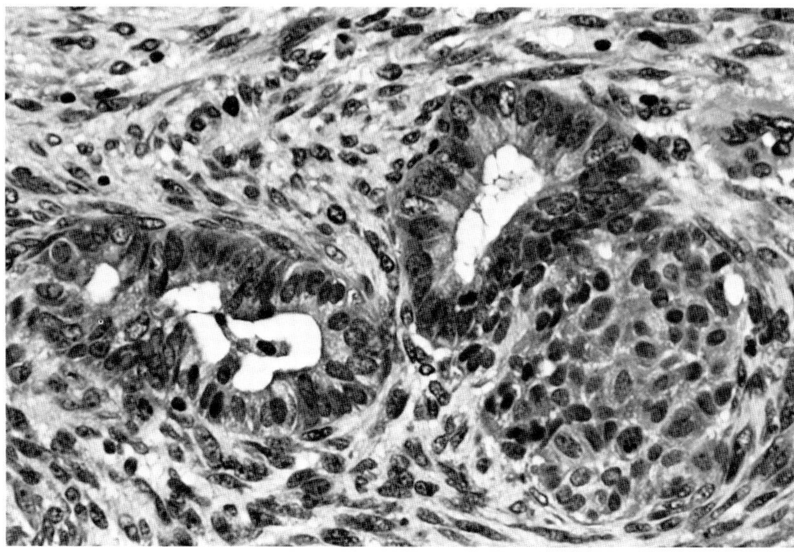

Fig. 7-35. Atypical polypoid adenomyoma. The glands are lined by cells with moderately atypical nuclei. Note the squamous morule. The cellular stroma is composed of smooth muscle cells with mildly atypical nuclei.

nority of cases. Occasional mitotic figures are usually present, but the mitotic rate is typically less than 2 MF/10 HPF.[181] In some cases, occasional glands are surrounded by a narrow cuff of cells of endometrial stromal type. In curettage specimens, the diagnostic fragments are usually admixed with normal proliferative or secretory endometrium, although occasionally, there may be associated endometrial hyperplasia or even adenocarcinoma, which may also involve and possibly originate in the adenomyoma.[181] The features of a lesion reported as an "atypical polypoid adenomyoma with carcinomatous transformation,"[186] are, in our opinion, those of a pure endometrial adenocarcinoma of villoglandular type. In hysterectomy specimens, APAs usually have a well-circumscribed noninvasive border with the adjacent endometrium and underlying myometrium.

DIFFERENTIAL DIAGNOSIS

The APA is sometimes misdiagnosed as an endometrial carcinoma. The latter, however, typically occurs in older women, and on gross examination may exhibit features inconsistent with an APA, such as large size, hemorrhage, necrosis, and myometrial invasion. The association of atypical glands and smooth muscle in APAs can be misinterpreted as invasion of the myometrium by adenocarcinoma or adenoacanthoma, especially in a curettage specimen. The glands, however, almost always lack frankly malignant features, and the smooth muscle is usually more cellular and more mitotically active and has a growth pattern that is more disorderly than that of normal myometrium. Finally, it is uncommon for large fragments of smooth muscle invaded by carcinoma to be present in a curettage specimen, particularly in the absence of obvious carcinoma separate from muscular tissue elsewhere in the specimen. Misinterpreting the mitotically active smooth mus-

cle stroma of APAs as sarcomatous can result in the misdiagnosis of MMMT or adenosarcoma. The last two tumors, however, usually lack prominent amounts of smooth muscle and adenosarcomas exhibit periglandular stromal condensation and intraglandular stromal papillae, which are absent in the APA. Additionally, the glandular component of the adenosarcoma is usually more cystic and less atypical than that of the APA. MMMTs, in contrast to APAs, have highly malignant epithelial and stromal components.

BEHAVIOR

Follow-up of the 40 reported cases treated by curettage or hysterectomy has shown no evidence of a malignant behavior. In most cases, however, the postcurettage follow-up has been short or hysterectomy was performed soon after diagnosis. The ultimate fate of the conservatively treated lesion remains uncertain. In several patients in whom a repeated curettage was performed, the lesion has persisted for as long as 4 years after the initial procedure.[181] In several other cases, a repeated curettage has revealed atypical endometrial hyperplasia, with or without squamous metaplasia, or an adenocarcinoma with squamous differentiation.

TREATMENT

The treatment depends on the age of the patient, her desire to retain fertility, and the severity of her symptoms. If she is menopausal or younger but has completed her family, or if bleeding is not controlled by polypectomy or curettage, a hysterectomy is justifiable. If the patient does not have intractable bleeding and desires to preserve her reproductive function, conservative management with repeated curettage can be attempted, and has been apparently curative in some cases; one patient had a successful pregnancy after conservative management. Because the APA may persist for a number of years and because its malignant potential, if any, is not yet known with certainty, patients who are managed conservatively should be followed with care.

REFERENCES

1. Bartsich EG, O'Leary JA, Moore JG: Carcinosarcoma of the uterus: a 50-year review of 32 cases (1917–1966). Obstet Gynecol 30:518, 1967

2. Chuang JT, Van Velden JJ, Graham JB: Carcinosarcoma and mixed mesodermal tumor of the uterine corpus: Review of 49 cases. Obstet Gynecol 35:679, 1970

3. Williamson EO, Christopherson WM: Malignant mixed mullerian tumors of the uterus. Cancer 29:585, 1972

4. Norris HJ, Roth E, Taylor HB: Mesenchymal tumors of the uterus. II. A clinical and pathologic study of 31 mixed mesodermal tumors. Obstet Gynecol 28:57, 1966

5. Norris HJ, Taylor HB: Mesenchymal tumors of the uterus. III. A clinical and pathologic study of 31 carcinosarcomas. Cancer 19:1459, 1966

6. Rachmaninoff N, Climie ARW: Mixed mesodermal tumors of the uterus. Cancer 19:1705, 1966

7. Masterson JG, Kremper J: Mixed mesodermal tumors. Am J Obstet Gynecol 104:673, 1969

8. Kempson RL, Bari W: Uterine sarcomas: classification, diagnosis, and prognosis. Hum Pathol 1:331, 1970

9. Schaepman-van Geuns EJ: Mixed tumors and carcinosarcomas of the uterus evaluated five years after treatment. Cancer 25:72, 1970

10. Mortel R, Koss LG, Lewis JL, Jr: Mesodermal mixed tumors of the uterine corpus. Obstet Gynecol 43:248, 1974

11. Barwick KW, LiVolsi VA: Malignant mixed mullerian tumors of the uterus: A clinicopathologic assessment of 34 cases. Am J Surg Pathol 3: 125, 1979

12. King ME, Kramer EE: Malignant mulle-rian mixed tumors of the uterus: a study of 21 cases. Cancer 45:188, 1980

13. Shaw RW, Lynch PF, Wade-Evans T: Mullerian mixed tumour of the uterine corpus: a clinical histopathological review of 28 patients. Br J Obstet Gynaecol 90:562, 1983

14. Lotocki R, Rosenshein NB, Grumbine F et al: Mixed mullerian tumors of the uterus: Clinical and pathologic correlations. Int J Gynaecol Obstet 20:237, 1982

15. Doss LL, Llorens AS, Henriquez EM: Carcinosarcoma of the uterus: a 40-year experience from the State of Missouri. Gynecol Oncol 18:43, 1984

16. Marchese MJ, Liskow AS, Crum CP et al: Uterine sarcomas: A clinicopathologic study, 1965–1981. Gynecol Oncol 18:299, 1984

17. Peters WA III, Kumar NB, Fleming WP et al: Prognostic features of sarcomas and mixed tumors of the endometrium. Obstet Gynecol 63:550, 1984

18. Macasaet MA, Waxman M, Fruchter RG et al: Prognostic factors in malignant mesodermal (mullerian) mixed tumors of the uterus. Gynecol Oncol 20:32, 1985

19. Wheelock JB, Krebs H, Schneider V et al: Uterine sarcoma: Analysis of prognostic variables in 71 cases. Am J Obstet Gynecol 151: 1016, 1985

20. George M, Pejovic MH, Kramar A et al: Uterine sarcomas: prognostic factors and treatment modalities—study on 209 patients. Gynecol Oncol 24:58, 1986

21. Kahanpaa KV, Wahlstrom T, Grohn P et al: Sarcomas of the uterus: a clinicopathologic study of 119 patients. Obstet Gynecol 67:417. 1986

22. Dinh TV, Slavin RE, Bhagavan BS et al: Mixed mullerian tumors of the uterus: a clinicopathologic study. Obstet Gynecol 74:388, 1989

23. Gagne H, Tetu B, Blondeau L, Raymond PE, Blais R: Morphologic prognostic factors of malignant mixed mullerian tumor of the uterus: a clinicopathologic study of 58 cases. Mod Pathol 2:433, 1989

24. Gallup DG, Gable DS, Talledo E, Otken LB, Jr: A clinical-pathologic study of mixed mullerian tumors of the uterus over a 16-year period—The Medical College of

Georgia experience. Am J Obstet Gynecol 161:533, 1989

25. Nielsen SN, Podratz KC, Scheithauer BW, O'Brien PC: Clinicopathologic analysis of uterine malignant mixed mullerian tumors. Gynecol Oncol 34:372, 1989

26. Podczaski E, Woomert CA, Stevens CW, Jr et al: Management of malignant, mixed mesodermal tumors of the uterus. Gynecol Oncol 32:240, 1989

27. Bitterman P, Chun B, Kurman RJ: The significance of epithelial differentiation in mixed mesodermal tumors of the uterus. A clinicopathologic and immunohistochemical study. Am J Surg Pathol 14:317, 1990

28. Larson B. Silversward C, Nilsson B. Pettersson F: Mixed mullerian tumours of the uterus—prognostic factors: a clinical and histopathologic study of 147 cases. Radiother Oncol 17:123, 1990

29. Schweizer W, Demopoulos R, Beller U, Dubin H: Prognostic factors for malignant mixed mullerian tumors of the uterus. Int J Gynecol Pathol 9:129, 1990

30. Silverberg SG, Major FJ, Blessing JA et al: Carcinosarcoma (malignant mixed mesodermal tumor) of the uterus. A gynecologic oncology group pathologic study of 203 cases. Int J Gynecol Pathol 9:1, 1990

31. Costa MJ, Khan R, Judd R: Carcinosarcoma (malignant mixed mullerian [mesodermal] tumor) of the uterus and ovary. Correlation of clinical, pathologic, and immunohistochemical features in 29 cases. Arch Pathol Lab Med 115:583, 1991

32. George E, Manivel JC, Dehner LP, Wick WR: Malignant mixed mullerian tumors: An immunohistochemical study of 47 cases, with histogenetic considerations and clinical correlation. Hum Pathol 22:215, 1991

33. Mosel A: Karzinosarkom des endometriums bei einer jungen frau mit Turner-syndrom. Geburtsh Frauenheilk 39:217, 1979

34. Chumas JC, Mann WJ, Tseng L: Malignant mixed mullerian tumor of the endometrium in a young woman with polycystic ovaries. Cancer 52: 1478, 1983

35. Press MF, Scully RE: Endometrial "sarcomas" complicating ovarian thecoma, polycystic ovarian disease and estrogen therapy. Gynecol Oncol 21:135, 1985

36. Altaras MM, Jaffe R, Cohen O et al: Role of prolonged excessive estrogen stimulation in the pathogenesis of endometrial sarcomas: two cases and a review of the literature. Gynecol Oncol 38:273, 1990

37. Amr SS, Tavassoli FA, Hassan AA et al: Mixed mesodermal tumor of the uterus in a 4-year-old girl. Int J Gynecol Pathol 5:371, 1986

38. Rodriguez-Escudero FJ Martin Mateos M, Burgos J et al: Malignant mixed mullerian tumor of the cervix in a 12-year-old girl. Eur J Gynaecol Oncol 9:5, 1988

39. Harlow BL, Weiss NS, Lofton S: The epidemiology of sarcomas of the uterus. JNCI 76:399, 1986

40. Norris HJ, Taylor HB: Postirradiation sarcomas of the uterus. Obstet Gynecol 26:689, 1965

41. Varela-Duran J, Nochomovitz LE, Prem KA et al: Postirradiation mixed mullerian tumors of the uterus: A comparative clinicopathologic study. Cancer 45:1625, 1980

42. Soper JT, McCarty KS Jr, Hinshaw W et al: Cytoplasmic estrogen and progesterone receptor content of uterine sarcomas. Am J Obstet Gynecol 150:342, 1984

43. Sutton GP, Stehman FB, Michael H et al: Estrogen and progesterone receptors in uterine sarcomas. Obstet Gynecol 68:709, 1986

44. Tseng L, Tseng JK, Mann WJ et al: Endocrine aspects of human uterine sarcoma: A preliminary study. Am J Obstet Gynecol 155:95, 1986

45. Young H, Damien M, Schwartz PE et al: Carcinosarcoma of the uterine cervix initially misinterpreted as high grade sarcoma. Hum Pathol 19:605, 1988

46. Peters WA III, Bagley CM, Smith MR: CA-125: use as a tumor marker with mixed mesodermal tumors of the female genital tract. Cancer 58:2625, 1986

47. Scioscia AL, Merino MJ, Haas M et al: Malignant mixed mullerian tumor of the uterus arising in association with a viable gestation. Obstet Gynecol 71: 1047, 1988

48. Maiman M, Remy JC, DiMaio TM et al: Uterine rupture secondary to a malignant mixed mesodermal (mullerian) tumor: a case report. Gynecol Oncol 30: 137, 1988

49. Uede T, Saito T, Minase T et al: A malig-

nant mixed mesodermal tumor of the uterine corpus with hypercatecholaminemia. Acta Pathol Jpn 40:293, 1990

50. Kawagoe K: A case of mixed mesodermal tumor of the uterus with alpha-fetoprotein production. Jpn J Clin Oncol 15:577, 1985

51. Abell MR, Ramirez JA: Sarcomas and carcinosarcomas of the uterine cervix. Cancer 31:1176, 1973

52. Hall-Craggs M, Toker C, Nedwich A: Carcinosarcoma of the uterine cervix: light and electron microscopic study. Cancer 48: 161, 1981

53. Waxman M, Waxman JS, Alinovi V: Heterologous malignant mixed mullerian tumor of the cervical stump. Gynecol Oncol 16:422, 1983

54. Miyazawa K, Hernandez E: Cervical carcinosarcoma: a case report. Gynecol Oncol 23:376, 1986

55. Zaloudek CJ, Norris HJ: Mesenchymal tumors of the uterus. p. 1. In Fenoglio CM, Wolff M (eds): Progress in Surgical Pathology. Vol. 3. Masson USA, New York, 1981

56. Manivel C, Wick MR, Sibley RK: Neuroendocrine differentiation in mullerian neoplasms. An immunohistochemical study of a "pure" endometrial small-cell carcinoma and a mixed mullerian tumor containing small-cell carcinoma. Am J Clin Pathol 86:438, 1986

57. Dictor M: Alpha-1-antitrypsin in a malignant mixed mesodermal tumor of the ovary. Am J Surg Pathol 5:543, 1981

58. Dictor M: Ovarian malignant mixed mesodermal tumor: The occurrence of hyaline droplets containing alpha-1-antitrypsin. Hum Pathol 13:930, 1982

59. Young RH, Kleinman GM, Scully RE: Glioma of the uterus. Report of a case with comments on histogenesis. Am J Surg Pathol 5:695, 1981

60. Schroder. R, Hillejahn A: Uber einen heterologen Kombinations—tumor des uterus. Zentralbl Gynaekol 44:1050, 1920

61. Gersell DJ, Duncan DA, Fulling KH: Malignant mixed mullerian tumor of the uterus with neuroectodermal differentiation. Int J Gynecol Pathol 8:169, 1989

62. DiSaia PJ, Morrow CP, Boronow R et al: Endometrial sarcoma: Lymphatic spread pattern. Am J Obstet Gynecol 130:104, 1978

63. Kahner S, Ferenczy A, Richart RM: Homologous mixed mullerian tumors (carcinosarcoma) confined to endometrial polyps. Am J Obstet Gynecol 121:278, 1975

64. Barwick KW, LiVolsi VA: Heterologous mixed mullerian tumor confined to an endometrial polyp. Obstet Gynecol 53:512, 1979

65. Klomp A, Smith LA, Pounder DJ: Malignant mixed mesodermal tumour of the uterus initially confined to a polyp. Aust NZ J Obstet Gynaecol 22:248, 1982

66. Bonazzi del Poggetto C, Virtanen I et al: Expression of intermediate filaments in ovarian and uterine tumors. Int J Gynecol Pathol 1:359, 1983

67. Marshall RJ, Braye SG: Alpha-1-antitrypsin alpha-1-antichymotrypsin, actin, and myosin in uterine sarcomas. Int J Gynecol Pathol 4:346, 1985

68. Ramadan M, Goudie RB: Epithelial antigens in malignant mixed mullerian tumors of endometrium. J Pathol 148:13, 1986

69. Geisinger KR, Dabbs DJ, Marshall RB: Malignant mixed mullerian tumors. An ultrastructural and immunohistochemical analysis with histogenetic considerations. Cancer 59:1781, 1987

70. Lisschitz-Mercer B, Czernobilsky B, Dgani R et al: Immunocytochemical study of an endometrial diffuse clear cell stromal sarcoma and other endometrial sarcomas. Cancer 59:1494, 1987

71. Mukai K, Varela-Duran J, Nochomovitz LE: The rhabdomyoblast in mixed mullerian tumors of the uterus and ovary: An immunohistochemical study of myoglobin in 25 cases. Am J Clin Pathol 74:101, 1980

72. Talerman A: Hyaline globules in ovarian mixed mesodermal (mullerian) tumors (letter). Hum Pathol 14:562, 1983

73. Liao SY, Choi BH: Expression of glial fibrillary acidic protein by neoplastic cells of mullerian origin. Virchows Arch [B] 52:185, 1986

74. Liao SY, Choi BH: The cultured cells of malignant mixed mullerian tumors and normal endometrium express glial fibrillary acidic protein: light and EM immunocytochemical study. Lab Invest 56:43A, 1987

75. Auerbach HE, LiVolsi VA, Merino MJ: Malignant mixed mullerian tumors of the uterus. An immunohistochemical study. Int J Gynecol Pathol 7: 123, 1988

76. Chung M, Mukai K, Teshima S et al: Expression of various antigens by different components of uterine mixed mullerian tumors. Acta Pathol Jpn 38:35, 1988

77. Meis JM, Lawrence WD: The immunohistochemical profile of malignant mixed mullerian tumor. Overlap with endometrial adenocarcinoma. Am J Clin Pathol 94:1, 1990

78. Evans HL: Endometrial stromal sarcoma and poorly differentiated endometrial sarcoma. Cancer 50:2170, 1982

79. Chou S, Fortune D, Beischer NA et al: Primary malignant fibrous histiocytoma of the uterus—ultrastructural and immunocytochemical studies of two cases. Pathology 17:36, 1985

80. Kindblom L, Seidal T: Malignant giant cell tumor of the uterus. A clinicopathologic, light- and electron-microscopic study of a case. Acta Pathol Microbiol Scand A 89:179, 1981

81. Fujii S, Kanzaki H, Konishi I, et al: Malignant fibrous histiocytoma of the uterus. Gynecol Oncol 26:319, 1987

82. Nogales FF, Gomez-Morales M, Raymundo C et al: Benign heterologous tissue components associated with endometrial carcinoma. Int J Gynecol Pathol 1:286, 1982

83. Spanos WJ Jr, Wharton JT, Gomez L et al: Malignant mixed mullerian tumors of the uterus. Cancer 53:311, 1984

84. Erickson DJ, Strittholt JT, Jones WH et al: Malignant mixed mullerian tumors of the uterus. Lab Invest 46:20A, 1982

85. Geszler G, Szpak CA, Harris RE et al: Prognostic value of peritoneal washings in patients with malignant mixed mullerian tumors of the uterus. Am J Obstet Gynecol 155:83, 1986

86. Kanbour AI, Buchsbaum HJ, Hall A, Kanbour AI: Peritoneal cytology in malignant mixed mullerian tumors of the uterus. Gynecol Oncol 33:91, 1989

87. Fleming WP, Peters WA III, Kumar NB et al: Autopsy findings in patients with uterine sarcoma. Gynecol Oncol 19:168, 1984

88. Perez CA, Askin F, Baglan RJ et al: Effects of irradiation on mixed mullerian tumors of the uterus. Cancer 43: 1274, 1979

89. Spanos WJ Jr, Peters M, Oswald MJ: Patterns of recurrence in malignant mixed mullerian tumor of the uterus. Cancer 57: 155, 1986

90. Rose PG, Boutselis JG, Sachs L: Adjuvant therapy for stage I uterine sarcoma. Am J Obstet Gynecol 156:660, 1987

91. Kohorn EI, Schwartz PE, Chambers JT et al: Adjuvant therapy in mixed mullerian tumors of the uterus. Gynecol Oncol 23:212, 1986

92. Grosh WW, Jones HW III, Burnett LS et al: Malignant mixed mesodermal tumors of the uterus and ovary treated with cisplatin-based combination chemotherapy. Gynecol Oncol 25:334, 1986

93. Piver MS, DeEulis TG, Lele SB et al: Cyclophosphamide, vincristine, adriamycin, and dimethyl-triazeno imidazole carboxamide (CYVADIC) for sarcomas of the female genital tract. Gynecol Oncol 14:319, 1982

94. Omura GA, Major FJ, Blessing JA et al: A randomized study of adriamycin with and without dimethyl triazenoimidazole carboxamide in advanced uterine sarcomas. Cancer 52:626, 1983

95. Sternberg WH, Clark WH, Smith RC: Malignant mixed mullerian tumor (mixed mesodermal tumor of the uterus). A study of twenty-one cases. Cancer 7:704, 1954

96. Chang WWL, Boyd CB, Ashraf M: An evolution of malignant mixed mullerian tumor. Diagn Gynecol Obstet 2:257, 1980

97. George E, Lillemoe T, Perrone T. Malignant mixed mullerian tumor versus high grade endometrial carcinoma: a comparative analysis of survival, abstracted. Modern Pathol 5:64A, 1992.

98. Abell MR: Papillary adenofibroma of the uterine cervix. Am J Obstet Gynecol 110:990, 1971

99. Vellios F, Ng ABP, Reagan JW: Papillary adenofibroma of the uterus: a benign mesodermal mixed tumor of mullerian origin. Am J Clin Pathol 60:543, 1973

100. Clement PB, Scully RE: Mullerian adenosarcoma of the uterus: a clinicopathologic analysis of ten cases of a distinctive type of

mullerian mixed tumor. Cancer 34:1138, 1974

101. Grimalt M, Arguelles M, Ferenczy A: Papillary cystadenofibroma of endometrium: A histochemical and ultrastructural study. Cancer 36:137, 1975

102. Silverberg SG: Adenomyomatosis of endometrium and endocervix—a hamartoma? Am J Clin Pathol 64:192, 1975

103. Roth LM, Pride GL, Sharma HM: Mullerian adenosarcoma of the uterine cervix with heterologous elements: a light and electron microscopic study. Cancer 37:1725, 1976

104. Sakamoto A, Sugano H: Mixed mesodermal tumor of the uterine body: relationship between histology and survival. Gann 67:263, 1976

105. Katzenstein AA, Askin FB, Feldman PS: Mullerian adenosarcoma of the uterus: An ultrastructural study of four cases. Cancer 40:2233, 1977

106. Philippe E, Schoetter F: A propos de l'adenosarcome mullerian et de l'adenofibrome uterin. Ann Anat Pathol 22:263, 1977

107. Damjanov I, Casey MJ, Maenza RM et al: Mullerian adenosarcoma of the uterus: ultrastructure before and after radiation therapy. Am J Clin Pathol 70:96, 1978

108. Bibro MC, Livolsi VA, Schwartz PE: Adenosarcoma of the uterus: Ultrastructural observations. Am J Clin Pathol 71:112, 1979

109. Borello DJ, Wood WG, Newman RL: Mullerian adenosarcoma: two additional cases with ultrastructural observations. Diagn Gynecol Obstet 1:275, 1979

110. Fox H, Harilal KR, Youell A: Mullerian adenosarcoma of the uterine body: a report of nine cases. Histopathology 3:167, 1979

111. Gloor E: Mullerian adenosarcoma of the uterus: clinicopathologic report of five cases. Am J Surg Pathol 3:203, 1979

112. Okagaki T, Brooker DC, Adcock LL et al: Mullerian adenosarcoma of the uterus with rapid progression: an ultrastructural study. Gynecol Oncol 7:361, 1979

113. Sampat MB, Krishnamurthy SC, Talwalkar GV: Mullerian adenosarcoma philloides of uterus. Report of a case and literature review. Ind J Cancer 16:74, 1979

114. Valdez VA, Planas AT, Lopez VF et al: Adenosarcoma of uterus and ovary: a clinicopathologic study of two cases. Cancer 43:1439, 1979

115. Ali M, Fayemi AO. Mullerian adenosarcoma of uterine cervix. Report of a case with rapidly fatal outcome. Diagnostic Gynecol Obstet 2:135, 1980

116. Baratz M, Gitstein SZ, David MP et al: Papillary cystadenofibroma of the endometrium. Acta Obstet Gynecol Scand 59:467, 1980

117. Martinelli G, Pileri S, Bazzocchi F et al: Mullerian adenosarcoma of the uterus: a report of 5 cases. Tumori 66:499, 1980

118. Orenstein HH, Richart RM, Fenoglio CM: Mullerian adenosarcoma of the uterus: literature review, case report, and ultrastructural observations. Ultrastruct Pathol 1:189, 1980

119. Ostor AG, Fortune DW: Benign and low grade variants of mixed mullerian tumour of the uterus. Histopathology 4:369, 1980

120. Vellios F: Papillary adenofibroma-adenosarcoma; the uterine cystosarcoma phyllodes. p. 205. In Fenoglio CM, Wolff M (eds): Progress in Surgical Pathology. Vol 1. Masson USA, New York, 1980

121. Dietze O, Hopfel-Kreiner I, Scharf O, Ortner A: Heterologes Mullersches Adenosarkom des uterus-ein seltener Tumor: Licht und elektronenmikroskopische Befunde, klinische Dignitat. Arch Gynecol 231:75, 1981

122. Mills SE, Sugg NK, Mahnesmith RC: Endometrial adenosarcoma with pelvic involvement following uterine perforation. Diagn Gynecol Obstet 3:149, 1981

123. Street B, Du Toit JP: Uterine adenosarcoma: report of a case with two further primary malignant tumors. Gynecol Oncol 11:252, 1981

124. Tang C, Toker C, Harriman B: Mullerian adenosarcoma of the uterine cervix. Hum Pathol 12:579, 1981

125. Zaloudek CJ, Norris HJ: Adenofibroma and adenosarcoma of the uterus: a clinicopathologic study of 35 cases. Cancer 48:354, 1981

126. Edinger DD, Safaii H, Tak W, et al: Cervical mullerian adenosarcoma: case report. Eur J Gynecol Oncol 3:69, 1982

127. Hanchard B, Coard K, Persaud V: Mullerian adenosarcoma of the uterus. West Indian Med J 31:41, 1982

128. Hidvegi DF, DeMay RM, Sorensen K: Uterine mullerian adenosarcoma with psammoma bodies. Cytologic, histologic and ultrastructural studies of a case. Acta Cytol 26:323, 1982

129. Miles PA, Greenburg H, Herrera GA et al: Mullerian adenofibroma of the endometrium: a report of a case with ultrastructural study. Diagn Gynecol Obstet 4:215, 1982

130. Czernobilsky B, Hohlweg-Majert P, Dallenbach-Hellweg G: Uterine adenosarcoma: a clinicopathologic study of 11 cases with a reevaluation of histologic criteria. Arch Gynecol 233:281, 1983

131. Hariri J: Mullerian adenosarcoma of the endometrium: review of the literature and report of two cases. Int J Gynecol Pathol 2:182, 1983

132. Segura-Fonseca JJ, Muikai K. Mullerian adenosarcoma of the uterus with heterologous component: case report with an immunohistochemical study of myoglobin. Pathologica 21:233, 1983

133. Altaras M, Cohen I, Cordoba M et al: Papillary adenofibroma of the endometrium: case report and review of the literature. Gynecol Oncol 19:216, 1984

134. Hilton P: Mullerian adenofibroma. Case report. Br J Obstet Gyncol 91:1261, 1984

135. Iwai M, Konishi I, Pujii S, et al: A light and electron microscopic study of mullerian adenofibroma of the uterus. Acta Obstet Gynaecol Japon 36:44, 1984

136. Yonemitsu N, Nakahara M, Sugihara H et al: A case of mullerian adenosarcoma of the uterus. Gan No Rinsho 30:105, 1984

137. Oda Y, Nakanishi I, Tateiwa T: Intramural mullerian adenosarcoma of the uterus with adenomyosis. Arch Pathol Lab Med 108:798, 1984

138. Bjerregaard B, Moll M, Gram NC: Mulleradenosarkom i uterus. Ugeskr Laeger 147:2305, 1985

139. Chen KTK: Rhabdomyosarcomatous uterine adenosarcoma. Int J Gynecol Pathol 4:146, 1985

140. Bahari CM, Gorodeski IG, Avidor I: Case report of two primary tumors: mullerian adenosarcoma and endometrial adenocarcinoma. Isr J Med Sci 22:127, 1986

141. Hirschfield L, Kahn LB, Chen S et al: Mullerian adenosarcoma with ovarian sex cord-like differentiation: a light- and electron-microscopic study. Cancer 57:1197, 1986

142. Piura B, Hagay ZJ, Goldstein J: Infected mullerian adenosarcoma of the endometrium. J Surg Oncol 34:235, 1987

143. Agdal H, Wilken-Jensen C: Adenosarcoma uteri. Acta Obstet Gynecol Scand 66:183, 1987

144. Baker TR, Piver MS, Lele SB, Tsukada Y: Stage I uterine adenosarcoma: a report of six cases. J Surg Oncol 37:128, 1988

145. Dekel A, Dicker D, Kugler D et al: Mullerian adenosarcoma of the uterus: report of a rare case and review of the literature. Gynecol Oncol 30:291, 1988

146. Hajnal-Papp R, Szilagyi I. Malignant mullerian tumours of the uterus. Arch Gynecol Obstet 241:209, 1988

147. Gal D, Kerner H, Beck D et al: Mullerian adenosarcoma of the uterine cervix. Gynecol Oncol 31:445, 1988

148. Clement PB: Mullerian adenosarcomas of the uterus with sarcomatous overgrowth. A clinicopathological analysis of 10 cases. Am J Surg Pathol 13:28, 1989

149. Clement PB, Scully RE: Mullerian adenosarcomas of the uterus with sex cord-like elements. A clinicopathological analysis of eight cases. Am J Clin Pathol 91:664, 1989

150. Gast MJ, Radkins LV, Jacobs AJ, Gersell D: Mullerian adenosarcoma with heterologous elements: diagnostic and therapeutic approach. Gynecol Oncol 32:381, 1989

151. Clement PB, Scully RE: Mullerian adenosarcoma of the uterus: a clinicopathological analysis of 100 cases with a review of the literature. Hum Pathol 21:363, 1990

152. Clement PB, Scully RE: Mullerian adenofibroma of the uterus with invasion of myometrium and pelvic veins. Int J Gynecol Pathol 9:363, 1990

153. Seltzer VL, Levine A, Spiegel G et al: Adenofibroma of the uterus: multiple recurrences following wide local excision. Gynecol Oncol 37:427, 1990

154. Agarwal PK, Husain N, Chandrawati [sic]:

Adenofibroma of uterus and endocervix. Histopathology 18:79, 1991

155. Lack EE, Bitterman P, Sundeen JT: Mullerian adenosarcoma of the uterus with pure angiosarcoma: case report. Hum Pathol 22:1289, 1991

156. Raymundo Garcia C, Toro Rojas M, Morales Jiminez CM et al: Uterine mullerian adenosarcoma with histiocytic (xanthomatous) mesenchymal component. Histopathology 6:363, 1991

157. Kaku T, Silverberg SG, Major FJ et al: Adenosarcoma of the uterus: a gynecologic oncology group clinicopathologic study of 31 cases. Int J Gynecol Pathol 11:75, 1992

158. Bocklage T, Lee KR, Belinson JL: Uterine mullerian adenosarcoma following adenomyoma in a woman on Tamoxifen therapy. Gynecol Oncol 44:104, 1992

159. Miller KN, McLure SP: Papillary adenofibroma of the uterus. Report of a case involved by adenocarcinoma and review of the literature. Am J Clin Pathol 97:806, 1992

160. Thompson M, Husemeyer R: Carcinofibroma—a variant of the mixed mullerian tumor. Br J Obstet Gynaecol 88:1151, 1981

161. Peters WM, Wells M, Bryce FC: Mullerian clear cell carcinofibroma of the uterine corpus. Histopathology 8:1069, 1984

162. Chen KTK, Vergon JM: Carcinomesenchymoma of the uterus. Am J Clin Pathol 75:746, 1981

163. Clement PB, Scully RE: Uterine tumors resembling ovarian sex-cord tumors. A clinicopathologic analysis of fourteen cases. Am J Clin Pathol 66:512, 1976

164. Tang C, Toker C, Ances IG: Stromomyoma of the uterus. Cancer 43:308, 1979

165. Mazur MT, Kraus FT: Histogenesis of morphologic variations in tumors of the uterine wall. Am J Surg Pathol 4:59, 1980

166. Caglar H, Traub B, Jenis EH et al: Plexiform or sex cord tumors resembling tumors of the uterus. Am J Obstet Gynecol 145:639, 1983

167. Fekete PS, Vellios F, Patterson BD: Uterine tumor resembling an ovarian sex-cord tumor: Report of a case of an endometrial stromal tumor with foam cells and ultrastructural evidence of epithelial differentiation. Int J Gynecol Pathol 4:378, 1985

168. Iwasaki I, Yu TJ, Takahashi A et al: Uterine tumor resembling ovarian sex-cord tumor with osteoid metaplasia. Acta Pathol Jpn 36: 1391, 1986

169. Kantelip B, Cloup N, Dechelotte P: Uterine tumor resembling ovarian sex cord tumors: report of a case with ultrastructural study. Hum Pathol 17:91, 1986

170. Malfetano JH, Hussain M: A uterine tumor that resembled ovarian sex-cord tumors: A low-grade sarcoma. Obstet Gynecol 74:489, 1989

171. Sullinger JC, Edgerton SM, Scully RE: Uterine tumors resembling ovarian sex-cord tumors. An immunohistochemical analysis (submitted).

172. Sullinger JC, Scully RE: Uterine tumors resembling ovarian sex-cord tumors: a clinicopathologic study of 92 cases (in preparation).

173. Morehead RP, Bowman MC: Heterologous mesodermal tumors of the uterus; report of a neoplasm resembling a granulosa cell tumor. Am J Pathol 21:53, 1945

174. Langley FA, Smith JP, Woodcock AS: Debatable uterine tumors. Acta Obstet Gynaecol Scand 32:143, 1953

175. Devaney K, Tavassoli FA: Immunohistochemistry as a diagnostic aid in the interpretation of unusual mesenchymal tumors of the uterus. Arch Pathol Lab Med 4:225, 1991

176. Lillemoe TJ, Perrrone T, Norris HJ, Dehner LP: Myogenous phenotype of epithelial-like areas in endometrial stromal sarcomas. Arch Pathol Lab Med 115:215, 1991

177. Franquemont DW, Frierson HF Jr, Mills SE: An immunohistochemical study of normal endometrial stroma and endometrial stromal neoplasms. Evidence for smooth muscle differentiation. Am J Surg Pathol 15:861, 1991

178. Kurman RJ, Norris HJ: Mesenchymal tumors of the uterus. VI. Epithelioid smooth muscle tumors including leiomyoblastoma and clear-cell leiomyoma. A clinical and pathologic analysis of 26 cases. Cancer 36: 1853, 1976

179. Kaminski PS, Tavassoli FA: Plexiform tumorlet: a clinical and pathological study of 15 cases with ultrastructural observations. Int J Gynecol Pathol 3:124, 1984

180. Mazur MT: Atypical polypoid adenomyomas of the endometrium. Am J Surg Pathol 5:473, 1981
181. Young RH, Treger T, Scully RE: Atypical polypoid adenomyoma of the uterus. A report of 27 cases. Am J Clin Pathol 86:139, 1986
182. Delprado WJ, Stevens SMB, Baird PJ: Atypical polypoid adenomyoma: a case report with ultrastructural examination. Pathology 17:522, 1985
183. Clement PB, Young RH: Atypical polypoid adenomyoma of the uterus associated with Turner's syndrome. A report of three cases, including a review of "estrogen-associated" endometrial neoplasms and neoplasms associated with Turner's syndrome. Int J Gynecol Pathol 6:104, 1987
184. Rollason TP, Redman CWE: Atypical polypoid adenomyoma—clinical histological and immunocytochemical findings. Eur J Gynaecol Oncol 9:444, 1988
185. Di Palma S, Santini D, Martinelli G: Atypical polypoid adenomyoma of the uterus. An immunohistochemical study of a case. Tumori 75:292, 1989
186. Staros EB, Shilkitus WF: Atypical polypoid adenomyoma with carcinomatous transformation: a case report. Surg Pathol 4:157, 1991
187. Kim K, Scully RE: Peritoneal keratin granulomas with carcinomas of endometrium and ovary and atypical polypoid adenomyoma of endometrium. Am J Surg Pathol 14:925, 1990
188. Clement PB, Scully RE: Uterine tumors with mixed epithelial and mesenchymal elements. Semin Diagn Pathol 5:199, 1988

8

Miscellaneous Primary Neoplasms and Metastatic Neoplasms

Philip B. Clement

PAPILLOMAS

SQUAMOUS PAPILLOMAS

The designation *squamous papilloma* has been used, predominantly in the older literature, to refer to papillary squamous lesions of the cervix with an appearance that has varied from benign to squamous cell carcinoma in situ.[1-7] The vast majority of these lesions would be currently classified as typical or dysplastic condyloma acuminatum, papillary squamous cell carcinoma in situ,[8] or verrucous carcinoma (see Ch. 2). In the most recent study of 21 cases of papillary squamous lesions of the cervix, for example, Qizilbash categorized 15 as condyloma, four as "true squamous papilloma," and two as verrucous carcinomas.[7] All the "squamous papillomas," however, contained multifocal areas of severe squamous dysplasia or carcinoma in situ, suggesting that they represented in situ papillary squamous carcinomas rather than papillomas. If true, noncondylomatous nondysplastic squamous papillomas of the cervix exist, they must be extremely rare, and such a diagnosis should be rendered only after the lesion has been completely examined microscopically to exclude the lesions in the differential diagnosis cited above.

MÜLLERIAN PAPILLOMAS

Müllerian papilloma, a rare benign epithelial tumor of the exocervix (or less commonly, the vagina), was once erroneously considered of mesonephric origin, but is now considered müllerian in nature.[9-12] In addition to their own case, Andrews et al. found 18 previously described cases in the literature.[11] These papillomas occur exclusively in children typically between 2 and 5 years of age (range 14 months to 9 years), although one case in an adult has been encountered[13]; vaginal bleeding or discharge are the usual symptoms. On clinical examination, the typically small (1 to 2 cm in diameter), friable, polypoid to papillary lesions involve the anterior or posterior lip or protrude through the external os. Microscopic examination reveals fine branching papillae typically lined by a single layer of benign-appearing epithelial cells that vary from flattened to cuboidal to columnar (Fig. 8-1). A focal lining of stratified squamous epithelium has been noted in some cases.[9] The fibrovascular cores of the papillae are variably edematous and often contain a variety of inflammatory cells. Psammoma bodies or osseous metaplasia have been rare findings within the stroma. A variety of features, including a superficial location, the presence of intracellular mucin in some

371

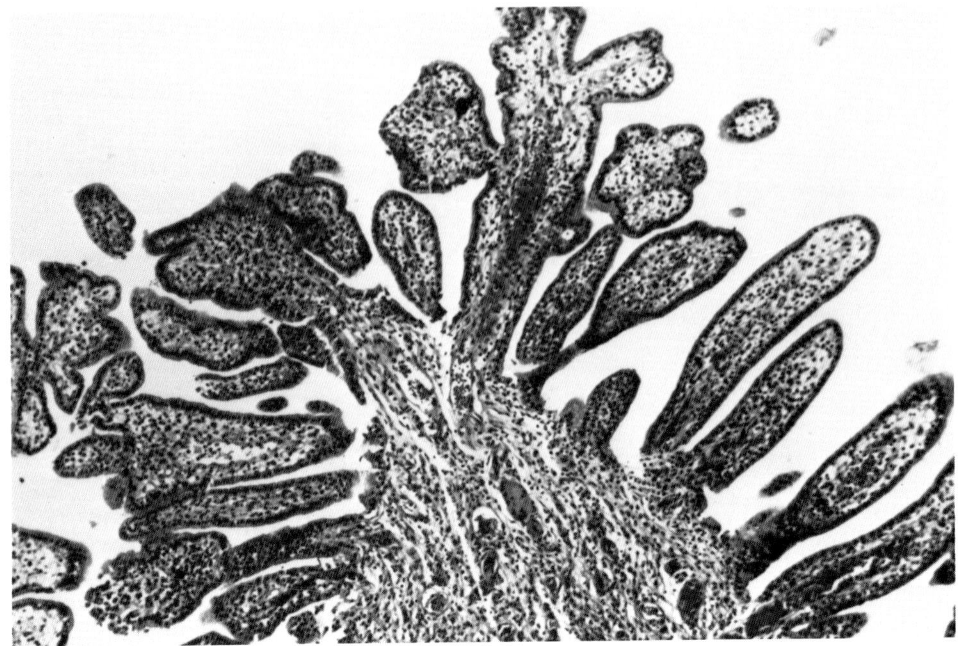

Fig. 8-1. Müllerian papilloma of cervix.

cases, a lack of association with typical mesonephric remnants, as well as ultrastructural findings, have established a müllerian origin. In all reported patients, follow-up has been uneventful or a local "recurrence" (possibly due to incomplete primary excision) has been treated successfully by re-excision. The differential diagnosis includes papillary endocervicitis (see Ch.1), villous and villoglandular papillary adenomas (see below), and villoglandular carcinomas (see Ch. 3).

VILLOUS AND VILLOGLANDULAR PAPILLARY ADENOMAS

A lesion closely related to the müllerian papilloma is the rare cervical villoglandular papillary adenoma, which has an architecture similar to that of a villoglandular papillary adenocarcinoma but contains uniformly well-differentiated cells[13] (Fig. 8-2). An occasional villoglandular tumor, however, has both benign and malignant components (see Ch. 3). Two cases of "villous adenoma" of the uterine cervix associated with underlying invasive carcinoma have been reported.[14, 15] In one of the cases, the invasive adenocarcinoma was well differentiated, with nuclear features similar to those of the villous portion of the tumor, whereas in the other case, the invasive portion of the tumor had more atypical nuclear features than the villous component. The benign and malignant components in both tumors were immunoreactive for carcinoembryonic antigen.

ADENOMATOID TUMORS

Adenomatoid tumors, benign tumors of mesothelial origin, are more common in the uterus[16–27a] than the number of cases in the literature (less than 100) would suggest; many are probably misinterpreted on gross examination as leiomyomas and not examined microscopically. Studies in which all

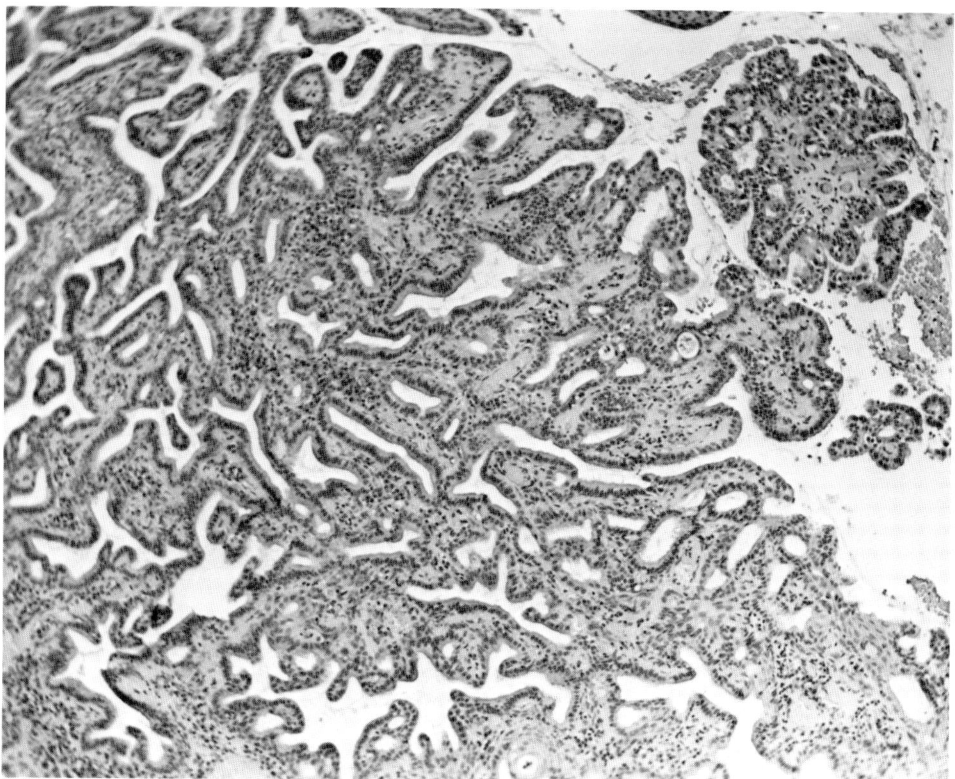

Fig. 8-2. Villoglandular adenoma of cervix.

myometrial nodules in consecutive hysterectomy specimens are sampled histologically indicate that the frequency of the tumors in such specimens is as high as 1.2 percent.[18] The tumors typically occur in women of reproductive age. Because of their usual small size, uterine adenomatoid tumors are typically an incidental pathologic finding, but occasional larger examples have been symptomatic.[20, 23–26] In one unique case, the presence of signet-ring-like cells within an endometrial curettage specimen was the presenting manifestation.[22] Occasional uterine tumors are accompanied by a similar tumor within the fallopian tube.[24]

On gross examination (Fig. 8-3), adenomatoid tumors are typically less than 4 cm in diameter; the mean diameter in one study was 2.1 cm.[19] Occasional cystic tumors, however, have been as large as 13 cm.[20, 23, 25, 26] The tumors most commonly form solitary masses in the fundus, often near a cornu. They typically involve the outer myometrium and are frequently subserosal (Fig. 8-3). Larger tumors may be transmural and, rarely, may extend into the endometrium.[22] Rare tumors have diffusely involved the myometrium.[27a] Occasional tumors are multiple and bilateral cornual tumors have been documented.[16, 18, 24] The sectioned surface is typically solid, gray-tan to gray-pink to yellow, and sometimes whorled or trabeculated, but usually less well circumscribed than a leiomyoma (Fig. 8-3). Small cysts may be appreciated on close inspection of the cut surface and occasionally within the overlying serosa. Rare tumors have been predominantly or entirely cystic, with fluid-filled locules of variable size separated by thin septa.[20, 23, 25, 26]

Microscopic examination typically shows the characteristic formations of adenomatoid tumor scattered irregularly on

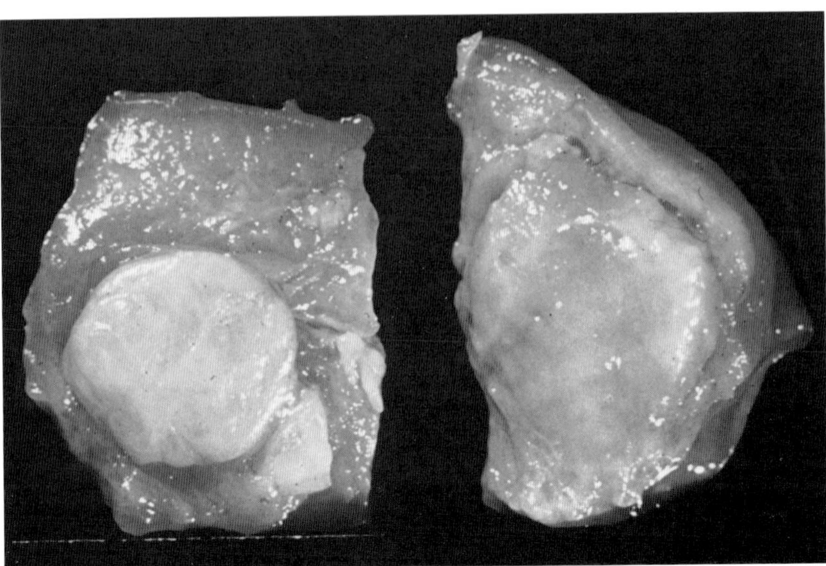

Fig. 8-3. An adenomatoid tumor within subserosal myometrium **(right)** and a uterine leiomyoma **(left)** for comparison. The adenomatoid tumor is less well circumscribed than the leiomyoma and lacks its characteristic whorled appearance.

a background of myometrial smooth muscle (Fig. 8-4). The periphery of the lesion may be well delineated in some cases, but it frequently is ill-defined. Rarely, an origin from the overlying mesothelium is seen.[20] Quigley and Hart encountered four patterns in their series of uterine tumors. One pattern usually predominated, although two or more patterns were frequent within a single tumor, as were transitions between the various patterns.[19] In the most common patterns (Fig. 8-5), anastomosing gland-like spaces are lined by cuboidal cells that often contain cytoplasmic vacuoles (adenoid pattern), or larger spaces are lined by flattened endothelium-like cells mimicking a vascular tumor (angiomatoid pattern). Much less commonly, polygonal cells with eosinophilic cytoplasm and occasional vacuoles grow in sheets, columns or plexiform cords ("solid" pattern) or numerous large cavities lined by flattened cells are separated by thin fibrous septa (cystic pattern). A rare papillary pattern resembles that seen in well-differentiated papillary mesotheliomas.[23, 27a] The intracellular vacuoles that may occur in several of the aforementioned

patterns of adenomatoid tumor may result in signet-ring–like cells, as mentioned above. The tumor cells in all the various patterns have bland, round to oval, mitotically inactive nuclei.

As noted above, the neoplastic elements in many cases are widely separated by hyperplastic myometrial smooth muscle potentially mimicking a leiomyoma on microscopic examination. In other cases, the stroma is loose and edematous or densely fibrous and hyalinized. Collections of lymphocytes, sometimes in the form of lymphoid follicles, are a common finding in the vicinity of the tumors[16, 20]; foamy histiocytes were prominent in one case.[21] In cases in which there is continuity with the uterine serosa, the latter may be focally replaced by tumor or exhibit papillary mesothelial hyperplasia, mesothelial inclusions, endosalpingiosis, fibrous adhesions, or combinations thereof.[19] Histochemical stains may be useful in confirming the presence of acid mucins (predominantly hyaluronic acid) within the vacuoles and lumina of the tumor, and in contrast to adenocarcinomas, an absence or paucity of

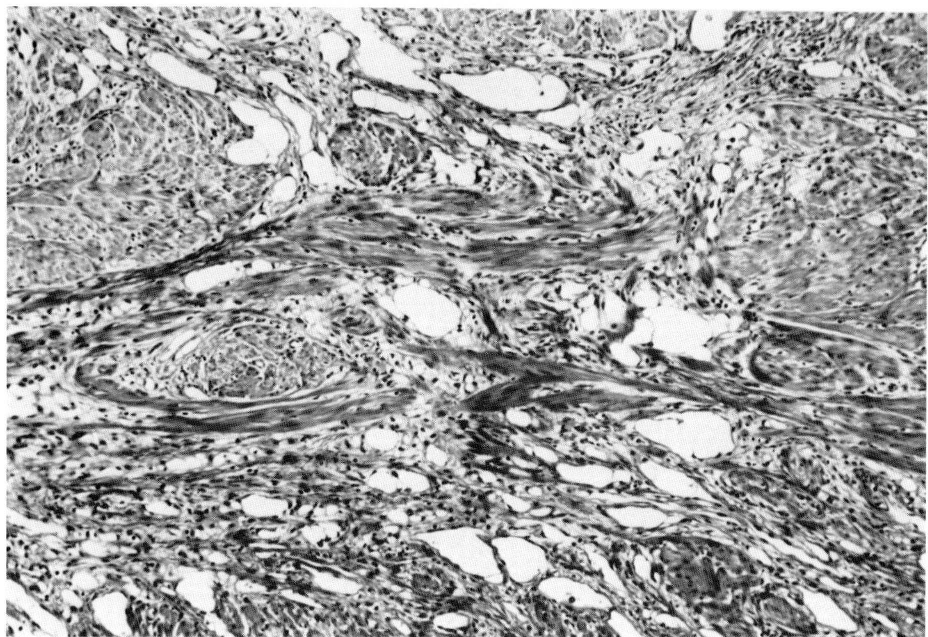

Fig. 8-4. Adenomatoid tumor infiltrating myometrial smooth muscle.

neutral mucins.[19, 27] The neoplastic cells are immunoreactive for cytokeratin and vimentin and have the typical ultrastructural features of mesothelial cells.[21–27]

The differential diagnosis of uterine adenomatoid tumor on gross examination includes leiomyoma, as well as adenomyosis, and, when the tumors are cystic, cystic

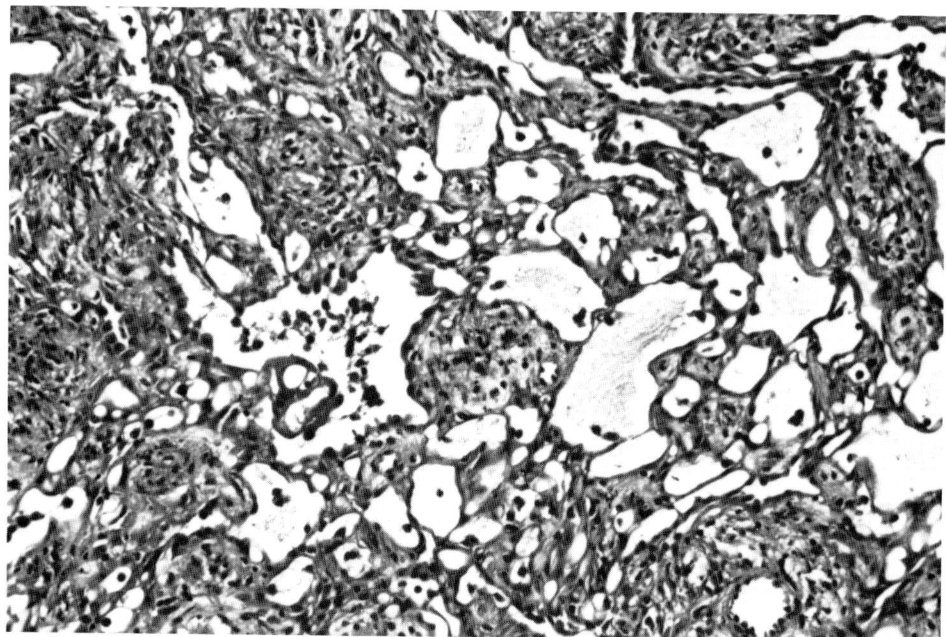

Fig. 8-5. Adenomatoid tumor.

lymphangioma and potentially other rare cystic lesions of the uterus (see Ch. 4) and pelvic peritoneum, such as peritoneal inclusion cysts (PICs). Although adenomatoid tumors may be grossly indistinguishable from leiomyomas, features favoring adenomatoid tumor over leiomyoma include a posterior, especially cornual, subserosal location, abnormalities of the overlying serosa, a color that is tan-gray to pink to yellow (rather than white), and a border that is not sharply circumscribed.[16, 19] On microscopic examination, the differential diagnosis includes leiomyoma (of both typical and epithelioid types), vascular tumors (hemangioma, lymphangioma), metastatic adenocarcinoma (particularly of signet-ring cell type), and, in the case of cystic tumors, PICs.[19, 22, 27] Although PICs may involve the uterine serosa and contain foci that closely resemble adenomatoid tumor,[28] they lack the characteristic mural location of the adenomatoid tumor. Awareness of the characteristic gross and microscopic features of adenomatoid tumors, together with the appropriate histochemical and immunohistochemical stains in problematic cases, will facilitate its distinction from the aforementioned lesions.

SMALL CELL UNDIFFERENTIATED (NEUROENDOCRINE) CARCINOMAS

SMALL CELL UNDIFFERENTIATED CARCINOMAS OF THE CERVIX

Small cell carcinomas of the cervix were originally considered a rare subtype of squamous cell carcinoma characterized by a highly malignant behavior. Although small cell squamous carcinomas exist (pp. 75 and 383), it has become apparent during the past 15 years that the majority of small cell carcinomas of the cervix express neuroendocrine differentiation.[29–86] In a minority of such tumors, squamous differentiation may also be present, as discussed below. The designations small cell undifferentiated carcinoma, neuroendocrine carcinoma, oat cell carcinoma, argyrophilic carcinoma, endocrine carcinoma, malignant carcinoid tumor, and malignant apudoma have been applied to these tumors. Because they are classified primarily on the basis of their appearance on routine light microscopy and because not all of them exhibit neuroendocrine differentiation, the term *small cell undifferentiated carcinoma* (SCUC) has generally been preferred. Conversely, occasional cervical carcinomas not of small cell type, such as rare adenosquamous carcinomas,[65, 87] have exhibited neuroendocrine differentiation on immunohistochemical or ultrastructural examination. The term *carcinoid tumor* should be avoided, except to refer to a well-differentiated tumor, resembling typical carcinoid tumors within the intestinal tract, with uniform nuclei and infrequent mitotic figures. It is questionable if such a tumor has been described within the cervix. Some tumors composed of larger cells arranged in insular and trabecular patterns (and with argentaffin granules in some cases) have resembled so-called poorly differentiated carcinoids. The "endocrine carcinomas of intermediate cell type" described by Silva et al. appear to fall into this category.[55] However, the prognosis of such tumors is similar to typical small cell carcinomas, and both are considered together in this discussion.

SCUCs may arise from argyrophilic cells, which have been demonstrated within the ectocervical or endocervical epithelium in 2 to 43 percent of normal subjects[88, 89] and as many as 35 percent of patients with SCUCs.[34] Some tumors, however, particularly those with an admixed squamous or adenocarcinomatous component, may originate from subcolumnar reserve cells.

Clinical Features

Approximately 250 SCUCs of the cervix have been described in the literature.[29–86] In most studies, they have accounted for approximately 2 percent of cervical carcinomas (range, 0.5 to 5 percent).[54] The clinical features of patients with SCUCs are similar to those of patients with squamous cell carcinomas. The age of individual patients has ranged widely (21 to 87 years), although in most series the median and mean ages are in the fifth decade. Four SCUCs have been encountered in pregnant women.[76] Most patients present with abnormal vaginal bleeding and have an obvious cervical mass on pelvic examination. Rare patients have presented with abdominal symptoms related to the presence of ovarian metastases.[84] The proportion of patients with SCUCs that have an abnormal Papanicolaou smear is smaller than in patients with squamous cell carcinoma, a feature attributed to the frequent absence of an associated in situ component, rapid growth of the tumor, or both.[71] An elevated serum carcinoembryonic antigen (CEA) level at presentation has been found in occasional patients.[39]

Approximately 75 percent of patients with SCUCs are clinical stage I or II, a figure similar to that for patients with squamous cell carcinoma. Many such patients, however, are of a higher stage if operative findings are considered. In one study of patients with clinical stage IB or IIA SCUCs undergoing pelvic lymph node dissection, 57 percent were found to have lymph node metastases; all patients with positive nodes had tumors larger than 2 cm.[69] In another series, however, 40 percent of stage IB tumors smaller than 3 cm had positive nodes.[70] In the most recent large study of SCUCs in the literature, 60 percent of patients were surgical stage III or IV.[76] Some patients have had ovarian metastases at presentation.[37, 84]

Despite the wide variety of hormones detectable immunohistochemically in SCUCs (see below), clinical or biochemical evidence of hormone production is rare. This observation suggests that the hormonal polypeptides are secreted in an inactive form, in insufficient levels to produce clinical syndromes, or are rapidly inactivated in the circulation.[55] Six patients have had Cushing's syndrome, some with documented elevations in serum adenocorticotropic hormone (ACTH), and in one, antidiuretic hormone (ADH)[29, 35, 42, 46, 49]; two patients have had hypoglycemia (one with elevated serum insulin)[31, 33]; three patients have had the carcinoid syndrome, one of whom had elevated serum levels of ACTH, cortisol, and human chorionic gonadotropin (hCG), and in another, there were elevated levels of somatostatin, ACTH, and serotonin[30, 62, 84]; one patient has had the syndrome of inappropriate ADH (SIADH) secretion (with elevated serum levels of ADH)[78]; one patient has had elevated serum and tumor levels of serotonin (but not the carcinoid syndrome)[77]; and one patient has had elevated serum levels of calcitonin.[73] The tumor from one of the patients with Cushing's syndrome was found to contain high levels of serotonin, ACTH, β-melanocyte-stimulating hormone (MSH), ACTH, histamine, and amylase.[42] Tumor extracts from four other SCUCs that were clinically nonfunctioning have contained one or more hormones including somatostatin, pancreatic polypeptide, calcitonin, vasointestinal polypeptide (VIP), ACTH, β-MSH, neuron-specific enolase (NSE), and insulin.[53, 86]

Gross and Microscopic Features

On gross examination (Fig. 8-6), SCUCs of the cervix are indistinguishable from squamous cell carcinomas. Many tumors are large ulcerating masses that frequently encompass and destroy the cervix and extend into the parametria, vagina, and occasionally, the corpus.

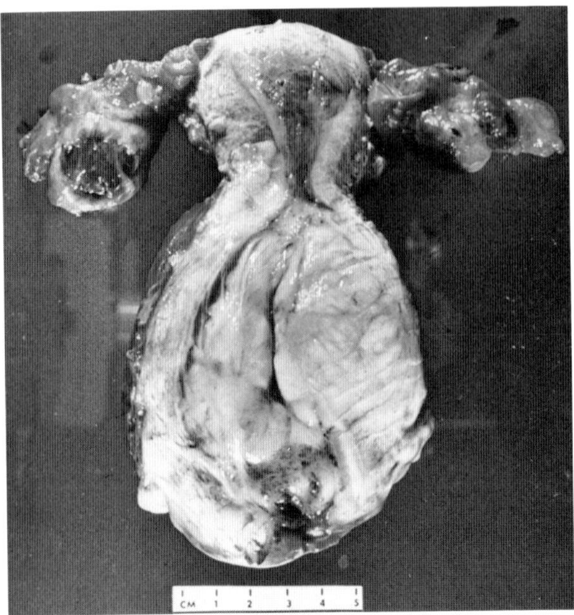

Fig. 8-6. Small cell undifferentiated carcinoma of cervix. The tumor expands the cervix and diffusely infiltrates its wall. (From Clement,[256] with permission.)

On microscopic examination, the tumors are typically densely cellular and exhibit a variety of patterns, frequently admixed, including solid sheets, ill-defined or sharply outlined nests, trabeculae, and single cells (Figs. 8-7 to 8-12). Small rosette-like or acinar structures (Fig. 8-11), sometimes containing periodic acid-Schiff (PAS)-positive material, may be present and when numerous impart a pseudoglandular pattern.[34, 55] As in pulmonary small cell undifferentiated carcinomas, both small (oat) and intermediate-type cells can be identified, with usually one cell type predominating. The small cells are oval to spindle in shape and contain scanty cytoplasm and hyperchromatic, molded nuclei with finely dispersed chromatin and indistinct nucleoli (Figs. 8-7 to 8-9). Nuclear detail is often obscured by intense hyperchromasia, smudged chromatin, and crush artifact.[67] The cells of intermediate type are round to polygonal and medium-sized with moderate amounts of pale, eosinophilic cytoplasm and ill-defined cell borders (Figs. 8-10 to 8-12); the cells may exhibit peripheral palisading[36, 55] (Fig. 8-12). Their round to oval nuclei are more

uniform than those of the small cells and exhibit a more coarse chromatin pattern; nucleoli may be prominent (Fig. 8-12). Mitotic figures are numerous within both the small and intermediate-type cells[55, 58, 67, 76]; in one study, two-thirds of cases had 20 to 50 mitotic figures per 10 high-power fields (MF/10 HPF), whereas the remaining cases had more than 50 MF/10 HPF.[76] Nuclear fragmentation (hematoxylin bodies)[81] and single-cell or confluent necrosis are frequently present. Foci of typical squamous cell carcinoma or adenocarcinoma (either of which may be in situ or invasive, or both) are present in as many as one-half of cases; these invasive components may be discrete or intimately admixed with the neoplastic small cells. The tumors typically have a delicate, fibrovascular stroma; a desmoplastic stromal response may occur but is uncommon. An inflammatory response is usually inconspicuous. Perivascular hematoxylin staining[67] and amyloid-like material within the stroma have been present in occasional cases. Lymphatic and vascular invasion is often prominent. The histologic appearance of

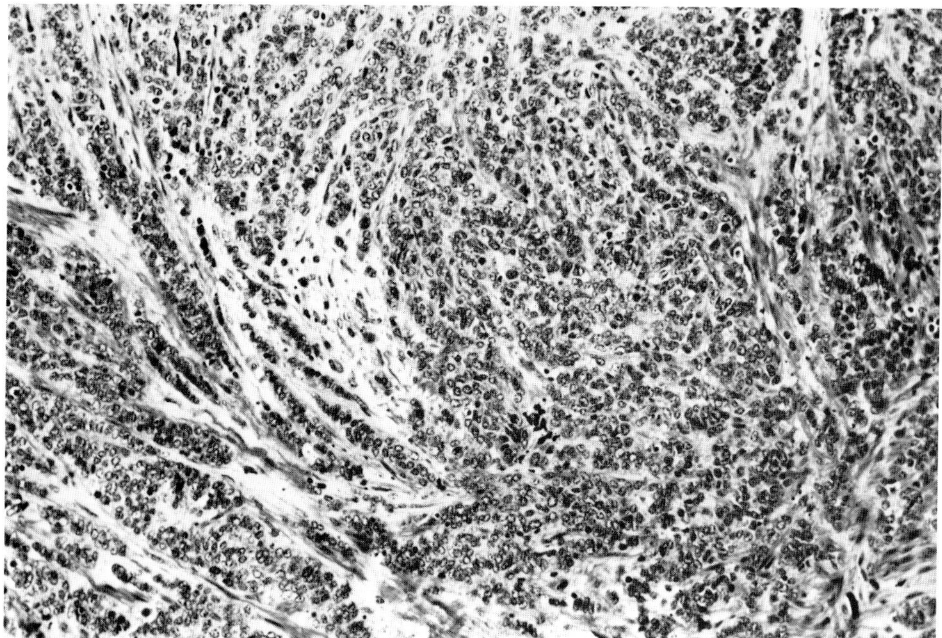

Fig. 8-7. Small cell undifferentiated carcinoma of cervix. The cellular tumor is composed of small cells with scanty cytoplasm arranged in sheets, nests, and ribbons, and as individually disposed cells within the sparse stroma.

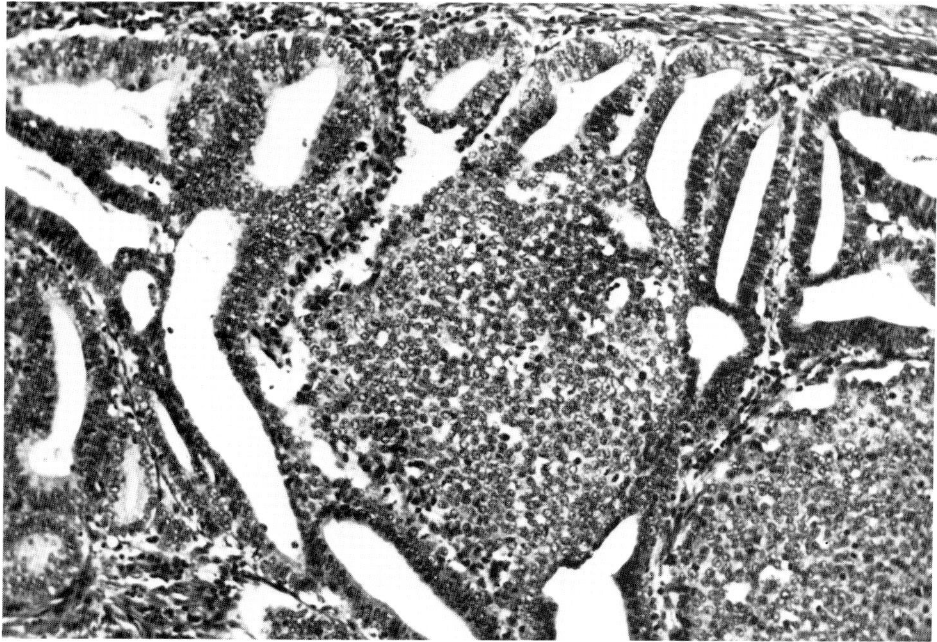

Fig. 8-8. Small cell undifferentiated carcinoma of cervix admixed with adenocarcinoma.

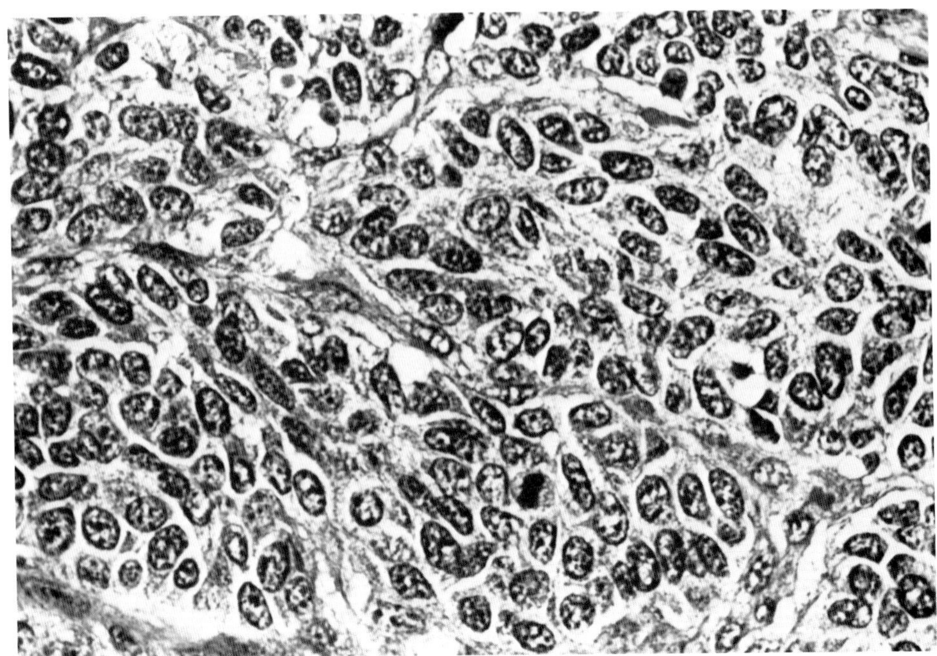

Fig. 8-9. Small cell undifferentiated carcinoma of cervix, higher-power view of tumor in Figure 8-7.

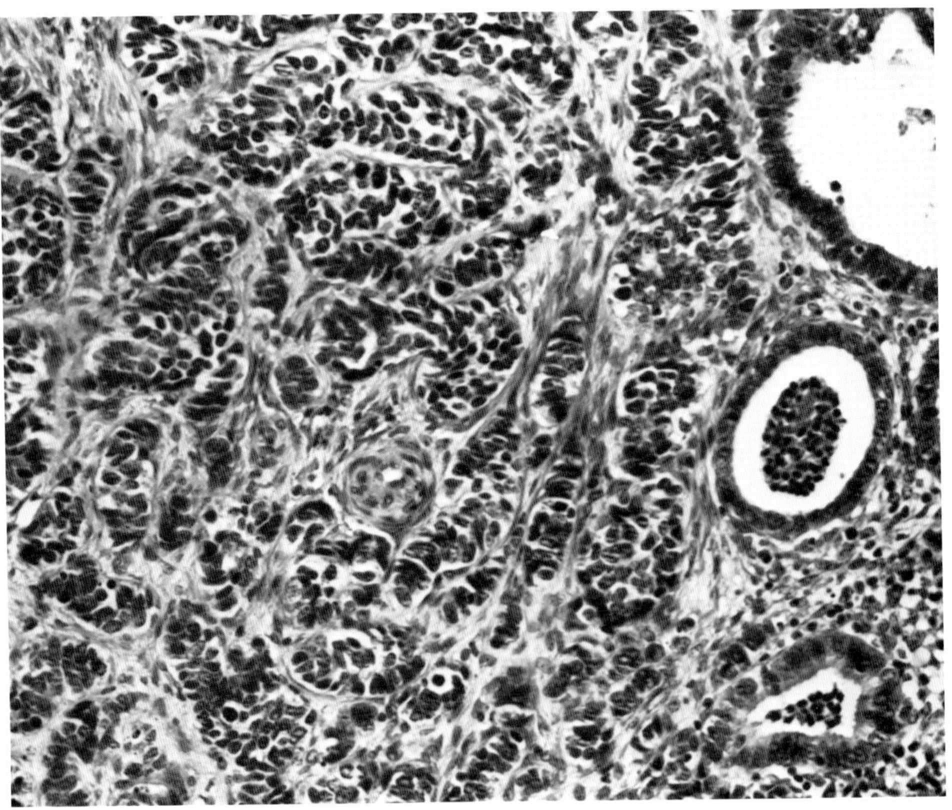

Fig. 8-10. Small cell undifferentiated carcinoma of cervix, intermediate cell type, with adjacent adenocarcinoma (extreme right). The cells are arranged in trabeculae.

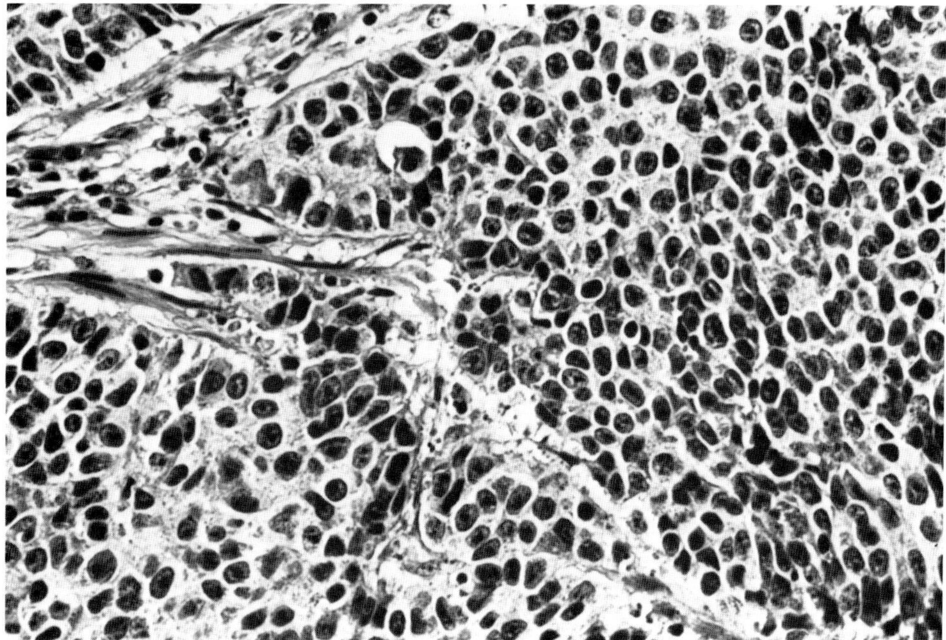

Fig. 8-11. Small cell undifferentiated carcinoma of cervix, intermediate cell type. The tumor cells have moderate amounts of pale cytoplasm that was argyrophilic and strongly immunoreactive for chromogranin (see Fig. 8-13). Note small acinus.

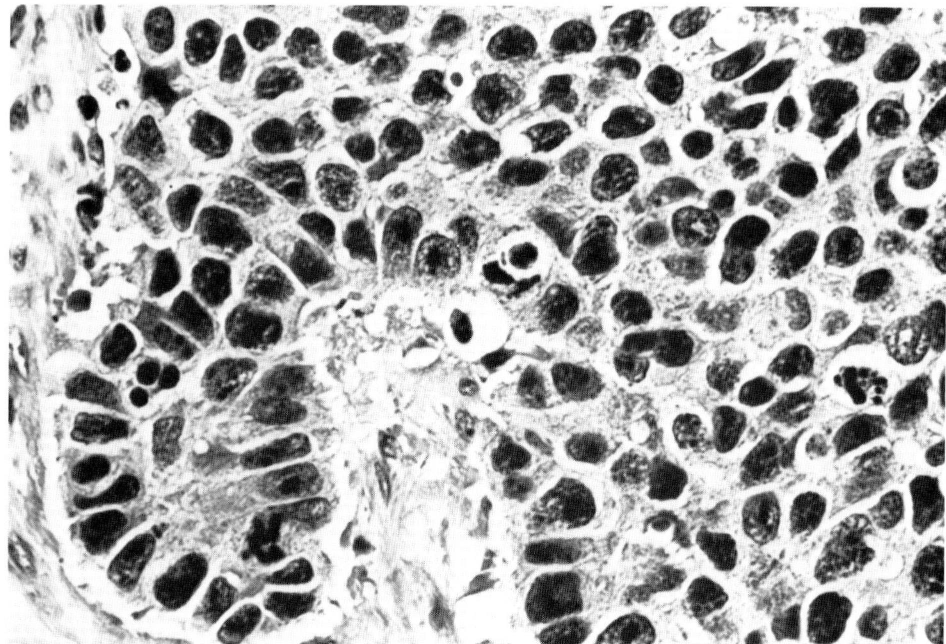

Fig. 8-12. Small cell undifferentiated carcinoma of cervix, intermediate cell type, higher power of tumor in Figure 8-11. Note peripheral nuclear palisading. Compared with the cells in Figure 8-9, the nuclei have coarser chromatin and some contain a prominent nucleolus.

metastatic or recurrent tumor is typically indistinguishable from that of the primary; occasional adenocarcinomas of the cervix have had a component of SCUC in recurrent or metastatic tumor that was not demonstrable within the primary tumor.[55]

Findings With Special Techniques

Most recent studies of SCUCs have shown that the majority of cases exhibit evidence of neuroendocrine differentiation, as determined by one or more techniques. The frequency with which the tumor cells contain arygyrophilic granules has varied from only a minority of cases to all the tumors in a particular series; the staining may be very focal and require prolonged search.[67] Argentaffin cells have been demonstrated in only very rare cases.[42, 45, 84] and appear to be more common in tumors of intermediate cell type. SCUCs have been shown to be variably immunoreactive for a wide variety of antigens, including cytokeratins (low- and high-molecular-weight), epithelial membrane antigen (EMA), CEA, NSE, chromogranin (Fig. 8-13), HNK-1, Leu-7, and synaptophysin, as well as for a variety of polypeptide and amine hormones, including ACTH, calcitonin, gastrin, serotonin, substance P, VIP, pancreatic polypeptide, and somatostatin.[41, 53, 55, 56, 63, 67, 74, 81] One example of a cervical SCUC was found to have an associated hyperplasia of benign-appearing cells within adjacent normal endocervical glands and glands showing adenocarcinoma in situ; the cells were argyrophilic and immunoreactive for NSE and chromogranin.[75]

The ultrastructural features of SCUCs have been well described elsewhere.[58, 67] As with similar tumors in the lung, the heterogeneity noted at the light microscopic level is reflected by electron microscopic examination. Dense-core granules can be demonstrated in most, but not all, SCUCs; they

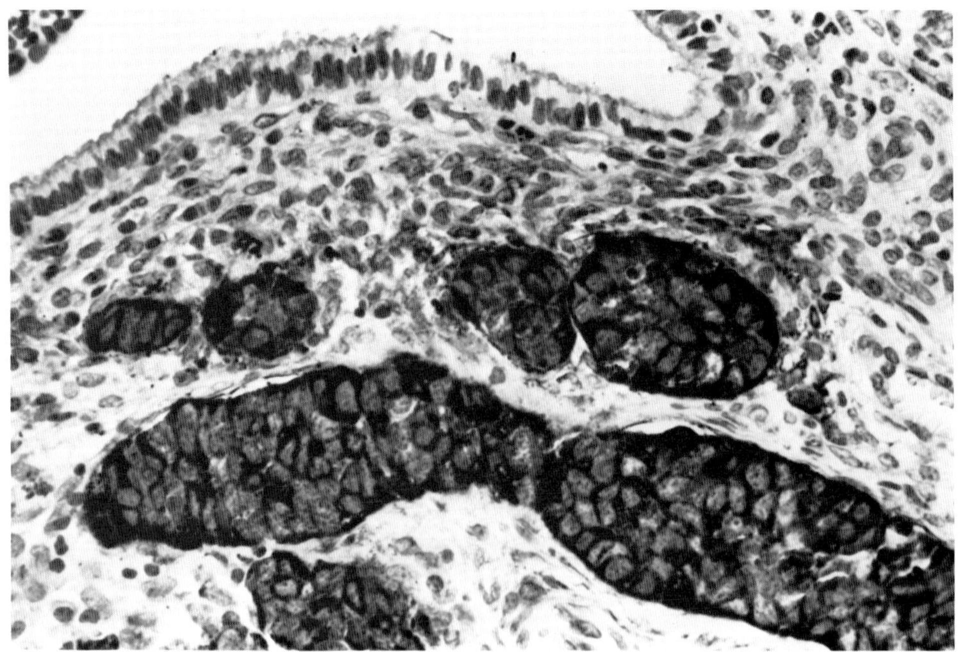

Fig. 8-13. Small cell undifferentiated carcinoma of cervix, intermediate cell type. The cells are intensely immunoreactive for chromogranin.

vary from scanty to numerous, and are often concentrated within dendritic cell processes. Absence of dense core granules may reflect sampling error, cyclic granule production and depletion, or dedifferentiation of the cells.[67] Microvilli, microfilaments, and poorly formed desmosomes with or without tonofilaments have also been observed, reflecting variable degrees of glandular or squamous differentiation that may not be appreciable histologically.[34, 42, 58, 67] In rare cases, both endocrine and exocrine features may be identified within the same neoplastic cells ("amphicrine carcinoma").[85]

Recently, an association between cervical SCUCs and human papillomavirus type 18 (HPV 18) has been found in most[81, 90, 91] but not all[92] studies. Combining the results of three studies, HPV 18 DNA or messenger RNA (mRNA) has been found in 62 percent of cases; in one study, the corresponding figure for SCUCs with neuroendocrine differentiation was 78 percent.[90] In another series, the presence of HPV 18 DNA was associated with a high frequency of lymph node metastases, and a significant association was found between the presence of aneuploidy, mitotic activity, and HPV 18 DNA.[81] HPV 16 has also been detected, but only in a small minority of cases,[81, 90] and in one series was confined to SCUCs showing squamous differentiation.[90] DNA ploidy analysis of 16 cases in one study revealed that 5 tumors were diploid and 11 were hyperploid,[76] whereas in another study of 6 cases, four tumors were peridiploid and two were aneuploid.[81] In a third study, all 14 cases were aneuploid.[82]

Differential Diagnosis

The differential diagnosis of cervical SCUCs includes other small cell malignant neoplasms that may involve the cervix, including small cell squamous carcinoma (SCSC), lymphoepithelioma-like carcinoma, adenoid basal carcinoma, lymphoma and leukemia, endometrial stromal sarcoma, and metastatic small cell carcinoma. The last three lesions, as well as neuroectodermal tumors, are in the differential diagnosis of endometrial SCUCs involving the endometrium (discussed below). All these tumors are discussed in detail elsewhere in this volume or later in this chapter. Although their distinction from SCUCs on histologic grounds alone may occasionally be difficult, particularly on a small biopsy specimen, routine light microscopic findings are usually diagnostic, and the histochemical, immunohistochemical, and ultrastructural findings will facilitate the diagnosis in problem cases. With respect to the differential diagnosis with SCSCs, a recent study found that a number of features favored a diagnosis of SCUC over SCSC, including a younger age (mean 36 years vs. 50 years for SCSC), an absence of squamous intraepithelial neoplasia (vs. 60 percent for SCSC), immunoreactivity for neuroendocrine markers combined with nonreactivity for cytokeratin (all tumors with this immunoprofile were SCUC), and the presence of HPV 18 DNA (60 percent vs. 36 percent for SCSC).[81] Despite these findings, significant overlap existed between the two groups of tumors, and the authors concluded that the distinction between SCUC and SCSC should be based primarily on their histologic features (see Ch. 2).

Behavior and Prognostic Factors

SCUCs, of both small and intermediate cell types, are highly aggressive neoplasms; this behavior appears independent of the presence or absence of neuroendocrine differentiation as demonstrated by special techniques.[67, 76] The tumors have a propensity to metastasize early and widely by both lymphatic and hematogenous routes, and involvement of regional and distant lymph nodes, lung, bone, brain, and liver is common. The disease-free interval is usually less than 2 years and almost 70 percent of recurrences were noted within 12 months of therapy in one study.[70] Approximately three-quarters of the patients reported in the literature have died from tumor progression or were alive with tumor at the time of reporting.

The best indicator is the surgical (pathologic) stage.[76] In one study, 8 of 11 patients with pathologic stage I or II disease survived 4 years (a survival rate similar to that of squamous cell carcinoma or adenocarcinoma in this site), whereas 22 of 23 patients with stage III or IV disease died of tumor.[76] Other potential adverse prognostic factors include lymph node involvement[63] and aneuploidy,[76, 81] although whether these factors have a prognostic effect independent of stage is not clear.[76] The presence of an admixed squamous or glandular component was associated with a better survival rate (35 percent vs. 8 percent) in one study,[76] but was not prognostically significant in two others.[67, 71] A DNA index of less than 1.5 was associated with prolonged survival in a recent series.[82] Factors not affecting prognosis in one study included mitotic rate, the presence of vascular invasion, and the number of quadrants involved by tumor.[76] Another study has shown a correlation between disease-free intervals and survival with primary tumor size. Median disease-free intervals and survival were 6 months and 13 months for patients with tumors greater than 2 cm; the corresponding figures for patients with tumors less than 2 cm were 30 months and 37 months.[69]

SMALL CELL CARCINOMA OF THE
ENDOMETRIUM

SCUCs of the endometrium are much less common that those of cervical origin; only 25 cases have been reported[94–104] (1 case was reported twice),[94, 100] but only 9 in

detail. Eight of the latter were postmenopausal (59 to 72 years of age), whereas the ninth was 23 years old. The mean age of patients with the small cell type of SCUC of the endometrium in a series of 14 cases (that included those of intermediate cell type) was 58.3 years.[103] The presenting manifestations are usually abnormal vaginal bleeding, or less commonly, pain, uterine enlargement, abnormal cytology, or combinations thereof. One patient presented with a paraneoplastic retinopathy.[104] At least 5 of the 9 patients had metastatic tumor at presentation, involving pelvic lymph nodes (three cases), the ovary (one case), or the vagina (one case). In one case, the SCUC was diagnosed on curettage after the patient had received chemotherapy for a well differentiated endometrial adenocarcinoma, and was interpreted as a dedifferentiated form of the latter tumor.[102] Six of the nine patients died of disease within 12 months, one patient developed a vaginal recurrence at 3 months, and the other two were alive with no evidence of tumor at 1 and 5 years. The 5- and 10-year survival rates in the series of 14 cases cited above were 64 percent.[103]

On gross examination, the tumors typically form bulky polypoid masses that fill the endometrial cavity and deeply invade the myometrium; one tumor, however, was confined to a polyp. Microscopically, the nine tumors reported in detail were typical small cell carcinomas of small (oat) cell type (Figs. 8-14 and 8-15); an unspecified number of the 14 cases in the series cited above were of intermediate-cell type.[103] Four of the tumors were admixed with another neoplasm, an adenosquamous carcinoma (two cases), a poorly differentiated adenocarcinoma (one case), and a malignant müllerian mixed tumor (one case). Similarly, we have found that approximately two-thirds of 15 personally studied small cell carcinomas of the endometrium have been associated with an adenocarcinoma of endometrioid type (Gilks et al.: un-

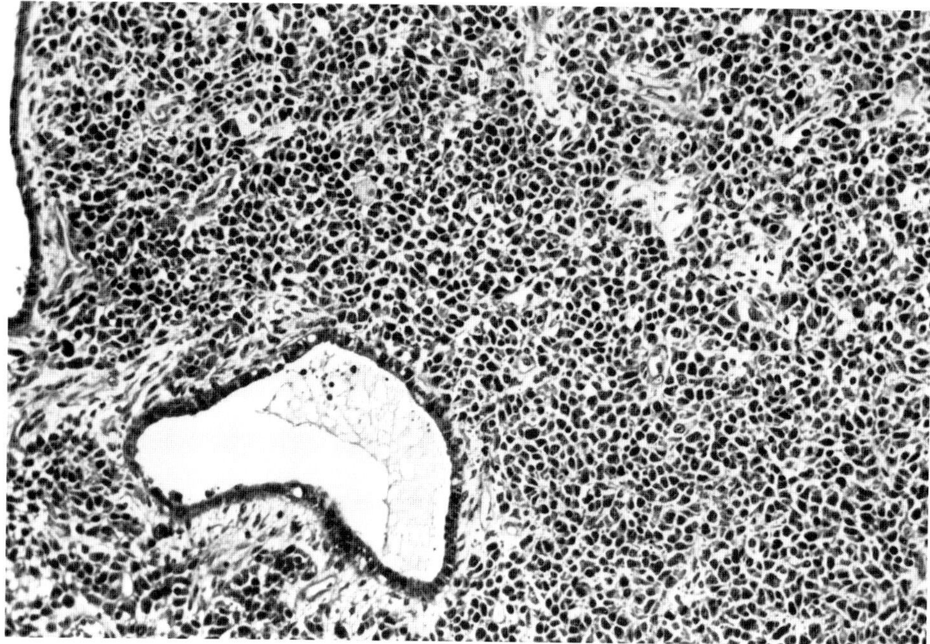

Fig. 8-14. Small cell undifferentiated carcinoma of endometrium.

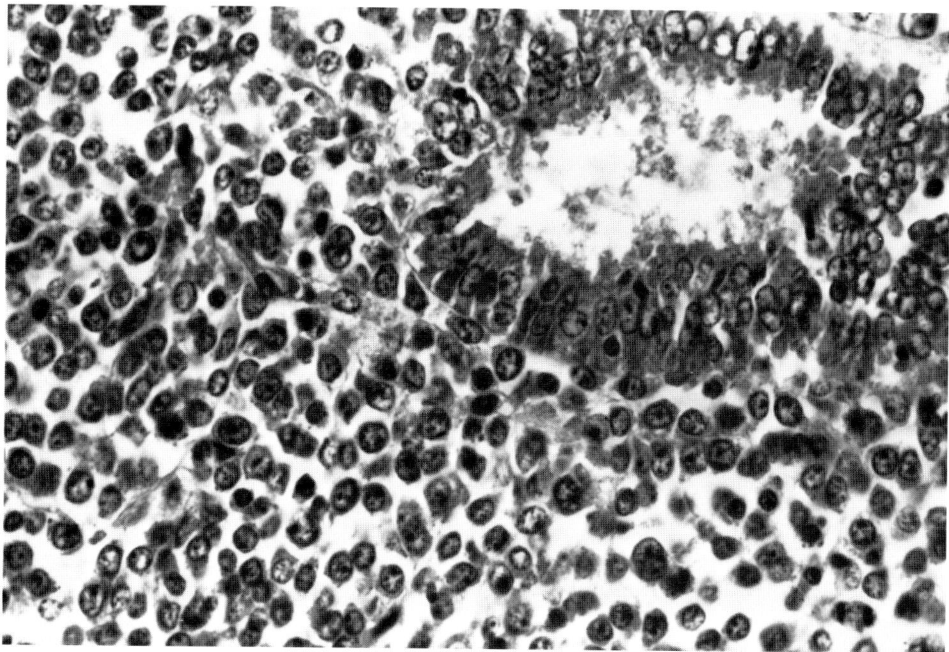

Fig. 8-15. Small cell undifferentiated carcinoma of endometrium, higher-power view of tumor in Figure 8-14.

published observations). The majority of the reported tumors have exhibited evidence of neuroendocrine differentiation with one or more special techniques (although not all tumors were similarly studied), including argyrophilia, immunoreactivity for one or more neuroendocrine markers (neuron-specific enolase, Leu-7, synaptophysin, bombesin, chromogranin, insulin), and dense core granules on ultrastructural examination. The differential diagnosis of these tumors has been noted above (see differential diagnosis of cervical SCUCs). Because endometrial SCUCs are much less common than cervical SCUCs, the former diagnosis should not be rendered until secondary involvement of the corpus by a cervical SCUC has been excluded.

GERM CELL TUMORS

Occasional tumors histologically identical to ovarian germ cell tumors have been encountered in the uterus. In these cases, the histogenesis of the tumors is not known with certainty, the tumors possibly arising from germ cells displaced during their embryonic migration, from somatic cells that have undergone aberrant differentiation, or from fetal remnants.

Yolk Sac Tumors

Yolk sac tumors (YSTs) of the uterus are rare. Five YSTs of the cervix (three of which also involved the vagina)[105, 106] and four of endometrial origin[107–110] have been reported. Three additional extragonadal pelvic YSTs were attached or adherent to the outer aspect of the uterus.[108] The cervical or cervicovaginal tumors have occurred in infants under years of age, whereas the endometrial and juxtauterine YSTs have occurred in women of reproductive age (17

to 42 years). The patients have typically presented with vaginal bleeding, pelvic pain, or combinations thereof; an elevated serum level of α-fetoprotein (AFP) was found in all of the cases in which this determination was performed. Eight of the 12 patients were apparently cured by excision of the tumor (usually hysterectomy) and chemotherapy; the remaining patients (one of whom did not receive chemotherapy) died of tumor progression within two years. On gross examination, cervical and endometrial YSTs are typically soft, friable, gray-tan polypoid mucosal masses that have ranged up to 6 cm in maximum dimension. The cervical stroma or myometrium is usually invaded, sometimes deeply. Histologic examination has revealed the typical patterns of YST (Fig. 8-16), usually with no other neoplastic elements. One of the juxtauterine YSTs, however, had an endometrioid-like glandular pattern and was associated with a teratoma.[108]

Teratomas

Approximately a dozen examples of a lesion interpeted as mature teratoma of the uterus have been described.[111–122] All the tumors occurred in women of reproductive age (26 to 45 years) who typically complained of abnormal vaginal bleeding or discharge. Gross examination has typically revealed a polypoid, sometimes pedunculated lesion within the endocervix or endometrium. The tumors have ranged from 2 to 6 cm in maximum dimension, with a sectioned surface that has varied from solid to predominantly solid or rarely, entirely cystic. Histological examination has revealed a haphazard or organoid admixture of mature tissues derived from at least two, but usually all three, germ layers. The differential diagnosis of mature teratoma includes heterotopic tissues of fetal origin (see Ch. 4). Indeed, it has been suggested that most, if not all, mature uterine "teratomas" repre-

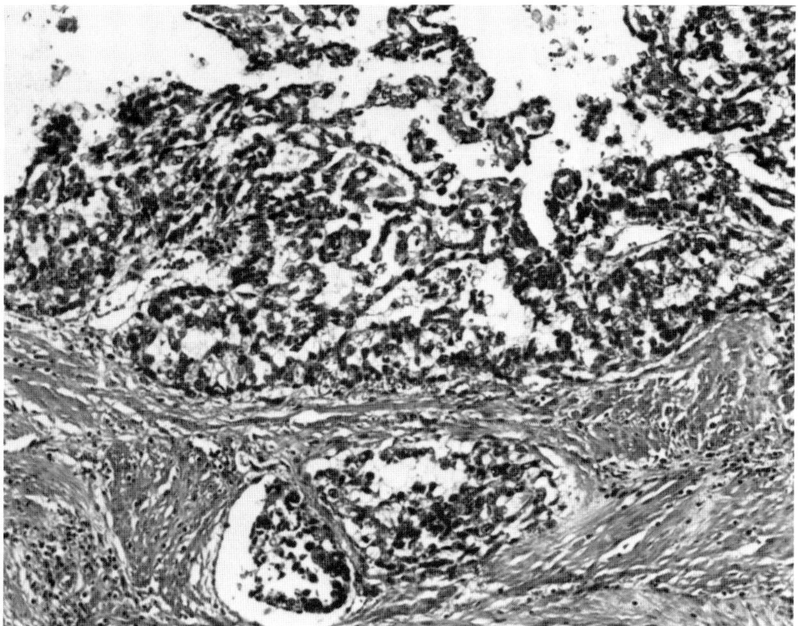

Fig. 8-16. Yolk sac tumor of uterine origin involving myometrium.

sent implants of fetal tissue rather than true neoplasms.[123]

In contrast to the foregoing, Ansah-Boateng et al.[124] have described what appears to be a bona fide case of immature teratoma of the uterus. A 37-year-old infertile woman, who presented with severe vaginal bleeding, was found to have a mass 10 cm in greatest dimension that filled the vagina, and was attached by a long pedicle to the endometrium. The tumor was composed of an admixture of grade 1 endometrial adenocarcinoma and immature teratoma, the latter consisting of a "significant" amount of immature neuroepithelium that, in contrast to PNETs, was associated with squamous and mucinous epithelium, cartilage, bone, and a tooth bud. Glial implants were found on the peritoneal surfaces of both ovaries. The patient was given postoperative irradiation, and was free of disease 2 years later. Henderickson and Kempson[125] have also encountered a case of immature teratoma with glial tissue that apparently arose in the uterus; no additional details were provided. A third tumor reported as an immature teratoma of the uterine cervix has features that we believe are more in keeping with a diagnosis of embryonal rhabdomyosarcoma.[126] The differential diagnosis of immature teratomas is with neuroectodermal tumors.

NEUROECTODERMAL TUMORS

Although some neuroectodermal tumors of the uterus may be of germ cell origin (representing monodermal teratomas), these tumors are considered separately here because in most cases, their histogenesis is not known with certainty. Some may be derived from neuroectodermal tissues of fetal origin (see Ch. 4), whereas other tumors, some of which have occurred in elderly women and in association with tumors of known müllerian origin, are likely of mesodermal origin, thereby representing a form of "neometaplasia."[127]

PRIMITIVE NEUROECTODERMAL TUMORS

Seven primitive neuroectodermal tumors (PNET) of the uterus have been described.[128–130] Five of the patients were postmenopausal, while two were adolescent, with an age range of 12 to 69 years (median 67 years). All the patients presented with abnormal vaginal bleeding, and in three cases, an enlarged uterus or a pelvic mass was palpable. One patient also had bone pain secondary to a tibial metastasis. At presentation, the tumor was confined to the uterine corpus in two patients (FIGO stage I) and involved the cervix in a third case (stage IIB). Two cases were stage IIC because of pelvic lymph node metastases and the final two cases were stage IVB because of omental or bony metastases. Follow-up data indicate that the prognosis of uterine PNETs correlates with the FIGO stage.[130] The two patients with stage I tumors had uneventful 5.5-year and 6-year follow-up intervals, whereas all but one of the patients with higher-stage disease died from tumor progression within 2 years of presentation.

On gross examination, all the uterine PNETs formed polypoid masses within the endometrial cavity, and in five cases, there was myometrial invasion, which was deep in four. In three cases, tumor extended inferiorly into the lower uterine segment (one case) or the cervix (two cases). The sectioned surfaces of the tumors were described as soft, fleshy, and gray to white. In each case, histologic examination revealed a primitive neuroectodermal tumor that typically exhibited a wide range of neural, glial, ependymal, and medulloepithelial differentiation (Figs. 8-17 and 8-18). In five cases, the tumors were pure, whereas two were admixed with another neoplasm, an endometrial stromal sarcoma in one, and in the other, a grade 1 endometrial adenocarcinoma. No other heterologous or teratomatous elements were identified in any of the tumors.

The differential diagnosis of uterine PNETs includes other neuroectodermal tumors discussed in this section, mature and

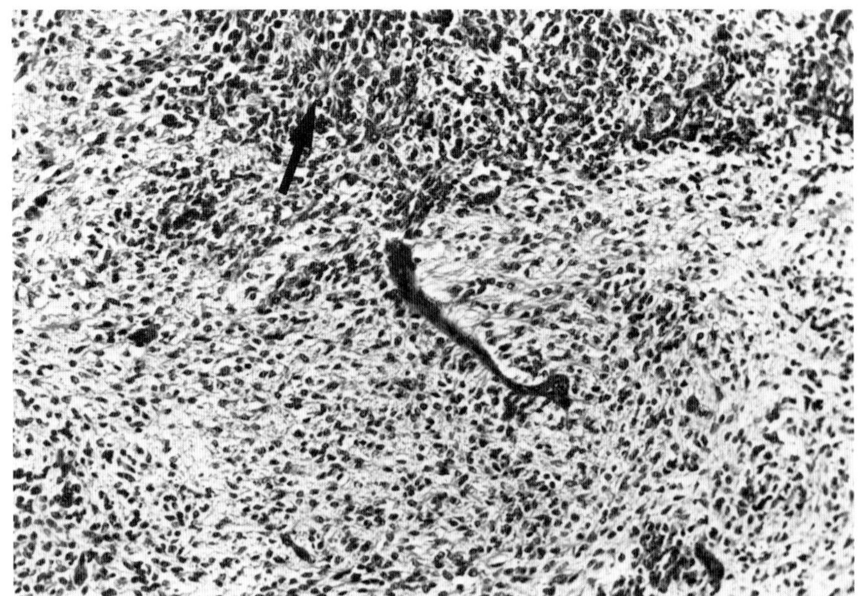

Fig. 8-17. Primitive neuroectodermal tumor of uterus with glial differentiation. Note pseudorosette (arrow).

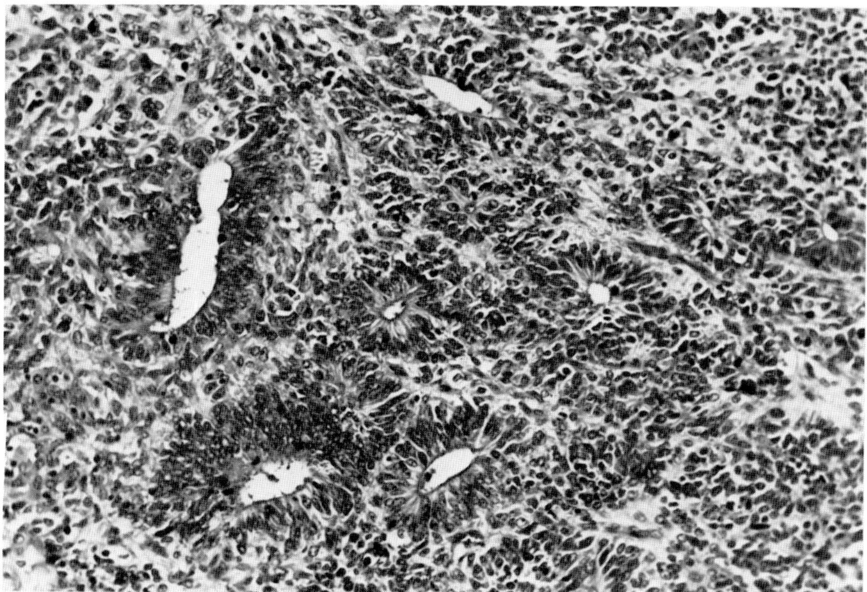

Fig. 8-18. Primitive neuroectodermal tumor of uterus with rosettes and tubules lined by primitive neuroepithelial cells.

immature teratomas with neuroectodermal differentiation (see above), and malignant mullerian mixed tumors with neuroectodermal differentiation (see Ch. 7). Fetal neuroectodermal remnants (see Ch. 4), in contrast to PNETs, are frequently microscopic and multifocal, consist predominantly or entirely of mature glial tissue, are occasionally associated with other heterotopic elements such as cartilage, bone, and adipose tissue (or in one case, refractile foreign material), and are frequently associated with a previous instrumental abortion.

UTERINE GLIOMAS

Two pure uterine gliomas have been reported. Young et al. described the case of a 15-year-old girl who underwent hysterectomy for intractable vaginal bleeding.[127] A polypoid tumor filled the endometrial cavity and invaded the myometrium (Fig. 8-19). Microscopic examination revealed a low-grade fibrillary astrocytoma (Fig. 8-20). The marked cellularity, mitotic activity,

and the diverse differentiation that characterize PNETs were absent. The patient was free of disease during a 6-year follow-up interval. The size of the lesion, its invasion of the myometrium, and a reliably negative coital history indicated that it was a true neoplasm that was unlikely to be of fetal derivation. Although not described in detail, a second case of endometrial glioma encountered by Liao and Choi was associated with metastatic nodules on the uterine serosa.[131]

OTHER NEUROECTODERMAL TUMORS

Schultz[132] has described an example of a "retinal anlage" tumor of the uterus in a 69-year-old woman who underwent curettage after 2 years of postmenopausal bleeding. The patient was treated with pelvic irradiation, but died of tumor progression 2 months later. At autopsy, the endometrial cavity was filled with a pedunculated mass measuring up to 3 cm. Its sectioned surface was predominantly black, and similar tu-

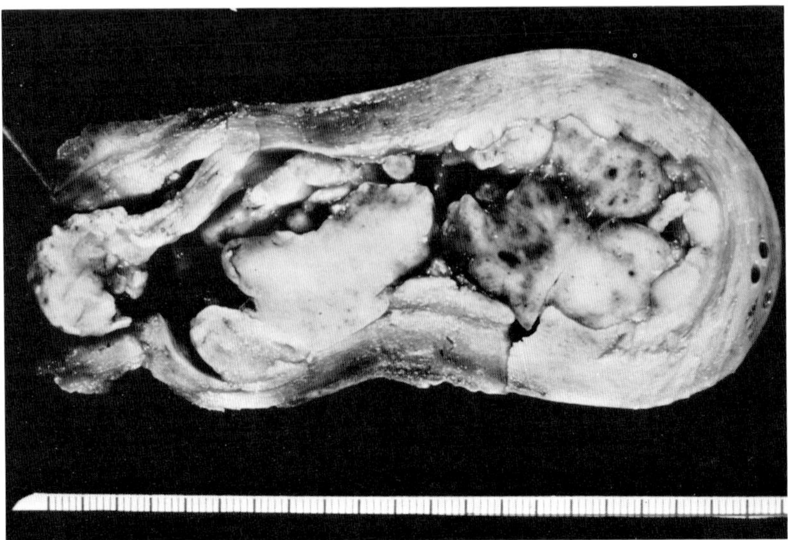

Fig. 8-19. Uterine glioma. Longitudinal section of uterus showing polypoid white tumor filling uterine cavity. (From Young et al.,[127] with permission.)

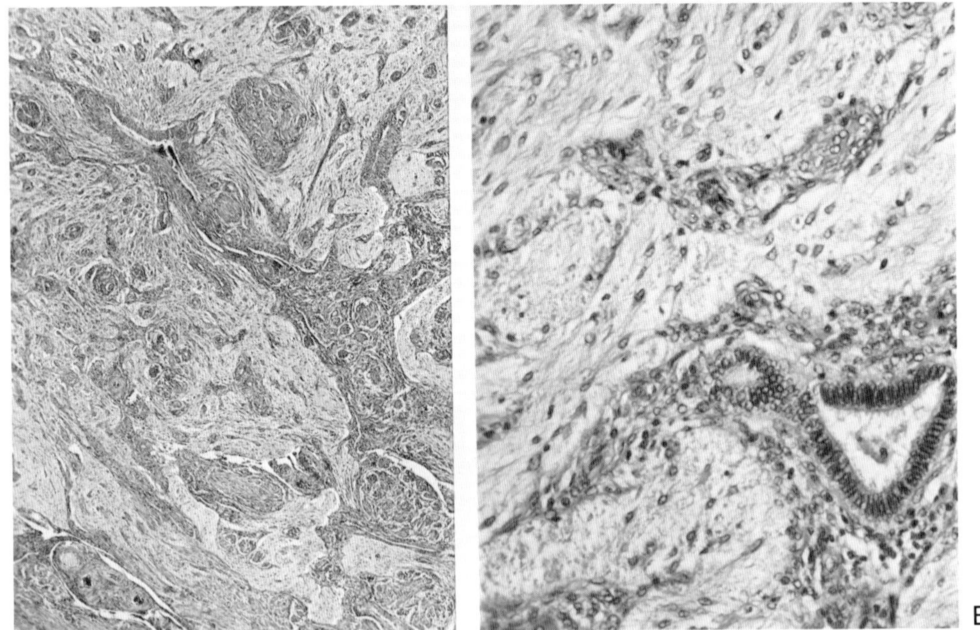

Fig. 8-20. Uterine glioma. Irregular confluent tongues of glial tissue invade the myometrium **(A)**, Endometrial gland and stroma are surrounded by glial tissue **(B)**.

mor involved the myometrium and the cervix. There was extensive metastatic tumor within the abdomen as well as the pleura. The predominant microscopic pattern was that of irregular acini, glomerulus-like structures, nests, and strands formed by large, cuboidal, melanin-laden cells. Other areas of the tumor had the appearance of a typical endometrial adenocarcinoma with squamous differentiation; several small foci of hyaline cartilage were also found.

A variety of tumors generally considered to arise from the neural crest (or peripheral nervous system) have also been rarely encountered in the uterine corpus or cervix. These include examples of neurofibromatosis,[133] benign paraganglioma of typical and melanotic types,[134, 135] malignant paraganglioma,[136] ganglioneuroma,[136] benign and malignant schwannoma,[138–140] granular cell tumors,[141] and "pigmented myomatous neurocristoma."[142] The latter lesion took the form of a focally pigmented, myometrial mass approximately 4 cm in diameter that was composed of pigmented and non-pigmented melanocytes in a matrix of altered smooth muscle cells.

TRANSITIONAL CELL TUMORS

Transitional cell tumors of the uterus are very rare. Of the five extraovarian Brenner tumors reported in women, one was an incidental finding in the uterine corpus in a hysterectomy specimen of a 55-year-old woman.[143] The 1.3 cm in diameter subserosal tumor had a homogeneous grayish tan cut surface and was microscopically indistinguishable from a typical benign Brenner tumor of the ovary.

Chen has recently described a transitional cell carcinoma arising in the corpus of a 71-year-old woman who presented with a 3-month history of vaginal spotting.[144] Gross examination of the hysterectomy specimen revealed a focally hemorrhagic, gray, friable tumor involving the endome-

trium and deeply invading the myometrium; a mass of 5.5 cm in greatest dimension was found with a similar appearance in the left paraovarian area. Microscopic examination of the uterine and paraovarian tumor revealed a grade II to III papillary transitional cell carcinoma similar to that occurring in the urinary tract. Scattered tumor cells contained intracytoplasmic mucin. Microscopic foci of transitional cell carcinoma were present within the mucosa of both fallopian tubes. The patient received postoperative radiation and was alive with no evidence of tumor 5 years later.

A similar case of transitional cell carcinoma has been reported arising within the endocervix, an origin consistent with the occasional occurrence of transitional cell metaplasia in this site. A 73-year-old woman underwent laparotomy for a pelvic mass; the right ovary was replaced by a cystic tumor 17 cm in greatest dimension.[84] Pathologic examination of the total abdominal hysterectomy and bilateral salpingo-oophorectomy specimen revealed a high-grade papillary transitional cell carcinoma (Figs. 8-21 and 8-22), deeply invading the wall of the cervix as well as cervical lymphatics; foci of in situ carcinoma were also found. The ovarian tumor had a similar histologic appearance, and was interpreted as metastatic from the cervical tumor.

WILMS' TUMOR

Two cases of uterine Wilms' tumor have been reported,[145, 146] and we are aware of several additional unreported examples (Fig. 8-23). The reported cases occurred in adolescent girls (13 and 14 years of age) who had normal kidneys on intravenous pyelogram. Both tumors were bulky polypoid, pedunculated masses that filled the vagina; one tumor was attached to the endocervix and the other to the endometrium. The endometrial tumor infiltrated the

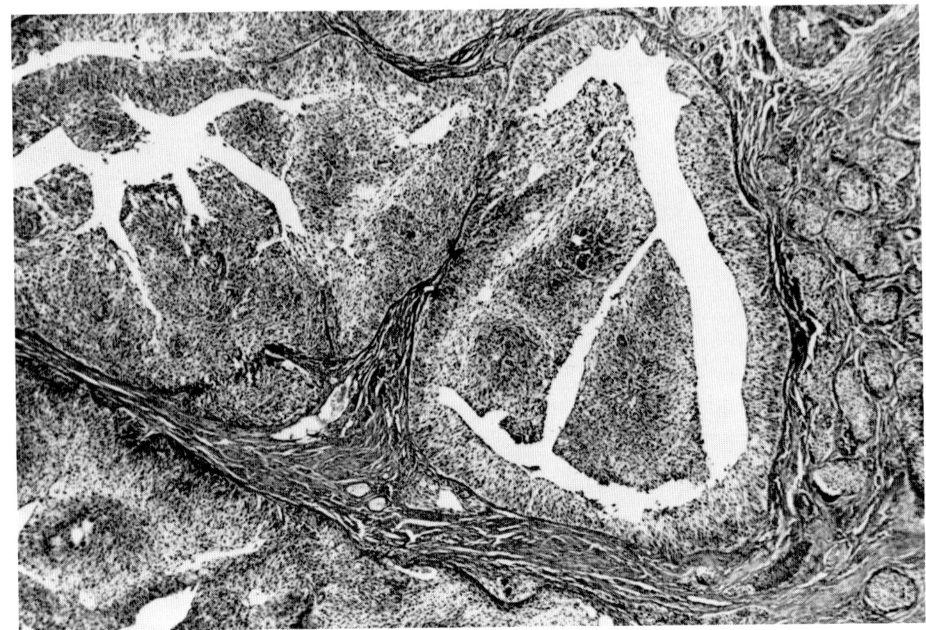

Fig. 8-21. Transitional cell carcinoma of cervix.

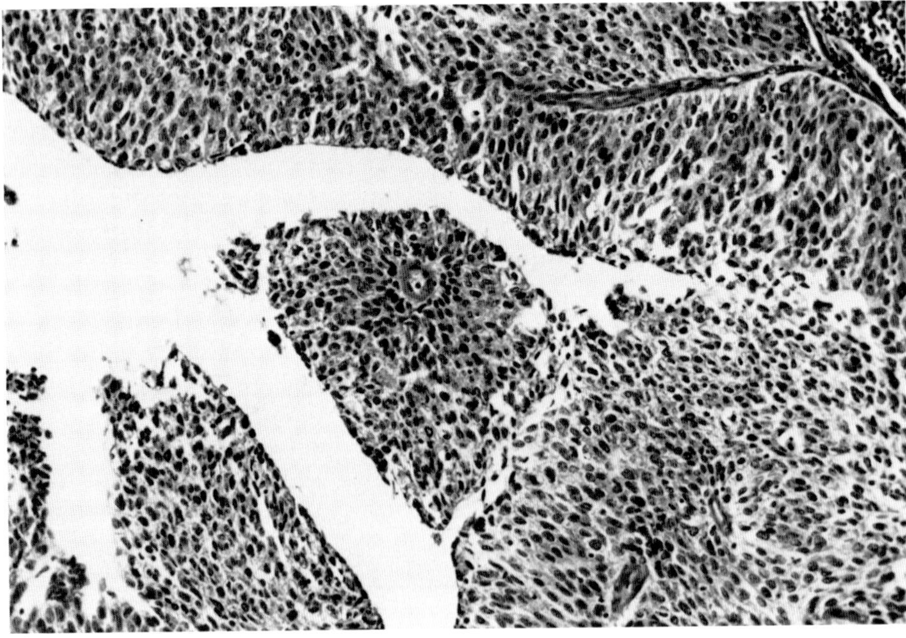

Fig. 8-22. Transitional cell carcinoma of cervix, higher-power view of Figure 8-21.

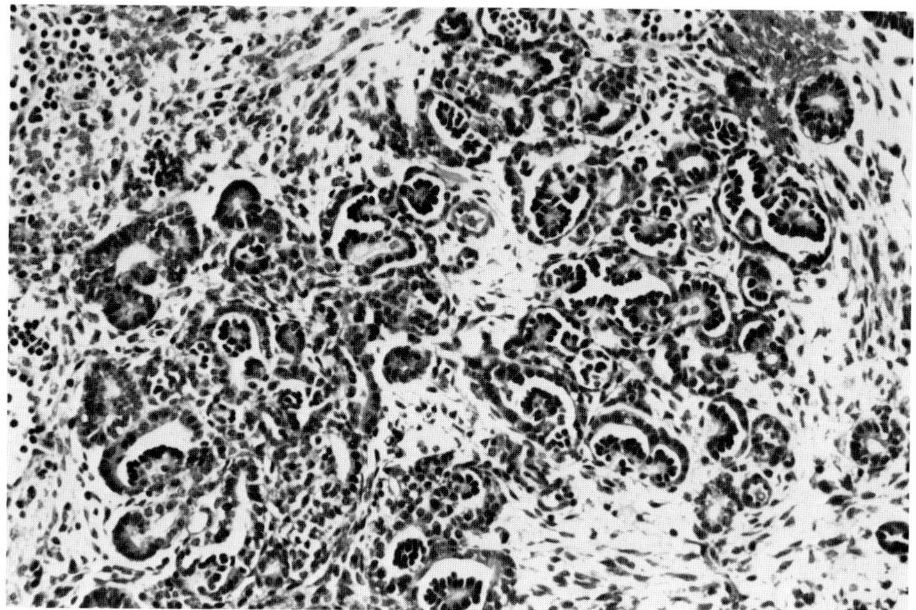

Fig. 8-23. Wilms' tumor of cervix.

Pouch of Douglas and the left broad ligament. No invasion was identified in the other case. Both tumors were typical Wilms' tumors on microscopic examination. Foci of both smooth and skeletal muscle were identified (two cases) as well as hyaline cartilage (one case). The patients had uneventful follow-up intervals of 5.7 and 9.6 years.

MALIGNANT MELANOMA

Approximately 35 cases of malignant melanoma have been reported as primary or probably primary within the cervix.[147–156] A cervical origin is consistent with the presence of melanin-containing cells, presumably melanocytes, demonstrated within the cervical epithelium in up to 3.5 percent of women.[157]

Patients with cervical melanoma have ranged in age from 26 to 74 years, although the majority have been between 50 and 70. Vaginal bleeding or discharge is the usual presenting complaint. In occasional pa-

tients, an abnormal Papanicolaou smear or manifestations related to blood-borne metastases have been the presenting feature; some patients have been asymptomatic. In one case, the cervical tumor (which had associated in situ changes) was preceded by multiple primary malignant melanomas of the vulva.[152] Clinical examination has usually revealed an exophytic polypoid cervical mass varying from several millimeters to 7 cm in size; in approximately one-half of the cases, brown to blue-black pigmentation of the tumor has been noted. In occasional cases the vagina either adjacent to or at a distance from the cervical tumor has also been involved.[147, 150, 156] Sixty percent of patients have had clinical evidence of tumor beyond the cervix at the time of diagnosis. Ninety percent of the reported patients with follow-up data have died of their disease, usually within 2 years of presentation.

On histologic examination (Figs. 8-24 and 8-25), the tumors do not differ significantly from melanomas in other sites, being composed of nests of polygonal to spindle-shaped cells (Fig. 8-24) containing mitoti-

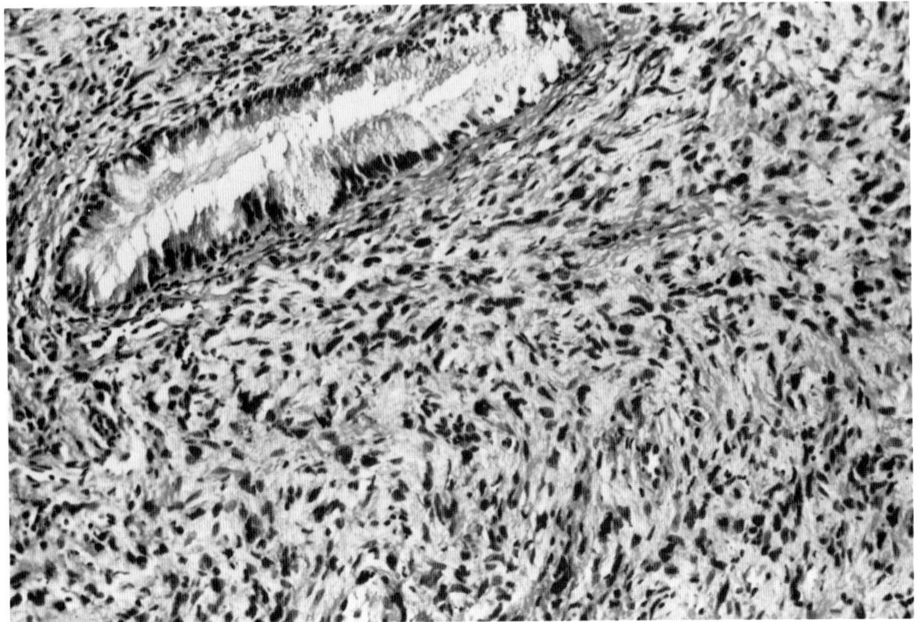

Fig. 8-24. Malignant melanoma of cervix composed of spindle-shaped cells. There was an associated in situ component within the overlying epithelium (see Fig. 8-25).

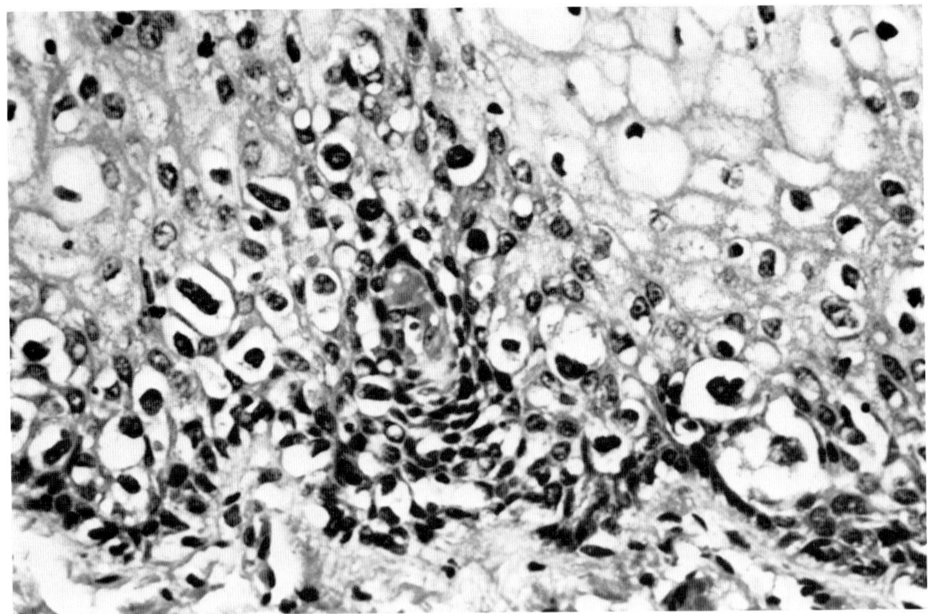

Fig. 8-25. In situ malignant melanoma within cervical squamous epithelium.

cally active pleomorphic nuclei and fine brown intracytoplasmic pigment. Occasional tumors, however, have been amelanotic.[147] In situ melanoma, typically of the lentiginous type (Fig 8-25), or melanosis within the adjacent mucosa provides evidence that the tumor is primary rather than metastatic, although these findings have been present in only a minority of reported cases.[151] In the absence of these adjacent changes, histologic distinction from metastatic melanoma may be difficult or impossible.

Primary melanoma of the cervix with a prominent spindle cell component (Fig. 8-24) should be distinguished from leiomyosarcoma. Features diagnostic or supportive of a diagnosis of spindle cell melanoma, rather than leiomyosarcoma, include the presence of melanin, in situ melanoma, immunoreactivity for S-100 and HMB 45 antigens, and absence of immunoreactivity for markers of smooth muscle differentiation. The neoplastic cells of alveolar soft part sarcoma, in contrast to those of melanoma, have uniform, mitotically inactive nuclei, and cytoplasm that contains PAS-positive diastase-resistant granules and crystals (see Ch. 6). The differential diagnosis of cervical melanoma also includes a number of benign melanotic lesions (see Ch. 1).

UTERINE INVOLVEMENT BY HEMATOPOIETIC AND HISTIOCYTIC DISORDERS

Malignant Lymphoma

Secondary involvement of the uterus in cases of disseminated lymphoma is not unusual. In one autopsy study, the cervix and corpus were involved in 6 percent and 10 percent, respectively, of women with intact reproductive organs.[158] Such involvement is usually not associated with clinical manifestations, but symptoms relating to the uterine disease (vaginal bleeding or discharge) have been the presenting complaint in a few cases.[159, 160] In most cases, the lymphoma is one of the more common types of non-Hodgkin's lymphoma, but rare examples of uterine involvement by disseminated Burkitt's lymphoma,[161] angiotropic lymphoma,[162] and Hodgkin's disease[163, 164] have been reported.

By contrast, the uterus is only rarely the initial site of involvement by lymphoma. Because local therapy is curative in most cases, most such tumors likely represent primary uterine lymphomas; occasional cases, however, may represent uterine involvement by occult, more widespread lymphomas. In one study of extranodal non-Hodgkin's lymphoma, only 0.5 percent were considered of uterine origin.[165] The following sections summarize the findings in the approximately 100 cases of primary or probably primary lymphoma of the uterus that have been reported since 1960.[166–198] Ninety percent of them have involved the cervix and the remainder, the corpus; in rare cases, both sites have been involved with no dominant mass.[175, 194] Uterine involvement by these tumors may be underdiagnosed by the pathologist because the lesions are unexpected in this site and because they can be confused with other types of malignant neoplasms or an inflammatory process.[183]

Clinical Features

Patients with uterine lymphomas range in age from 15 to 90 years; in the largest study in the literature,[183] median and mean ages of 41 and 44 years were found in patients with cervical tumors. The most common presenting symptom, whether the lymphoma involves the cervix or corpus, is vaginal bleeding, which can be severe. Less common presenting complaints are vaginal discharge, dyspareunia, or perineal, pelvic, or abdominal pain.[200] One patient had severe anemia and jaundice secondary to cold-re-

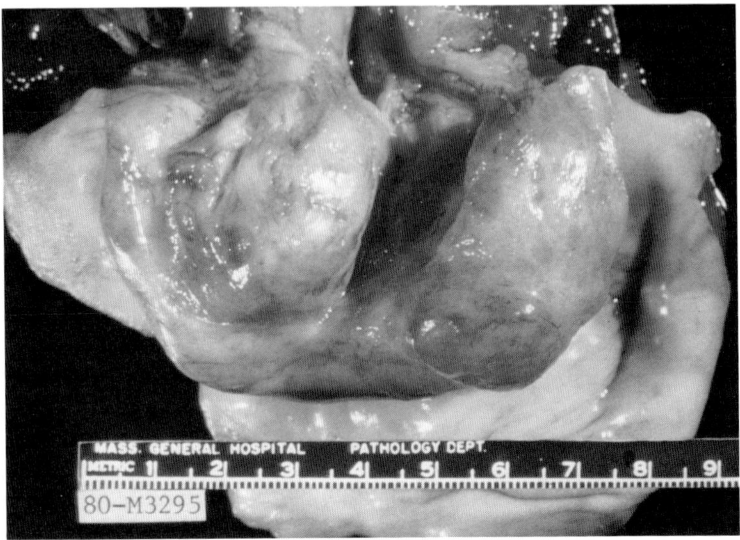

Fig. 8-26. Malignant lymphoma of cervix. The cervix is enlarged and nodular.

acting autoantibody-mediated hemolytic anemia.[187] Occasional patients have been asymptomatic, and the tumor has been detected by a cervicovaginal smear. Andrews et al.[161] estimated that only 10 to 40 percent of cases of cervical lymphoma are associated with a positive smear, presumably because the lymphomas usually do not cause ulceration. In some cases, the smear is interpreted as abnormal or positive for malignancy, but in others, a specific diagnosis of lymphoma has been made.[177, 186] Pelvic examination in patients with cervical lymphomas will usually disclose an obvious mass;

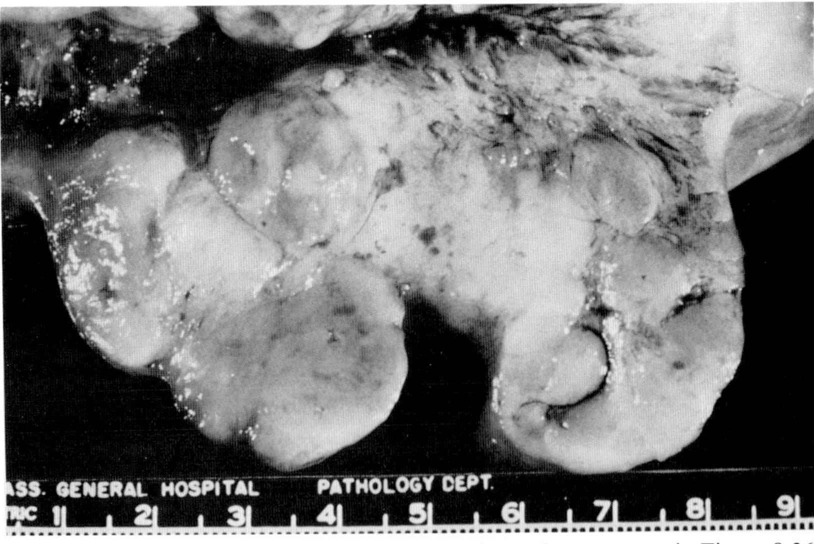

Fig. 8-27. Malignant lymphoma of cervix, sectioned surface of tumor seen in Figure 8-26. Homogeneous fleshy tumor involves entire thickness of cervical wall. (From Harris and Scully,[183] with permission.)

in cases of lymphoma involving the corpus, a pelvic mass or an enlarged uterus may be palpable.[164, 175]

Pathologic Features

On gross examination, cervical lymphomas typically result in a diffusely enlarged, barrel-shaped cervix (Figs. 8-26 and 8-27); local structures including the vagina, paracervical tissues, pelvic side walls, lower uterine segment, rectum, urinary bladder, and ureters (with consequent hydronephrosis) may be involved.[174, 183] Mucosal ulceration is rare. Occasionally the tumor is a solitary or multinodular submucosal mass or is polypoid, sometimes forming a fungating exophytic mass. Lymphomas of the corpus may form a polypoid endometrial mass, diffusely coat the endometrium, or grow as one or more myometrial or endomyometrial infiltrative masses up to 18 cm in diameter[169, 173, 175, 183] (Fig. 8-28). The sectioned surfaces of uterine lymphomas are usually described as fleshy, rubbery or firm, and homogeneous white to tan to yellow; areas of hemorrhage, necrosis, or both, however, may be present.

The majority of uterine lymphomas are of the diffuse large cell type.[200] In the series of Harris and Scully, 67 percent were of the diffuse large cell type, 28 percent were follicular lymphomas (follicular, predominantly small cleaved type; follicular mixed small-cleaved and large cell type; or follicular, predominantly large cell type), and one (5 percent) was a Burkitt's lymphoma (malignant lymphoma, small noncleaved cell type).[183] Other subtypes of uterine lymphoma have also been rarely reported, including small noncleaved cell, non-Burkitt's type,[190] diffuse small cleaved cell type,[182] diffuse mixed small and large cell type,[184] and Hodgkin's disease.[166, 168, 170, 173]

The microscopic appearance of the lymphomas is generally similar to that seen in nodal and other extranodal sites (Figs. 8-29

to 8-31). In the cervix, there is often a band of uninvolved stroma just below the typically intact surface epithelium (Fig. 8-29). The lymphomas usually deeply invade the wall of the cervix in the form of single or multiple large circumscribed nodules with pushing margins[183] (Fig. 8-29). In cases of follicular lymphoma, there is often perivascular spread (Fig. 8-29). The normal endocervical glands are frequently surrounded and entrapped by the neoplastic cells. There is often prominent sclerosis (Fig. 8-30A), resulting in epithelial-like patterns that range from individual cells, cords, or groups of cells separated by fine fibrils to dense bands of collagen in which scattered

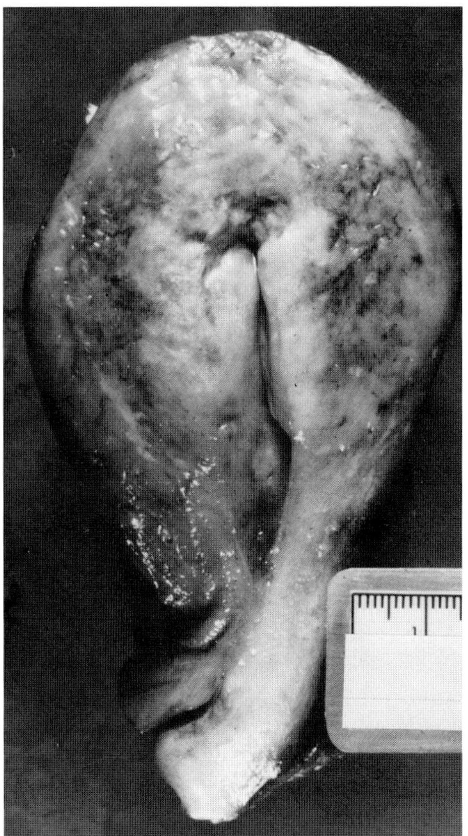

Fig. 8-28. Malignant lymphoma of the corpus. Fleshy tumor diffusely infiltrates the endometrium and myometrium.

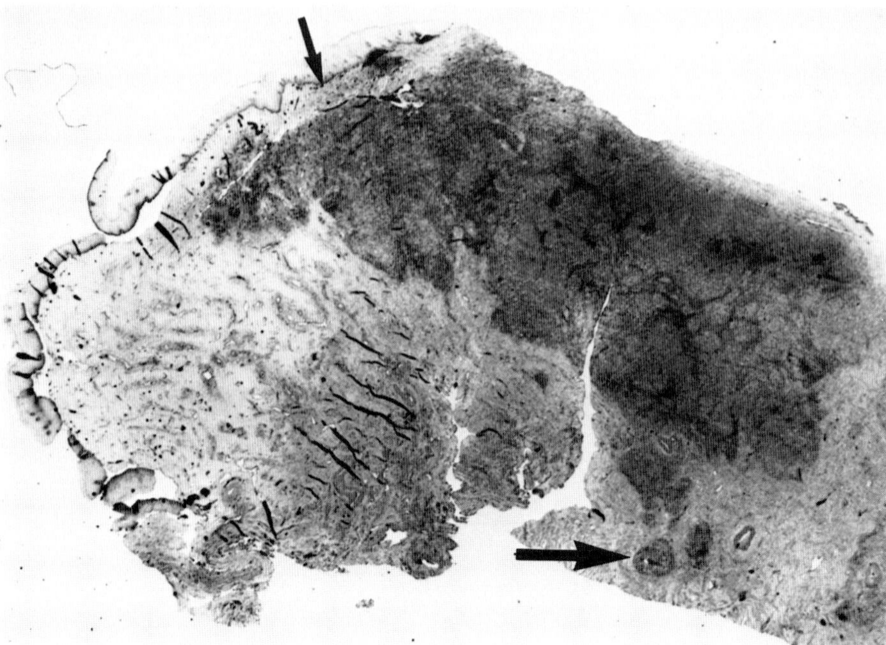

Fig. 8-29. Malignant lymphoma of cervix. Note narrow band of uninvolved stroma (small arrow) beneath surface epithelium, deep invasion, and perivascular tumor (large arrow).

neoplastic cells are embedded. In the sclerotic areas, the neoplastic cells are frequently spindle-shaped, resembling fibroblasts. An infiltrate of benign lymphocytes and, often, plasma cells is frequently present immediately beneath the epithelium and at the periphery of the neoplastic infiltrate; the latter, however, is otherwise monomorphous, in contrast to the population of cells in lymphoma-like lesions (see Ch. 1). Ulceration, hemorrhage, and necrosis are rare. The appearance is similar in lymphomas involving the corpus, although in occasional cases the tumor is sharply delimited to the endometrium without myometrial involvement and sclerosis is uncommon.[183] With the exception of one T-cell lymphoblastic lymphoma,[188] the few uterine lymphomas on which immunophenotyping studies have been reported have been of B-cell lineage.[183, 187, 189, 190]

Differential Diagnosis

Uterine lymphomas must be distinguished not only from other malignant small cell neoplasms, such as small cell (neuroendocrine) carcinomas, but also from lymphoma-like lesions in the cervix and corpus. In cases in which the cells are spindle shaped, the question of a sarcoma may be raised. Decidual transformation of the endocervical stroma has also been rarely confused with lymphoma. Distinguishing a lymphoma from these lesions may be difficult, particularly in a small biopsy specimen if the tissue is not optimally fixed and processed. Unlike carcinoma, which tends to invade with obliteration of normal structures, lymphoma tends to infiltrate with relative preservation of the normal endocervical and endometrial glands, typically sparing the subepithelial stroma. However, these features are often not ap-

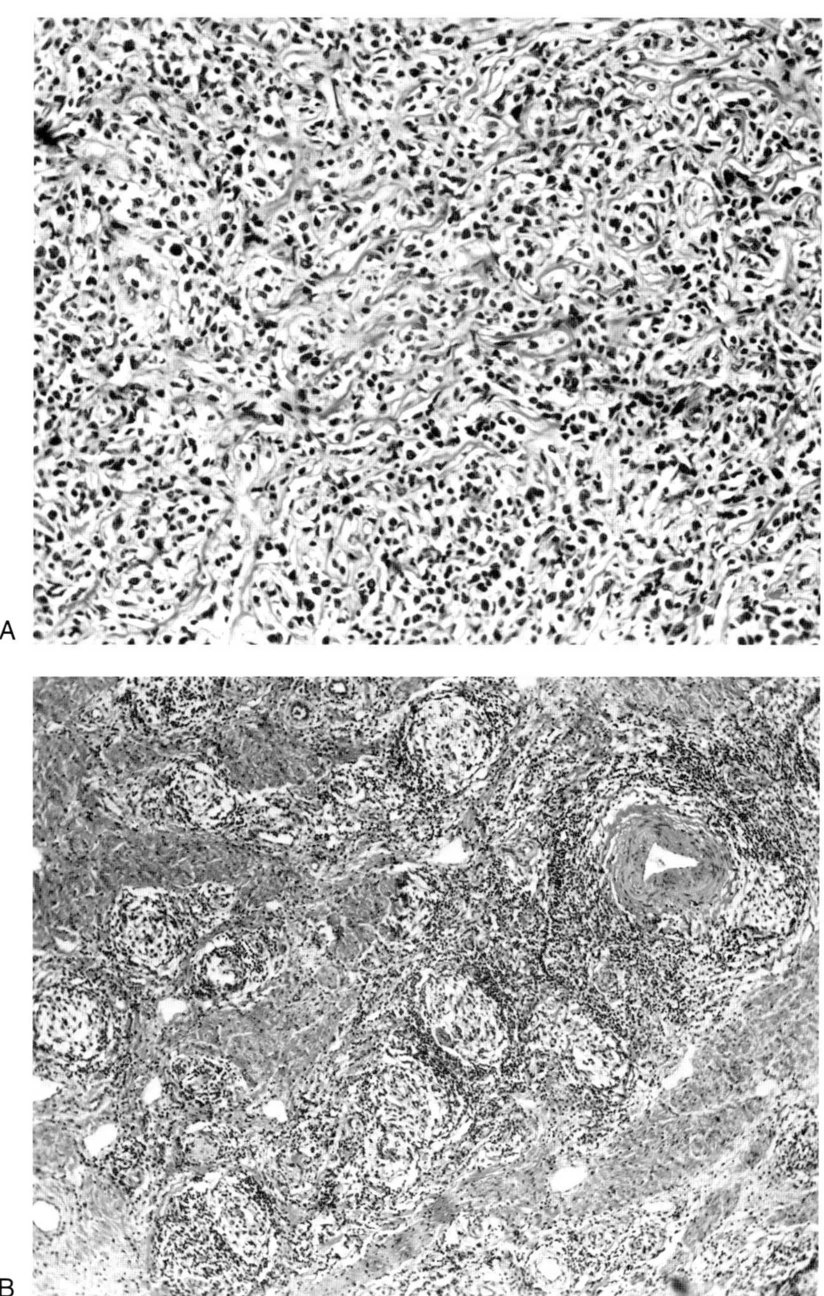

Fig. 8-30. Malignant lymphoma of cervix, diffuse large cell type with focal follicular areas. **(A)** Area of the tumor with a diffuse pattern and prominent sclerosis. **(B)** Area with follicular pattern.

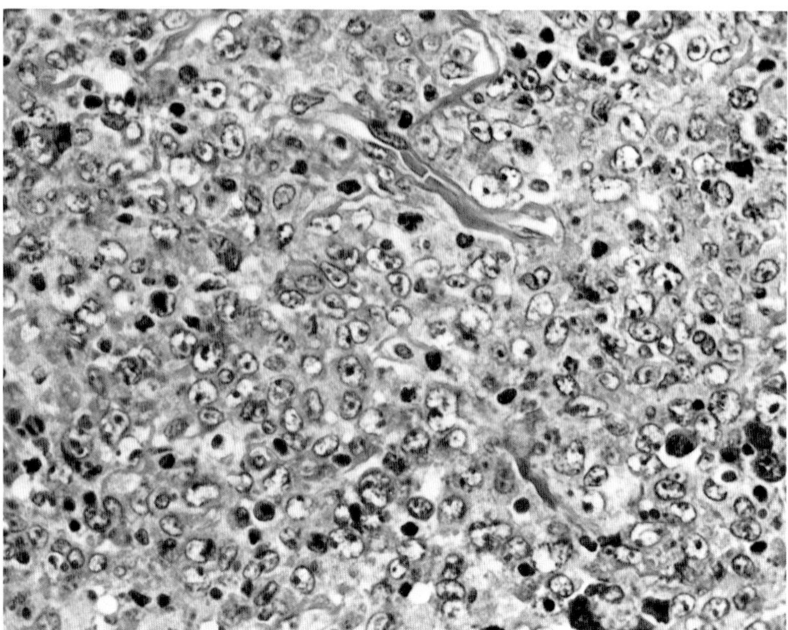

Fig. 8-31. Malignant lymphoma of cervix, diffuse large cell type, composed of large noncleaved cells typical of most primary cervical lymphomas.

preciable in a small biopsy; in most cases, the distinction between the two entities depends on a careful evaluation of the cytologic features. The cells of small cell carcinomas have molded nuclei and nuclear chromatin that is finely granular or smudged, whereas the cells of lymphoma lack nuclear molding and have more coarsely clumped chromatin. Rosette-like structures or focal squamous or glandular differentiation within the tumor are features that may be encountered in a small cell carcinoma, but not lymphoma. Associated in situ squamous or adenocarcinoma may be helpful circumstantial evidence in favor of carcinoma. The rare lymphoepithelioma-like carcinoma of the cervix[201] (see Ch. 2), which resembles its nasopharyngeal counterpart, can be confused with either a malignant lymphoma or with a lymphoma-like lesion. Cohesive nests or trabecular arrangements of cells are findings that help exclude lymphoma. Special techniques may also facilitate the differential diagnosis between lymphoma and a small cell or lym-

phoepithelioma-like carcinoma. Imprint preparations may show singly dispersed cells of lymphoma compared to the cohesive cellular aggregates of carcinomas. Immunoreactivity for leukocyte common antigen is found in most lymphomas, whereas immunoreactivity for keratin and epithelial membrane antigen is found in most carcinomas. Electron microscopic examination may also be helpful, although it is rarely needed.

The presence of an admixture of small cleaved cells and large noncleaved cells, a focal nodular pattern, and focal perivascular infiltration are features helpful in establishing a diagnosis of lymphoma when sclerosis and elongation of the nuclei in a lymphoma produce a resemblance to a sarcoma, including endometrial stromal sarcoma. In addition, the latter, unlike lymphomas, are characterized by cells that bear a close resemblance to normal endometrial stromal cells as well as a network of uniform small vessels resembling those of a proliferative endometrium. Immunoreactivity for vimentin and one or more smooth muscle markers obviously favors a diagnosis of sarcoma (see Ch. 6) over lymphoma.

Behavior

Malignant lymphomas of the uterus have a favorable prognosis, particularly compared with lymphomas presenting within the ovaries.[183, 184, 196] In the series of 21 uterine lymphomas reported by Harris and Scully,[183] 16 had disease confined to a single extranodal site (Ann Arbor stage IE), three had positive pelvic or abdominal nodes or both (stage IIE), and two had ovarian and abdominal nodal involvement (stage IV). In most cases, patients were treated by hysterectomy and postoperative radiation or chemotherapy, or both; five patients received no therapy other than hysterectomy. The overall and relapse-free 5-year survival rates were 77 percent and 70 percent respectively for the entire group of patients.[183] The stage of the disease was the most important single factor in predicting survival, with overall and relapse-free 5-year survival rates of 93 percent and 84 percent for stage IE tumors; none of the patients with stage IE disease who received definitive local initial therapy relapsed. By contrast, only one of four patients with higher stage tumors survived. These observations have been confirmed in a more recent series which included 43 stage IE tumors, 38 collected from the literature (including 13 from the Harris-Scully series) and 5 newly reported cases.[196] In this study, there was only one treatment failure among 28 patients (followed for at least 2 years) in whom the treatment included radiation.

The effect of histologic type on survival was more difficult to assess in the Harris-Scully study because of the high concordance between histologic type and stage. All patients with tumors that had a predominantly nodular pattern survived, but all such patients had stage IE disease. Among diffuse lymphomas, a better prognosis was seen among those with a significant component of large cleaved cells, compared to those with large non-cleaved cells, small noncleaved cells, or immunoblasts.

UTERINE INVOLVEMENT BY
LEUKEMIA

Leukemic infiltration of the uterus is common at autopsy, being present in 40.8 percent of women in one study.[202] In another autopsy study, there was uterine involvement in 25 percent of patients with acute lymphoblastic leukemia, with corresponding figures of 11 percent, 14 percent, and 4 percent in patients with acute myelogenous leukemia, chronic lymphocytic leukemia, and chronic granulocytic leukemia respectively.[203] Similarly, leukemic cells have been found in cervicovaginal smears in as many as 28 percent of leukemic patients.[204] Less commonly, leukemic infiltration of the uterus in patients with leukemia has been associated with symptoms, usually abnormal bleeding,[205–211] or less commonly pain,[207–209] a cervical mass,[205, 207, 209, 210] or combinations thereof.

In contrast to the foregoing, the uterus is only rarely the initial site of clinically recognized involvement by leukemia. Approximately 15 cases of myelogenous leukemia have presented as granulocytic sarcomas of the uterus.[173, 183, 212–219a] The patients have been 32 to 71 years of age, with a mean age in the sixth decade, and have typically presented with abnormal vaginal bleeding, sometimes accompanied by abdominal pain. In three of these patients, cervicovaginal smears contained malignant cells. One was considered positive for malignant lymphoma or leukemia[215] and in another, the diagnosis of lymphoma was suggested.[213] With the exception of one case in which uterine involvement was confined to the corpus,[218] the cervix has been involved in all of the cases. In approximately one-half of the latter, the process has also involved the vagina, the corpus, the parametrium, or the vulva. Further investigations in some cases has revealed concurrent involvement of sites outside the female genital tract, including lymph nodes, gastrointestinal tract, or bone marrow. Although most of these women did not have leukemic cells in the peripheral blood at presentation, most developed acute myelogenous leukemia during the course of their disease.

On gross examination, granulocytic sarcomas of the cervix have appeared as nodules, ulcers, or large masses, often extending into the vagina or paracervical tissues. The tumors have ranged from gray-tan to gray-blue to green in color.[183] On microscopic examination, the immature granulocytes, like the neoplastic cells of uterine lymphomas, tend to infiltrate around, rather than destroy, normal structures. The histologic appearance is similar to that of granulocytic sarcoma in other sites (Fig. 8-32).

In the majority of these cases, the correct diagnosis was not rendered on the initial biopsy; the most common misdiagnosis was malignant lymphoma, or less commonly small cell carcinoma or sarcoma. Indeed, granulocytic sarcomas of the cervix may be difficult or impossible to differentiate from lymphoma on routinely stained sections.[183] As in other sites, histologic recognition of the myeloid cells frequently requires the use of chloroacetate esterase stain or immunohistochemical stain for lysozyme, or both. These procedures should thus be performed in cases of diffuse neoplastic infiltrates in the cervix that exhibit patterns and cellular features consistent with leukemic involvement.

The treatment for patients with granulocytic sarcomas of the uterus has varied widely and included surgical excision or radiation, or a combination of these. However, therapy was frequently not specifically directed against granulocytic sarcoma or myeloid leukemia. One patient treated with radiation and chemotherapy entered

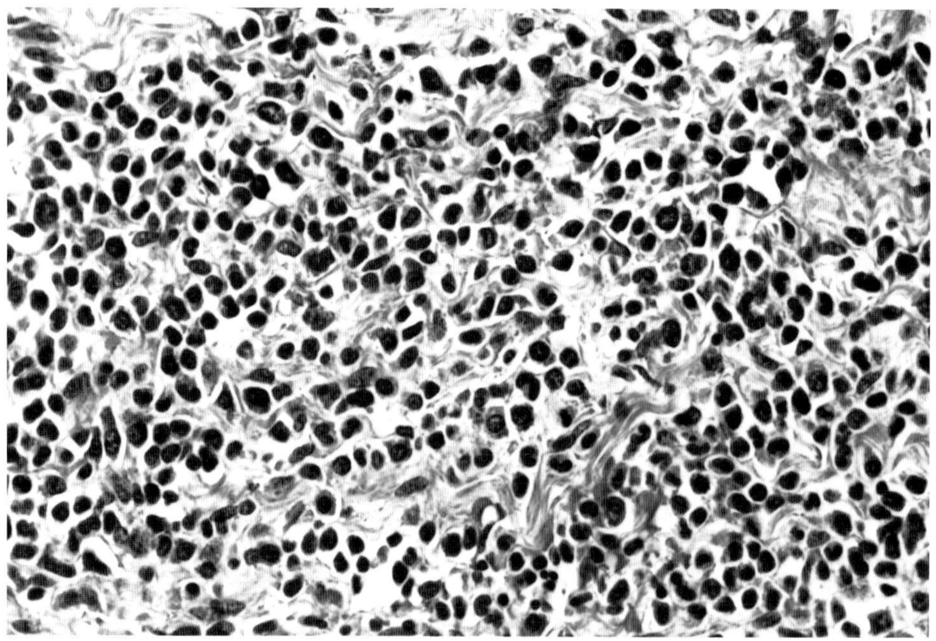

Fig. 8-32. Granulocytic sarcoma of cervix.

complete remission, two patients were alive with disease 3 months[213] and 1 year[183] after presentation, and five patients died of disease several days to 32 months after presentation.[173, 212, 215] One patient achieved complete remission following chemotherapy but relapsed at 18 months and died of acute myeloid leukemia at 2 years. The prognosis, therefore, is poor, but the outcome could possibly be improved with accurate diagnosis on the initial biopsy and earlier institution of appropriate therapy.[200]

PLASMACYTOMA

The uterus is involved in only 1 percent of cases of multiple myeloma (Fig. 8-33) and uterine involvement as the initial manifestation of disease is very rare.[220] In one unusual case, however, the initial diagnosis of plasma cell neoplasia was made in a 55-year-old woman after a cervical smear showed primitive plasmacytoid cells, and

biopsy of a polypoid endocervical mass showed a malignant plasmacytic infiltrate.[220] Further investigation revealed monoclonal immunoglobulin in the serum, as well as bone lesions and marrow involvement indicating multiple myeloma. The patient was treated with chemotherapy but died 4 months after initial presentation. At autopsy, tumor involved the bone marrow, liver, spleen, adrenals, kidneys, lymph nodes, lungs, and appendix, but no residual plasma cell tumor was found in the uterus.[220]

MYELOFIBROSIS

Involvement of the uterus in other forms of myeloproliferative disorders is rare. Ferry and Young[200] have seen one case of primary myelofibrosis in which there was extensive myeloid metaplasia in the myometrium.

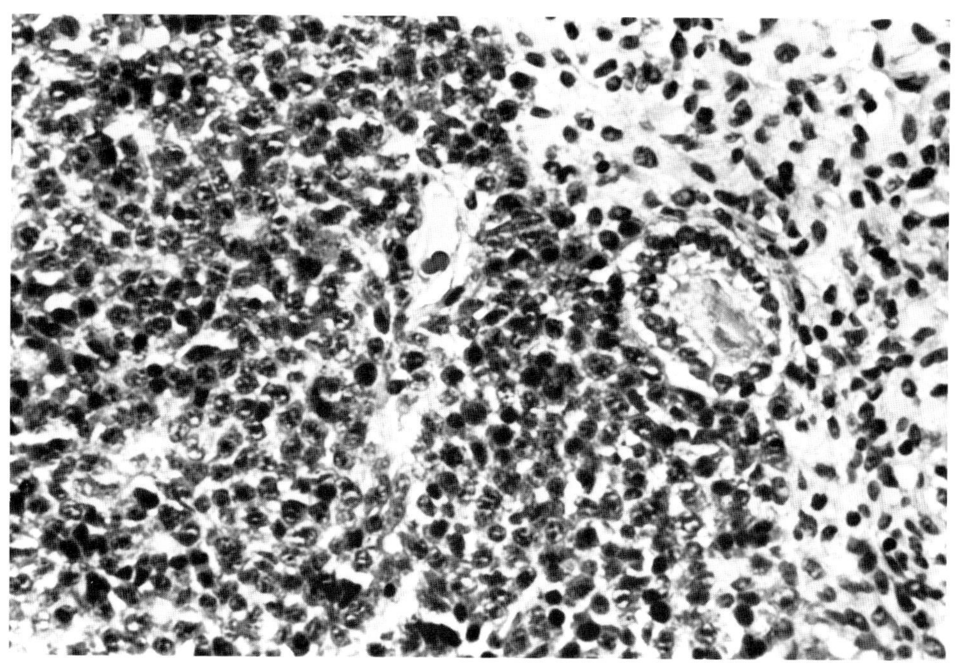

Fig. 8-33. Multiple myeloma involving endometrium. Dense collections of immature plasma cells are present within the endometrial stroma.

UTERINE INVOLVEMENT BY HISTIOCYTIC DISORDERS

As shown in a recent study by Axiotis et al.,[221] involvement of the female genital tract by Langerhans cell histiocytosis (LCH) (histiocytosis X, eosinophilic granuloma) is rare. In more than 80 percent of such patients, vulvovaginal lesions precede, follow, or are synchronous with extragenital multiorgan involvement, diabetes insipidus, or both. In the remainder, LCH is confined to the genital organs, at least for the period of observation. In the seven patients in the latter category included in the review cited above, three had uterine involvement.[222–224] In one of these cases, a 38-year-old woman presented with indurated vulvar ulcers; a curettage revealed that the endometrium was "heavily infiltrated" by eosinophils. There was no evidence of disease 6 years after partial vulvectomy.[222] In another case, a 29-year old woman presented with vulvar ulcers, followed by vaginal, cervical, and endometrial involvement.[223] The patient was treated by cervicectomy and irradiation but was then lost to follow-up. In the third patient with uterine LCH, a 33-year-old woman was found to have a cervical ulcer; a cervicectomy was performed and she had no evidence of further disease during the 3-year follow-up period.[224]

Murray and Fox[225] recently described a case of cervical involvement by Rosai-Dorfman disease (sinus histiocytosis with massive lymphadenopathy). A 37-year-old woman underwent hysterectomy for menorrhagia; there were no abnormal findings on physical examination, including an absence of lymphadenopathy. Within the uterus was a fleshy endocervical mass, 5 cm in maximum dimension, that on microscopic examination had the typical features of Rosai-Dorfman disease. The lesional cells, which included large histiocytes containing mature lymphocytes within their cytoplasm, infiltrated between the endocervical stromal cells. The characteristic microscopic features of these histiocytic disorders should facilitate their distinction from uterine involvement by granulomatous or lipogranulomatous inflammation and malakoplakia (see Chs. 1 and 4).

METASTATIC CARCINOMAS

GENITAL TRACT CARCINOMA

Secondary tumor involvement of the uterus is usually a result of contiguous spread from a carcinoma arising elsewhere in the genital tract, such as direct extension of vaginal or tubal carcinomas, or ingrowth of ovarian carcinomas that have involved the uterine serosa or cul-de-sac. In such cases, the primary tumor is usually clinically apparent. Rarely, however, the presence of microscopic fragments of tumor within a curettage or biopsy specimen is the presenting manifestation of luminal or lymphatic spread from an ovarian, tubal, or peritoneal carcinoma; in other cases, patients with an occult ovarian or tubal carcinoma have a cervical mass that clinically mimics a primary carcinoma in this site.[226–230] For these reasons, and because primary papillary serous carcinomas of the uterus are rare (in the endocervix)[231] to uncommon (in the endometrium), direct spread from a papillary serous carcinoma from the upper genital tract should be considered before rendering a diagnosis of primary uterine papillary serous carcinoma.

EXTRAGENITAL CARCINOMAS

Extragenital carcinomas rarely metastasize to the uterus; Kiaer and Holm-Jensen[232] collected 179 such cases from the world literature in 1972. Potential metastatic routes to the uterus include hematogenous and retrograde lymphatic spread, and transperitoneal seeding with either transtubal luminal spread or ingrowth from the serosa or cul-de-sac. The uterine involvement is usually a manifestation of disseminated spread in a patient with a known primary tumor, and in such cases the diagnosis is usually straightforward. Rarely, however, the uterine tumor is the presenting manifestation of an extragenital carcinoma, and in such cases, misdiagnosis of the lesion as a primary uterine cancer is more likely. Morphologic features that should suggest the possibility or even probability of a metastasis (Figs. 8-34 to 8-37) include an appearance on clinical or macroscopic examination that is atypical for a primary carcinoma, a lack of associated precancerous changes or an in situ carcinoma, tumor confined to the myometrium or endocervical stroma with a normal overlying surface epithelium, a multinodular growth pattern, a permeative growth pattern within the endometrial (Fig. 8-34) or endocervical stroma with tumor entrapping normal glands, and unusually prominent involvement of lymphatics (Figs. 8-34 and 8-35) or blood vessels. Specific extragenital primary tumors should be considered when there are histological features that are unusual for a primary uterine neoplasm, such as a prominent signet-ring cell component (breast, stomach) (Fig. 8-36), an Indian-file arrangement of the tumor cells (breast), and copious necrotic debris within the lumina of the neoplastic glands, so-called dirty necrosis (colon).[233] Metastatic lobular carcinoma of the breast, in particular, can cause major diagnostic problems, with a permeative growth of small uniform cells within the endometrial stroma that can simulate an endometrial stromal sarcoma.[233] When such cells are rare, they can even be misinterpreted as non-neoplastic stromal cells.

The following sections summarize the literature pertaining to metastatic carcinomas involving the cervix and the uterine corpus as encountered in surgical specimens; the former site appears to be more commonly

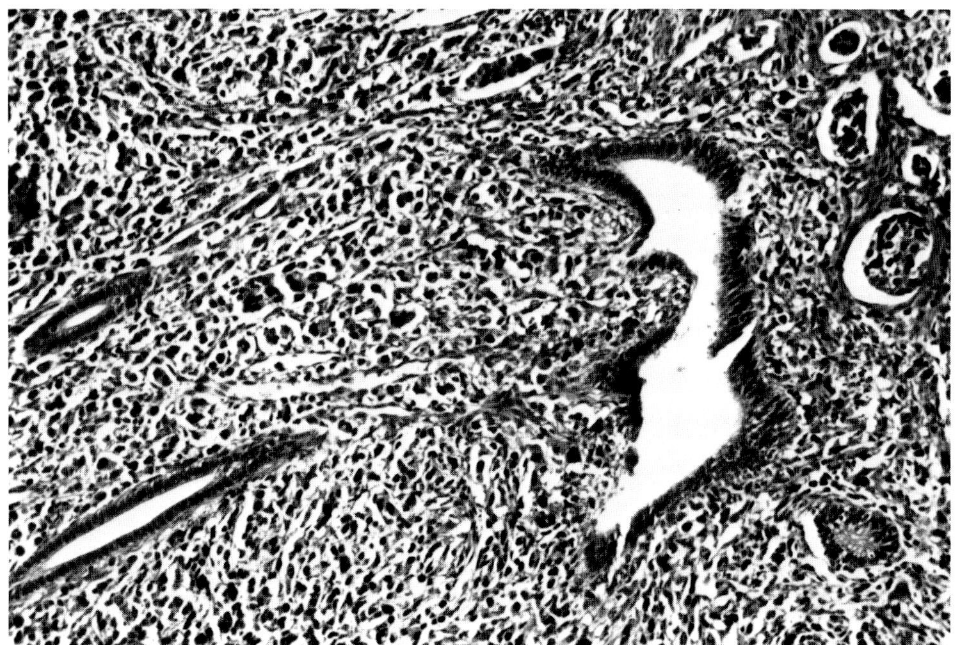

Fig. 8-34. Metastatic adenocarcinoma to endometrium from a gastric adenocarcinoma. The tumor cells infiltrate the endometrial stroma and surround benign glands. Lymphatic invasion is present (extreme right).

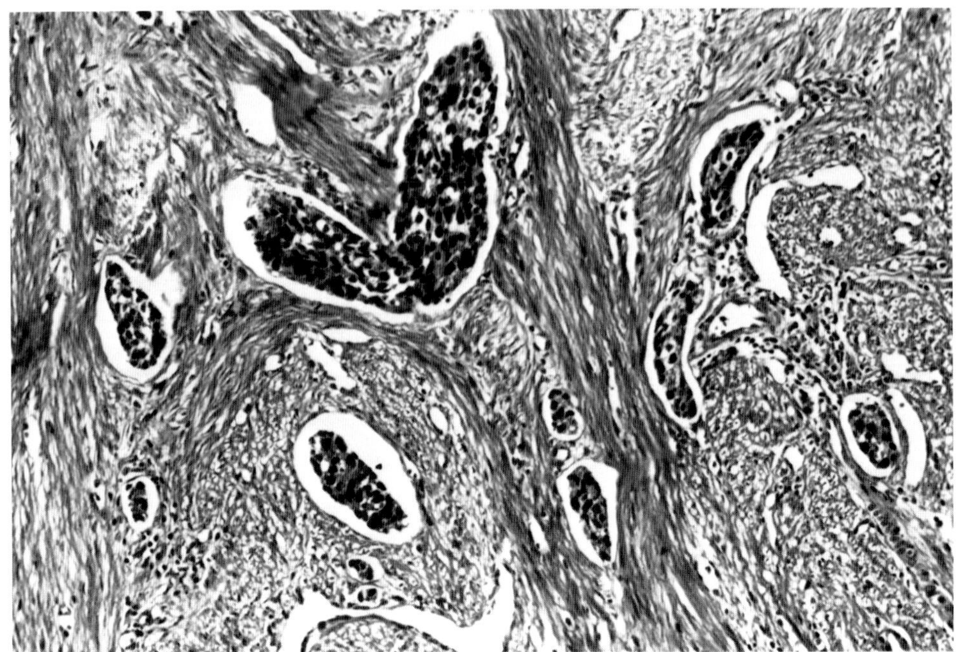

Fig. 8-35. Metastatic adenocarcinoma to myometrium from a gastric adenocarcinoma (same case as illustrated in Fig. 8-34). Note prominent lymphatic involvement.

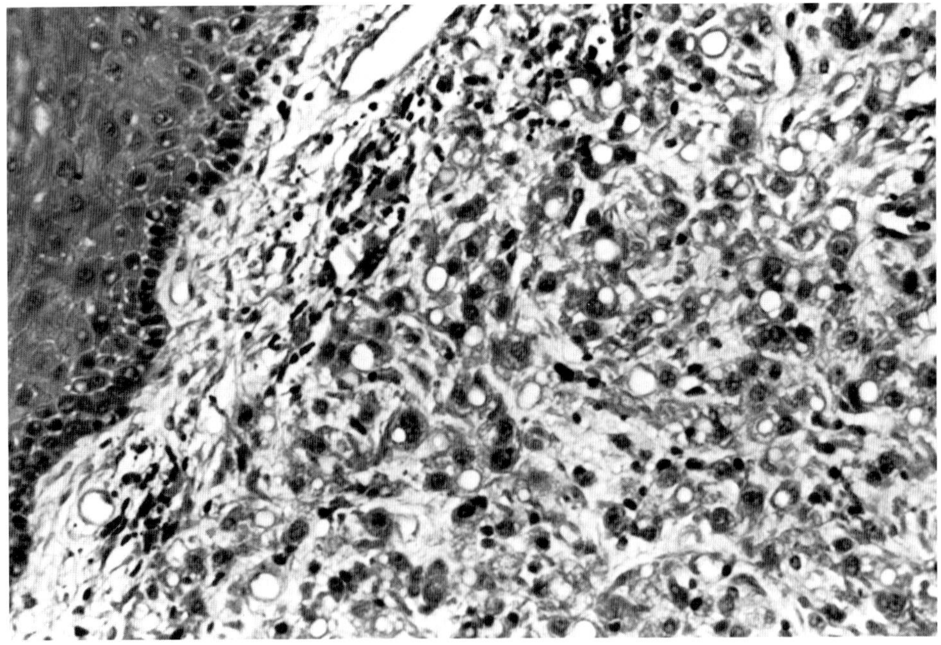

Fig. 8-36. Metastatic lobular carcinoma of breast to ectocervix. Note signet-ring cells.

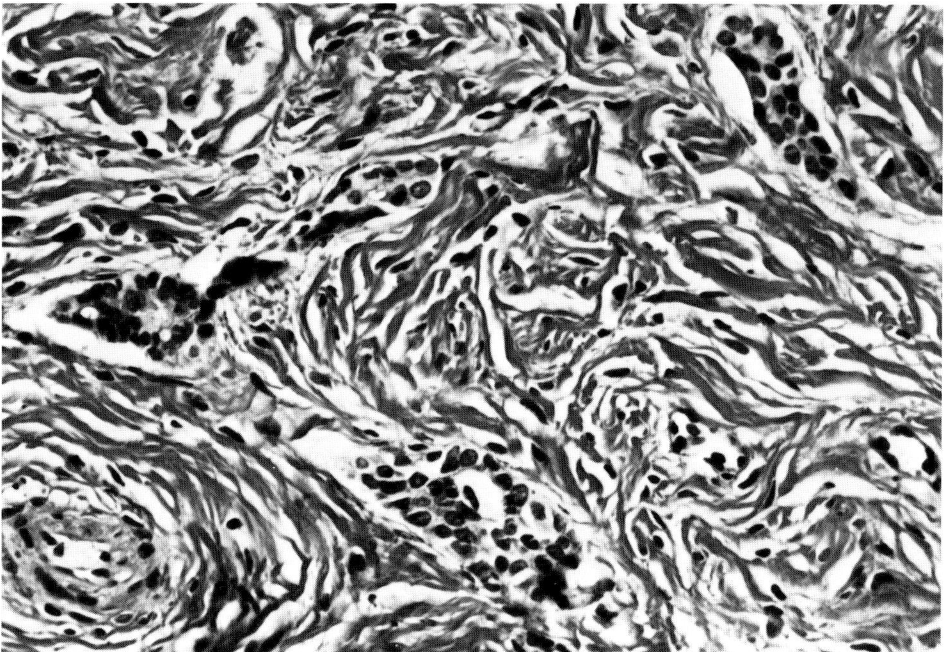

Fig. 8-37. Metastatic lobular carcinoma of breast to cervix. The cells have bland nuclear features and form small tubules. The lesion was initially misdiagnosed as hyperplasia of mesonephric remnants.

involved. In a literature review in 1982, Takeda et al.[234] found that in cases in which the location in the uterus was specified, the sole site of uterine spread was the cervix in 60.6 percent of cases, the corpus alone was involved in 21.2 percent of cases, while both sites were involved in 18.2 percent of cases.

Cervical Involvement

Extragenital carcinomas that most commonly metastasize to the cervix arise in the breast, stomach, and colon. Yazigi et al.[235] recently analyzed 24 cases of breast carcinoma metastatic to the cervix collected from the literature. In 80 percent of cases, the cervical metastases were detected following treatment of the breast carcinoma, with a median interval of 1 year; the longest reported interval was 9 years. In the remaining cases, the cervical and breast tumors were detected simultaneously with the exception of one patient in whom detection of the cervical metastasis preceded that of the primary tumor by 2 months. The patients typically presented with vaginal bleeding and malignant cells were detected on cervicovaginal smears in four of six cases. Only 5 patients had macroscopic evidence suggestive of a neoplasm. Almost 90 percent of the patients had evidence of metastatic disease in other sites; the endometrium, myometrium, or both were frequently involved. The histological appearance of the tumor within the cervix typically mimics that of the primary tumor, including the frequent presence of an Indian file arrangement of the cells, and in some, signet-ring cells (Fig. 8-36). Six of 21 patients with follow-up data were alive at the time of reporting, whereas 14 of the remaining 15 died of tumor progression; the median survival from the time of diagnosis of the cervical metastases was 12 months.

Approximately 30 cases of gastric carcinoma metastatic to the cervix have been reported (Figs. 8-34 and 8-35); most have been of signet-ring cell type.[229, 236–240] In approximately one-half of the cases, the findings of signet-ring cells on cervicovaginal Papanicolaou smears or the presence of similar cells (or conventional adenocarcinoma) within cervical biopsy specimens have been the presenting manifestation of the gastric carcinoma. Ovarian Krukenberg tumors have also been present in some cases.[239]

Approximately 30 cases of carcinoma of the colon or rectum with spread to the cervix have been described.[226, 228, 229, 237, 238, 241–243] With the exception of one case reported by Way,[226] in which a primary carcinoma of the sigmoid colon presented as an ulcerating mucosal lesion of the cervix, the cervical metastases were diagnosed at intervals of 3 to 60 months following colectomy, and were usually a manifestation of extensive recurrent tumor within the pelvis.

Of four cases of lung carcinoma metastatic to the cervix in which the histologic type was specified, three were anaplastic small cell carcinomas[244] and one was an adenocarcinoma.[238] Rare examples of carcinomas of the pancreas,[245] gallbladder,[246] kidney,[229] renal pelvis,[229] urinary bladder,[247] as well as malignant melanoma[238] and an appendiceal carcinoid tumor,[248] have metastasized to the cervix. In addition, we have recently encountered a case of malignant mesothelioma of the peritoneum that was associated with a small, grossly visible metastatic implant on the endocervical mucosa.

Uterine Corpus Involvement

The largest study of metastases to the uterine corpus from extragenital cancer was by Kumar and Hart[233] in 1983; of their 63 cases, 20 were encountered in surgical material, the remainder at autopsy. The surgical cases consisted of metastatic carcinoma in 9 hysterectomy specimens and 11 endometrial curettage specimens (these patients did not have a subsequent hysterectomy). In the former group, tumor was typically confined to the myometrium (8 of 9 cases); in the ninth case, both the endometrium and myometrium were involved. Myometrial leiomyomas also contained metastatic tumor, and in occasional cases, the metastatic tumor in the myometrium was confined to the leiomyoma.[233, 249] Similarly, in occasional tumors metastatic to the endometrium, the tumor may be confined to an endometrial polyp.[250] In the study by Kumar and Hart, there was synchronous ovarian involvement by metastatic tumor in 62 percent of surgical cases.

The histologic types of carcinoma metastatic to the corpus are similar to those involving the cervix, the majority of cases arising from the breast, colon, and stomach, in order of frequency. Malignant melanomas are the next most common group.[234, 251–255] In several such cases, endometrial tumor has been the presenting manifestation of the skin lesion[254]; in other cases, the uterine involvement was the first evidence of recurrent tumor after intervals of up to 8 years after removal of the primary melanoma.[234, 251, 253, 255] Metastases to the corpus have also rarely originated from carcinomas of the pancreas, lung, urinary bladder, and thyroid gland.[233] The appendiceal carcinoid tumor noted above also metastasized to the endometrium.[248]

REFERENCES

1. Marsh MR: Papilloma of the cervix. Am J Obstet Gynecol 64:281, 1952
2. Greene RR, Peckham BM: Squamous papillomas of the cervix. Am J Obstet Gynecol 67:883, 1954
3. Kistner RW, Hertig AT: Papillomas of the uterine cervix—their malignant potential. Obstet Gynecol 6:147, 1955

4. Kazal HL, Long JP: Squamous cell papillomas of the uterine cervix. A report of 20 cases. Cancer 11:1049, 1958

5. Pitkin RM, Kent TH: Papillary squamous lesions of the uterine cervix. A difficult problem in diagnosis. Am J Obstet Gynecol 85:440, 1963

6. Gilbert EF, Palladino A: Squamous papillomas of the uteirine cervix. Review of the literature and report of a giant papillary carcinoma. Am J Clin Pathol 46:115, 1966

7. Qizilbash AH: Papillary squamous tumors of the uterine cervix. A clinical and pathological study of 21 cases. Am J Clin Pathol 61:508, 1974

8. Randall MH, Andersen WA, Mills SE, Kim JC: Papillary squamous cell carcinomas of the uterine cervix: a clinicopathological study of nine cases. Int J Gynecol Pathol 5:1, 1986

9. Selzer I, Nelson HM: Benign papilloma (polypoid tumor) of the cervix uteri in children. Report of 2 cases. Am J Obstet Gynecol 84:165, 1962

10. Janovski HA, Kasdon EJ: Benign mesonephric papillary and polypoid tumors of the cervix in childhood. J Pediatr 63:211, 1963

11. Andrews CF, Jourdain L, Damjanov I: Benign cervical mesonephric papilloma of childhood. Report of a case studied by light and electron microscopy. Diagn Gynecol Obstet 3:39, 1981

12. Ulbright TM, Alexander RW, Kraus FT: Intramural papilloma of the vagina. Evidence of mullerian histogenesis. Cancer 48:2260, 1981

13. Young RH, Scully RE: Invasive adenocarcinoma and related tumors. Semin Diagn Pathol 7:205, 1990

14. Michael H, Sutton G, Hull MT, Roth LM: Villous adenoma of the uterine cervix associated with invasive adenocarcinoma: a histologic, ultrastructural, and immunohistochemical study. Int J Gynecol Pathol 5:163, 1986

15. Alvaro T, Nogales F: Villous adenoma and invasive adenocarcinoma of the cervix (letter). Int J Gynecol Pathol 7:96, 1988

16. Youngs LA, Taylor HB: Adenomatoid tumors of the uterus and fallopian tube. Am J Clin Pathol 48:537, 1967

17. Honore LH: Uterine mesothelioma. Am J Obstet Gynecol 135:162, 1979

18. Tiltman AJ: Adenomatoid tumours of the uterus. Histopathology 4:437, 1980

19. Quigley JC, Hart WR: Adenomatoid tumors of the uterus. Am J Clin Pathol 76:627, 1981

20. Iwasaki I, Yu TJ, Tamaru J, Asanuma K: A cystic adenomatoid tumor of the uterus simulating lymphangioma grossly. Acta Pathol Jpn 35:989, 1985

21. Suzuki T, Yoshida Y, Kaku T et al: Adenomatoid tumor of the uterus. Arch Pathol Lab Med 109:1049, 1985

22. Carlier MT, Dardick I, Lagace AF, Sreeram V: Adenomatoid tumor of the uterus: presentation in endometrial curettings. Int J Gynecol Pathol 5:69, 1986

23. Bisset DL, Morris JA, Fox H: Giant cystic adenomatoid tumor (mesothelioma) of the uterus. Histopathology 12:555, 1988

24. Srigley JR, Colgan TJ: Multifocal and diffuse adenomatoid tumor involving uterus and fallopian tube. Ultrastruct Pathol 12:351, 1988

25. Palacios J, Manrique AS, Villaespesa AR et al: Cystic adenomatoid tumor of the uterus. Int J Gynecol Pathol 10:296, 1991

26. De Rosa G, Boscaino A, Terracciano LM, Giordano G: Giant adenomatoid tumors of the uterus. Int J Gynecol Pathol 11:156, 1992

27. Goddard MJ, Grant JW: Adenomatoid tumours: a mucin histochemical and immunohistochemical study. Histopathology 20:57, 1992

27a. Livingstone EG, Guis MS, Pearl ML et al: Diffuse adenomatoid tumor of the uterus with a serosal papillary cystic component. Int J Gynecol Pathol 11:288, 1992

28. Jones EG, Donovan AJ: Adenomatoid tumor of the ovary versus mesothelial reaction. Am J Obstet Gynecol 92:694, 1965

29. Berthelot P, Benhanou JP, Fauvert R: Hypercorticisme et cancer de l'uterus. Presse Med 69:189, 1961

30. Driessens J, Clay A, Adenis L, Demaille A. Tumeur cervico-uterine et syndrome biologique de carcinoidose. Arch Anat Pathol 12:200, 1964

31. Shames JM, Dhurandhar NR, Blackard

WG: Insulin-secreting bronchial carcinoid tumor with widespread metastases. Am J Med 44:632, 1968

32. Albores-Saavedra J, Poucell S, Rodriguez-Martinez HA: Primary carcinoid of the uterine cervix. Patologia 10:185, 1971

33. Kiang DT, Bauer GE, Kennedy BJ: Immunoassayable insulin in carcinoma of the cervix associated with hypoglycemia. Cancer 31:801, 1973

34. Tateishi R, Wada A, Hayakawa K et al: Argyrophil cell carcinomas (apudomas) of the uterine cervix. Light and electron microscopic observation of 5 cases. Virchows Arch [A] 366:257, 1975

35. Jones HW III, Plymate S, Gluck FB et al: Small cell nonkeratinizing carcinoma of the cervix associated with ACTH production. Cancer 38:1629, 1976

36. Albores-Saavedra J, Larraza O, Poucell S, Rodriguez Martinez HA: Carcinoid of the uterine cervix. Additional observations on a new tumor entity. Cancer 38:2328, 1976

37. Daw H: Carcinoid of the cervix. Postgrad Med J 53:272, 1977

38. Van Hagell JR Jr, Donaldson ES, Wood EG et al: Small cell cancer of the uterine cervix. Cancer 40:2243, 1977

39. Warner TFCS: Carcinoid tumor of the uterine cervix. J Clin Pathol 31:990, 1978

40. Mackay B, Osborne B, Wharton JT: Small cell tumor of cervix with neuroepithelial features. Ultrastructural observations in two cases. Cancer 43:1138, 1979

41. Albores-Saavedra J, Rodriguez-Martinez HA, Larraza-Hernandez O: Carcinoid tumors of the cervix. Pathol Annu 14:273, 1979

42. Matsuyama M, Inoue T, Ariyoshi Y et al: Argyrophil carcinoma of the uterine cervix with ectopic production of ACTH, beta-MSH, serotonin, histamine, and amylase. Cancer 44: 1813, 1979

43. Habib A, Kaneko M, Cohen CJ, Walker G: Carcinoid of the uterine cervix. A case report with light and electron microscopic studies. Cancer 43:535, 1979

44. Jacobs AJ, Marchevsky A, Gordon RE et al: Oat cell carcinoma of the uterine cervix in a pregnant woman treated with cis-diamminedichloroplatinum. Gynecol Oncol 9:405, 1980

45. Johannessen JV, Capella C, Solcia E et al: Endocrine cell carcinoma of the uterine cervix. Diagn Gynecol Obstet 2:127, 1980

46. Lojek MA, Fer MF, Kasselberg AG et al: Cushing's syndrome with small cell carcinoma of the uterine cervix. Am J Med 69:140, 1980

47. Hsu C, Ma L, Wong LC, Chan CW: Nonendocrine carcinoid tumour of the uterine cervix: aspects of diagnosis and treatment. Case Report. Br J Obstet Gynaecol 88: 1056, 1981

48. Mullins JD, Hilliard GD: Cervical carcinoid ("argyrophil cell" carcinoma) associated with an endocervical adenocarcinoma: A light and ultrastructural study. Cancer 47:785, 1981

49. Pazdur R, Bonomi P, Slayton R et al: Neuroendocrine carcinoma of the cervix: implications for staging and therapy. Gynecol Oncol 12:120, 1981

50. Stahl R, Demopoulos RI, Bigelow B: Carcinoid tumor within a squamous cell carcinoma of the cervix. Gynecol Oncol 11:387, 1981

51. Stassart J, Crum CP, Yordan EL et al: Argyrophilic carcinoma of the cervix: A report of a case with coexisting cervical intraepithelial neoplasia. Gynecol Oncol 13:247, 1982

52. Hariri J, Rasmussen EA, Hage E: Carcinoid tumor of the uterine cervix. Acta Obstet Gynecol Scand 62:539, 1983

53. Inoue T, Yamaguchi K, Suzuki H et al. Production of immunoreactive polypeptide hormones in cervical carcinoma. Cancer 53:1509, 1984

54. Scully RE, Aguirre P, DeLellis RA: Argyrophilia, serotonin, and peptide hormones in the female genital tract and its tumors. Int J Gynecol Pathol 3:51, 1984

55. Silva EG, Kott MM, Ordonez HG: Endocrine carcinoma intermediate cell type of the uterine cervix. Cancer 54:1705, 1984

56. Yamasaki M, Tateishi R, Hongo J et al: Argyrophil small cell carcinomas of the uterine cervix. Int J Gynecol Pathol 3:146, 1984

57. Yoshida A, Yoshida H, Fukunishi R, Inohara R: Carcinoid tumor of the uterine cervix. A light and electron microscopic study. Virchows Arch [A] 402:331, 1984

58. Groben P, Reddick R, Askin F: The pathologic spectrum of small cell carcinoma of the cervix. Int J Gynecol Pathol 4:42, 1985
59. Inoue M, Ueda G, Hakajima T: Immunohistochemical demonstration of neuron-specific enolase in gynecologic malignant tumors. Cancer 55:1686, 1985
60. Miles PA, Herrera GA, Mena H, Trujillo I: Cytologic findings in primary malignant carcinoid tumor of the cervix, including immunohistochemistry and electron microscopy performed on cervical smears. Acta Cytol 29:1003, 1985
61. Fujii S, Konishi I, Ferenczy A et al: Small cell undifferentiated carcinoma of the uterine cervix: histology, ultrastructure, and immunohistochemistry of two cases. Ultrastruct Pathol 10:337, 1986
62. Stockdale AD, Leader M, Phillips RH, Henry K: The carcinoid syndrome with multiple hormone secretion associated with a carcinoid tumour of the uterine cervix. Case report. Br J Obstet Gynaecol 93:397, 1986
63. Ulich TR, Liao S, Layfield L et al: Endocrine and tumor differentiation markers in poorly differentiated small-cell carcinoids of the cervix and vagina. Arch Pathol Lab Med 110:1054, 1986
64. Turner WA, Gallup DG, Talledo OE et al: Neuroendocrine carcinoma of the uterine cervix complicated by pregnancy: case report and review of the literature. Obstet Gynecol 67:80S, 1986
65. Barrett RJ II, Davos I, Leuchter RS, Lagasse LD: Neuroendocrine features in poorly differentiated and undifferentiated carcinomas of the cervix. Cancer 60:2325, 1987
66. Muraoka S, Takahashi T, Ando M et al: Minute carcinoid tumor of the uterine cervix associated with microinvasive adenocarcinoma, with reference to its histogenesis. Acta Pathol Jpn 37:1183, 1987
67. Gersell DJ, Mazoujian G, Mutch DG, Rudloff MA: Small-cell undifferentiated carcinoma of the cervix. A clinicopathologic, ultrastructural, and immunocytochemical study of 15 cases. Am J Surg Pathol 12:684, 1988
68. Seidel R Jr, Steinfeld A. Carcinoid of the cervix: natural history and implications for therapy. Gynecol Oncol 30:114, 1988
69. Sheets EE, Berman ML, Hrountas CK et al: Surgically treated, early-stage neuroendocrine small-cell cervical carcinoma. Obstet Gynecol 71:10, 1988
70. Van Hagell JR, Jr, Powell DE, Gallion HH et al: Small cell carcinoma of the uterine cervix. Cancer 62:1586, 1988
71. Walker AN, Mills SE, Taylor PT: Cervical neuroendocrine carcinoma: a clinical and light microscopic study of 14 cases. Int J Gynecol Pathol 7:64, 1988
72. Husain AN, Gattuso P, Abraham K, Castelli MJ: Synchronous adenocarcinoma and carcinoid of the uterine cervix: immunohistochemical study of a case and review of literature. Gynecol Oncol 33:125, 1989
73. Tsukamoto N, Hirakawa T, Matsukuma K et al: Carcinoma of the uterine cervix with variegated histological patterns and calcitonin production. Gynecol Oncol 33:395, 1989
74. Ueda G, Shimizu C, Shimizu H et al: An immunohistochemical study of small-cell and poorly differentiated carcinomas of the cervix using neuroendocrine markers. Gynecol Oncol 34:164, 1989
75. Chang JKC, Tsui WMS, Tung SY, Ching RCT: Endocrine cell hyperplasia of the uterine cervix. A precursor of neuroendocrine carcinoma of the cervix? Am J Clin Pathol 92:825, 1989
76. Silva EG, Gershenson D, Sneige N et al: Small cell carcinoma of the uterine cervix: pathology and prognostic factors. Surg Pathol 2:105, 1989
77. Hirahatake K, Hareyama H, Kure R et al: Cytologic and hormonal findings in a carcinoid tumor of the uterine cervix. Acta Cytol 34:119, 1990
78. Kothe MJC, Prins JM, De Wit R et al: Small cell carcinoma of the cervix with inappropriate antidiuretic hormone secretion. Case report. Br J Obstet Gynaecol 97:647, 1990
79. Miller B, El-Torky M, Photopulus G: Simultaneous small cell carcinoma of the cervix and adenocarcinoma of the ovary. Gynecol Oncol 39:99, 1990
80. Ramsay IN, Gardiner DS: Small cell undif-

ferentiated carcinoma of the cervix. Case report. Br J Obstet Gynaecol 97:1046, 1990

81. Ambros RA, Park J, Shah K, Kurman RJ: Evaluation of histologic, morphometric, and immunohistochemical criteria in the differential diagnosis of small cell carcinomas of the cervix with particular reference to human papillomavirus types 16 and 18. Mod Pathol 4:586, 1991

82. Miller B, Dockter M, El Torky M, Photopulos G. Small cell carcinoma of the cervix: a clinical and flow-cytometric study. Gynecol Oncol 42:27, 1991

83. O'Hanlan KA, Goldberg GL Jones JG et al: Adjuvant therapy for neuroendocrine small cell carcinoma of the cervix: review of the literature. Gynecol Oncol 43:167, 1991

84. Young RH, Gersell DJ, Roth LM, Scully RE: Ovarian metastases from cervical carcinomas other than pure adenocarcinoma: a report of 12 cases with clinical manifestations. Cancer (in press)

85. Hammar SP, Insalaco SJ, Lee RB et al: Amphicrine carcinoma of the uterine cervix. Am J Clin Pathol 97:516, 1992

86. Ueda G, Yamasaki M: Neuroendocrine carcinoma of the uterus, p. 309. In Sasano N (ed): Current Topics in Pathology. Vol. 85: Gynecological Tumors. Springer-Verlag, New York, 1992

87. Miles PA, Herrera GA, Greenberg H, Rawding-Patterson G: Primary carcinoid tumor of the uterine cervix presenting as an adenosquamous carcinoma. Diagn Gynecol Obstet 4:327, 1982

88. Fox H, Kazza B, Langley FA: Argyrophil and argentaffin cells in the female genital tract and in ovarian mucinous cysts. J Pathol 88:479, 1964

89. Fetissof F, Serres G, Arbeille B et al: Argyrophilic cells and ectocervical epithelium. Int J Gynecol Pathol 10:177, 1991

90. Stoler MH, Mills SE, Gersell DJ, Walker AN: Small-cell neuroendocrine carcinoma of the cervix: a human papillomavirus type 18-associated cancer. Am J Surg Pathol 15:28, 1991

91. Wolber RA Clement PB: In situ DNA hybridization of cervical small cell carcinoma and adenocarcinoma using biotin-labeled human papillomavirus probes. Mod Pathol 4:96, 1991

92. Pao CC, Lin C, Tseng C et al: Human papillomaviruses and small cell carcinoma of the uterine cervix. Gynecol Oncol 43:206, 1991

93. Ueda G, Yamasaki M, Inoue M et al: Immunohistochemical demonstration of HNK 1-defined antigen in gynecologic tumors with argyrophilia. Int J Gynecol Pathol 5:143, 1986

94. Olson H, Twiggs L, Sibley R: Small-cell carcinoma of the endometrium: light microscopic and ultrastructural study of a case. Cancer 50:760, 1982

95. Bannatyne P, Russell P, Wills EJ: Argyrophilia and endometrial carcinoma. Int J Gynecol Pathol 2:235, 1983

96. Kumar NB: Small cell carcinoma of the endometrium in a 23-year-old woman: light microscopic and ultrastructural study. Am J Clin Pathol 81:98, 1984

97. Kristensen PB, Paulsen SM: Simultaneous presentation of small-cell carcinoma involving the ovary and uterine endometrium. J Submicrosc Cytol 17:97, 1985

98. Paz RA, Frigerio B, Sundblad AS, Eusebi V: Small-cell (oat cell) carcinoma of the endometrium. Arch Pathol Lab Med 109:270, 1985

99. Bertarelli C, Cattani MG, Magni E, Eusebi V: Carcinoma a piccole cellule dell'endometrio con differenziazione ghiandolare e squamosa. Pathologica 78:79, 1986

100. Manivel C, Wick MR, Sibley RK: Neuroectodermal differentiation in mullerian neoplasms. An immunohistochemical study of a "pure" endometrial small-cell carcinoma and a mixed mullerian tumor containing small-cell carcinoma. Am J Clin Pathol 86:438, 1986

101. Tohya T, Miyazaki K, Katabuchi, H et al: Small cell carcinoma of the endometrium asociated with adenosquamous carcinoma: a light and electron microscopic study. Gynecol Oncol 25:363, 1986

102. Tenti P, Camevali L, Paulli M et al: Dedifferentiating endometrial adenocarcinoma. Report of case. Eur J Gynaecol Oncol 10:292, 1989

103. Abeler VM, Kjorstad KE, Nesland JM: Undifferentiated carcinoma of the endometrium. A histopathologic and clinical study of 31 case. Cancer 68:98, 1991

104. Campo E, Brunier MN, Merino MJ: Small

cell carcinoma of the endometrium with associated ocular paraneoplastic syndrome. Cancer 69:2283, 1992

105. Zaczek T. Mesonephric carcinoma of the cervix uteri in an 11-month-old girl treated by hysterectomy. Am J Obstet Gynecol 85:176, 1963

106. Copeland LJ, Sneige N, Ordonez NG et al: Endodermal sinus tumor of the vagina and cervix. Cancer 55:2558, 1985

107. Pileri S, Martinelli G, Serra L, Bazzocchi F: Endodermal sinus tumor arising in the endometrium. Obstet Gynecol 56:391, 1980

108. Clement PB, Young RH, Scully RE: Extraovarian pelvic yolk sac tumors. Cancer 62:620, 1988

109. Ohta M, Sakakibara K, Mizuno K et al: Successful treatment of primary endodermal sinus tumor of the endometrium. Gynecol Oncol 31:357, 1988

110. Joseph MG, Fellows FG, Hearn SA: Primary endodermal sinus tumor of the endometrium. Cancer 65:297, 1990

111. Mann W. Zwei seltene Geschwulste des Corpus uteri mit Bemerkungen zu ihrer Enstehungsweise. Virchows Arch [A] 273:663, 1929

112. Hellendall H. Ein intramurales Teratom des Corpus uteri mit Durchbruch in die Uterushohle und Haarabgang durch die Scheide. Zentralbl Gynakol 54:2398, 1930

113. Lackner JE, Krohn L: Report of a case of teratoma of the uterus. Am J Obstet Gynecol 25:735, 1933

114. Nicholson GW: Studies on tumour formation. Guys Hosp Rep 105:157, 1956

115. Forster VR: Teratoma adultum cervicis uteri. Gynaecologia 134:164, 1952

116. Pyrah RD, Redman TF: Teratoma of the uterus with an associated congenital anomaly. J Pathol 95:291, 1968

117. Mold JW: Benign solid teratoma of the uterus. J Pathol 99:173, 1969

118. Dallenbach-Hellweg G, Wittlinger H: Benign solid teratoma of the uterus. Beitr Pathol Bd 158:307, 1976

119. Mihailovici A, Radulescu D, Bendescu M, Paraschiv L: Teratoma of the uterine cervix. Morphol Embryol 135:191, 1976

120. Martin E, Scholes J, Richart RM, Fenoglio CM: Benign cystic teratoma of the uterus. Am J Obstet Gynecol 135:429, 1979

121. Hanai J, Tsuji M: Uterine teratoma with lymphoid hyperplasia. Acta Pathol Jpn 31:153, 1981

122. Iwanaga S, Ishii H, Nagano H et al: Mature cystic teratoma of the uterine cervix. Asia-Oceania J Obstet Gynaecol 16:363, 1990

123. Tyagi SP, Saxena K, Rizvi R, Langley FA: Foetal remnants in the uterus and their relation to other uterine heterotopia. Histopathology 3:339, 1979

124. Ansah-Boateng Y, Wefls M, Poole DR: Coexistent immature teratoma of the uterus and endometrial adenocarcinoma complicated by gliomatosis peritonei. Gynecol Oncol 21:106, 1985

125. Hendrickson MR, Kempson RL: p. 211. In Surgical Pathology of the Uterine Corpus. WB Saunders, Philadelphia, 1980

126. Cortes J, Llompart M, Rossello JJ et al: Immature teratoma primary of the uterine cervix. Eur J Gynaecol Oncol 11:37, 1990

127. Young RH, Kleinman GM, Scully RE: Glioma of the uterus. Report of a case with comments on histogenesis. Am J Surg Pathol 5:695, 1981

128. Hendrickson MR, Scheithauer BW: Primitive neuroectodermal tumor of the endometrium: report of two cases, one with electron microscopic observations. Int J Gynecol Pathol 5:249, 1986

129. Rose PG, O'Toole RV, Keyhani-Rofagha S, Qualman S, Boutselis JG: Malignant peripheral primitive neuroectodermal tumor of the uterus. J Surg Oncol 35:165, 1987.

130. Daya D, Lukka H, Clement PB: Primitive neuroectodermal tumors of the uterus: a report of four cases. Hum Pathol 23:1120, 1992

131. Liao SY, Choi BH: Expression of glial fibrillary acidic protein by neoplastic cells of mullerian origin. Virchows Arch 52:185, 1986

132. Schulz DM: A malignant melanotic neoplasm of the uterus, resembling the "retinal anlage" tumors. Report of a case. Arch Pathol 28:524, 1957

133. Gersell DJ, Fulling KH: Localized neurofibromatosis of the female genitourinary tract. Am J Surg Pathol 13:873, 1989

134. Young TW, Thrasher TV: Nonchromaffin paraganglioma of the uterus. A case report. Arch Pathol Lab Med 106:608, 1982

135. Tavassoli FA: Melanotic paraganglioma of the uterus. Cancer 58:492, 1986

136. Beham A, Schmid C, Fletcher COM et al: Malignant paraganglioma of the uterus. Virch Arch A 420:453, 1992

137. Fingerland A: Ganglioneuroma of the cervix uteri. J Pathol 47:631, 1938

138. Gwavava NJ, Traub AI: A neurilemmoma of the cervix. Br J Obstet Gynaecol 87:444, 1980

139. Junge J, Horn T, Bock J: Primary malignant schwannoma of the uterine cervix. Case report. Br J Obstet Gyanecol 96:111, 1989

140. Terzakis JA, Opher E, Melamed J et al: Pigmented melanocytic schwannoma of the uterine cervix. Ultrastruct Pathol 14:357, 1990

141. Gal R, Halpern M, Kessler E: Granular cell myoblastoma (GCM) of cervix and vulva. A clinical and immunohistochemical study, abstracted. In Seventeenth International Congress of the International Academy of Pathology, Dublin, Ireland, September 1988

142. Martin PC, Pulitzer DR, Reed RJ: Pigmented myomatous neurocristoma of the uterus. Arch Pathol Lab Med 113:1291, 1989

143. Arhelger RB, Bocian JJ: Brenner tumor of the uterus. Cancer 38:1741, 1976

144. Chen KTK: Extraovarian transitional cell carcinoma of female genital tract (letter). Am J Clin Pathol 94:670, 1990

145. Bittencourt AL, Britto JF, Fonseca LE Jr: Wilms' tumor of the uterus: The first report of the literature. Cancer 47:2496, 1981

146. Bell DA, Shimm DS, Gang DL: Wilms' tumor of the endocervix. Arch Pathol Lab Med 109:371, 1985

147. Yu HC, Ketabchi M: Detection of malignant melanoma of the uterine cervix from Papanicolaou smears. A case report. Acta Cytol 31:73, 1987

148. Holmquist ND, Torres J: Malignant melanoma of the cervix: report of a case. Acta Cytol 32:252, 1988

149. Owens OJ, Pollard K, Khoury GG et al: Case report: primary malignant melanoma of the uterine cervix. Clin Radiol 39:33, 1988

150. Chua S, Viegas OAC, Wee A, Ratnam SS: Malignant melanomas of the cervix. Gynecol Obstet Invest 27:107, 1989

151. Mordel H, Mor-Yosef S, Ben-Baruch N, Anteby SO: Malignant melanoma of the uterine cervix: Case report and review of the literature. Gynecol Oncol 32:375, 1989

152. Podczaski E, Abt A, Kaminski P et al: A patient with multiple, malignant melanomas of the lower genital tract. Gynecol Oncol 37:422, 1990

153. Santoso JT, Kucera PR, Ray J: Primary malignant melanoma of the uterine cervix: two case reports and a century's review. Obstet Gynecol Surv 45:733, 1990

154. Vleugels MPH, Brolmann HAM, van Beek M: Primary melanoma of the cervix uteri, an avis rara? Acta Obstet Gynecol Scand 69:259, 1990

155. Pinedo F, Ingelmo JM, Miranda P, et al: Primary malignant melanoma of the uterine cervix: case report and review of the literature. Gynecol Obstet Invest 31:121, 1991

156. Khoo US, Collins RJ, Ngan HYS: Malignant melanoma of the female genital tract. Pathology 23:312, 1991

157. Cid JM: La pigmentation melanique de l'endocervix. Ann Anat Pathol 4:617, 1959

158. Lathrop JC: Malignant pelvic lymphomas. Obstet Gynecol 30:137, 1967

159. Johnson CE, Soule EH: Malignant lymphoma as a gynecologic problem. Report of five cases including one primary lymphosarcoma of the cervix uteri. Obstet Gynecol 9:149, 1957

160. Maeda T, Kamegai H, Mori H: Malignant lymphoma presenting as initial sympton in the uterus. Br J Obstet Gynaecol 95:1195, 1988

161. Andrews SJ, Hernandez E, Woods J, Cook B: Burkitt's-like lymphoma presenting as a gynecologic tumor. Gynecol Oncol 30:131, 1988

162. Davey D, Munn R, Smith LW, Cibull ML: Angiotrophic lymphoma. Presentation in uterine vessels with cytogenetic studies. Arch Pathol Lab Med 114:879, 1990

163. Hung LHY, Kurtz DM: Hodgkin's disease of the endometrium. Arch Pathol Lab Med 109:952, 1985

164. Raggio ML, Bostrom SG, Harden EA: Hodgkin's lymphoma of the uterus presenting as refractory pelvic inflammatory disease. J Reprod Med 33:827, 1988

165. Freeman C, Berg JW, Cutler SJ: Occurrence and prognosis of extranodal lymphomas. Cancer 29:252, 1972
166. Retikas DG: Hodgkin's sarcoma of the cervix. Report of a case. Am J Obstet Gynecol 80:1104, 1960
167. Welch JW, Hellwig CA: Reticulum cell sarcoma of the uterine cervix. Obstet Gynecol 22:293, 1963
168. Nasiell M: Hodgkin's disease limited to the uterine cervix. Acta Cytol 8:16, 1964
169. Fox H, More JRS: Primary malignant lymphoma of the uterus. J Clin Pathol 18:723, 1965
170. Anderson GG: Hodgkin's disease of the uterine cervix. Report of a case. Obstet Gynecol 29:170, 1967
171. Stransky GC, Acosta A, Kaplan AL, Friedman JA: Reticulum cell sarcoma of the cervix. Obstet Gynecol 41:183, 1973
172. Wright CJE: Solitary malignant lymphoma of the uterus. Am J Obstet Gynecol 117:114, 1973
173. Chorlton I, Karnei RF Jr, King FM, Norris HJ: Primary malignant reticuloendothelial disease involving the vagina, cervix, and corpus uteri. Obstet Gynecol 33:735, 1974
174. Cihak RW, Hamada J: Primary reticulum cell sarcoma of the uterus. Cancer 33:1039, 1974
175. Gall JA, Sartino G, Deutsch M: Primary reticulum cell sarcoma of the uterus. Oncology 31:157, 1975
176. Carr I, Hill AS, Hancock B, Neal FE: Malignant lymphoma of the cervix uteri: histology and ultrastructure. J Clin Pathol 29:680, 1976
177. Delgado G, Smith JP, Luis D, Gallagher S: Reticulum-cell sarcoma of the cervix. Am J Obstet Gynecol 125:691, 1976
178. Whitaker D: The role of cytology in the detection of malignant lymphoma of the uterine cervix. Acta Cytol 20:510, 1976
179. Krumerman M, Chung A: Solitary reticulum cell sarcoma of the uterine cervix with initial cytodiagnosis. Acta Cytol 22:46, 1978
180. Steinfeld AD: Histiocytic lymphoma of the cervix. Gynecol Oncol 8:97, 1979
181. Tunca JC, Reddi PR, Shah SH, Slack ST: Malignant non-Hodgkin's-type lymphoma of the cervix uteri occurring during pregnancy. Gynecol Oncol 7:385, 1979
182. Volpe R, Tirelli U, Tumolo S et al: Stage II_E diffuse small cleaved cell lymphoma of the cervix. Pathologica 75:887, 1983
183. Harris NL, Scully RE: Malignant lymphoma and granulocytic sarcoma of the uterus and vagina. A clinicopathologic analysis of 27 cases. Cancer 53:2530, 1984
184. Komaki R, Cox JD, Hansen RM et al: Malignant lymphoma of the uterine cervix. Cancer 54:1699, 1984
185. Gharpure KJ, Mahesh D, Bhargava MK: Malignant lymphoma of the uterine cervix—a report of two cases with review of literature. Indian J Cancer 22:296, 1985
186. Taki I, Aozasa K, Kurokawa K: Malignant lymphoma of the uterine cervix. Cytologic diagnosis of a case with immunocytochemical corroboration. Acta Cytol 29:607, 1985
187. Barr BMAM, Reijnders FJL, Keuning JJ et al: Primary malignant lymphoma of the uterine cervix associated with cold-reacting autoantibody-mediated hemolytic anemia. Acta Haematol 75:232, 1986
188. Cunningham D, Gilchrist NL, Lee ED et al: T-cell lymphoblastic lymphoma of the uterus complicated by Chlamydia trachomatis pneumonia. Postgrad Med J 62:55, 1986
189. Cardillo MR, Manente L, Ambrad O et al: Immunohistochemical study in a case of primitive lymphoma of the uterine cervix. Eur J Gynaecol Oncol 8:607, 1987
190. Mann R, Roberts WS, Gunasakeran S, Tralins A: Primary lymphoma of the uterine cervix. Gynecol Oncol 26:127, 1987
191. Strang P, Sorbe B, Sundstrom C: Primary aneuploid lymphoma of the uterine cervix: a case report. Gynecol Oncol 30:302, 1988
192. Johnston C, Senekjian EK, Ratain MJ, Talerman A: Conservative management of primary cervical lymphoma using combination chemotherapy: a case report. Gynecol Oncol 35:391, 1989
193. Khoury GG, Robinson A: Lymphoma of uterine cervix. Eur J Surg Oncol 15:65, 1989
194. Matsuyama T, Tsukamoto N, Kaku T et al: Primary malignant lymphoma of the uterine corpus and cervix. Report of a case with immunocytochemical analysis. Acta Cytol 33:228, 1989
195. Sandvei R, Lote K, Svendsen E, Thunold

S: Successful pregnancy following treatment of primary malignant lymphoma of the uterine cervix. Gynecol Oncol 38:128, 1990

196. Muntz HG, Ferry JA, Flynn D et al: Stage IE primary malignant lymphomas of the uterine cervix. Cancer 68:2023, 1991

197. Pasini F, Iuzzolino P, Santo A et al: A primitive lymphoma of the uterine cervix. Case report. Eur J Gynecol Oncol 12:107, 1991

198. Perren T, Farrant M, McCarthy K, Harper P, Wiltshaw E: Lymphomas of the cervix and upper vagina: a report of five cases and a review of the literature. Gynecol Oncol 44:87, 1992

199. Kashimura M, Kusano S, Hamagaki K, Sato Y: Primary malignant lymphoma of the endometrium: report of a case and review of the literatures. Acta Obstet Gynaecol Jpn 43:1731, 1991

200. Ferry JA, Young RH: Malignant lymphoma, pseudolymphoma, and hematopoietic disorders of the female genital tract. Pathol Annu 26:227, 1991

201. Mills SE, Austin MB, Randal ME: Lymphoepithelioma-like carcinoma of the uterine cervix. A distinctive, undifferentiated carcinoma with inflammatory stroma. Am J Surg Pathol 9:883, 1985

202. Lucia SP, Mills H, Lowenhaupt E, Hunt ML: Visceral involvement in primary neoplastic diseases of the reticulo-endothelial system. Cancer 5:1193, 1952

203. Barcos M, Lane W, Gomez GA et al: An autopsy study of 1206 acute and chronic leukemias (1958 to 1982). Cancer 60:827, 1987

204. Ceelen GH, Sakurai M: Vaginal cytology in leukemia. Acta Cytol 6:370, 1962

205. Hauptman H, Taussig FJ: Leucemic infiltration of the female internal genitalia as a cause of vaginal bleeding. Am J Obstet Gynecol 39:70, 1940

206. Israel SL, Mutch JC: Leukemic infiltration of female genitalia. A gynecologic entity. Obstet Gynecol 7:425, 1956

207. Hartford CE: Bleeding from the uterus caused by chloroma. Report of a case. Obstet Gynecol 31:166, 1968

208. Pascoe HR: Tumors composed of immature granulocytes occurring in the breast in chronic granulocytic leukemia. Cancer 25:697, 1970

209. Steinbock GS, Morrisseau PM, Vinson RK: Acute obstructive renal failure secondary to granulocytic sarcoma (chloroma). Urology 27:268, 1986

210. Arulkumaran S, Koh CH, Pang M et al: Chronic myeloid leukemia presenting as a gynecological emergency. Gynecol Oncol 28:111, 1987

211. Mikhail MS, Runowicz CD, Kadish AS, Romney SL: Colposcopic and cytologic detection of chronic lymphocytic leukemia. Gynecol Oncol 34:106, 1989

212. Seo IS, Hull MT, Pak HY: Granulocytic sarcoma of the cervix as a primary manifestation. Cancer 40:3030, 1977

213. Kapadia SB, Krause JR, Kanbour AI, Hartsock RJ: Granulocytic sarcoma of the uterus. Cancer 41:687, 1978

214. Ersboll J, Petri J, Jensen KH, Hansen MM: Granulocytic sarcoma preceding acute myeloid leukaemia. Scand J Haematol 24:435, 1980

215. Spahr J, Behm FG, Schneider V: Preleukemic granulocytic sarcoma of cervix and vagina. Initial manifestation by cytology. Acta Cytol 26:55, 1982

216. Abeler V, Kjorstad KE, Langholm R, Marton PF: Granulocytic sarcoma (chloroma) of the uterine cervix: report of two cases. Int J Gynecol Pathol 2:88, 1983

217. Cassi E, Tosi A, De'Paoli A et al: Granulocytic sarcoma without evidence of acute leukemia: 2 cases with unusual localization (uterus and breast) and 1 case with bone localization. Haematologica 69:464, 1984

218. Meis JM, Butler JJ, Osborne BM, Manning JT: Granulocytic sarcoma in nonleukemic patients. Cancer 58:2697, 1986

219. Banik S, Grech AB, Eyden BP: Granulocytic sarcoma of the cervix: an immunohistochemical, histochemical, and ultrastructural study. J Clin Pathol 42:483, 1989

219a. Friedman HD, Adelson MD, Elder RC, Lemke SM: Granulocytic sarcoma of the uterine cervix—Literature review of granulocytic sarcoma of the female genital tract. Gynecol Oncol 46:128, 1992

220. Figueroa JM, Huffaker AK, Diehl E: Malignant plasma cells in cervical smear. Acta Cytol 22:43, 1978

221. Axiotis CA, Merino MJ, Duray PH: Langerhans cell histiocytosis of the female genital tract. Cancer 67:1650, 1991
222. Issa PY, Salem PA, Brihi E, Azoury RS: Eosinophilic granuloma with involvement of the female genitalia. Am J Obstet Gynecol 137:608, 1980
223. Schwartz A, Zich P: Eosinophilic histiocytic granuloma of the vulva and cervix. Sb Lek 91:1, 1989
224. Hadinec V, Namestek S, Vanata J: Eosinophilic granuloma of the cervix uteri. Cesk Gynekol 49:266, 1984
225. Murray J, Fox H: Rosai-Dorfman disease of the uterine cervix. Int J Gynecol Pathol 10:209, 1991
226. Way S: Carcinoma metastatic in the cervix. Gynecol Oncol 9:298, 1980
227. McComas BC, Farnum JB, Donaldson RC: Ovarian carcinoma presenting as a cervical metastasis. Obstet Gynecol 63:593, 1984
228. Korhonen M, Stenback F: Adenocarcinoma metastatic to the uterine cervix. Gynecol Obstet Invest 17:57, 1984
229. Lemoine NR, Hall PA: Epithelial tumors metastatic to the uterine cervix. A study of 63 cases and review of the literature. Cancer 57:2002, 1986
230. Danielian PJ: Ovarian metastatic carcinoma presenting as a primary cervical carcinoma. Acta Obstet Gynecol Scand 69:265, 1990
231. Gilks CB, Clement PB: Papillary serous carcinomas of the uterine cervix: a report of three cases. Mod Pathol 5:426, 1992
232. Kiaer W, Holm-Jensen S: Metastases to the uterus. Five cases diagnosed on the basis of curettings. Acta Pathol Microbiol Scand A 80:835, 1972
233. Kumar NB, Hart WR: Metastases to the uterine corpus from extragenital cancers. A clinicopathologic study of 63 cases. Cancer 50:2163, 1982
234. Takeda M, Diamond SM, DeMarco M, Quinn DM: Cytologic diagnosis of malignant melanoma metastatic to the endometrium. Acta Cytol 22:503, 1978
235. Yazigi R, Sandstad J, Munoz AK: Breast cancer metastasizing to the uterine cervix. Cancer 61:2558, 1988
236. Kashimura M, Kashimura Y, Matsuyama T et al: Adenocarcinoma of the uterine cervix metastatic from primary stomach cancer: cytologic findings in six cases. Acta Cytol 27:54, 1983
237. Zhang Y, Zhang P, Wei Y: Metastatic carcinoma of the cervix uteri from the gastrointestinal tract. Gynecol Oncol 15:287, 1983
238. Mazur MT, Hsueh S, Gersell DJ: Metastases to the female genital tract. Analysis of 325 cases. Cancer 53:1978, 1984
239. Atobe Y, Yoshimura T, Kako H et al: Gastric cancer diagnosed by biopsy of the uterine cervix. Gynecol Oncol 26:135, 1987
240. McGill F, Adachi A, Karimi N et al: Abnormal cervical cytology leading to the diagnosis of gastric cancer. Gynecol Oncol 36:101, 1990
241. Esposito JM, Zarou DM, Zarou GS: Extragenital adenocarcinoma metastatic to the cervix uteri: A diagnostic problem. Am J Obstet Gynecol 92:792, 1965
242. Daw E: Extragenital adenocarcinoma metastatic to the cervix uteri. Am J Obstet Gynecol 114:1104, 1972
243. Abell MR, Gosling JRG: Gland cell carcinoma (adenocarcinoma) of the uterine cervix. Am J Obstet Gynecol 83:729, 1962
244. Takeda M, King DE, McHenry MJ et al: Lung cancer metastatic to the uterine cervix, abstracted. Acta Cytol 25:442, 1981
245. Boysen TH, McCloskey JF, Scheffey LC: Carcinoma of the pancreas with metastasis to the cervix uteri. Am J Obstet Gynecol 61:923, 1951
246. Hall PA, Lemoine NR, Ryan JF: Carcinoma of the gall bladder metastatic to the cervix. Case report. Br J Obstet Gynaecol 93:1187, 1986
247. Brady LW, O'Neill EA, Farber SH: Unusual sites of metastases. Semin Oncol 4:59, 1977
248. Post RC, Cohen T, Blaustein AU, Shenker L: Carcinoid tumor metastatic to the cervix and corpus uteri. Obstet Gynecol 27:171, 1966
249. Banooni F, Labes J, Goodman PA: Uterine leiomyoma containing metastatic breast carcinoma. Am J Obstet Gynecol 111:427, 1971

250. Sullivan LG, Sullivan JL, Fairey WF: Breast carcinoma metastatic to endometrial polyp. Gynecol Oncol 39:96, 1990
251. Casey JH, Shapiro RF: Metastatic melanoma presenting as primary uterine neoplasm: a case report. Cancer 33:729, 1974
252. Wood C: Metastatic melanoma simulating a primary endometrial tumor. Am J Obstet Gynecol 131:820, 1978
253. Jaffrey IS, Lefkowitz L, Lestch SD, Weiss DR: Metastatic melanoma presenting as abnormal uterine bleeding: a case report. Mt Sinai J Med 43:180, 1976
254. Bauer RD, McCoy CP, Roberts DK, Fritz G: Malignant melanoma metastatic to the endometrium. Obstet Gynecol 63:264, 1984
255. Nagy P, Csaba I, Kadas I: Malignant melanoma metastatic to the endometrium. Cytologic findings in a direct endometrial sample. Acta Cytol 34:382, 1990
256. Clement PB: Miscellaneous primary and metastatic tumors of the uterine cervix. Semin Diagn Pathol 7:228, 1990

9

Pathology of Trophoblastic Disease

Janice M. Lage and Robert H. Young

Almost nothing that trophoblast does or does not do should surprise anyone who has had any experience with this tissue.

Arthur T. Hertig, M.D.
Human Trophoblast, 1968

The placental villus is the functional unit of the placenta. The villous structure consists of a mesenchymal core with overlying trophoblast (Fig. 9-1). The mesenchymal core contains fetal blood vessels, scattered macrophages (Hofbauer cells), and stromal cells. There are two generic categories of trophoblast: *villous trophoblast* and *extravillous trophoblast.* The villous trophoblast is composed of two layers: syncytiotrophoblast (or syncytium) in the outer layer facing the maternal intervillous space, and cytotrophoblast (Langhans' layer) in the inner layer adjacent to the villous stroma. The immature villus has a small component of intermediate trophoblast (Fig. 9-1).

Extravillous trophoblast consists of the trophoblast that is not in direct contact with the villi. Extravillous trophoblast populates the extraplacental membranes (chorion laeve), endomyometrial implantation site, maternal spiral arteries, and placental trophoblastic columns. The extraplacental membranes are composed of three layers: amnion, chorion laeve, and decidua (superficial maternal endometrium). The implantation site trophoblast consists mainly of intermediate trophoblasts with some syncytiotrophoblasts.

TYPES OF TROPHOBLAST

To date, three types of trophoblast have been characterized: syncytiotrophoblast (ST), cytotrophoblast (CT), and intermediate trophoblast (IT).[1-9]

SYNCYTIOTROPHOBLAST

ST is present on villi, as scattered cells in the endomyometrial placental implantation site, and, rarely, in spiral arteries. ST is derived from the fusion of mature CT, resulting in a syncytium that forms a continuous layer covering the villous surfaces. At the implantation site, ST forms discrete multinucleated cells. ST is characterized hormonally by human chorionic gonadotropin (hCG) production that varies with the gestational age.

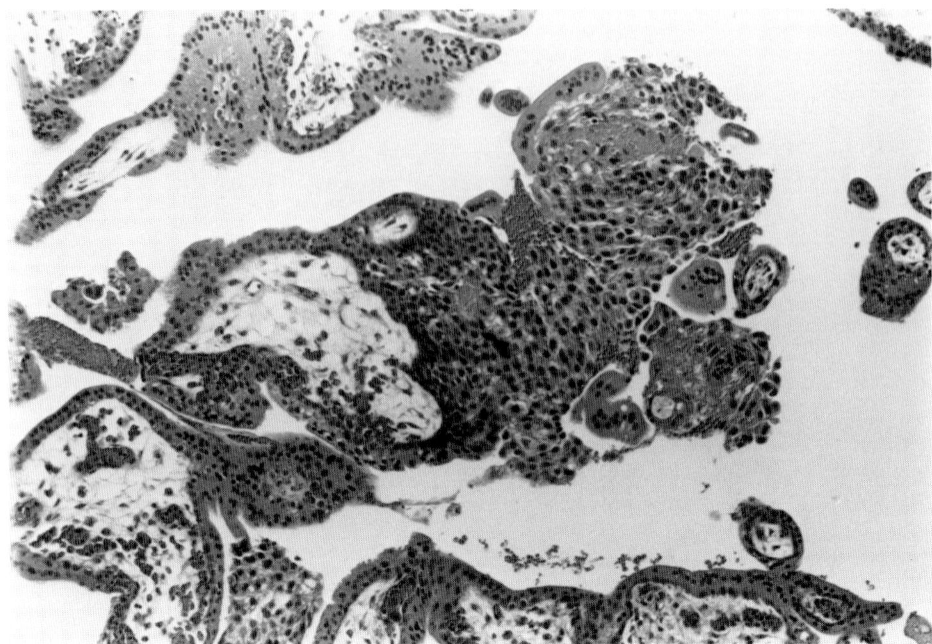

Fig. 9-1. Normal, immature chorionic villus (center) with polar proliferation of cytotrophoblast (adjacent to villous stroma), intermediate trophoblast (forming large, central mass), and syncytiotrophoblast (multinucleated cells covering intermediate trophoblast).

By immunostaining, ST is strongly hCG positive in the first trimester, moderately positive in the second trimester, and only slightly positive by term.[9] The opposite is true for human placental lactogen (hPL). ST of immature placentas is weakly positive for hPL but by term shows strong hPL positively.[9] ST reacts with antibodies to both low- and high-molecular-weight cytokeratins.

On microscopic examination, the nuclei of ST are small and uniform, with bland vesicular chromatin. Nucleoli are inconspicuous, but small eosinophilic nucleoli may be found in immature ST. ST is most easily recognized by its abundant violaceous to amphophilic granular cytoplasm. ST has a dense brush border, apparent by light microscopy. Since both benign and malignant ST are incapable of cell division, there are no mitotic figures in these cells.

Cytotrophoblast

CT forms the inner layer of trophoblast overlying the villi and is most prominent in early placentas. It becomes less conspicuous as the placenta matures; only occasional villous CT cells remain in the normal term placenta. There are scattered CT at the implantation site throughout gestation.

In contrast to ST, the cells of CT are mononucleate, with well-defined cytoplasmic borders. Their nuclei are larger than those of ST, and the chromatin is more clumped. Nucleoli are generally inconspicuous and, if visible, are small and eosinophilic. The cytoplasm is clear to granular, slightly eosinophilic, and moderate in amount. Mitotic activity may be observed in the CT of early gestation, declining markedly in the normal placenta by the end of the second trimester. Unlike ST, the immunophenotype of CT does not depend on the stage of gestation. CT is not immunoreactive for hCG or hPL but is keratin positive.

INTERMEDIATE TROPHOBLAST

The third type of trophoblast, IT, is characterized both by specific uteroplacental location and by hormone production. On the basis of electron microscopic features, IT has ultrastructural characteristics intermediate between those of the germinative CT and the mature ST.[6, 8] On microscopic examination, it is generally uninucleate, but it may be binucleate or multinucleate. The nucleus is large and may be lobulated or vesicular. The nuclear chromatin is more dense and basophilic than that of the other trophoblast, and nucleoli, although uncommon, may be present. IT is characterized by its dense amphophilic to eosinophilic cytoplasm. At the implantation site, this dense cytoplasm serves to distinguish IT from the surrounding decidualized endometrial stromal cells.

IT is strongly keratin positive throughout gestation. Immunoreactivity for hPL is strongest in mid-gestation with moderate positivity in the first and third trimesters.[9] Antibodies to β-hCG give a weakly positive reaction in all trimesters.[9] The recognition of distinct electron microscopic and immunohistochemical phenotypes of the IT served to set the stage for the separate subclassification of pathologic lesions composed of IT.

TYPES OF GESTATIONAL TROPHOBLASTIC DISEASE

Gestational trophoblastic lesions may be divided into two basic groups: those with villi and those without (Table 9-1). The former includes *hydatidiform moles,* both partial and complete. A variant of hydatid-

Table 9-1. Types of Gestational Trophoblastic Disease

With villi
  Hydatidiform mole
    Complete mole
    Partial mole
  Invasive mole
  Persistent mole
  Chorangiocarcinoma

Without villi
  Placental site nodules
  Placental site trophoblastic tumor
  Choriocarcinoma

iform mole is the *invasive mole,* in which molar villi invade the uterine wall. *Retained molar villi,* or persistent mole, is a descriptive term denoting residual molar villi in a curettage or hysterectomy specimen obtained subsequent to the initial uterine evacuation.

In the category of trophoblastic lesions devoid of villi are choriocarcinoma and the placental site proliferations consisting of placental site nodules and plaques and placental site tumors. Table 9-2 presents the World Health Organization (WHO) nomenclature for gestational trophoblastic lesions.

HYDATIDIFORM MOLES

Biology

Although both complete hydatidiform mole (CM) and partial hydatidiform mole (PM) contain hydropic villi, these pla-

Table 9-2. World Health Organization Classification of Gestational Trophoblastic Lesions

Hydatidiform mole
  Complete
  Partial
Invasive hydatidiform mole
Choriocarcinoma
Placental site trophoblastic tumor
Trophoblastic lesions, miscellaneous
  Exaggerated placental site
  Placental site nodule or plaque
Unclassified trophoblastic lesion

cental lesions have genetic,[10–16] morphologic[11–13, 17, 18] and clinical differences.[11, 12–19] Seminal cytogenetic studies disclosed that the genomic DNA of a CM is solely paternal (androgenetic).[10] Although this uniparental genomic DNA lacks any maternal component, it has the normal diploid content of 46 chromosomes. Elegant experiments in mice have shown that paternal DNA appears to control the formation of the placenta, whereas the maternal DNA appears to be more involved in embryonic development.[20, 21] These findings are consistent with what occurs in a CM in which the conceptus exists in the form of a placenta without any associated fetal tissue.

Subsequent molecular studies have shown that the maternal mitochondrial DNA is conserved in hydatidiform moles.[22] The androgenetic origin of CM has been confirmed by molecular diagnostic studies using restriction fragment-length polymorphisms[23] and DNA fingerprinting.[24] In Japan, novel molecular diagnostic studies assaying hypervariable regions of specific gene loci using polymerase chain reaction (PCR) have detected early CM by the absence of maternal alleles and homozygosity for paternal alleles in placental villi.[25] Where there is only a suspicion of CM by ultrasonography, chorionic villous sampling could provide tissue for diagnosis.

Flow cytometric studies[26–30] of both fresh and fixed placental tissues have furthered our understanding of molar gestations by providing an inexpensive assay of the total genomic DNA content (Fig. 9-2). As most CM are diploid or tetraploid and most PM triploid, knowledge of the DNA content of a hydatidiform mole may be extremely useful in guiding the histopathologic classification[30] (Table 9-3).

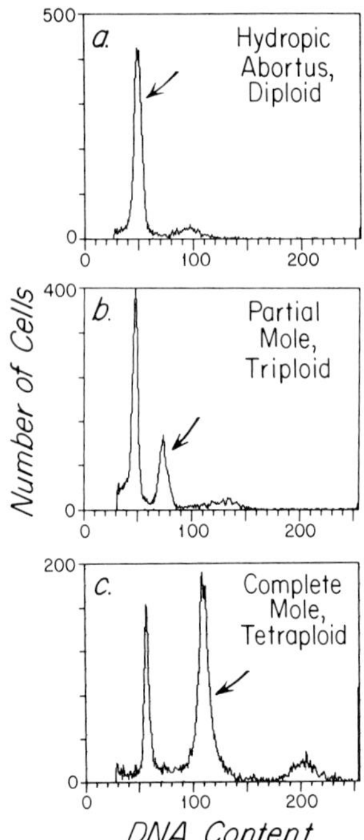

Fig. 9-2. Composite DNA histograms generated from fresh placental tissues. Diploid hydropic abortus represented in **(A)**, triploid partial mole in **(B)**, and tetraploid complete mole in **(C)**. (From Lage et al.,[30] with permission.)

Epidemiology

Hydatidiform moles, both partial and complete, occur in women in the reproductive age group. Hydatidiform mole has a reported frequency of 1 : 4,500 deliveries in the United States,[31] 1 : 1,300 in Israel,[32] and 1 : 85 to 1 : 373 in Indonesia.[33] In a recent large study, the average age of women with both CM and PM was 28 years, ranging from 14 to 53 years.[30] No significant difference was found between the ages of women with PM as compared with CM. Risk factors for both CM and PM include (1) personal or family history of previous gestational trophoblastic disease, (2) two or more previous spontaneous miscarriages, (3) infertility, and (4) smoking.[34] There is no association between the risk of CM or PM and the following factors: induced abortions, age at first pregnancy, alcohol consumption, or blood group type A women married to blood group O men.[34] The fre-

Table 9-3. Gross, Microscopic, and Genetic Distinctions Among Complete Hydatidiform Mole, Partial Hydatidiform Mole, and Hydropic Abortus

	Complete Mole	Partial Mole	Hydropic Abortus
Amount of placental tissue compared to norm for gestational age	Voluminous, excessive, (5- to 10-fold increase)[a]	Moderately increased (2-fold)	Scant tissue: far less than normal
Villous trophoblast	Diffusely hyperplastic	Focally hyperplastic	Attenuated
Villous population	Spectrum of sizes	Two populations	Spectrum of sizes
Fetal tissue	None	Present and abnormal	Usually none
Trophoblast atypia	Prominent	Rarely present	None
Villous cavitation	Many villi	Some villi	Few villi
Mean maximum villous diameter	0.71 cm	0.53 cm	0.28 cm
DNA content by flow cytometry	Diploid/tetraploid[b]	Triploid[b]	Diploid[b]
Chromosome number by cytogenetic analysis	46	69	46+/− a few

[a] Excludes first trimester complete moles.
[b] See text for exceptions.

quency of CM increases with maternal age.[31, 32]

Clinical Signs and Symptoms

The most common clinical presentation for both groups is vaginal bleeding.[19, 35–37] Those with CM may pass tissue vaginally, present with uterine size greater than expected for gestational age, or have signs or symptoms ascribable to abnormally elevated serum β-hCG levels, including prominent ovarian theca lutein cysts, preeclampsia occurring early in gestation, hyperemesis gravidarum, hyperthyroidism, or, pulmonary trophoblastic emboli.[36] More than 50 percent of women with CM are anemic at presentation.[36]

The symptomatology of women with PM is similar to that of women with CM, but in milder form.[37] The presenting signs or symptoms of patients with PM are vaginal bleeding (72.8 percent), absent fetal heart beat (14.8 percent), excessive uterine size (3.7 percent), small uterine size (3.7 percent), and toxemia (2.5 percent); a few are asymptomatic (2.5 percent).[35] Pre-eclamp-

sia tends to occur later in the course of PM than CM but may be equally severe.[37] On examination, uterine size is less than expected for dates in most patients. The most common pre-evacuation diagnosis of women with PM is missed or incomplete abortion.[35, 37]

Women with CM often have markedly elevated serum β-hCG for the gestational age. In a recent study, the median serum β-hCG for women with CM was 356,500 mIU/ml, in the range of 24,000 to 2,190,600 mIU/ml.[30] By contrast, most women with PM had a normal to slightly elevated serum β-hCG for gestational age: the median serum β-hCG was 65,851 mIU/ml, the range of 133,000 to 778,100 mIU/ml.[30] Pre-evacuation β-hCG values in PM are significantly lower as compared with CM.[30]

The diagnosis of hydatidiform mole, both partial and complete, may be first suspected on the basis of obstetric ultrasonography.[38–42] Although ultrasonographic diagnosis of molar pregnancy is accurate in the later stages, diagnosis in early pregnancy is fraught with difficulties. Missed abortion with hydropic degeneration, for example, may simulate hydatidiform mole.[40, 41] Correlation of fetal heart rates with β-hCG levels has provided alternative diagnostic criteria. Fetal heart rates have been detected in 99 percent of normal pregnancies when the serum β-hCG values were above 82,350 mIU/ml.[42] Conversely, absence of the fetal heart movement and a serum β-hCG value greater than 82,350 mIU/ml were strongly correlated with hydatidiform moles in an analysis of 39 women.[42] In cases with recognizable fetal tissues, a serum β-hCG greater than 2 SD above that expected for gestational age was associated with PM.[42]

Early pregnancy intervention based on abnormal ultrasonographic findings forces the pathologist to diagnose hydatidiform mole much earlier in gestation than was previously required. The recognition of clinically silent "early" hydatidiform moles among elective terminations requires ongoing vigilance for unsuspected cases, necessitating careful gross examination of curettings from early conceptuses, adequate sampling of tissues, and recognition of subtle histopathology.[43]

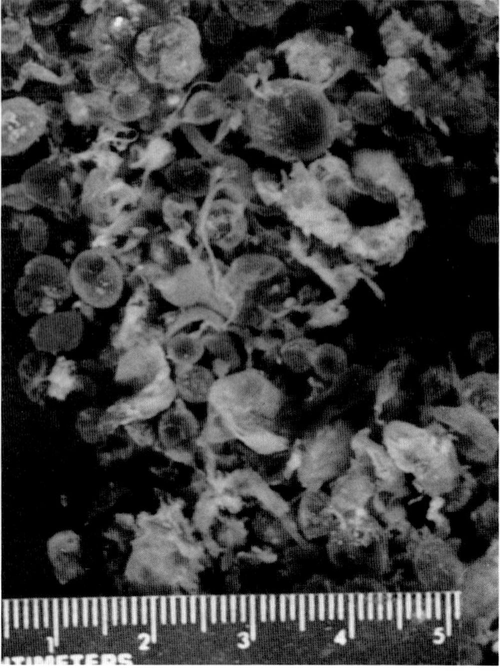

Fig. 9-3. Gross photograph of fresh, intact hydropic villi of complete hydatidiform mole. Note spectrum of villous sizes.

Complete Hydatidiform Mole

Gross Examination. The complete hydatidiform mole is an abnormal placenta characterized by gross and microscopic villous hydrops (Table 9-3). When fresh, swollen villi are filled with translucent fluid and visible grossly (Fig. 9-3). Fetal tissues are lacking. In a recent study, the maximum diameter of the villous vesicles in CM averaged 0.71 cm and ranged from 0 cm (no vesicles found) to 1.6 cm.[30] Often the curettage procedure causes villous disruption, with subsequent collapse of many villi. In the past, CM was a diagnosis readily made by the first person who saw the specimen, generally the clinician. The pathologist confirmed the diagnosis. Villous hydrops was extensive, curetted tissue voluminous, and trophoblast hyperplasia prominent on microscopy. Today, when the uterus is evacuated early in gestation, prompted by an abnormal obstetric ultrasound, the tissue volume is increased only slightly over that of a normal gestation, and the diagnosis is often missed by both the clinician and pathologist as villous hydrops may be inapparent.

Microscopic Examination. On microscopic examination, the hallmarks of the fully developed CM are easily recognized: villous hydrops, and excessive trophoblastic proliferation (trophoblast hyperplasia) (Fig. 9-4). Central cisterns or cavities are present within the edematous stroma of the larger villi (Fig. 9-4); in fully developed CM, there is diffuse villous cavitation. The number of cavitated villi is proportional to the age of the CM. In "younger" CM, villous stromal edema may not have culminated in cavitation and the diagnosis rests on recognition of an excessive amount of villous and extravillous trophoblast.

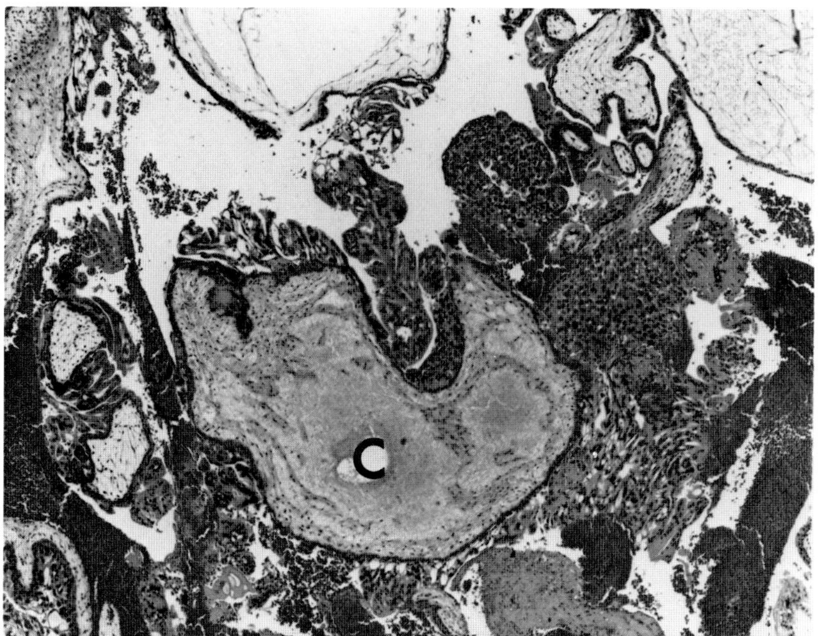

Fig. 9-4. Hydropic villi of complete hydatidiform mole with central cavitation (C) of large villi and extensive hyperplasia of both villous and extravillous trophoblast.

The trophoblast of a CM is abnormal in geometry, quantity, and quality. In the normal placenta, trophoblast proliferation is orderly, localized, and directional. The growing trophoblast forms a cap at one end of the villus (polar), aiming toward the uterine implantation site (Fig. 9-1). Away from the polar cap, only two layers of trophoblast overlie the villus: a single layer of inner CT, and an outer layer of ST. In the region of the polar cap, the trophoblast proliferation is orderly: the inner CT layer is maintained, although stratified; an interposed mass of IT proliferates toward the implantation site, and the ST faces the intervillous space. In a CM, there is total loss of trophoblast polarity, with the proliferative trophoblast encircling the entire villus (Fig. 9-4).

The excessive quantity of trophoblast in CM is distinctive. A diagnosis of CM requires increased trophoblastic proliferation (trophoblast hyperplasia), which, in mature CM, involves the majority of villi. Gener-

ally, both villous CT and ST are hyperplastic, although the ST may predominate in some cases. Hyperplastic ST forms lacy, delicate mounds protruding from the villous surface (Fig. 9-5). As in normal early ST, the cytoplasm of the hyperplastic ST is often markedly vacuolated. Nuclear atypia tends to be minimal in ST. CT hyperplasia in CM varies from slight to moderate and may be associated with striking nuclear pleomorphism with enlarged hyperchromatic forms.

The abundance and atypicality of extravillous trophoblast, both in the intervillous space and at the implantation site, are further evidence of trophoblast hyperplasia in CM. This IT, and to a lesser degree, the villous CT, is the most provocative, showing marked cytologic atypicality: spectacular increases in nuclear and cytoplasmic size and marked nuclear atypia with dense, hyperchromatic chromatin (Fig. 9-5). In cytogenetic studies of molar trophoblast, nuclear polyploidy has been documented.[44]

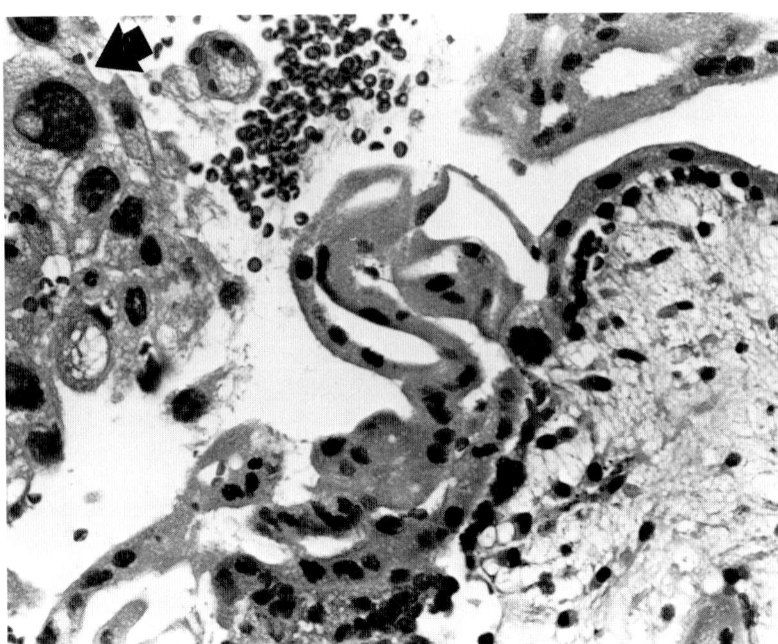

Fig. 9-5. Complete hydatidiform mole showing molar villus with hyperplasia of syncytiotrophoblast and marked cytologic atypia of extravillous trophoblast (arrow).

Commonly, the villi of CM have no residual fetal blood vessels. If present, the blood vessels contain karyorrhectic debris without intact fetal normoblasts. Occasionally, residual stromal vessels have primitive nucleated red blood cells (derived from the yolk sac) containing dense amphophilic cytoplasm. Prominent fetal red blood cells are uncommon in CM and should suggest the possibility of PM or twin gestation. The villous stroma of a CM contains karyorrhectic debris.

The CM does not contain the fetal tissue that is commonly associated with PM. When fetal tissues are found in association with a diagnostic CM, a twin gestation is suggested. In a large series of CM, 3.5 percent were twin gestations composed of a CM and a co-twin with normal fetus and normal placenta.[30] In a review of such gestations, fetal outcomes were viable child (27 percent), intrauterine death (46 percent), nonviable fetus (23 percent), and malignant degeneration (4 percent).[45]

The villous outline of CM is different from that of PM or hydropic abortus. When intact, the mature CM contains totally spherical hydropic villi (Fig. 9-3). In curettage specimens, the villi collapse; the residuum of a cistern is denoted by a sharp, curved demarcation in the marginal villous stroma adjacent to a central cleft (an appearance analogous to that of a deflated balloon).

In CM, some villi exhibit an unusual clustering of clublike, exophytic projections (Fig. 9-6), a finding that suggests the diagnosis of CM. These outwardly scalloped processes of villous stroma are lined by trophoblast. Since they are exophytic, tangential sectioning does not result in stromal trophoblastic inclusions.

Early Complete Hydatidiform Mole. The diagnosis of CM in the first trimester (especially 5 to 8 weeks gestational age) requires an increased index of suspicion. The difficulty with early CM lies in the paucity and focality of trophoblast hyperplasia, in

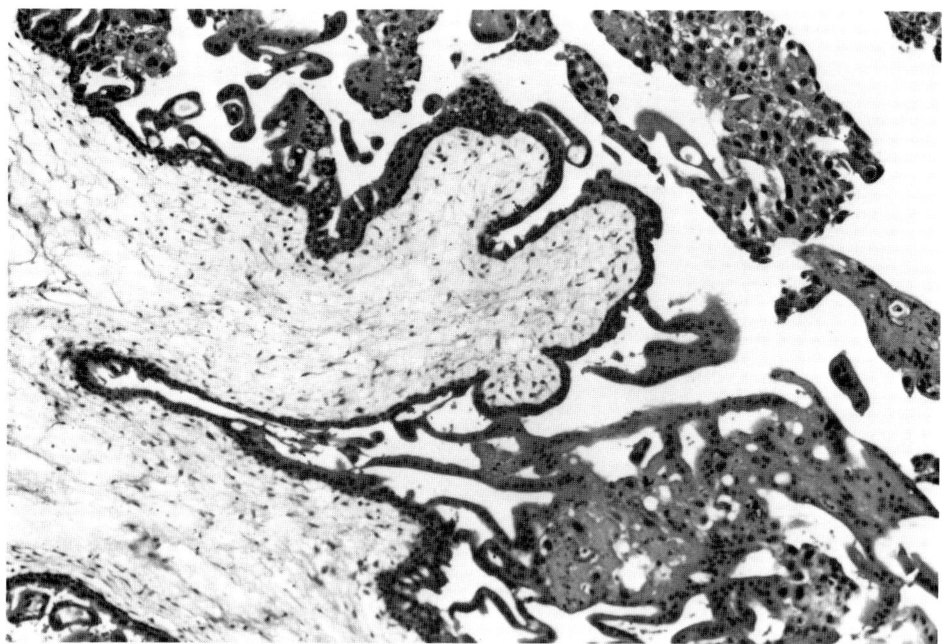

Fig. 9-6. Complete hydatidiform mole with club-shaped villous projections, villous stromal edema, and extensive villous and extravillous trophoblast hyperplasia.

some cases involving less than 5 to 10 percent of villi. Most villi have a "normal" appearance. Only a few are slightly enlarged, and the trophoblast hyperplasia is circumferential (Fig. 9-7), lacking a polar cap (Fig. 9-1).

The diagnosis may be first suggested by stratification of villous trophoblast (Fig. 9-8) or cytologic atypicality in extravillous trophoblast. Villous stromal changes are subtle, and stromal cisterns with sharp margins are generally inapparent. The villous outline may have clublike projections. Karyorrhectic debris in villous stroma and blood vessels documents the absence of a viable fetus. Any abnormality suggesting possible CM should prompt microscopic examination of the entire specimen in an attempt to find pathognomonic villi.

Prognostic Factors, Grading, and Trophoblast Hyperplasia. Early investigations of CM demonstrated that the degree of trophoblast hyperplasia combined with the degree of cytologic atypicality were

predictive of clinical outcome.[46, 47] Further studies, however, concluded that assessment of the quantity and quality of the trophoblast was not predictive of outcome in CM.[48] The earlier studies were performed before recognition of the partial molar phenotype and included a mixture of

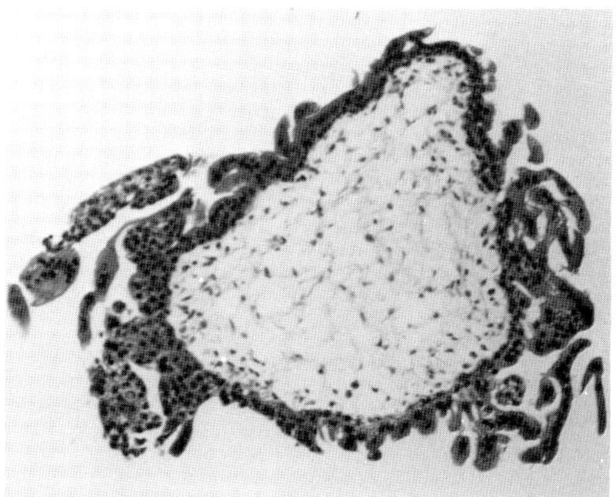

Fig. 9-7. Immature villus of "early" complete hydatidiform mole with prominent, circumferential, trophoblast hyperplasia. Villous stroma is edematous.

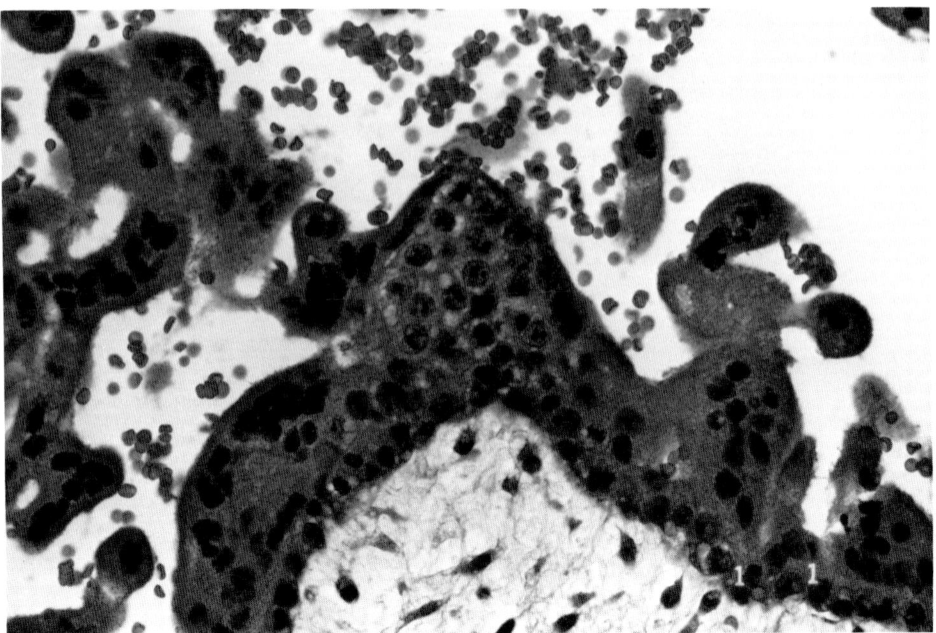

Fig. 9-8. Cytotrophoblast stratification in "early" complete hydatidiform mole. Note extensive syncytiotrophoblastic proliferation.

both PM and CM. A recent study of 153 CM demonstrated that microscopic grading or "grouping" based on the original criteria of Hertig and Sheldon[46] could not predict clinical outcome.[49] Although there has been some suggestion that the presence of fibrinoid deposits in sharp curettings obtained at the initial molar evacuation may be predictive of persistent disease,[50] these observations must be confirmed by additional studies.

Flow Cytometry in Complete Hydatidiform Mole. Flow cytometric studies of both fresh and fixed CM have demonstrated a wider spectrum of nuclear DNA content than previously indicated by cytogenetic studies. While most CM are diploid, flow cytometric analyses have revealed cases of triploid, tetraploid, haploid, and aneuploid CM.[15, 28–30, 51–53] Enzyme analyses or molecular evaluations, or both, have demonstrated retention of the predominance of paternal versus maternal genomic DNA.[15, 51] Even among these chromosom-

ally anomalous gestations, it appears that the relative increase in paternal DNA plays a significant role in initiating and maintaining the CM.

Extrauterine Sites. While the vast majority of hydatidiform moles, both partial and complete, are intrauterine, one can find a mole at any site suitable for an ectopic pregnancy. In a series of 2,100 women with gestational trophoblastic disease, 0.8 percent involved the fallopian tube.[54] Of 16 tubal cases, 5 (31 percent) were PM, 5 (31 percent) were CM, and 6 (38 percent) were choriocarcinoma. Of the five women with tubal CM, four had spontaneous remission. Pulmonary metastases appeared 1 month after salpingo-oophorectomy in the fifth woman, who attained complete remission after four courses of chemotherapy.[55]

Clinical Management of Complete Hydatidiform Mole. Initial treatment for complete molar pregnancy is removal of molar tissue by uterine evacuation or, if the patient desires sterility, by hysterectomy.

Most patients are treated by suction evacuation with curettage; the initial uterine evacuation is curative for most.[36] Standard follow-up in the United States is by measurement of serum β-hCG weekly until negative and then monthly for 6 months.[19]

Patients are instructed to avoid conception during the follow-up period. If the β-hCG level fails to decline for 3 consecutive weeks or begins to rise at any point, clinical evaluation is undertaken. Following exclusion of a new, normal pregnancy, the elevation of β-hCG implies persistent gestational trophoblastic disease and chemotherapy is initiated. A common step in the evaluation of women with persistent gestational trophoblastic disease is a repeat dilatation and curettage (D&C). Uterine curettings usually show residual molar villi with or without implantation site trophoblast and decidua. It has been suggested that curettings containing residual molar villi without decidua reflect abnormal villous implantation (i.e., accreta).[56]

There was some initial evidence that in women with heterozygous (dispermic) complete moles, persistent disease developed more commonly as compared with homozygous (monospermic) complete moles.[57] Subsequent studies have found no difference between the rates of persistence following homozygous versus heterozygous CM.[51] Some studies have reported that aneuploid nuclear DNA content determined by flow cytometric analysis was predictive of persistent trophoblastic disease in CM.[52] Others have found no such association.[30, 58]

Rates of persistence following CM are correlated with certain risk factors pertaining to the antecedent CM. Risk factors of known significance include pre-evacuation hCG greater than 100,000 mIU/ml, uterine size greater than gestational age, theca lutein cysts greater than 6 cm in diameter, associated medical factors (preeclampsia, hyperthyroidism, trophoblastic embolization), maternal age over 40 years, and previous molar pregnancy.[36] After molar evacuation, women in the high-risk group have a 31 percent risk of local uterine invasion and 8.8 percent risk of metastases, with corresponding frequencies of 3.4 percent and 0.6 percent in the low-risk group.[59] The lungs and vagina are the most frequent metastatic sites.

In reports from some large trophoblastic disease centers, persistence rates for CM range from 8.3 to 45 percent.[51, 52, 59–65] The rate cited depends on the referral patterns of the centers reporting as well as the diagnostic criteria used to define persistence. At some centers, a diagnosis of persistence is based on a predicted time course for hCG remission, and women with continued hCG production after a designated point are diagnosed as having persistent disease. Reported persistence rates tend to be higher in gestational trophoblastic disease centers in the United States because (1) high-risk patients are more likely to be sent to trophoblast centers for initial clinical management and (2) patients diagnosed as having persistence are referred to trophoblast centers for treatment. In Great Britain, where virtually all patients are initially followed and treated at trophoblastic disease centers, reported rates of persistence tend to be lower, with estimated rates of 8.3 percent[65] and 18 percent[51] in recent publications. Probably the "true" rate of persistence for nonselected cases is 10 to 20 percent.[49]

At some centers, prophylactic chemotherapy in women with high-risk CM has decreased the rates of persistence among this group from 47 percent to 14 percent.[66] Prophylactic chemotherapy has not significantly altered the persistence rates among women with low-risk CM (7.7 percent versus 5.6 percent).[66]

Invasive Mole (Chorioadenoma Destruens). In 5 to 10 percent of women with CM, molar villi invade the myometrium in a manner similar to placenta increta, a finding termed *invasive mole* (chorioadenoma destruens).[56] PM may also be invasive, but much less commonly than CM. In women with an antecedent hydatidiform mole and persistent trophoblastic disease, the lack of residual villous tissue in a repeat uterine curettage and a negative metastatic workup imply a diagnosis of invasive mole. Only rarely is this confirmed pathologically (Fig. 9-9), since hysterectomy is not required for treatment. The management in persistent molar disease, including invasive mole, depends on clinical staging parameters that include extent of disease and serum β-hCG values, as well as the patient's desire to preserve fertility.

Chemotherapy for Persistent Disease. In general, medical treatment of persistent disease consists of systemic chemotherapy with surgery and radiotherapy as adjuvant modalities.[36, 67] Chemotherapy begins with single-agent methotrexate with citrovorum factor rescue or with actinomycin D. If unsuccessful, a multiagent drug regimen is given, often consisting of actinomycin D, cis-platinum, etoposide, cyclophosphamide, and/or vincristine in various combinations.[36, 67] The exact drugs used may

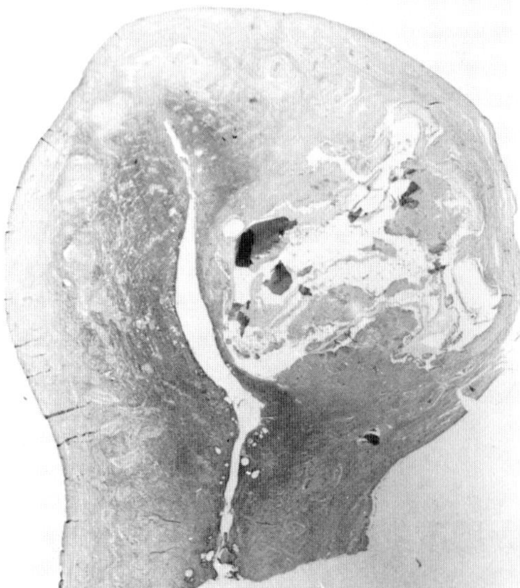

Fig. 9-9. Hysterectomy specimen with invasive complete hydatidiform mole. Molar villi penetrate deep into the myometrium.

vary in different settings with some centers adding other agents. Cure rates for persistent trophoblastic disease following CM approach 100 percent.[49, 51]

Postmolar Choriocarcinoma. In a small percentage of patients with persistent gestational trophoblastic disease, approximately 1 to 2 percent at most, uterine curettage will reveal choriocarcinoma (CCA). The frequency increases to 6 to 8 percent when associated with invasive mole.[68] In a recent series of 153 women with CM treated at a large trophoblastic disease center during the years of 1980 to 1990, there were no cases of postmolar CCA.[49] Perhaps this recent reduction in the frequency of postmolar CCA is a result of earlier diagnosis, increased sensitivity of immunoassays for β-hCG, and more efficacious chemotherapeutic management of molar gestations.

The diagnosis of CCA should be made with caution, as it will alter clinical treatment. To make this diagnosis, the entire specimen must be examined microscopically. Criteria for CCA include abundant biphasic trophoblast, endomyometrial invasion, and complete absence of villous tissue (see section on Diagnosis of Choriocarcinoma in Uterine Curettings). A diagnosis of "molar villi" should be made, even if there is only a single residual villus or villus fragment. One may comment on markedly atypical trophoblast admixed with villous tissue, but a diagnosis of CCA is not appropriate in such specimens. In general, treatment of postmolar CCA consists of multiple cycles of multiagent chemotherapy. Cure rates for postmolar CCA are quite high, approaching 90 to 100 percent.[67]

Recurrent Gestational Trophoblastic Disease. Recurrent (repeat) gestational trophoblastic disease is a new episode of gestational trophoblastic disease that develops subsequent to previous complete gonadotropin remission after chemotherapy for a trophoblastic disease.[69, 70] Such patients have a re-elevation of serum β hCG after three consecutive negative weekly β-hCG values. In one large study, women with recurrent gestational trophoblastic disease were staged clinically and divided into three groups: (1) nonmetastatic disease, (2) good-prognosis metastatic disease, and (3) poor-prognosis metastatic disease.[70] The good-prognosis metastatic category included women with lung or vaginal metastases, serum β-hCG levels less that 40,000 mIU/Ml, and short duration of disease. The poor-prognosis category included brain, liver, or kidney metastases, hCG level greater than 40,000 mIU/ml, or gestational tumor after a term gestation. In a series of women treated between 1968 and 1985 at a large trophoblastic disease center in the United States, 100 percent cure rates were achieved after nonmetastatic recurrences or good-prognosis metastatic disease.[70] Only 50 percent of those with poor-prognosis metastatic disease were cured after intensive chemotherapy and, often, extirpative surgery. However, survival rates have improved recently with 83 percent survival rate in women with recurrent disease treated after 1978 at the same institution.[70] This increased survival rate was attributed to the availability of additional chemotherapeutic agents. Women with one episode of recurrence have a 28 to 50 percent probability of subsequent trophoblastic disease episode.[69, 70]

Partial Hydatidiform Mole

Genetics. The PM, like the CM, is a pathologic placenta resulting from an abnormal fertilization. In PM, maternal haploid genomic DNA is retained (23 chromosomes), but instead of fertilization with one haploid paternal DNA set, two haploid paternal sets are added by dispermy or diplospermy (46 chromosomes).[11–14, 16, 26, 27, 30, 51] The total genomic DNA consists of three haploid sets, termed triploid (69 chromosomes). The conceptus has a predominance of paternal versus maternal DNA but, unlike the CM, which lacks maternal genomic DNA, the clinical and phenotypic expressions of PM are mollified by the retained maternal DNA. Careful cytogenic and histopathologic studies have elucidated a specific phenotype for the triploid PM.[11, 17, 37]

Gross Examination. On gross examination, the villous vesicles of PM are slightly smaller than those of CM. In a recent study of 49 PM, the maximum villous vesicle diameter was 0.51 cm, with a range of 0 cm (no vesicles identified) to 1.8 cm.[30] The population of enlarged villi stand out against a background population of normal sized villi (Fig. 9-10). This dichotomy of villous sizes is characteristic of PM and may be recognized on gross examination. Fetal tissues are often found.

Microscopic Examination. Although the PM was initially considered an "incomplete form" of CM, it is now known that the phenotype of the PM is quite distinct from CM. The hallmarks of PM are two populations of villi with focal villous hydrops and focal trophoblast hyperplasia[11, 17, 37] (Table 9-3). The two populations of villi consist of (1) some that are enlarged and hydropic, containing occasional central cisterns; and (2) some that are normal to sclerotic or hyalinized, appearing appropriate to small in size for the gestational age (Fig. 9-10). Within one specimen, the villi tend to be equally divided into small or large villi, with very few intermediate in size.

On low-power examination, the larger villi have scalloped villous outlines (Fig. 9-10). This scalloping results in trophoblastic incursions or invaginations that, on cross-sectioning, form rings of trophoblast within the villous stroma (Fig. 9-10). The villous stroma is edematous, focally culminating in true cavitation, but the degree of villous cavitation or cistern formation is much less than in CM, and villous cavitation is not a diagnostic criterion for PM. Most PM will have 5 to 10 or more cavitated villi, if adequately sampled; as in CM,

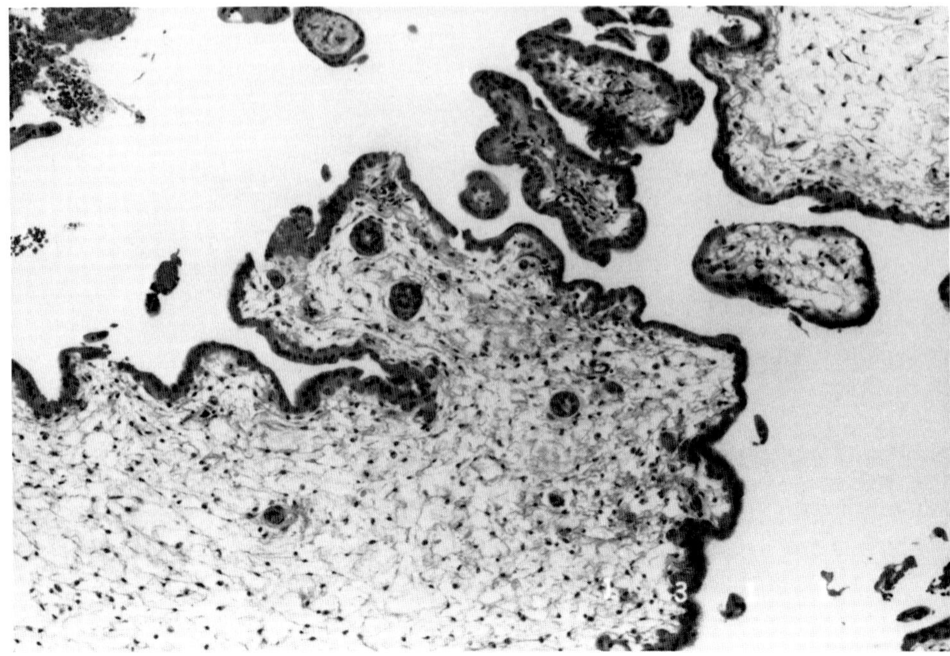

Fig. 9-10. Partial hydatidiform mole with two distinct populations of villi. The largest villus shows scalloped outline and trophoblastic invaginations, resulting in stromal trophoblastic inclusions. Note marked difference in size between large and small villi.

the degree of villous cavitation increases with the gestational age. An early PM may not exhibit villous cavitation. Conversely, if most of the villi are cavitated, PM is an unlikely diagnosis, and CM should be excluded.

In addition to focal villous hydrops, a second diagnostic criterion for PM is focal trophoblast hyperplasia (Fig. 9-11), involving ST in particular (Fig. 9-12). Scattered villi contain small piles of ST, forming lacy outpouchings; often, the same villus has a second focus of hyperplastic trophoblast on the opposite side. Another common finding is trophoblastic notches, or knuckles of ST extending from the villous surfaces (Fig. 9-13); they tend to be multiple. Tangential sectioning isolates these notches from their underlying villous attachments, cluttering the intervillous spaces. These trophoblastic notches are not pathognomonic for PM, as they are also seen in nonmolar triploid placentas in which the extra haploid DNA set

is maternally derived. Otherwise, such nonmolar triploids have no other features in common with PM.

The older PM often shows a striking abnormality in the configuration of the villous vasculature.[17] These anomalous endothelium-lined vessels become thin-walled and form oddly shaped, ectatic, "mazelike" anastomosing channels (Fig. 9-14). The surrounding stroma appears slightly hyperplastic. In some ways, these vessels resemble arteriovenous-lymphatic malformations (Fig. 9-15). It is rare to find these irregular ectatic channels in villi other than those associated with karyotypic abnormalities, and their presence should suggest PM. Mazelike vessels are particularly common in late second-trimester triploid PM.

The nature of the fetal tissues in PM is dependent on the age of the gestation, whether intervening fetal death has occurred, and the extent of tissue sampling. The vast majority of PM contain macro-

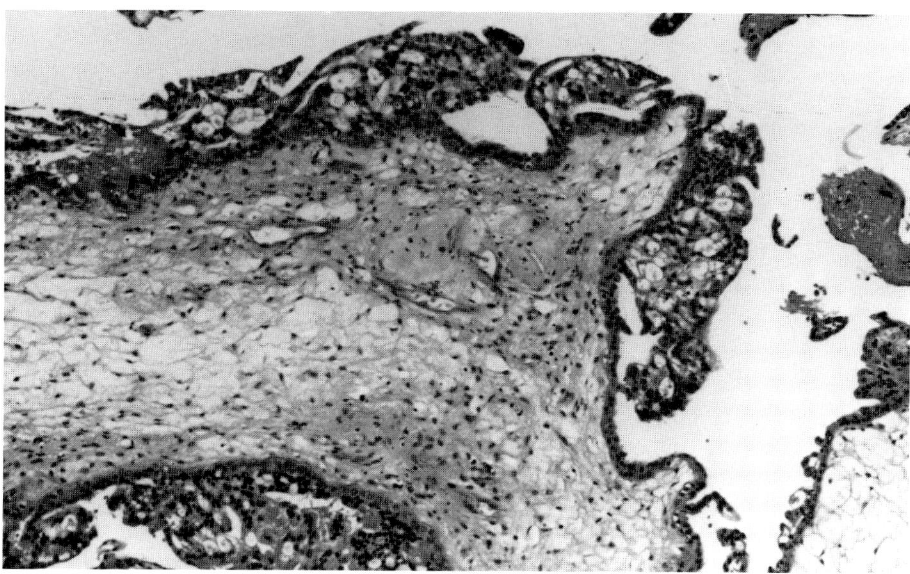

Fig. 9-11. Partial hydatidiform mole with exuberant trophoblast hyperplasia. Villous stroma is edematous with central clearing. Scattered trophoblastic knuckles dot surface of adjacent villus (lower right).

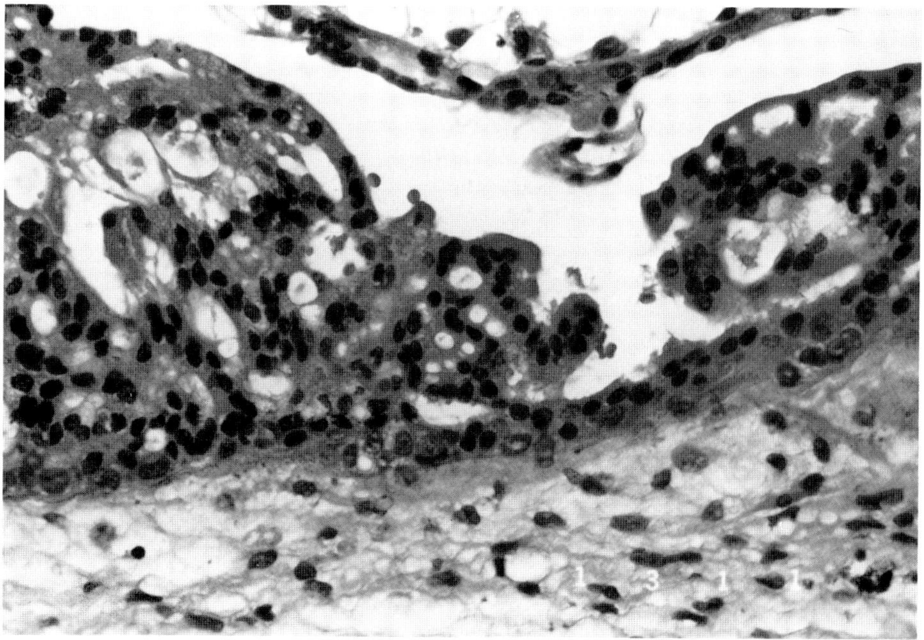

Fig. 9-12. Partial hydatidiform mole, illustrating lacy appearance of hyperplastic syncytiotrophoblast. Same case as Figure 9-11.

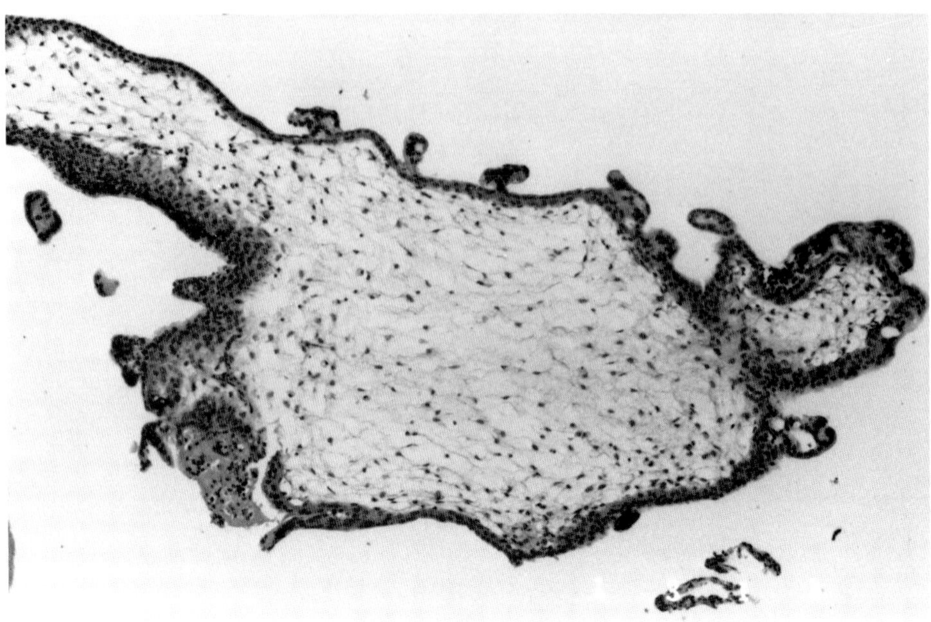

Fig. 9-13. Partial hydatidiform mole with prominent trophoblastic knuckles involving circumference of villus. Stroma is slightly cellular.

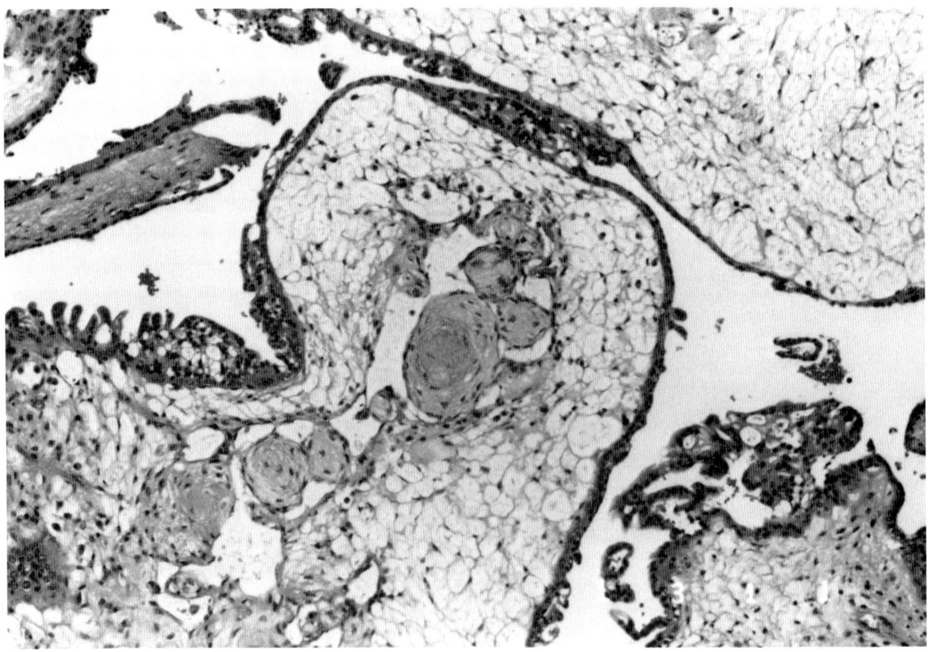

Fig. 9-14. Partial hydatidiform mole with enlarged villus containing bizarre, anastomosing vascular channels in villous stroma. Note syncytiotrophoblastic hyperplasia and villous stromal edema in larger villi. A small sclerotic villus is apparent at the upper left.

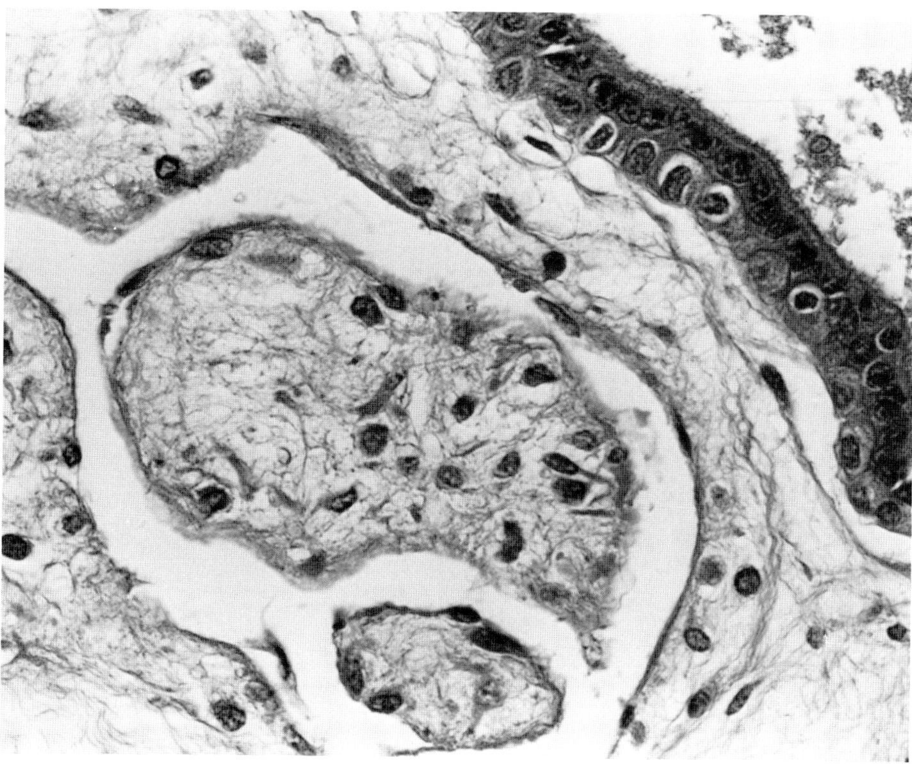

Fig. 9-15. Higher-power view of Figure 9-14 illustrating bizarre, mazelike, endothelium-lined, vascular channels of partial hydatidiform mole. In other sections, these channels contained well-formed nucleated red blood cells.

scopically or microscopically identifiable fetal tissues. Since some degree of fetal development occurs, fetal red blood cells, whether nucleated or not, are identified in stromal vessels. In rare instances, liveborn malformed infants have been delivered at term. Fetal malformations include unilateral or bilateral partially fused digits (syndactyly), generally involving fingers 3-4 and toes 2-3-4, and gastrointestinal tract (omphalocele, atresia), cardiovascular and central nervous system anomalies.[71, 72] Sustained fetal viability is not possible.

Flow Cytometry and Cytogenetic Studies. While the vast majority of PM assayed are triploid or near-triploid (greater than 90 percent), flow cytometric and cytogenetic studies indicate that a few are diploid, haploid, tetraploid, or aneu-

ploid.[12, 28, 29, 30, 73] The relative preponderance of paternal versus maternal DNA has been confirmed in some of these anomalous cases.[51, 73] The histomorphology of the genetically "anomalous" PM is similar to triploid PM. There are two populations of villi with focal trophoblast hyperplasia, although villous scalloping and trophoblastic inclusions are less conspicuous. There may be a lower frequency of persistent trophoblastic disease following these anomalous PM.[30]

A "Third Type" of Hydatidiform Mole? A third type of hydatidiform mole with a diploid karyotype was initially posited by Szulman and Surti.[11] These moles are generally classified as PM based on morphologic similarities to triploid PM, including focal villous hydrops and lack of extensive trophoblast hyperplasia.[11, 30] This unique mole may require a separate category because, unlike any other mole, it has the normal amount of both maternal and paternal DNA (biparental). In a specimen described by Vejerslev et al.,[74] the fetus survived to 22 weeks gestational age, and a diploid biparental genetic origin of the placenta was confirmed.

Differential Diagnosis: Partial Mole Versus Complete Mole With Coexistent Normal Twin. A misdiagnosis of PM may result if the diagnosis is based solely on the presence of a normal fetus, infant, or fetal tissue in conjunction with a molar placenta.[75–78] Many of the latter combinations are CM with a coexisting normal twin gestation,[30] whereas others may be early CM with less trophoblast hyperplasia than usually apparent in the more mature CM. The recognition of two separate gestations is aided by previous obstetric ultrasound examination or receipt of an intact specimen by hysterectomy, or both (Fig. 9-16).

Table 9-4 presents diagnostic criteria for distinguishing CM with coexisting twin from PM in curettings. CM with twin is characterized by an admixture of normal well-vascularized villi (with trophoblast maturation consistent with the fetal gestational age) interspersed with molar villi exhibiting marked circumferential trophoblast hyperplasia.

Rare cases of massive placentomegaly with marked villous hydrops and diploid DNA content have been associated with Beckwith-Wiedemann syndrome.[79] One example reported as diploid PM had features suggestive of fetal Beckwith-Wiedemann syndrome.[80] Whereas massive placento-

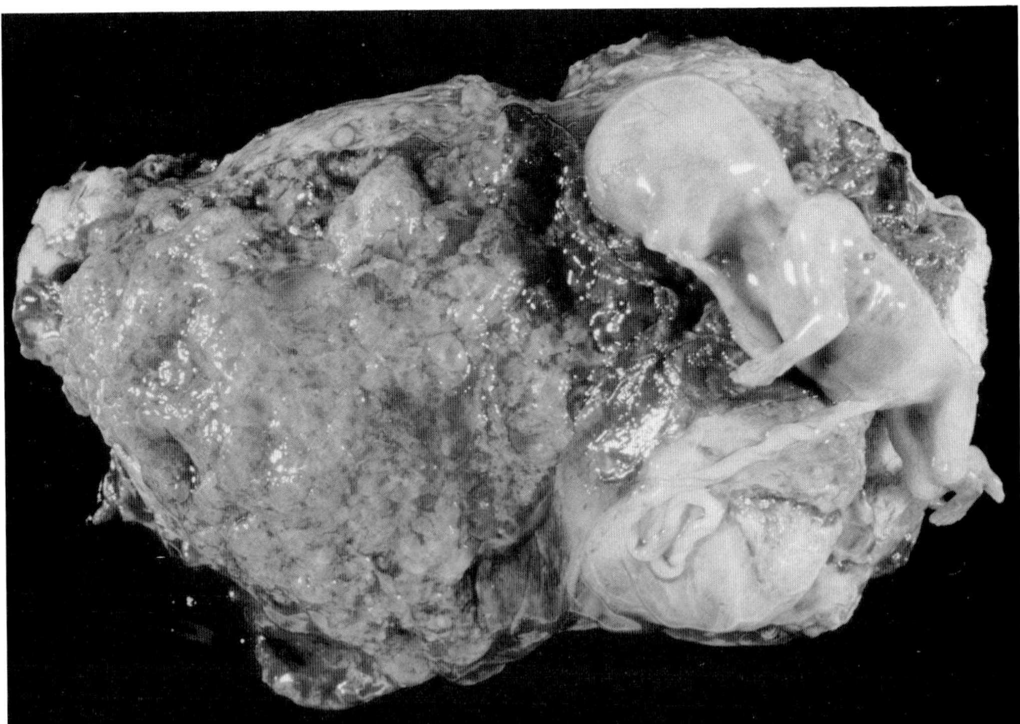

Fig. 9-16. Hysterectomy for complete hydatidiform mole and coexisting normal twin gestation. Copious molar villi far exceed the volume of villi in the normal placental disc of the co-twin. (From Lage et al.,[30] with permission.)

Table 9-4. Differential Diagnosis of Complete Mole With Normal Twin Versus Partial Hydatidiform Mole

	Complete Mole and Coexistent Twin	Partial Mole
Trophoblast hyperplasia	Marked on some villi, totally absent on others	Focal hyperplasia, never marked
Villous scalloping and trophoblastic inclusions	Absent	Present
Fetal tissues	Present	Present, usually with anomalies
Trophoblastic notches	Absent	Present
Trophoblast atypia	Moderate to prominent	Never prominent
Villous cavitation	Present in many villi, conspicuous	Focal, but less conspicuous
Mazelike villous vessels	Absent	May be present

megaly and villous hydrops without trophoblast hyperplasia may not be pathognomonic for the Beckwith-Wiedemann syndrome, there appears to be some genetic linkage between these placentas and the anomalies associated with this syndrome. The differential diagnosis of PM versus hydropic abortus is presented in the section on hydropic abortus.

Clinical Management of Partial Mole. The clinical management of PM is essentially the same as for CM. At some centers, monitoring of serial hCG measurements are continued for only 3 months after complete gonadotropin remission. Persistent gestational trophoblastic disease is diagnosed by the same criteria as for CM, but sequelae after PM are much less common.[30, 35, 37, 51, 64, 65] Rates of persistence have ranged from 0 to 10 percent[11–13, 19, 28, 35, 81, 82] and are correlated with the referral patterns of the reporting center. Persistence rates tend to be higher at gestational trophoblastic disease centers, where high-risk patients and patients with persistent disease are more likely to be referred for treatment.[83] At these centers, persistence rates range from 5 to 10 percent.[35, 81] Much lower persistence rates of 0[51] to 0.5 percent[65] have been reported from Great Britain. Very rarely, PM may invade the myometrium and metastasize. Only rare cases of CCA after PM have been reported.[65, 84] Chemotherapeutic require-

ments in treatment of persistence after PM are usually much less than that for CM.[30]

HYDROPIC ABORTUS

General Considerations

A review of molar conceptuses would be incomplete without a discussion of one of the most common obstetric specimens, the hydropic abortus (HA). The HA is a morphologically abnormal placenta with gross or microscopic villous hydrops. Fetal tissues are not usually present, although nucleated fetal red blood cells may remain in the villous capillaries. Often, these gestations are associated with karyotypic abnormalities. Early publications on PM included many conceptuses with karyotypic abnormalities[12] not generally associated with the currently recognized PM phenotype, suggesting that examples of HA were included in these early studies.

Since the clinical and ultrasonographic features of the HA and hydatidiform moles overlap, the final diagnosis rests with the pathologist. A diagnosis of either type of hydatidiform mole, CM or PM, will initiate many months of hormonal surveillance and require contraceptive measures—a significant hardship for those with infertility. Conversely, no hormonal surveillance will follow a diagnosis of HA as this diagnosis implies no risk of gestational trophoblastic disease.

Gross Examination

The HA is characterized by swelling of villi recognized ultrasonographically, grossly or microscopically (Fig. 9-17). In a recent series, the maximum villous size in HA was 0.28 cm, range 0 to 1.9 cm.[30] This villous hydrops may be as extreme in maximum dimension as in CM, but usually only a few villi are this large, the rest being small. In our experience, massive hydrops of some villi is particularly common in other genetic abnormalities, including trisomy 18 and the Beckwith-Wiedemann syndrome.[79]

Microscopic Examination

The specimen must be adequately sampled for microscopic examination; in diffi-cult cases, the entire specimen should be examined. The quantity of villous tissue in the entire sample is crucial. The diagnosis of hydatidiform mole, partial or complete, is extremely unlikely if the entire sample has been examined microscopically and all of the villous tissue (chorionic vesicle) is contained within only one tissue block. The average HA has villous tissues on only one to three slides.

Secondly, the spectrum of villous sizes is helpful in distinguishing HA from PM. The HA displays a full spectrum of villous sizes. This spectrum, apparent on each slide, is formed by an admixture of small, sclerotic villi, normal-size villi and large, edematous villi (Fig. 9-17).

The attenuated trophoblast of the HA is in contradistinction to the focal trophoblast hyperplasia of the PM. The most edematous villi of HA are characterized by ballooning degeneration with extremely thin overlying trophoblast. The villi may contain central cisterns, most commonly from the chorion leave. Usually, there are no fe-

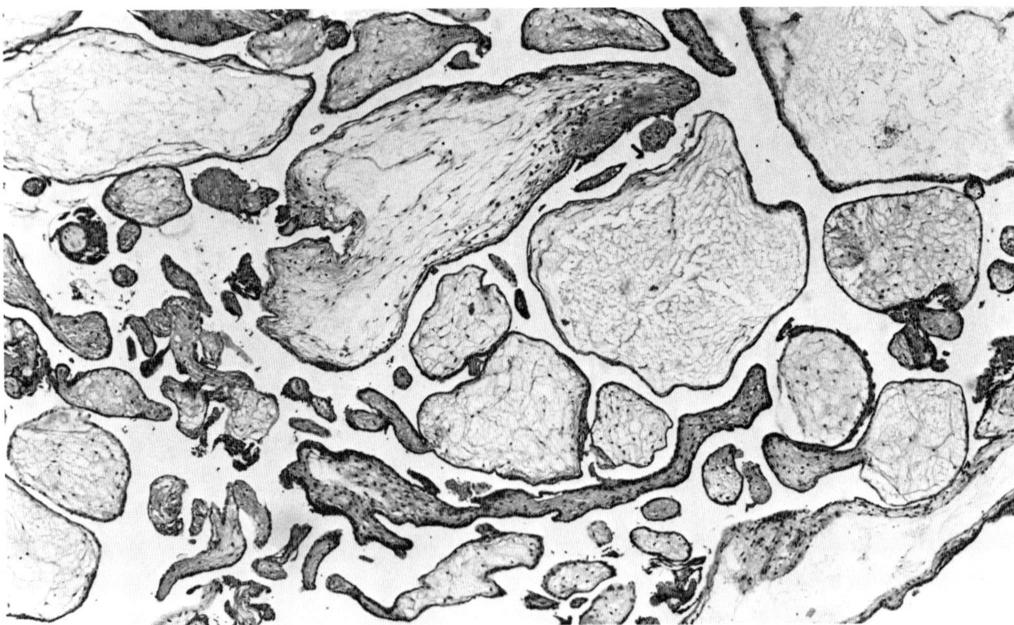

Fig. 9-17. Hydropic abortus with edematous, focal villous cavitation and attenuation of overlying trophoblast. Note spectrum of villous sizes. (From Lage,[43] with permission.)

tal tissues, either intact or fragmented, or well-preserved nucleated red blood cells within the villous capillaries.

Differential Diagnosis: Hydropic Abortus Versus Partial Mole

The greatest diagnostic difficulty is distinguishing between HA and PM, as HA is usually not confused with a CM, the trophoblast hyperplasia in the latter being conspicuous. The most helpful morphologic criteria for diagnosing HA are presented in Table 9-5, and include (1) small amount of tissue, (2) attenuated trophoblast, and (3) full spectrum of villous sizes. The results of both flow cytometry, which may be performed on fresh or formalin-fixed paraffin-embedded tissues, or cytogenetics, which must be anticipated in advance because fresh tissues are required, may be very helpful in separating these lesions (Fig. 9-2). Studies of HA have indicated that the majority are diploid or near-diploid.[30] More than 90 percent of PM are triploid[30]; among triploid gestations, more than 86 percent are PM.[30, 85] Of all triploid gestations, only 11 to 14 percent are HA.[30, 85] The nuclear DNA ploidy of a difficult case may serve as a guide to the right diagnosis. When in doubt, the clinician should be notified that PM cannot be excluded, and hormonal surveillance should be undertaken.

GESTATIONAL CHORIOCARCINOMA

CCA is the most malignant trophoblastic lesion and, before the advent of modern chemotherapy, it was one of the most lethal human tumors, with a crude death rate of 85 percent when treated by surgery alone.[86, 87] Apart from its association with villi in rare cases arising in a term placenta,[88–94] CCA is devoid of villi.[95]

Epidemiology

A tumor of trophoblast, by definition gestational CCA is derived from a conceptus. Reported frequencies of CCA in the United States range from 1 : 19,920 livebirths,[96] 1 : 24,096 pregnancies[96] to 1 : 40,000 deliveries.[31] Compared with whites, CCA is more common in blacks and other races, with relative risks of 2.1 and 1.8, respectively.[96] For reasons that remain unclear, gestational trophoblastic tumors and CCA are more common in third-world countries than in more developed nations. The incidence of CCA varies widely throughout the world: 1 : 570 to 1 : 1,650 deliveries in Indonesia,[33] to 1 : 30,000 deliveries in Great Britain.[65] The prevalence of CCA among Asian, African, and Latin American women is 20 to 40 times higher than among women from North America, Europe, and Australia.[33, 97–100]

Seminal studies conducted by Hertig and

Table 9-5. Differential Diagnosis Between Partial Hydatidiform Mole and Hydropic Abortus

	Partial Hydatidiform Mole	Hydropic Abortus
Quality of villous tissue	Large, increased for gestational age	Scant, decreased for gestational age
Spectrum of villous sizes	Two populations only: large and small	Full spectrum from small to large
Quality of trophoblast	Focally hyperplastic	Attenuated
Villous outline	Scalloped	Round or normal
Trophoblastic notches	Present	Absent
Fetal tissues	Present, usually	Absent, usually
DNA content	Triploid	Diploid

Mansell revealed that 50 percent of CCA cases were preceded by CM, 25 percent by abortion, 22.5 percent by a normal pregnancy, and 2.5 percent by ectopic pregnancy.[47] In that study, CCA followed 1/160,000 normal gestations, 1/15,386 abortions, 1/5,333 ectopic gestations, and 1/40 molar gestations.[47] That CCA will follow CM in 2.5 percent may represent the extreme,[46, 49, 61, 101] since in a more recent study of 153 women with CM treated at a large trophoblastic disease center, none developed CCA.[49]

Rarely, CCA is discovered unexpectedly in a term placenta.[89, 91, 102, 103] In one case, CCA was diagnosed on pathologic examination of a term abruptio placenta in a woman found to have clinically unsuspected metastatic disease[93] (Figs. 9-18 and 9-19).

Whereas the nature of the antecedent pregnancy may vary based on the patient's geographic location, its strong association with a previous CM seems to cross international lines. Other clinical factors have been identified. In a case-control study, CCA was associated with low body mass index, low-calorie dieting, light menstrual flow, menarche after age 12, family or personal history of dizygotic twins, more than one marriage, and infrequent intercourse.[104] These risk factors pertained to women with previous hydatidiform mole as well as other antecedent pregnancy types.

Clinical experience indicates that CCA is derived from the antecedent pregnancy, a conclusion confirmed histologically in tumors arising within normal placentas.[89–93, 102, 103] Another possibility is that the tumor is the initial and only product of a new fertilization event, termed *CCA ab initio*. Few, if any such specimens have been authenticated.

With the advent of chromosomal banding to study DNA heteromorphisms and DNA restriction fragment-length polymorphism assays, the genetic origin of CCA can be identified in both fresh and fixed tissues.

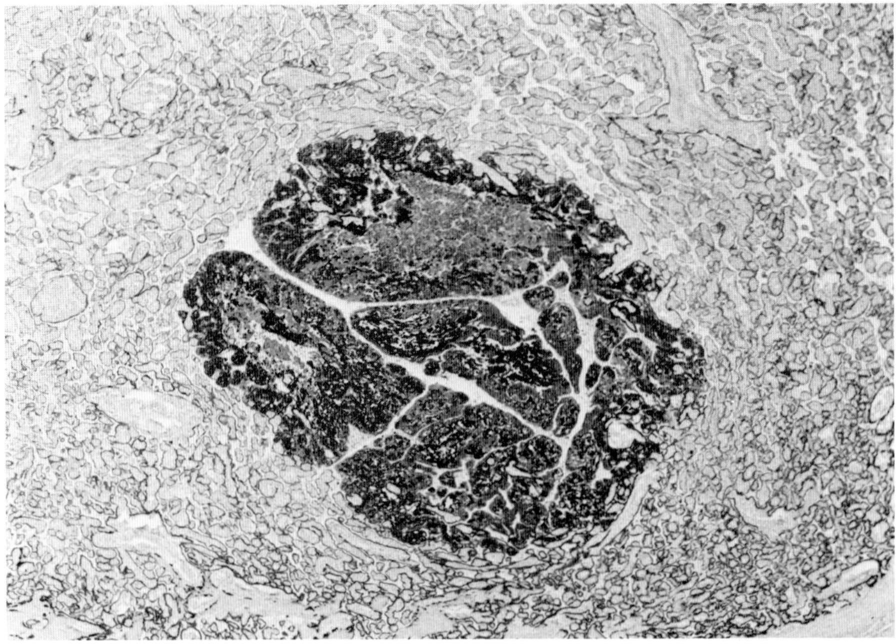

Fig. 9-18. Choriocarcinoma in a term placenta. Multiple small white tumor nodules were present on gross examination. Immunoreactivity to keratin antibodies highlights the tumor. Centers of tumor nests are necrotic. (From Lage and Roberts,[93] with permission.)

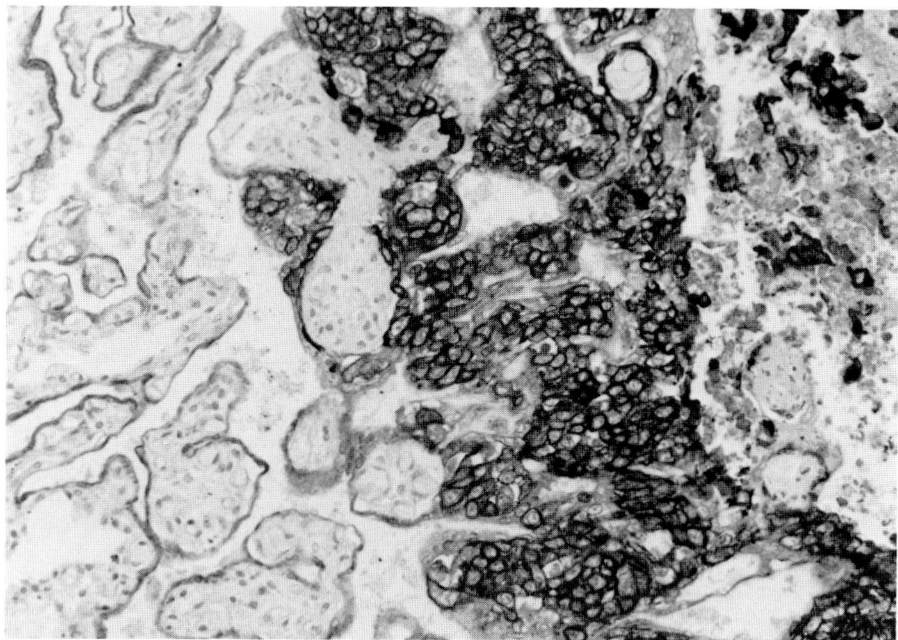

Fig. 9-19. High-power magnification of Figure 9-18 depicting choriocarcinoma proliferating from the surfaces of normal villi. Some villi have normal trophoblast alternating with malignant trophoblast. Necrotic tumor on the right. Immunoperoxidase stain with antibodies to keratin. (From Lage and Roberts,[93] with permission.)

Initial studies have validated the concept that CCA is derived from an antecedent gestation.[105–107] Restriction fragment length polymorphism analysis of two cases indicated that CCA may follow both heterozygous and homozygous CM.[107] Further studies are needed to evaluate the role of molar zygosity in affecting risk for subsequent CCA.

There appears to be some association between parental blood group type and the frequency of CCA, an association strongest for blood types A and O.[108–110] Yet, in women with CCA the products of the antecedent gestations appear to show no proclivity for a given blood group type. Red blood cell RhO(D) antigen was expressed in a post-term CCA arising in a RhO(D)-negative woman, and the tumor induced RhO(D) sensitization.[111]

Increased prevalence of Y chromosomal material has been found in DNA from CCA.[112] This is in contradistinction to the marked decrease in the frequency of Y chromosomal material in CM, the most common antecedent to CCA. It remains unclear whether women with 46,XY CM are at greater risk of the development of CCA than are women with 46,XX CM.

Clinical Signs and Symptoms

The presenting symptoms of CCA generally reflect the involved organ system: vaginal bleeding from uterine tumors is by far the most common.[94, 113] As CCA is apt to enter the bloodstream, a normal function of trophoblast, dissemination is common. The lung is the most frequent metastatic site. Other sites include brain, liver, kidney, intestinal tract, and skin.[67, 94, 113–118] Most women with post-term CCA have metastases at the initial diagnosis.[113] CNS lesions lead to dysfunction from embolic stroke, subarachnoid hemorrhage, subdural or intracerebral hematoma, or a hemorrhagic intraspinal mass.[114] Other manifestations of metastases include hemoptysis, hematemesis, and bluish nodules in skin and mucous membranes.[113, 115–117]

Unfortunately, in patients without a previous history of CM, the possibility of CCA is often not entertained, and valuable time lost before the diagnosis is made. Unusual presentations have been reported, and CCA has masqueraded as a number of diseases.[117] In some, tumor is diagnosed at postmortem examination, and organs from donors with unsuspected CCA have been unknowingly transplanted into recipients, sometimes with fatal results.[119]

CCA may be initially diagnosed in the mother or infant. Metastases to the infant are uniformly lethal.[116] In one series summarizing the world's literature, evaluation of 11 women revealed no evidence of CCA in three, even though their children had died of metastatic CCA.[116]

Gross Examination

If a hysterectomy is performed, gross examination of the uterus may reveal large tumor nodules (Fig. 9-20) or be totally unremarkable.[114] CCA is typically characterized by red to dark brown hemorrhagic nodules with extensive destructive myometrial invasion. A superficial tumor may project into the endometrial cavity (Fig. 9-21). Occasional lesions may be light tan in color with less hemorrhage and necrosis.[117] In some cases, there is no residual uterine lesion despite widespread metastases. Metastatic nodules are generally well circumscribed and deep red.[114,117]

Microscopic Examination

On microscopic examination, the extent of necrosis, hemorrhage and infarction surpasses that of any other tumor. The diagno-

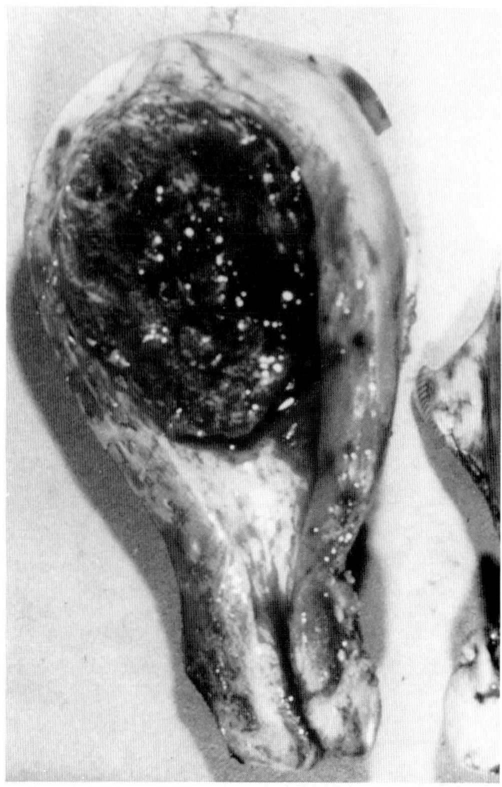

Fig. 9-20. Uterus with large pedunculated choriocarcinoma showing extensive hemorrhage and necrosis.

sis requires a proliferation of malignant ST and CT (Figs. 9-22 and 9-23). The tumor is biphasic, with multinucleated ST juxtaposed to mononucleated trophoblast, CT and/or IT. Often a plexiform network is formed by large sheets of CT alternating with ST and, occasionally, IT. While the CT or IT may simulate a number of malignant tumors, the presence of admixed ST facilitates the diagnosis (Figs. 9-22 and 9-23). With its multinucleation and dense amphophilic to violaceous cytoplasm, the ST is usually not confused with any other cell type. The ST may form lacunae containing maternal red blood cells recapitulating the blood lakes of the previllous blastocyst.

Although most pathologists consider all trophoblast to show significant nuclear pleomorphism and atypicality, the malig-

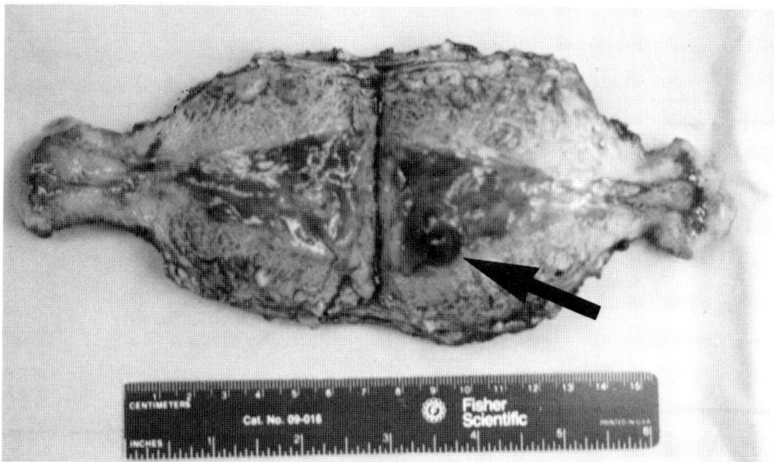

Fig. 9-21. Bivalved uterus removed from a woman 3 months postpartum demonstrating a single polypoid nodule of choriocarcinoma (arrow). Liveborn infant had negative serum human chorionic gonadotropin on examination (age 3 months) and has remained well. Mother attained complete gonadotropin remission after hysterectomy and single course of chemotherapy. Placenta of infant was buried after delivery.

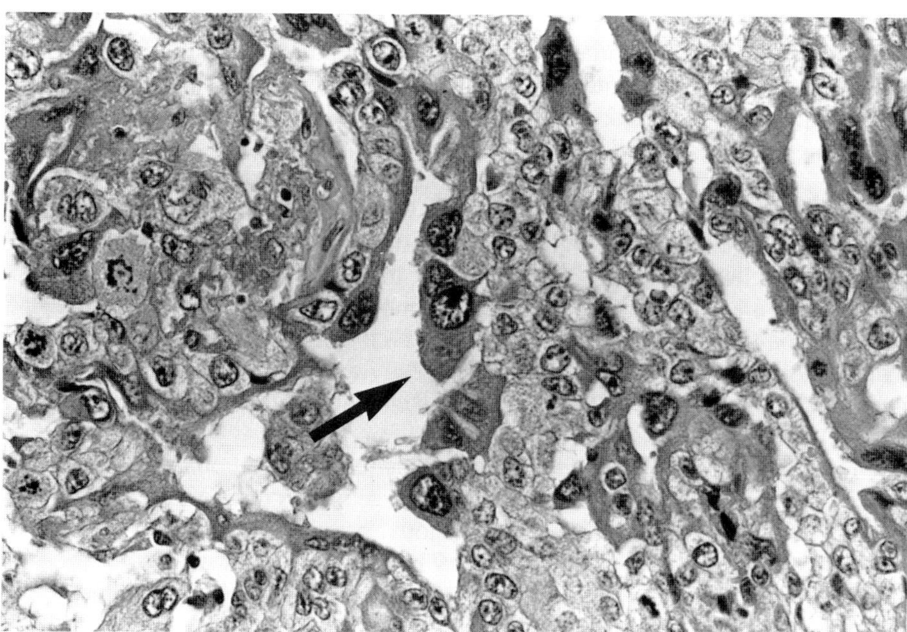

Fig. 9-22. Choriocarcinoma composed of central blood-lake lined by intermediate trophoblast (arrow), surrounded predominantly by cytotrophoblast with scattered syncytiotrophoblast.

forgotten; gestational CCA may occur anywhere an ectopic pregnancy might be found, including ovary, fallopian tube, or abdominal cavity.[54, 115, 124]

Diagnosis of Choriocarcinoma in Uterine Curettings. The diagnosis of CCA in uterine curettings may be life-saving. Some authorities flatly refuse to make a diagnosis on the basis of uterine curettings. Others acknowledge that occasions arise in which the diagnosis is appropriate. Even with a thorough understanding of the histopathology of trophoblastic lesions, this is treacherous territory, and mistakes are likely.

Classification of Trophoblast in Curettings. In a classic publication on the interpretation of trophoblastic processes obtained by uterine curettage, Elston and Bagshawe[125] offered the following diagnostic terminology:

1. Villous trophoblast.
2. Simple trophoblast.
3. Trophoblast with an appearance suspicious of CCA.
4. Trophoblast diagnostic of CCA.

The interpretation of specimens containing *villous trophoblast* is contingent on evaluation of the villous portion of the specimen: normal villi, HA, PM, or CM.

Simple trophoblast is defined as small amounts of undifferentiated trophoblast in the absence of villous tissue.[125] The early trophoblast of a normal blastocyst is composed of primitive cells that invade normal tissues and that normally have a strikingly "malignant" appearance, including nuclear enlargement and hyperchromasia. After embryonic death, superimposed degenerative changes induce further cytologic atypia. These atypical trophoblastic cells exfoliate and become entrapped in thrombi and may be misdiagnosed as CCA.

A diagnosis of simple trophoblast requires that the entire sample be examined, that only scant trophoblastic cells are found (usually in a few foci on only a couple of slides at most), and that there is minimal

differentiation toward CT or ST. Nucleoli are not prominent. As vascular invasion by normal benign trophoblast is the rule, its presence does not imply malignancy.

The third category, *suspicious trophoblast*, is defined by moderate to large amounts of trophoblast with clear differentiation into ST and CT/IT. No villous tissue is present, and there is endomyometrial invasion. While such curettings are suspicious for CCA, a definite diagnosis is not possible. Further interpretation requires correlation with the clinical history and review of any pathology from the antecedent conceptus. In the series of Elston and Bagshawe,[125] all patients with a previous normal pregnancy and simple or suspicious trophoblast on curettings developed malignant or metastatic trophoblastic disease with a 31 percent mortality despite chemotherapy. Fifty-three percent of those with a previous molar gestation developed malignant or metastatic disease. In the latter group, chemotherapy was far more successful, with only one death.

Definitive *diagnosis of CCA* in uterine curettings requires (1) differentiation of tumor cells into diagnostic ST and CT/IT, (2) large sheets of tumor, (3) invasion of endomyometrium, and (4) absence of villous tissue.

Avoidance of Pitfalls. A spontaneous abortion is the most common event prompting a misdiagnosis of CCA. When avillous trophoblast is present on initial sections, it is essential that the entire specimen be submitted for microscopic examination. Identification of any villous tissue excludes a diagnosis of CCA. The previous pregnancy history must be known in full. In a few instances, we have puzzled over a diagnosis of avillous trophoblast only to find out that a curettage specimen containing normal villi had been processed at a different hospital the previous day.

In one study, women with simple or suspicious avillous trophoblast and a nonmolar antecedent gestation had a threefold increased risk of the development of CCA as compared with those whose antecedent pregnancy was molar.[125] In either case, hormonal assay of β-hCG and clinical evaluation is recommended.

Retained implantation site trophoblast, particularly when following a molar gestation or second trimester spontaneous abortion, may pose a significant diagnostic dilemma; this problem is discussed below.

CCA is most often overlooked in the clinical setting of persistent *vaginal bleeding postpartum* (Fig. 9-20). Most commonly, curettage reveals retained placental fragments with ghost villi. CCA should be suspected whenever there are *large sheets of CT and ST/IT,* and *no villi.* Endomyometrial invasion by masses of avillous CT and ST/IT confirms the diagnosis. As is true in spontaneous abortions, the entire sample must be examined microscopically before making a definitive diagnosis. The clinician should be notified of preliminary findings, as prompt diagnosis is vital.

Treatment. CCA is treated aggressively with multiagent chemotherapy; radiotherapy and operative treatment serve as adjuvant modalities. As with most malignant tumors, early diagnosis and treatment before dissemination are associated with higher survival rates. Hysterectomy in women with postmolar metastatic CCA will contain no tumor in more than 50 percent of cases.[115]

Survival in CCA appears to be related directly to tumor burden, as poorer survival is correlated with high serum β-hCG value, brain or liver metastases, and duration of symptoms related to untreated tumor (often prolonged in post-term CCA).[67] In many, death is related to hemorrhage.[122] In a study of 196 women with gestational CCA treated at a large trophoblastic disease center during 1962 to 1980, 49 (25 percent) died.[122] Evaluation of 31 fatal cases at autopsy revealed no correlation between the amount of chemotherapy and the distribution or number of metastatic lesions.[122] Although chemotherapy has resulted in clear improvement in survival rates, it is not without associated risks. Therapy-induced fatal acute myeloid leukemia has been reported following treatment.[67] Five-year survival rates in CCA are 81 percent for all women, and 71 percent for those with metastatic tumor.[126]

CHORANGIOCARCINOMA, AN
UNCLASSIFIED TROPHOBLASTIC
LESION

A case report in 1988 by Jauniaux et al.[127] described an extremely unusual and interesting placental lesion found in a near-term placenta. They termed this incidental finding *chorangiocarcinoma.*[127] Microscopically, this well-circumscribed lesion had nonhydropic villi with pronounced stromal vascular proliferation. The histologic appearance was distinguished from a benign placental chorangioma only by virtue of the finding of villi lined by malignant trophoblast. The trophoblast was an admixture of ST and CT with marked nuclear atypia and hCG immunostaining of the "peripheral trophoblast," presumably ST.[127] Maternal hCG titers were normal antenatally and postpartum. There were no malignant sequelae in either the mother or the healthy infant. This unique lesion showed no villous hydrops and therefore cannot be classified with the hydatidiform moles. It is most similar to CCA in a term placenta; however, abnormal villous stroma has not been found in placental choriocarcinomas. Further studies to determine the natural history of this rare lesion are needed, since a similar benign outcome has been reported after some placental choriocarcinomas.[89]

LESIONS OF INTERMEDIATE TROPHOBLAST

Proliferations and tumors of the IT of the placental site may pose significant diagnostic problems for the surgical pathologist, particularly in curettage specimens. These lesions include the *exaggerated placental site*,[128] a florid form of the process of normal infiltration of IT at the placental site; a recently described benign lesion, designated *placental site nodule or plaque*,[129] and the neoplasm of IT, *placental site trophoblastic tumor*.[130] Before these lesions are discussed the features of normal intermediate trophoblast will be briefly reviewed because some of the features of normal IT (Figs. 9-25 to 9-28) are also seen in proliferation or neoplasms of IT.

The term *IT* was introduced to describe a distinctive type of trophoblastic cell that shares some features with CT and ST and appears to represent a transition between them.[9,131] IT cells, often associated with fibrin (Fig. 9-26), are typically mononucleate (Figs. 9-25 and 9-26) but may be binucleate or multinucleate (Fig. 9-28). The mononucleate cells vary in shape from round or polyhedral to spindle shaped. Their cytoplasm is typically abundant and eosinophilic or amphophilic and may contain scattered small vacuoles. The nuclei may vary in size and shape and are occasionally strikingly hyperchromatic (Fig. 9-28), with coarsely granular chromatin. Cytoplasmic nuclear invaginations may be seen. IT cells stain immunohistochemically for both cytokeratins and human placental lactogen,[131, 132] a feature of diagnostic help in the recognition of both normal IT and lesions, both proliferative and neoplastic, composed of IT cells. For example, it may be difficult to distinguish IT cells from decidual cells and smooth muscle cells at the implantation site, but staining of cells for cytokeratin and human placental lactogen identifies them as IT.

Exaggerated Placental Site

The normal placental site is infiltrated by a profuse number of IT cells (Figs. 9-27 and 9-28). On occasion, these cells extensively involve the underlying myometrium, and

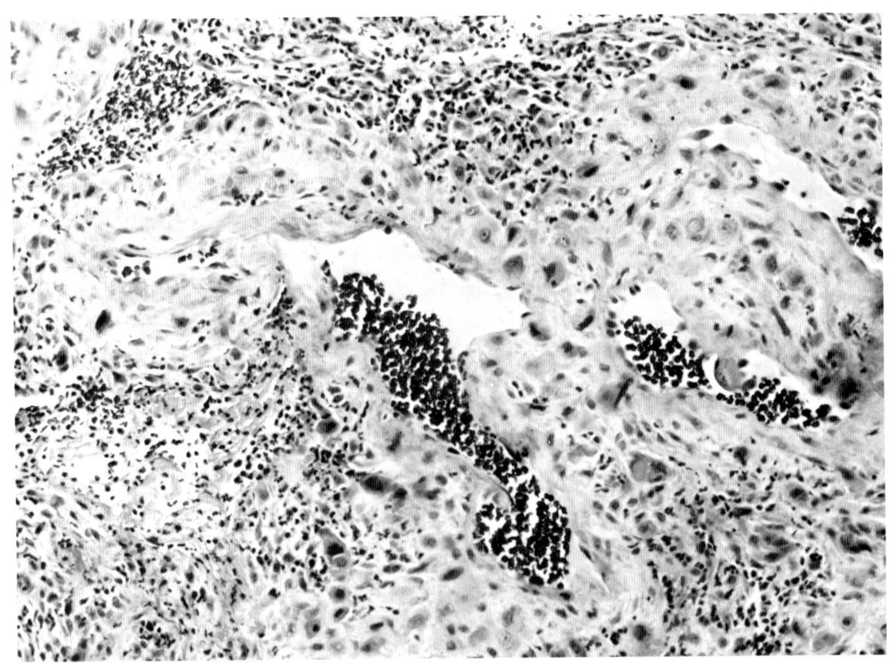

Fig. 9-25. Normal intermediate trophoblast. Cells have abundant cytoplasm and are infiltrating the walls of several blood vessels.

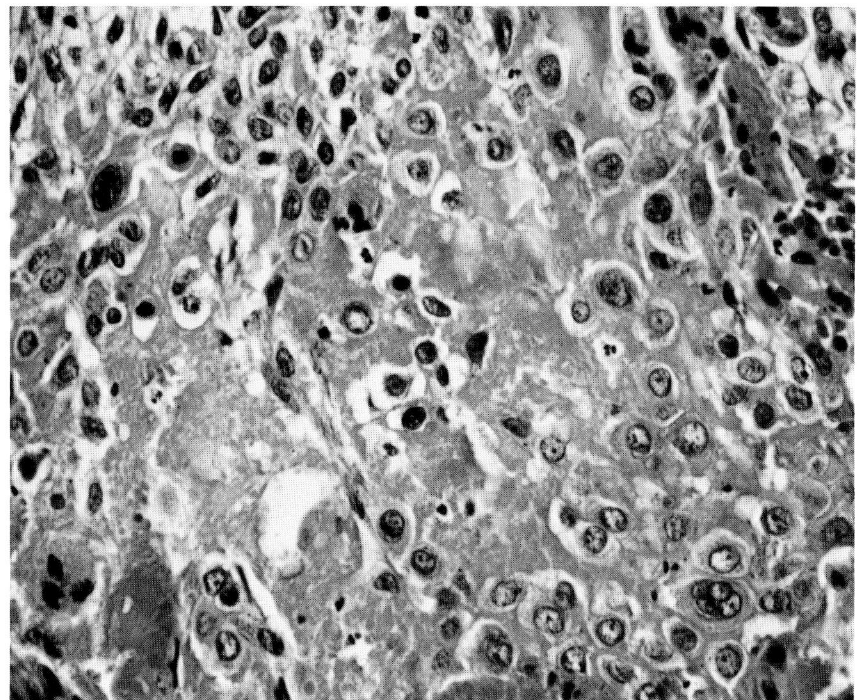

Fig. 9-26. Normal intermediate trophoblast. Cells are associated with fibrinoid material.

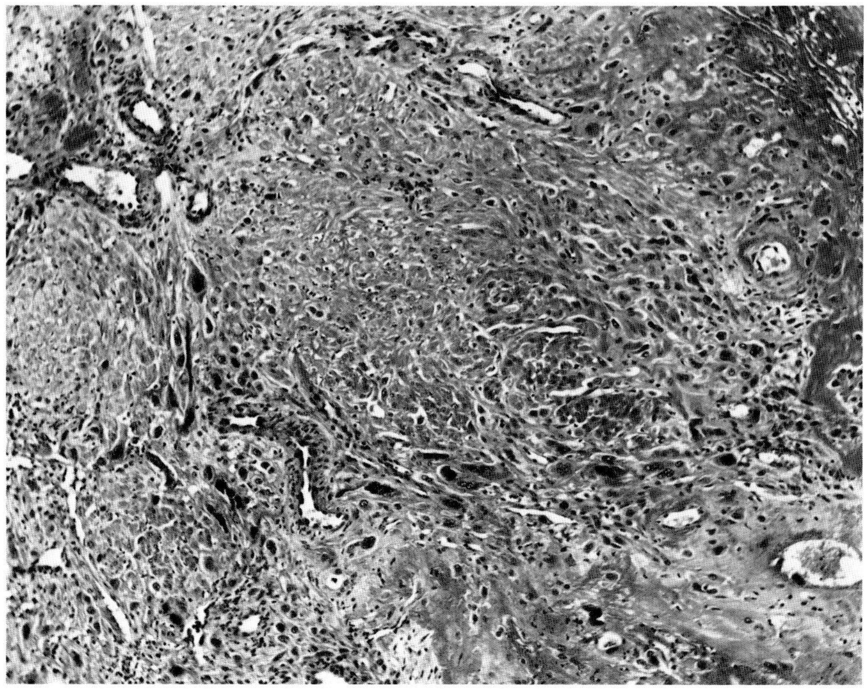

Fig. 9-27. Normal placental site. Intermediate trophoblast cells infiltrate muscle bundles of the superficial myometrium.

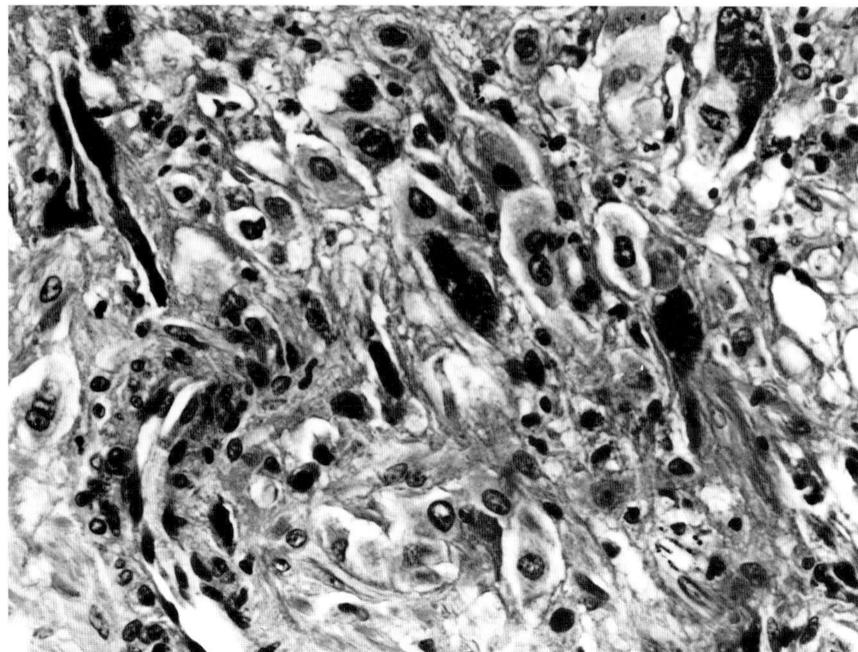

Fig. 9-28. Intermediate trophoblast cells at placental site. Note the enlarged hyperchromatic nuclei and occasional multinucleated cells.

because of their occasional nuclear atypia sometimes produce a worrisome histologic appearance (Fig. 9-29). This process was designated *syncytial endometritis* by Ewing[133] and has more recently been frequently referred to as *exaggerated placental site reaction.*[86] In the WHO classification, the term *exaggerated placental site* is preferred. The cells of this lesion have the typical features of IT cells, specifically abundant eosinophilic or amphophilic cytoplasm, and irregular, often hyperchromatic, nuclei, some of which may be multiple. The trophoblast cells are admixed to varying degrees with normal myometrial cells, decidual cells, inflammatory cells, and fibrin, which is often conspicuous.

Since the exaggerated placental site is composed largely of IT cells, the major problem in the differential diagnosis is its distinction from a placental site trophoblastic tumor. This may be difficult, particularly in a curettage specimen. If the cells of the process appear bland with little or no mi-

totic activity and are not arranged confluently to form a mass, a benign diagnosis is probable. The presence of more than an occasional mitotic figure, large confluent aggregates of the trophoblast cells, massive muscle infiltration, or any combination of these findings warrants a diagnosis of placental site trophoblastic tumor (PSTT). The presence of villi, particularly nonmolar villi, in a patient with a PSTT, although it occurs,[134] is very unusual. It is occasionally impossible to make a certain diagnosis. One may have to suggest a careful follow-up examination, which should include a subsequent uterine curettage as well as measurements of the levels of hCG and hPL, although the results may be negative in the presence of disease. The IT cells in an exaggerated placental site reaction may be confused with decidual cells, but the latter have pale basophilic cytoplasm and paler, more uniform, nuclei than do those of IT; also, the invasive properties of IT are not a feature of decidual cells. Immunocyto-

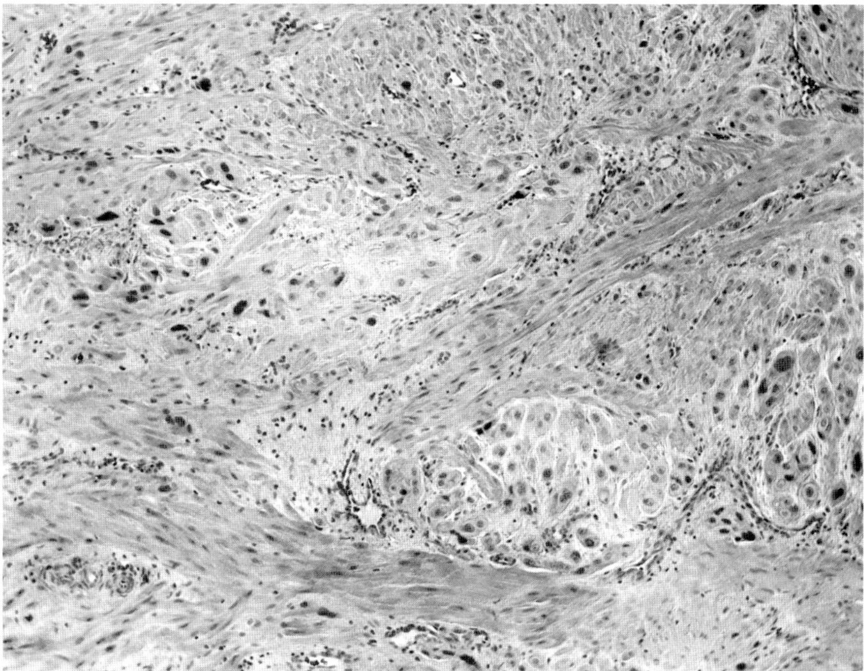

Fig. 9-29. Exaggerated placental site. There is an extensive permeation of the myometrium by intermediate trophoblast cells that focally form aggregates of moderate size.

chemical staining for cytokeratin and hPL is helpful in distinguishing these cells, as IT cells are positive for both hPL and cytokeratin, whereas decidual cells are negative.

PLACENTAL SITE NODULE AND PLAQUE

It has recently been recognized that a distinctive form of IT proliferation of the placental site that may be nodular or plaque-like occurs, and the above designations have been proposed for them.[129] This lesion (Figs. 9-30 to 9-39) generally occurs in women in the reproductive age group but is occasionally discovered in the early post-menopausal years. In most cases it has been an incidental finding in a patient whose symptoms are attributable to another process. The interval from the most recent known pregnancy may be quite long.

In one series, it ranged up to 8 years (average 3 years) in the 13 cases in which this information was available.[129] Two of the 20 patients in that series had undergone tubal ligation 3 and 4 years before presentation, and 3 had a history of hydaditidiform mole. Although usually found in an endometrial curettage specimen, the lesion may be found in an endocervical specimen, or incidentally in a hysterectomy specimen. In one series of 20 cases the lesion was grossly visible in only 5 cases, measuring a maximum of 2.5 cm.[129] Although generally located in the endometrium above the lower uterine segment, approximately one-third of the lesions are found in the lower uterine segment or upper endocervix. The findings in one study suggest a predilection for the lower uterine segment, as 63 percent of lesions were confined to that site and an additional 18 percent at least partially involved the lower uterine segment.[135] Microscopic examination discloses single (Fig. 9-29) or

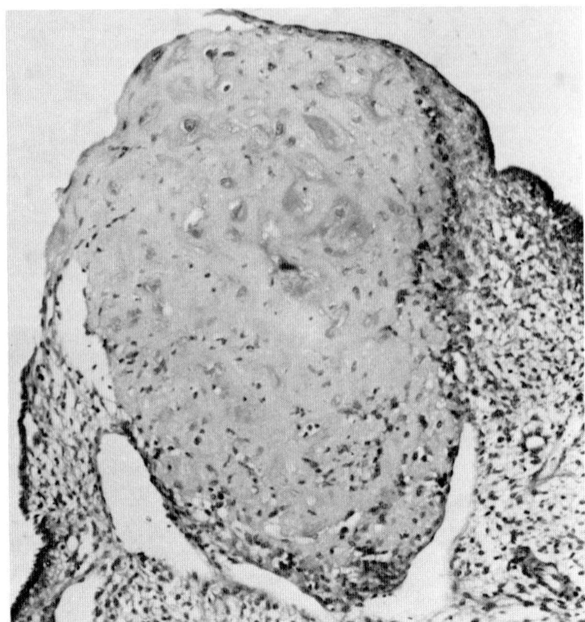

Fig. 9-30. Placental site nodule. Oval aggregate of intermediate trophoblast cells occupies the superficial endometrium. Note the hyalinization.

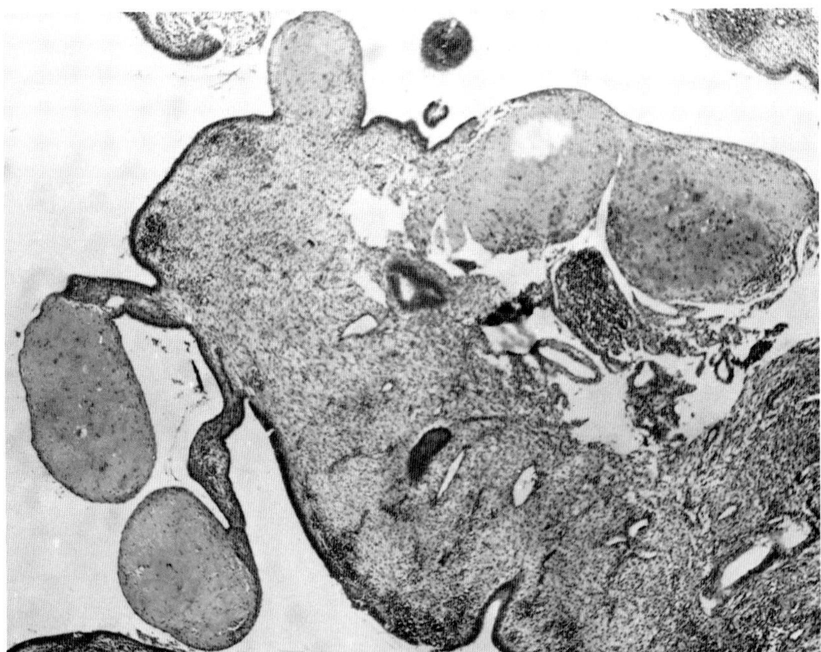

Fig. 9-31. Placental site nodules. Multiple nodules are present in the endometrium, with several forming pedunculated nodules.

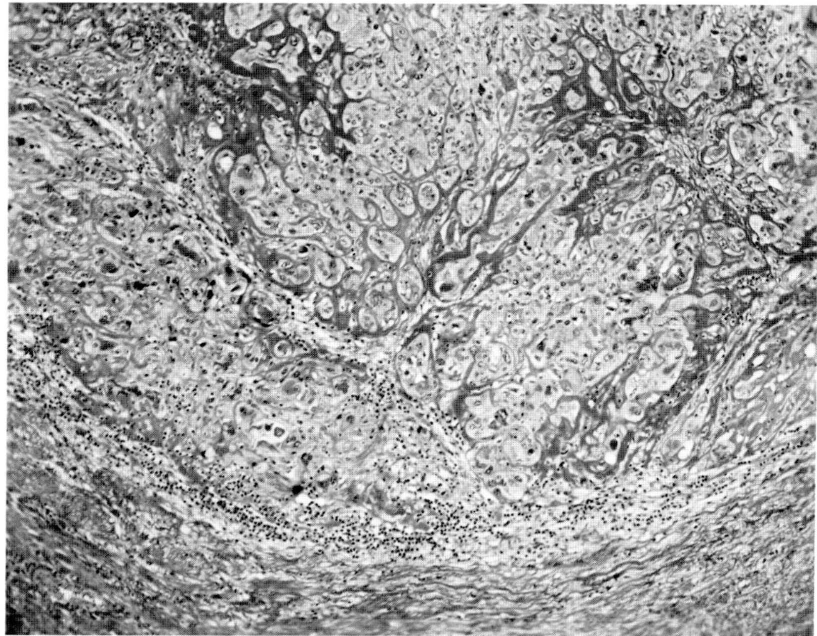

Fig. 9-32. Placental site nodule. Note well-circumscribed border of the lesion (bottom).

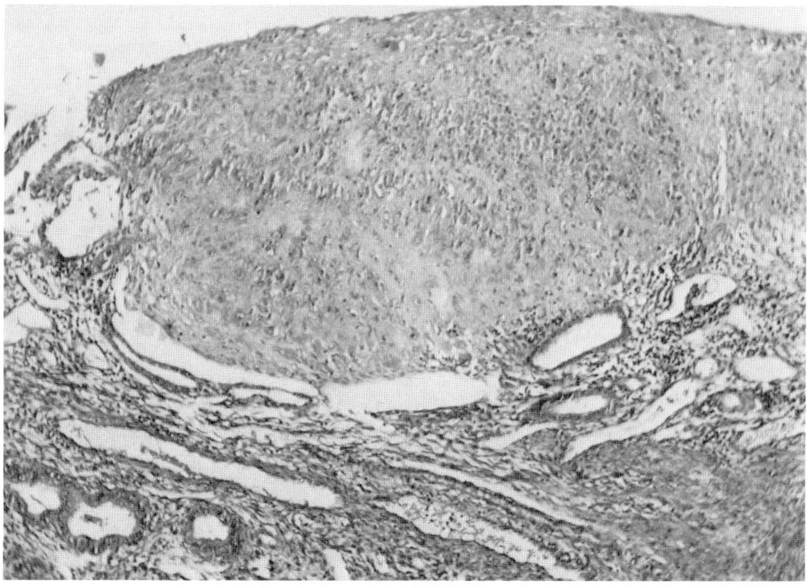

Fig. 9-33. Placental site plaque. This lesion is an elongated proliferation on the surface of the endometrium.

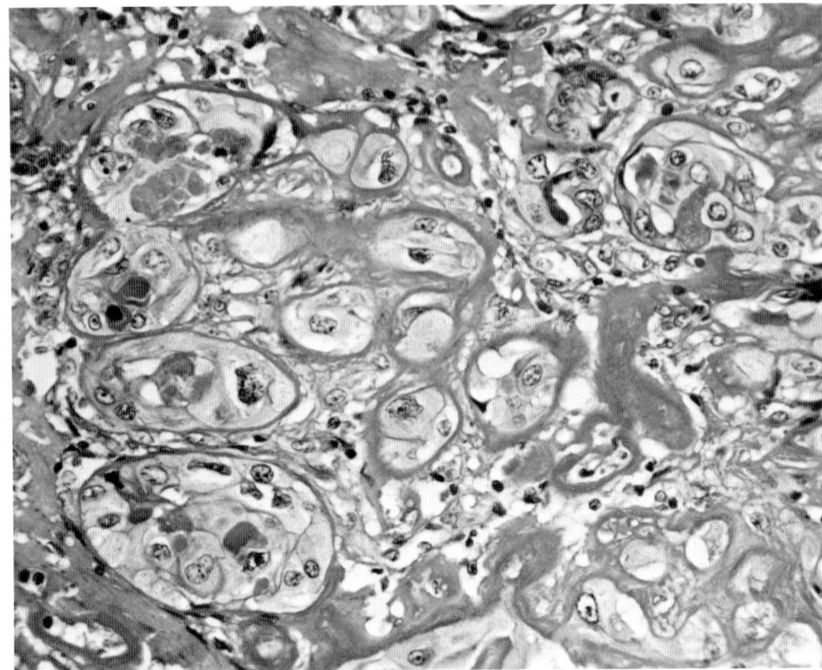

Fig. 9-34. Placental site nodule. Cells have abundant cytoplasm and slightly irregular nuclei without mitotic activity. Note hyaline material present between a number of the cells.

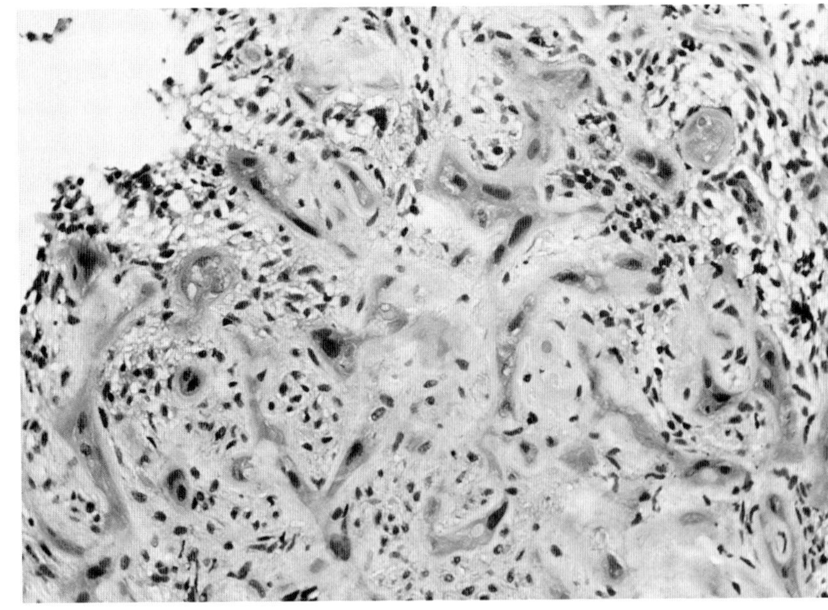

Fig. 9-35. Placental site nodule. Cells are growing as single cells, small clusters, and cords.

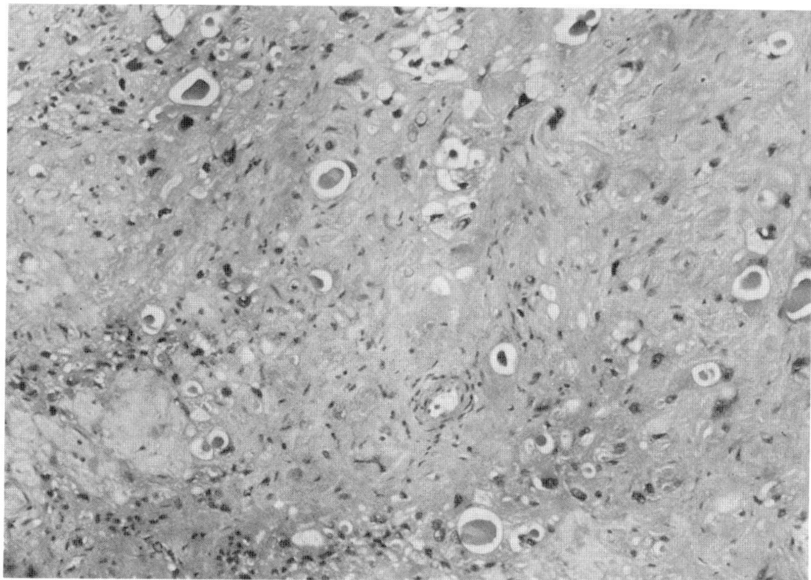

Fig. 9-36. Placental site nodule. Note extensive hyalinization and many vacuolated cells containing eosinophilic hyaline bodies.

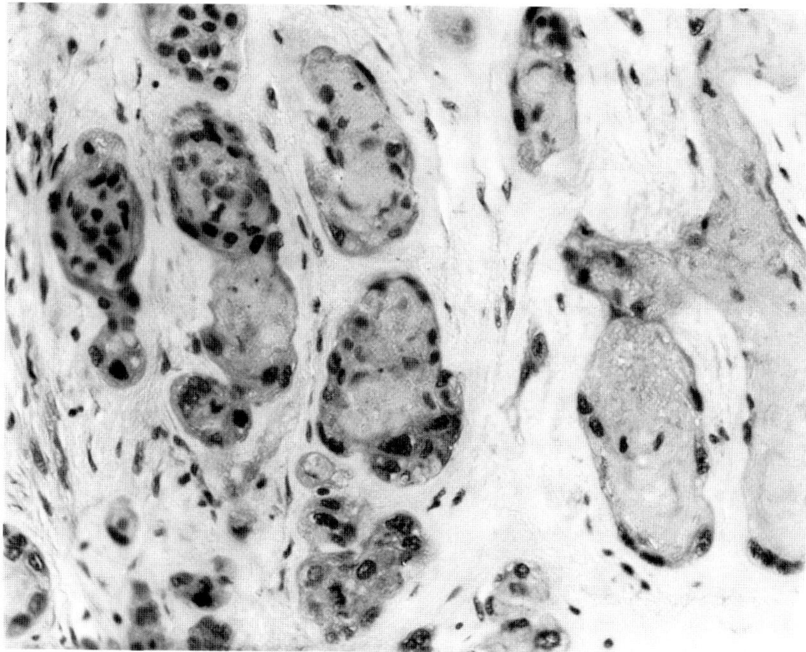

Fig. 9-37. Placental site nodule. Small cellular clusters of intermediate trophoblast with associated fibrin may simulate nests of squamous cells.

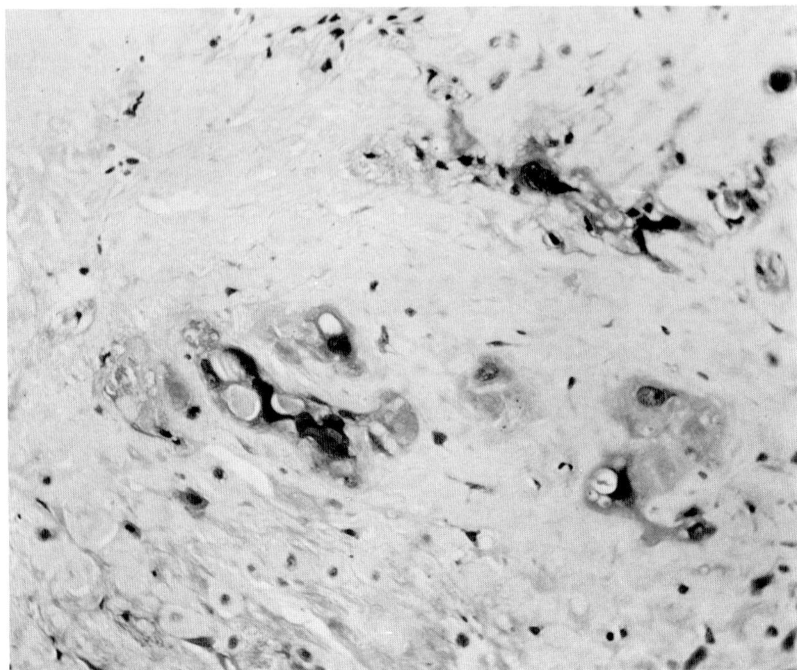

Fig. 9-38. Placental site nodule. Cells have hyperchromatic irregular nuclei and are widely scattered in a hyalinized stroma.

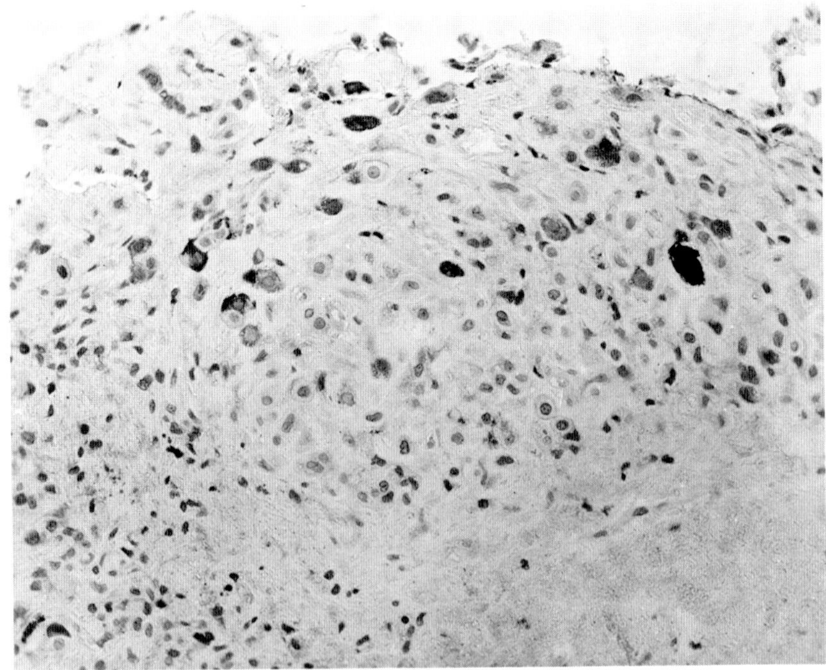

Fig. 9-39. Placental site nodule. Scattered cells stain positively for human placental lactogen (immunohistochemical preparation).

multiple (Fig. 9-30), almost always well-circumscribed (Figs. 9-30 and 9-32), oval or rounded nodules, sometimes with lobulated margins. Less commonly they form elongated structures parallel to the surface of the endometrium (Fig. 9-33). The lesion may be on the surface of the endometrium, within it, within the adjacent myometrium, or in superficial endocervical tissue. They are typically densely eosinophilic with hyalinized material surrounding single cells, small irregular clusters of cells (Fig. 9-35), or rounded nests of cells (Fig. 9-34). Sometimes the hyalinization is most pronounced centrally and is surrounded by a cellular zone. Foci of necrosis are present in almost one-half of the cases. In about 10 percent of the cases, the nodules undergo focal cystic degeneration.[129] Although typically essentially well circumscribed, small rounded pseudopods often project from the periphery of the nodules (Fig. 9-35). The pseudopods are often associated with brightly eosinophilic fibrinlike material that is sometimes suggestive of keratin and the impression of a squamous lesion may result (Fig. 9-37). The lesions are occasionally associated with evidence of a remote pregnancy in the form of necrotic or hyalinized chorionic villi. Immunohistochemical stains show that the cells stain for cytokeratin and for hPL, lesser numbers of cells usually staining for the latter (Fig. 9-39). Focal staining for hCG is occasionally seen.

The cells resemble IT cells that are degenerative in appearance with abundant amphophilic cytoplasm and one or more irregular, often lobulated nuclei. The nuclei vary from hyperchromatic (Fig. 9-38) to pale and vesicular. Mitotic figures are typically absent with rare ones present in only about 20 percent of the cases. The cells are generally haphazardly arranged singly, in clusters or cords (Fig. 9-35). Occasionally they are relatively evenly distributed throughout the lesion. In some cases, the cytoplasm is scanty, clear, or vacuolated. The vacuolated cytoplasm may contain rounded eosinophilic hyaline bodies of varying sizes (Fig. 9-36).

The distinction of a placental site nodule from a placental site trophoblastic tumor is generally easy in a hysterectomy specimen, because of the small size of the former, its circumscription, extensive hyalinization, and lack of mitotic figures (Table 9-6). This distinction is occasionally difficult, however, in a curettage specimen, because placental site trophoblastic tumors may contain areas that closely resemble the placental site nodule and occasionally have sharp instead of infiltrating borders. In these cases, the degenerative appearance of the cells and the lack or rarity of mitotic figures aid in making the correct diagnosis. It is important to distinguish between the two lesions because there is no evidence that placental site nodules and plaques have a malignant potential. In a recent series of 20 cases, uneventful follow-up of 1 to 7 years was obtained in 14 cases, including 5 in whom the only treatment was D&C.[129] The above features, and the absence of squamous differentiation, help distinguish placental site nodules and plaques from the rare hyalinizing squamous cell carcinoma of the cervix.[128] It should be remembered that placental site nodules may have nests

Table 9-6. Comparison of Pathologic Features of Placental Site Nodule/Plaque and Placental Trophoblastic Tumor

Placental Site Nodule/Plaque	Placental Site Trophoblastic Tumor
Usually a focal microscopic finding	Usually a gross or large microscopic mass
Circumscribed with occasional minimal infiltration	Almost always infiltrates myometrium
Nodular or plaquelike	Diffuse and ill defined
Typically hyalinized	Occasionally focally hyalinized
Mitotic figures absent or rare	Mitotic figures always present

that superficially resemble those of a squamous cell carcinoma (Fig. 9-37). In addition, we have seen one case in which a placental site nodule and placental site trophoblastic tumor were present in the same specimen. Placental site nodules have sometimes been misinterpreted as hyalinized decidua, but decidual cells have more basophilic cytoplasm than do IT and have more distinct cell membranes. In addition, the nuclei of decidual cells do not exhibit the pleomorphism and hyperchromasia of IT. Finally, decidual cells do not stain immunohistochemically for cytokeratin or human placental lactogen. The placental site nodule and plaque differs from an exaggerated placental site in its distinctive shapes, circumscription, extensive hyalinization, and lack of association with a current or recent pregnancy.

PLACENTAL SITE TROPHOBLASTIC TUMOR

Both Marchand[136] and Ewing[133] recognized that occasional trophoblastic disorders did not fit into the categories of hydatidiform mole, choriocarcinoma, or "syncytial endometritis." Marchand introduced the term *atypical chorioepithelioma* for what in retrospect appears, in some cases at least, to have been placental site trophoblastic tumor; Ewing[133] later subdivided the atypical chorioepithelioma into *syncytial endometritis* and *syncytioma*. The latter designation was applied to a process that resembled syncytial endometritis but had "more definite characteristics of a neoplasm." Other terms used for this lesion have included *atypical choriocarcinoma,*[137] and *trophoblastic pseudotumor.*[138] The latter designation was proposed because follow-up of 11 cases of this lesion disclosed no recurrences after hysterectomy or even curettage alone despite the frequent presence of blood vessel invasion and, in one case, direct spread outside the uterus. It

subsequently became clear, however, that occasional examples of this lesion metastasized and accordingly, in 1981 the term *placental site trophoblastic tumor* (PSTT) was proposed for it[130] and has met with relatively wide acceptance. PSTT should be separately classified from CCA because its morphologic features, biologic behavior, and response to chemotherapy differ markedly from those of CCA.

PSTT, as expected, typically occurs in women in the reproductive age group, with an average age of about 28 years,[140–142] but two lesions occurred in postmenopausal patients, one of whom was 5 years postmenopausal.[139, 143] The age of the patients has ranged from 19 to 53 years of age. Amenorrhea of up to 1 year's duration, menorrhagia, and metrorrhagia of varying duration are common presenting symptoms. In approximately 5 percent of cases, there is a history of a spontaneous abortion or a hydatidiform mole. A history of a hydatidiform mole is much less common, however, than in cases of CCA. Uterine enlargement is frequently evident on pelvic examination; when accompanied by amenorrhea and a positive pregnancy test, as found in approximately one-third of cases, it often suggests the erroneous diagnosis of a normal pregnancy. A diagnosis of missed abortion may be made when the uterus decreases in size under observation in association with vaginal bleeding. A rare patient has presented with spontaneous uterine perforation but, more often, perforation is a complication of uterine curettage. Two patients have presented with virilization and had ovarian stromal hyperthecosis which was considered to result from the elevated hCG levels in these cases.[144, 145] Another patient had erythrocytosis that disappeared after the tumor was removed,[146] as did hyperprolactinemia present in another case.[147] The serum levels of hCG are almost always lower than those in patients with choriocarcinoma, being normal in approximately 23 percent of cases, slightly elevated in 46 percent and moderately elevated in 31 percent.[128]

An unusual complication that has been reported in a few cases is the nephrotic syndrome.[143, 148, 149] In two cases that we studied, renal biopsies revealed a distinctive glomerular lesion (Fig. 9-40), characterized by the presence of conspicuous intracapillary deposits that contained abundant fibrinogen-related material as well as IgM.[148] In these two cases, there was laboratory evidence of disseminated intravascular coagulation and it seems likely that chronic intravascular coagulation resulting from factors released by the tumor had a major role in the pathogenesis of the renal lesion. Such a role is supported by the typical resolution of the renal disorder after hysterectomy.

The gross appearance of PSTT is variable. In most cases, examination of the uterus reveals a visible mass, although occasionally most of the lesion has been removed by curettage and no residual tumor is appreciable. The mass may be largely polypoid, sometimes filling the endometrial cavity, or predominantly infiltrative of the myometrium, which may be perforated. In several cases the tumor has invaded the cervix, and it has occasionally resulted in a polypoid endocervical mass. Most of the masses appear to be well circumscribed, but occasionally the border with the underlying myometrium is ill-defined or there is diffuse uterine enlargement without a discrete mass. Sectioning typically reveals tan, white, or yellow tissue, which is usually soft (Fig. 9-41); foci of hemorrhage may be present, but the diffuse hemorrhagic appearance of the typical choriocarcinoma is rare (Fig. 9-42). One tumor had a large central cyst.[149] Although the tumors are usually confined to the uterus, they may grow through the wall of the uterus to involve an ovary.[138, 147, 150]

Microscopic examination reveals an ill-defined mass of polyhedral, rounded, or occasionally spindle-shaped cells, most of which are mononucleate but some of which are binucleate or multinucleate (Figs. 9-43 to 9-45). The multinucleate cells occasionally have the features of syncytiotro-

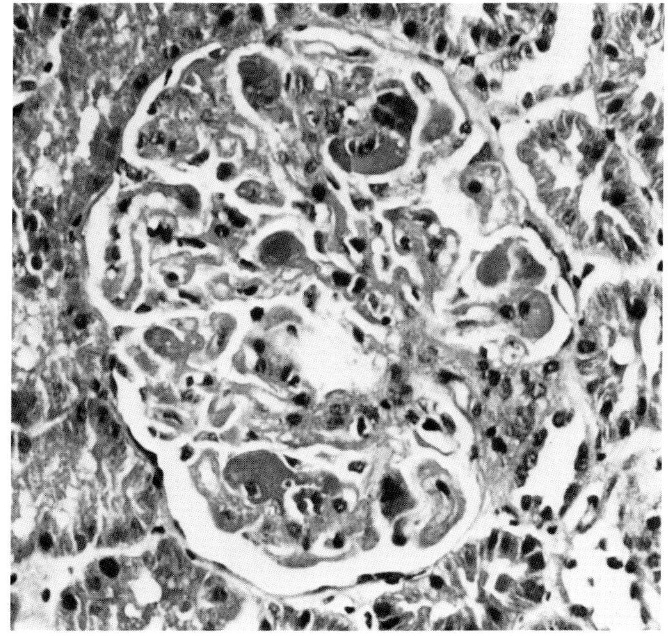

Fig. 9-40. Renal glomerulus in patient with placental site trophoblastic tumor. Glomerular capillary loops contain dense material that was eosinophilic.

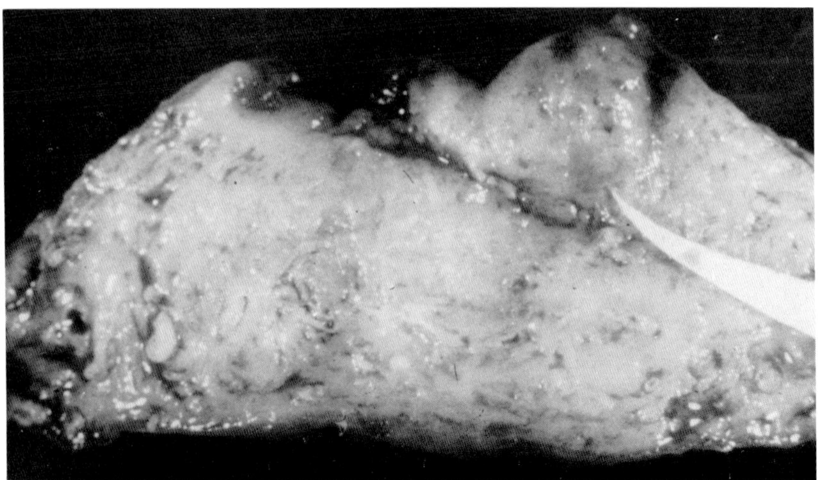

Fig. 9-41. Placental site trophoblastic tumor. The tumor (arrow) was tan, merging imperceptibly with the subjacent myometrium.

phoblast cells (Fig. 9-46) but typically do not. The cytoplasm is typically abundant and amphophilic, but it may be eosinophilic or rarely clear. The nuclei may vary considerably in size, shape and staining properties; some are small, round and pale, whereas others are large, convoluted, and hyperchromatic or smudgy. Nucleoli are usually visible and may be prominent. Intranuclear cytoplasmic pseudoinclusions may be seen. The mitotic count averages approximately two per 10 high-power fields (HPF) and only occasionally exceeds five; abnormal mitotic figures are not uncommon (Fig. 9-45). The mass may be infiltrated with chronic inflammatory cells, but the latter are rarely, if ever, conspicuous. The neoplasm characteristically infiltrates the myometrium in the form of single cells or cellular aggregates dissecting between individual muscle fibers and bundles of fibers (Fig. 9-43), but an occasional tumor invades with a pushing border and has the hyalinization more characteristic of a placental

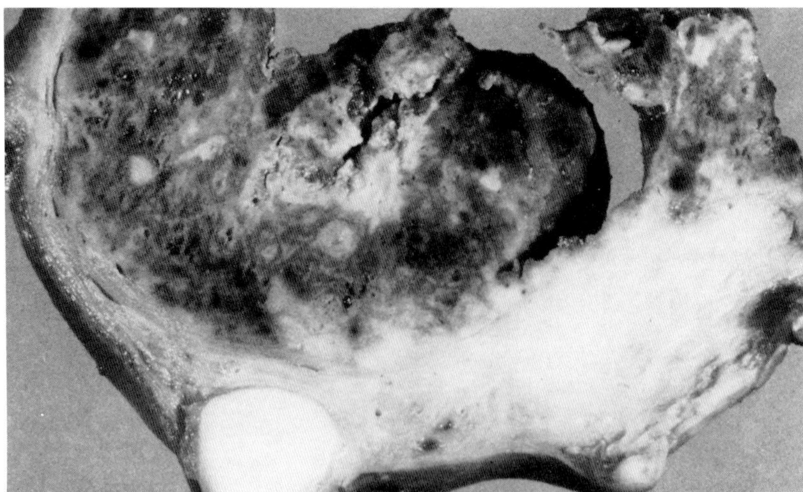

Fig. 9-42. Placental site trophoblastic tumor. The tumor was unusual because of extensive hemorrhage.

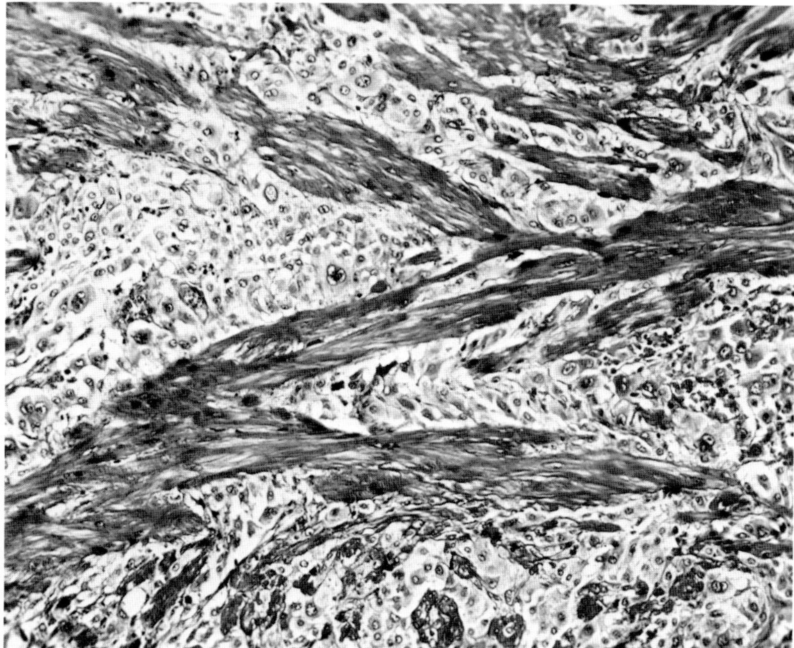

Fig. 9-43. Placental site trophoblastic tumor. Tumor cells infiltrate the muscle fibers of the myometrium. (From Young and Scully,[140] with permission.)

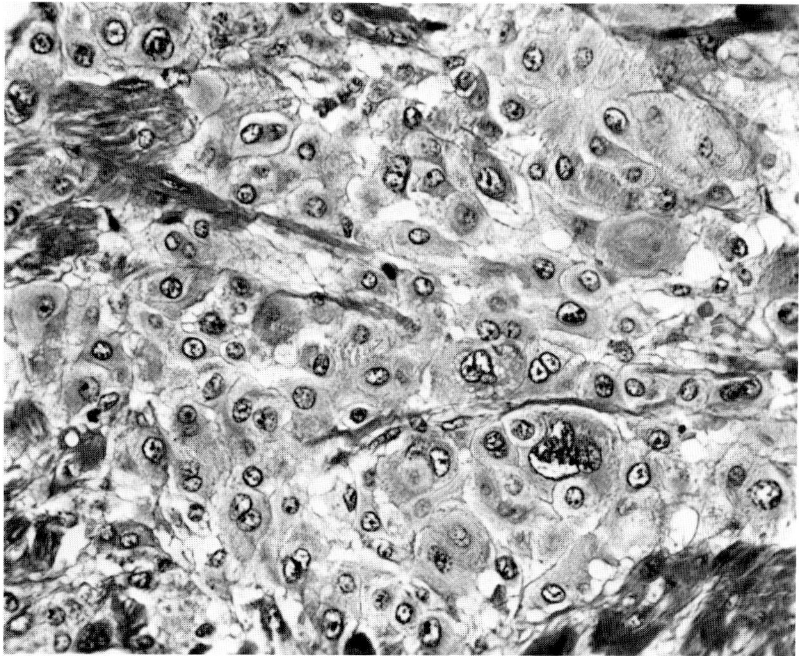

Fig. 9-44. Placental site trophoblastic tumor. Tumor cells have abundant cytoplasm and well-defined cytoplasmic membranes. The nuclei are predominantly mononucleate, but a few are multinucleate. (From Young and Scully,[140] with permission.)

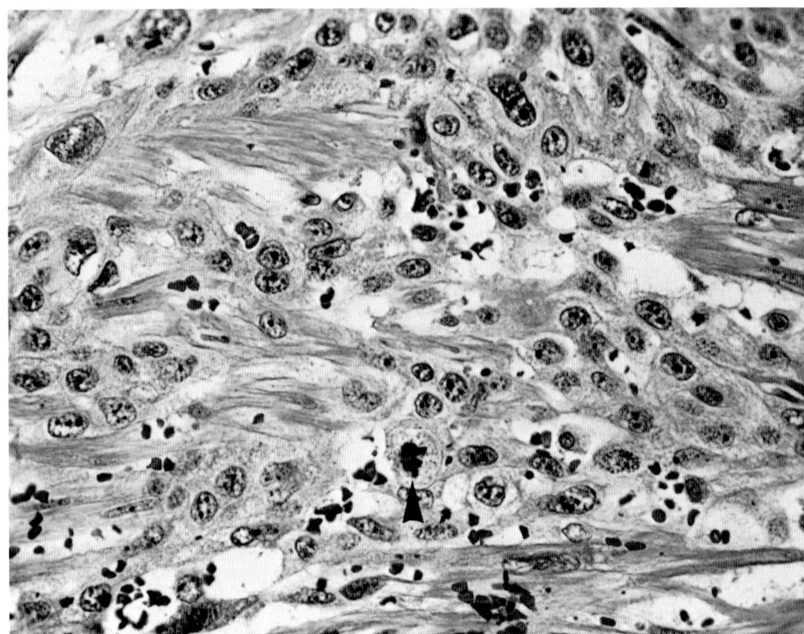

Fig. 9-45. Placental site trophoblastic tumor, which was clinically malignant. Note the mitotic figure (arrow).

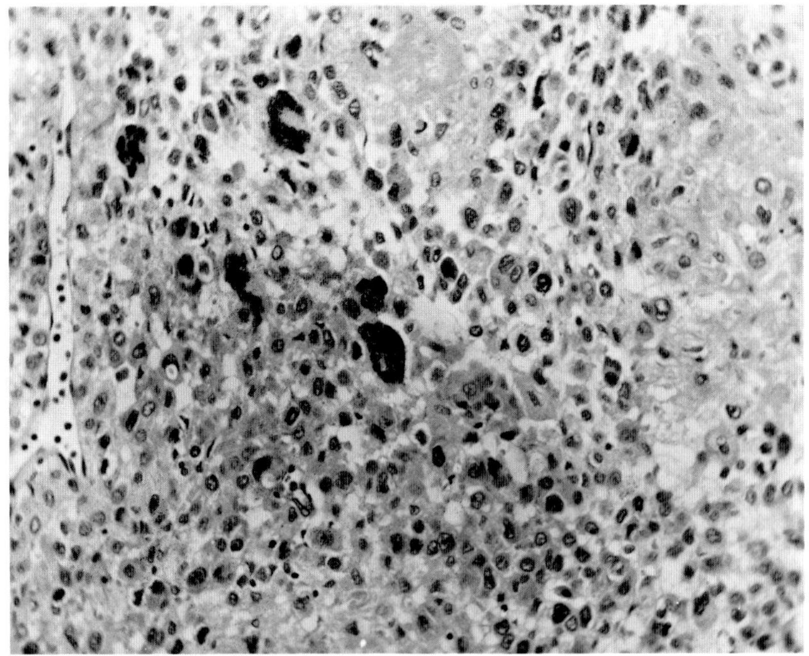

Fig. 9-46. Placental site trophoblastic tumor. The tumor contains scattered syncytiotrophoblast giant cells.

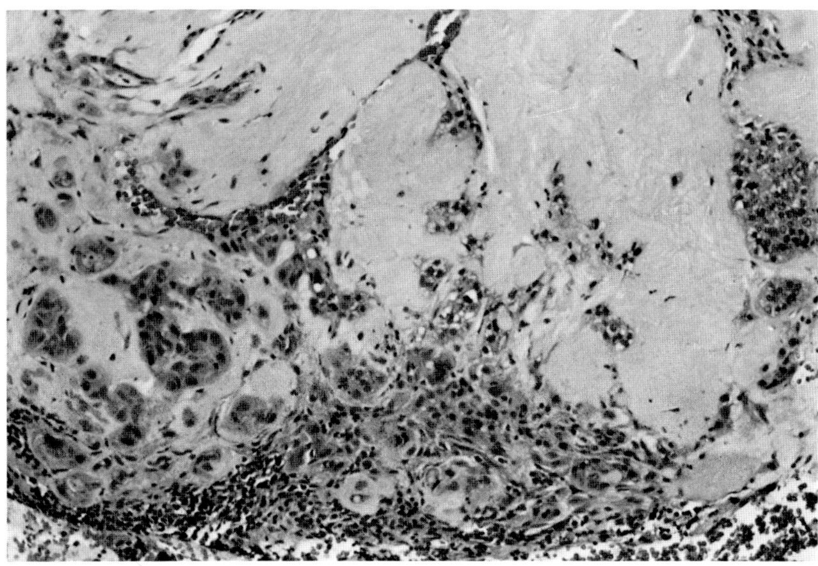

Fig. 9-47. Placental site trophoblastic tumor. The tumor is relatively well circumscribed (bottom) and is extensively hyalinized, two features that are more typical of placental site nodule.

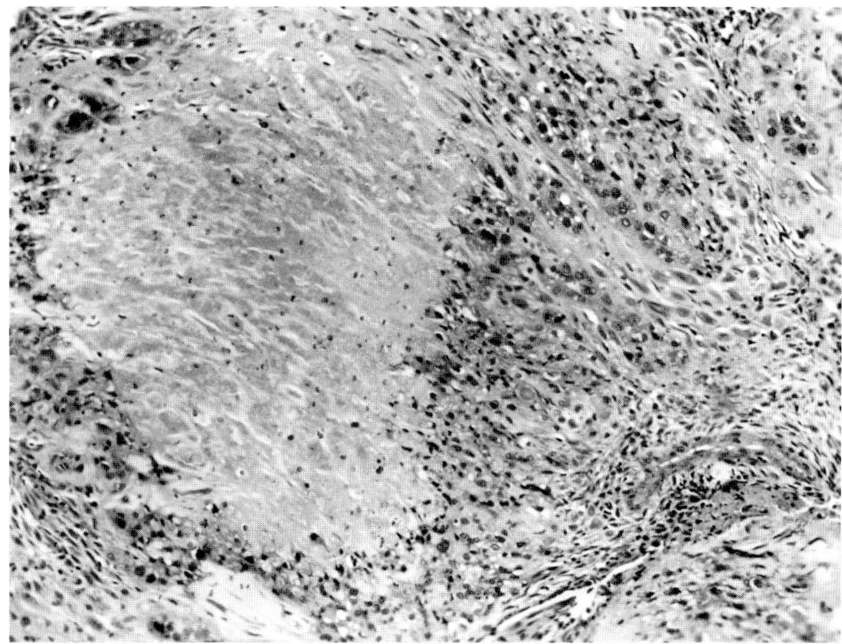

Fig. 9-48. Placental site trophoblastic tumor with focal necrosis.

site nodule (Fig. 9-47). The tumors may exhibit foci of necrosis (Fig. 9-48), but this is usually not conspicuous. The muscle fibers may exhibit degenerative changes. The tumor cells invade the uterine wall to the serosa in approximately one-third of the cases, occasionally extending to the endocervix. They are frequently seen in clumps within the lumens of blood vessels or may replace their walls. Commonly, the vessel walls are partly or completely replaced by fibrin, and the tumor cells line the lumen of the vessel (Fig. 9-49). The patterns of myometrial and vascular invasion closely simulate those of the physiologic infiltration of IT at the placental site. In occasional cases, fibrinlike material is diffusely distributed throughout large areas of the tumor (Fig. 9-50). In some cases foci of fibrin associated with small clusters of cells may superficially suggest squamous cells with keratin (Fig. 9-51), particularly when they are present at the edge of the tumor. The endometrium adjacent to a PSTT may be the site of a decidual reaction, the Arias-Stella phenomenon, or both.

PSTT displays a characteristic immunostaining pattern for hCG, hPL, and cytokeratin, which may may be helpful in distinguishing this lesion from choriocarcinoma and certain nontrophoblastic tumors with which it may be confused. In most cases of PSTT, staining for both cytokeratin and hPL is diffuse (Fig. 9-52), but hCG is present only focally.[151] The light microscopic and immunohistochemical similarities between the cells of the PSTT and the IT cells of the normal placental site indicate that the former are the neoplastic counterpart of the latter.

On ultrastructural examination, the cells of PSTTs are usually attached to one another by well-formed desmosomes and typically have electron-dense cytoplasm that contains moderate numbers of mitochondria, dilated rough endoplasmic reticulum, scattered single strands of rough endoplasmic reticulum, and free ribosomes.[150, 152–158]

Some cells contain vesicles of smooth endoplasmic reticulum, Golgi complexes, and pools of glycogen. The free surfaces of the cells have microvilli that are less numerous and more blunt than those of ST cells. In most reported cases, the cells have contained large bundles of paranuclear intermediate filaments. Ploidy studies have shown a triploid peak in one case[159] and a diploid peak in three others.[142, 143]

PSTT must be distinguished from an exaggerated placental site, a placental site nodule, decidua, and other trophoblastic and nontrophoblastic tumors. Differentiation from an exaggerated placental site has already been discussed. PSTT lacks the characteristic, usually orderly, admixture of cytotrophoblast and syncytiotrophoblast seen in the typical CCA. Also, the former usually invades the myometrium by splitting muscle bundles and fibers, whereas the latter forms a hemorrhagic mass that invades and destroys the myometrium in a massive fashion. The distinctive pattern of vascular invasion of a PSTT is also not a feature of CCA, nor is the fibrinoid material present in vascular walls and occasionally throughout the tumor. Hemorrhage is usually much more extensive in a choriocarcinoma than in a PSTT. Immunocytochemical staining for hCG and hPL is also helpful in this differential diagnosis. In contrast to the staining of the PSTT, hPL has a focal distribution, and hCG a diffuse pattern of staining in a choriocarcinoma. In several of the malignant PSTTs we have studied, however, the staining pattern was atypical, resembling that of CCA. Experience with poorly differentiated PSTTs has been too limited to conclude that all of them will be readily distinguishable from the occasional choriocarcinomas that lack the usual orderly biphasic pattern; indeed, some of the multinucleate cells within PSTTs are indistinguishable from ST cells. It is possible that intermediate forms exist between PSTT and CCA. As, in our experience, some CCA have areas that resemble PSTT,

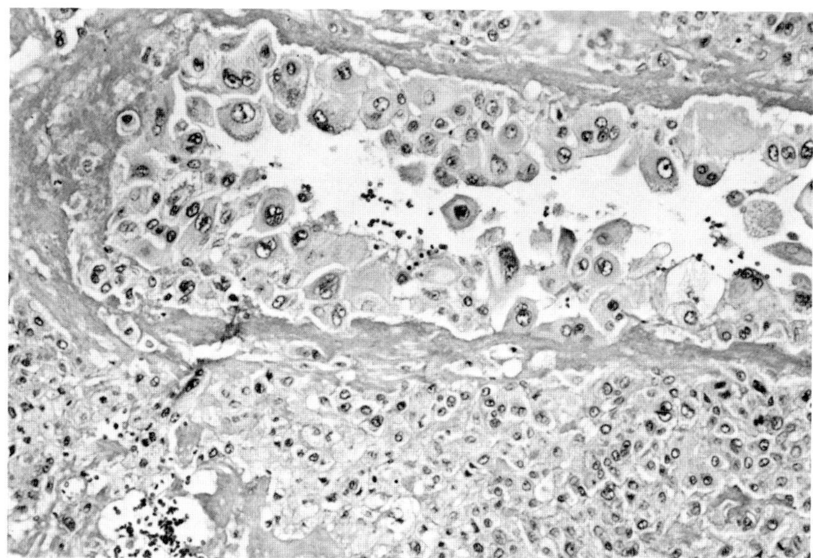

Fig. 9-49. Placental site trophoblastic tumor. Tumor cells line the intima of a blood vessel. The wall of the blood vessel has been transformed into a mesh of fibrin. (From Young et al.,[148] with permission.)

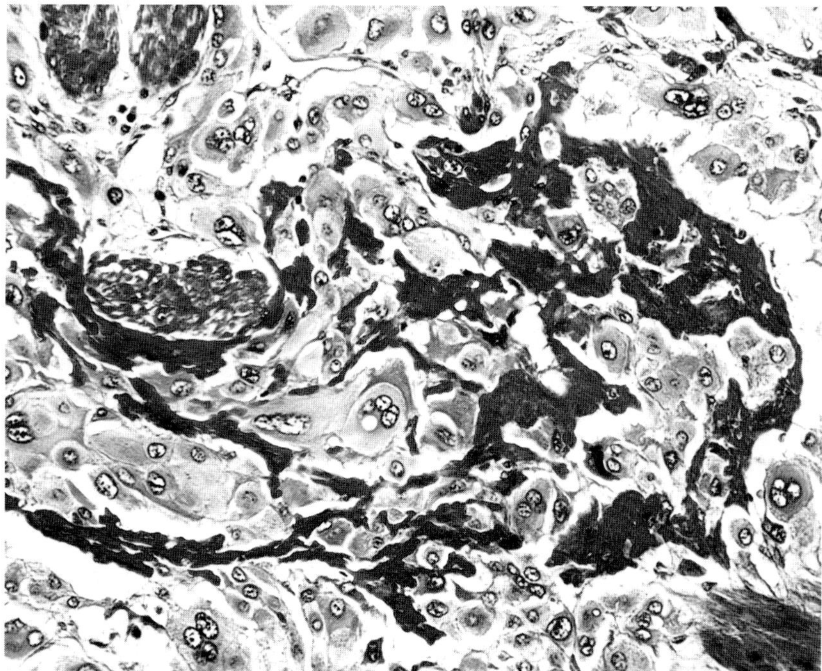

Fig. 9-50. Placental site trophoblastic tumor. Prominent dark-staining material represents fibrin that was conspicuous within this neoplasm from a patient with the nephrotic syndrome. (From Young et al.,[148] with permission.)

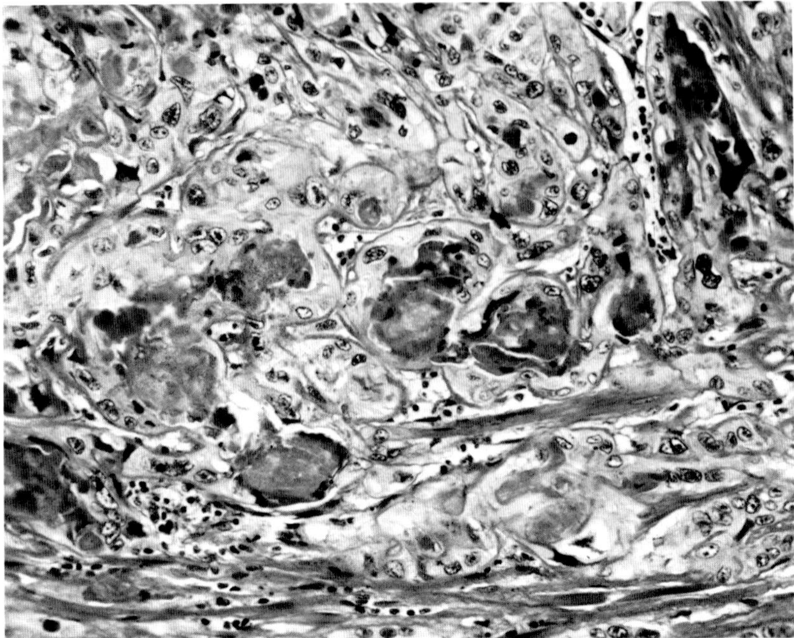

Fig. 9-51. Placental site trophoblastic tumor. Several small relatively well-delineated foci of dark-staining material, representing fibrin, associated with clusters of tumor cells, impart a superficial resemblance to clusters of squamous cells with keratinization.

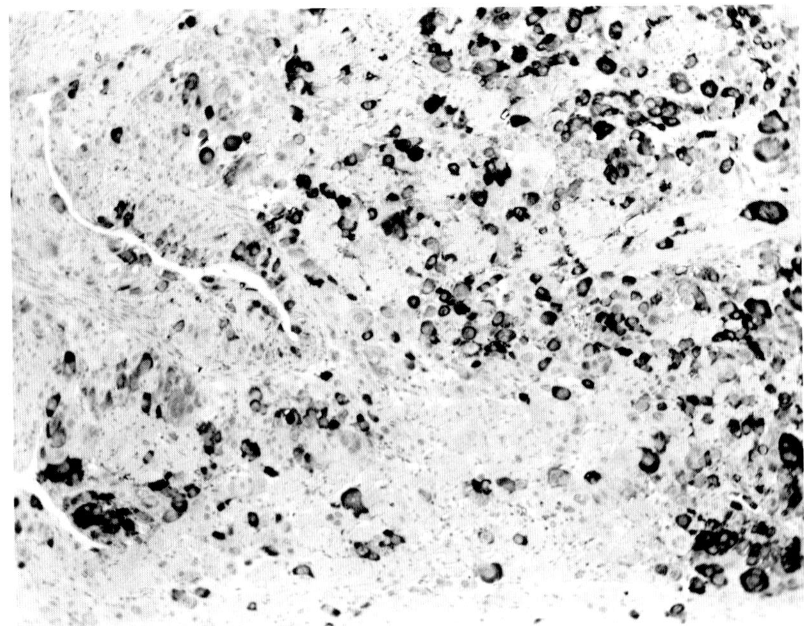

Fig. 9-52. Placental site trophoblastic tumor. Most tumor cells stain positively for human placental lactogen (immunohistochemical preparation).

sampling obviously may limit the confident distinction between these two neoplasms. For this reason, the definite diagnosis of PSTT probably should not be made until a hysterectomy specimen has been thoroughly examined. One reported case of "PSTT" is suspect for this reason, particularly as the serum hCG level was unusually high.[160] Another case of "PSTT" probably best fits in the category of CCA.[161]

PSTTs may also be confused with sarcomas, particularly epithelioid leiomyosarcomas, which are also composed of cells that often have copious dense cytoplasm. However, the clinical setting, associated symptoms and pattern of growth of the PSTT usually differ from those of a leiomyosarcoma. Immunohistochemical staining may be helpful in problem cases because smooth muscle tumors are negative for hCG and hPL.

Uterine carcinomas, particularly a rare form of squamous cell carcinoma of the cervix characterized by necrosis and hyalinization, of which we have seen several examples, may resemble a PSTT, particularly in a biopsy specimen.[128] The hyaline areas in these cases may suggest the fibrinoid material of a PSTT. The additional presence of more typical foci of invasive squamous cell carcinoma or adjacent carcinoma in situ and keratinization should be searched for in an attempt to resolve this problem in differential diagnosis. It should be remembered that the reverse mistake, the simulation of a squamous cell carcinoma by a PSTT may occur (Fig. 9-51). Areas within a PSTT in which the cells have clear cytoplasm may also resemble a clear cell carcinoma, but the latter diagnosis is rarely a serious consideration. The clinical and laboratory features in cases of PSTT, including the young age of the patient, a history of amenorrhea, occasionally following an abortion or a hydatidiform mole, and a sometimes elevated hCG level differ from those of most patients with a uterine carcinoma. More specifically, the microscopic features of the PSTT, including its characteristic mode of spread in the myometrium, its distinctive manner of vascular invasion, as well as associated changes in the adjacent endometrium suggestive of a high progesterone level should permit differentiation from nontrophoblastic tumors. Immunohistochemical staining for hCG and hPL is of great value in the exceptional case in which differentiation from nontrophoblastic lesions cannot be accomplished with routine staining methods. Poorly differentiated carcinomas are only rarely positive for hPL and hCG.

Approximately 60 PSTTs have now been reported.[134, 138, 139, 141–150, 152–171] Two patients died as a result of uterine perforation.[138, 141] In 15 to 20 percent of the remainder, the tumor has behaved in a malignant fashion with metastases. The tumors that have spread have usually had mitotic counts of 4 or more per 10 HPF. By contrast, to the best of our knowledge, only one tumor with a benign follow-up of 1 year or longer has had more than 5 MF/10 HPF.[142] One malignant tumor with only 2 MF/10 HPF metastasized to the lungs 5 years after hysterectomy,[170] and another exhibited lymph node metastases 18 months after hysterectomy,[141] establishing the metastatic potential of tumors with low mitotic counts and the necessity for long-term follow-up of all patients with this tumor. Spread to the lungs has been quite common when the tumors metastasize (Fig. 9-53); involvement of the liver and central nervous system is also relatively common. It should be emphasized that a curettage specimen of a PSTT may not be representative of the entire tumor, as there has been considerable variation in the mitotic count and occasionally in other cytologic features from one area to another. Additional differences between some of the fatal tumors and those that have been clinically benign include a greater extent of necrosis and the

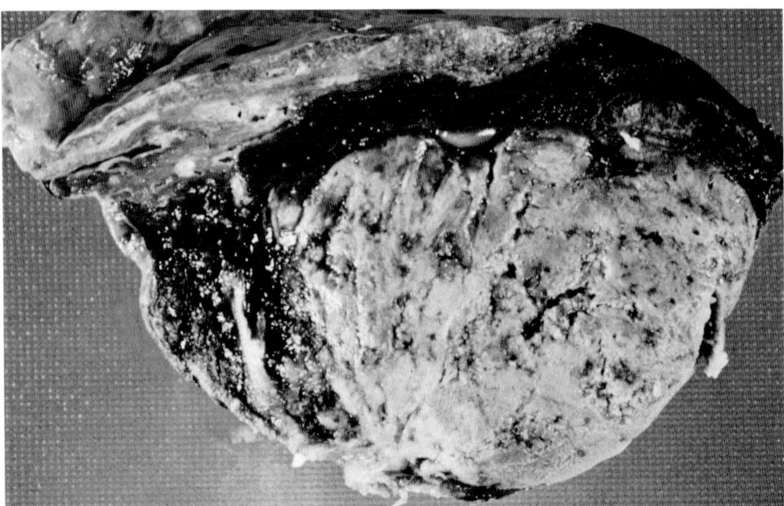

Fig. 9-53. Placental site trophoblastic tumor metastatic to lung.

presence of many cells with clear rather than amphophilic cytoplasm in the former. From the clinical viewpoint, Lathrop et al.[142] concluded from their review that patients with a good prognosis were younger and had had fewer pregnancies than did those with tumors that metastasized.

A hysterectomy is the optimal initial therapy of a PSTT. The uneventful outcome in occasional cases in which curettage was the only therapeutic procedure indicates that the tumor may regress if incompletely excised and that conservative therapy may be considered if the tumor does not have microscopic features indicating a significant risk of malignant behavior, and if the patient has a strong desire for childbearing, is aware of the risk involved, and can be followed adequately. Careful monitoring of the levels of hCG, hPL, and possibly other trophoblastic tumor markers as well as radiologic investigations for lymphatic and hematogenous tumor spread are indicated after hysterectomy to detect recurrence at an early stage. Additional D&Cs as well as monitoring of tumor markers are indicated when conservative management is chosen. It must be reempha-

sized, however, that the hCG levels may be low and are not helpful as they are in monitoring the course of choriocarcinoma. The tendency for the uterus to rupture easily should be borne in mind when a D&C is being performed. Various combinations of chemotherapeutic agents have typically not been curative in the few cases in which they have been used for residual or metastatic disease, in contrast to the effectiveness of chemotherapy in the treatment of choriocarcinoma. McLellan et al.[139] reported the case of a patient with lung metastases that did not respond to therapy with VP-16, actinomycin D, and methotrexate. However, after a change to cisplatin and cyclophosphamide, there was a complete resolution of disease and the patient was free of disease 16 months after the completion of chemotherapy. There was significant regression of pulmonary metastases in another patient who received etoposide, methotrexate, and actinomycin D alternating weekly with cyclophosphamide and vincristine.[147] Radiation therapy has been beneficial in controlling disease in one patient with lymph node metastases and paravaginal recurrence.[141]

REFERENCES

1. Wislocki GB, Bennett HS: The histology and cytology of the human and monkey placenta with special reference to the trophoblast. Am J Anat 73:335, 1943
2. Wislocki GB: The histology and cytochemistry of the basal plate and septae placentae of the normal human placenta delivered at full term, abstracted. Anat Rec 109:359, 1951
3. Wislocki GB: Succinic dehydrogenase, esterases and protein-linked sulfhydryl groups in human placenta. Anat Rec 115:380, 1953
4. Dallenbach-Hellweg G, Nette G: Morphological and histochemical observations on trophoblast and decidua of the basal plate of the human placenta at term. Am J Anat 115:309, 1964
5. Latta JS, Beber CR: The differentiation of a special form of trophoblast in the human placenta. Am J Obstet Gynecol 74:105, 1957
6. Terzakis JA: The ultrastructure of normal human first trimester placenta. J Ultrastruct Res 9:268, 1963
7. Tighe JR, Garrod PR, Curran RC: The trophoblast of the human chorionic villus. J Pathol 93:559, 1967
8. Wynn RM: Cytotrophoblastic specializations: an ultrastructural study of the human placenta. Am J Obstet Gynecol 114:339, 1972
9. Kurman RJ, Main CS, Chen HC: Intermediate trophoblast—a distinctive form of trophoblast with specific morphological, biochemical and functional features. Placenta 5:349, 1984
10. Kajii T, Ohama K: Androgenetic origin of hydatidiform mole. Nature 268:633, 1977
11. Szulman AE, Surti U: The syndromes of hydatidiform mole. I. Cytogenetic and morphologic correlations. Am J Obstet Gynecol 131:665, 1978
12. Vassilakos P, Riotton G, Kajii T: Hydatidiform mole: two entities: a morphologic and cytogenetic study with some clinical considerations. Am J Obstet Gynecol 127:167, 1977
13. Ohama K, Ueda K, Okamoto E et al: Cyto-genetic and clinicopathologic studies of partial moles. Obstet Gynecol 68:259, 1986
14. Jacobs PS, Szulman AE, Funkhouser J et al: Human triploidy: relationship between parental origin of the additional haploid complement and development of partial hydatidiform mole. Ann Hum Genet 46:223, 1982
15. Vejerslev LO, Dissing J, Hansen HE et al: Hydatidiform mole: genetic origin in polypoid conceptuses. Hum Genet 76:11, 1987
16. Jacobs PA, Hunt PA, Matsuura JS et al: Complete and partial hydatidiform mole in Hawaii: cytogenetics, morphology and epidemiology. Br J Obstet Gynaecol 89:258, 1982
17. Szulman AE, Surti U: The syndromes of hydatidiform mole. II. Morphologic evolution of the complete and partial mole. Am J Obstet Gynecol 132:20, 1978
18. Czernobilsky B, Barash A, Lancet M: Partial moles: a clinicopathologic study of 25 cases. Obstet Gynecol 59:75, 1982
19. Berkowitz RS, Goldstein DP: Diagnosis and management of primary hydatidiform mole. Obstet Gynecol Clin 15:491, 1988
20. Surani MAH, Barton SC, Norris ML: Nuclear transplantation in the mouse: heritable differences between parental genomes after activation of embryonic genome. Cell 45:127, 1986
21. McGrath J, Solter D: Completion of mouse embryogenesis requires both the maternal and paternal genomes. Cell 37:179, 1984
22. Azuma C, Saji F, Tokugawa Y et al: Application of gene amplification by polymerase chain reaction to genetic analysis of molar mitochondrial DNA: the detection of anuclear empty ovum as the cause of complete mole. Gynecol Oncol 40:29, 1991
23. Ko TM, Hsieh CY, Ho HN et al: Restriction fragment length polymorphism analysis to study the genetic origin of complete hydatidiform mole. Am J Obstet Gynecol 164:901, 1991
24. Saji F, Tokugawa Y, Kimura T et al: A new approach using DNA fingerprinting for the determination of androgenesis as a cause of hydatidiform mole. Placenta 10:399, 1989
25. Fukuyama R, Takata M, Kudoh J et al:

DNA diagnosis of hydatidiform mole using the polymerase chain reaction. Hum Genet 87:216, 1991

26. Lage JM, Driscoll SG, Yavner DL et al: Hydatidiform moles: application of flow cytometry in diagnosis. Am J Clin Pathol 89:596, 1988

27. Fisher RA, Lawler SD, Ormerod MG et al: Flow cytometry used to distinguish between complete and partial hydatidiform moles. Placenta 8:249, 1987

28. Hemming JK, Quirke P, Womack C et al: Diagnosis of molar pregnancy and persistent trophoblastic disease by flow cytometry. J Clin Pathol 40:615, 1987

29. Lage JM, Weinberg DS, Yavner DL, Bieber FR: The biology of tetraploid hydatidiform moles: histopathology, cytogenetics and flow cytometry. Hum Pathol 20:419, 1989

30. Lage JM, Mark SD, Roberts DJ et al: A flow cytometric study of 137 fresh hydropic placentas: correlation between types of hydatidiform moles and nuclear DNA ploidy. Obstet Gynecol 79:403, 1992

31. Yen S, MacMahon B: Epidemiologic features of trophoblastic disease. Am J Obstet Gynecol 101:126, 1968

32. Matalon M, Modan B: Epidemiologic aspects of hydatidiform mole in Israel. Am J Obstet Gynecol 112:107, 1972

33. Poen HT, Djojopranoto M: The possible etiologic factors of hydatidiform mole and choriocarcinoma. Am J Obstet Gynecol 92:510, 1965

34. Parazzini F, Mangili G, La Vecchia C et al: Risk factors for gestational trophoblastic disease: a separate analysis of complete and partial hydatidiform moles. Obstet Gynecol 78:1039, 1991

35. Berkowitz RS, Goldstein DP, Bernstein MR: Natural history of partial molar pregnancy. Obstet Gynecol 66:667, 1983

36. Berkowitz RS, Goldstein DP, DuBeshter B, Bernstein MR: Management of complete molar pregnancy. J Reprod Med 32:634, 1987

37. Szulman AE, Surti U: The clinicopathologic profile of the partial hydatidiform mole. Obstet Gynecol 59:597, 1982

38. Fine C, Bundy AL, Berkowitz RS et al: Sonographic diagnosis of partial hydatidiform mole. Obstet Gynecol 73:414, 1989

39. Reid MH, McGahan JP, Oi R: Sonographic evaluation of hydatidiform mole and its look-alikes. AJR 140:307, 1983

40. Woodward RM, Filly RA, Callen PW: First trimester molar pregnancy. Nonspecific ultrasonographic appearance. Obstet Gynecol 55:31S, 1980

41. Munyer TP, Callen PW, Filly RA et al: Further observations on the sonographic spectrum of gestational trophoblastic disease. J Clin Ultrasound 9:349, 1981

42. Romero R, Horgan JG, Kohorn EI et al: New criteria for the diagnosis of gestational trophoblastic disease. Obstet Gynecol 66:553, 1985

43. Lage JM: Diagnostic dilemmas in gynecologic pathology. Semin Diagn Pathol 7:146, 1990

44. Habibian R, Surti U: Cytogenetics of trophoblasts from complete hydatidiform moles. Cancer Genet Cytogenet 29:271, 1987

45. Berrebi A, Mercier B, Sarramon MR et al: Un nouveau cas de mole hydatidiforme survenant dans l'un des oeufs d'une grossese gemellaire. Rev Fr Gynecol Obstet 83:439, 1988

46. Hertig AT, Sheldon WH: Hydatidiform mole: a pathologico-clinical correlation of 200 cases. Am J Obstet Gynecol 53:1, 1947

47. Hertig AT, Mansell H: Tumors of the female sex organs. Part 1. Hydatidiform mole and choriocarcinoma. p. 7. In Atlas of Tumor Pathology. Sect. 9, fasc. 33. Armed Forces Institute of Pathology, Washington DC, 1956

48. Elston CW, Bagshawe KD: The value of histological grading in the management of hydatidiform mole. J Obstet Gynaecol Br Commonw 79:717, 1972

49. Genest DG, Laborde O, Berkowitz RS et al: A clinicopathologic study of 153 cases of complete hydatidiform mole (1980–1990): histologic grade lacks prognostic significance. Obstet Gynecol 78:402, 1991

50. Rice LW, Genest DR, Berkowitz RS et al: Pathologic features of sharp curettings in complete hydatidiform mole. Predictors of persistent gestational trophoblastic disease. J Reprod Med 36:17, 1991

51. Lawler SD, Fisher RA, Dent J: A prospective genetic study of complete and partial hydatidiform moles. Am J Obstet Gynecol 164:1270, 1991

52. Martin DA, Sutton GP, Ulbright TM et al: DNA content as a prognostic index in gestational trophoblastic neoplasia. Gynecol Oncol 34:383, 1989

53. Vejerslev LO, Fisher RA, Surti U, Walke N: Hydatidiform mole: cytogenetically unusual cases and their implications for the present classification. Am J Obstet Gynecol 157:180, 1987

54. Muto MG, Lage JM, Berkowitz RS et al: Gestational trophoblastic disease of the fallopian tube. J Reprod Med 36:57, 1991

55. Govender NS, Goldstein DP: Metastatic tubal mole and coexisting intrauterine pregnancy. Obstet Gynecol 49:67s, 1977

56. Ober WB: Pathology of trophoblastic diseases. Hum Reprod 2:143, 1987

57. Wake N, Fujino T, Hoshi S et al: The propensity to malignancy of dispermic heterozygous moles. Placenta 8:319, 1987

58. Hemming JD, Quirke P, Womack C et al: Flow cytometry in persistent trophoblastic disease. Placenta 9:615, 1988

59. Berkowitz RS, Goldstein DP: Management of molar pregnancy and gestational trophoblastic tumors. p. 425. In Knapp RC, Berkowitz RS (eds): Gynecologic Oncology. New York, Macmillan, 1986

60. Curry SL, Hammond CV, Tyrey L et al: Hydatidiform mole: Diagnosis, management, and long-term follow-up of 347 patients. Obstet Gynecol 45:1, 1975

61. Lurain JR, Brewer JI, Torok EE et al: Natural history of hydatidiform mole after primary evacuation. Am J Obstet Gynecol 145:591, 1983

62. Hatch KD, Shingleton HM, Austin JM et al: Southern Regional Trophoblastic Disease Center, 1972–1977. South Med J 71:1334, 1978

63. Morrow CP: Postmolar trophoblastic disease: diagnosis, management and prognosis. Clin Obstet Gynecol 27:211, 1984

64. Wong LC, Ma HK: The syndrome of partial mole. Arch Gynecol 234:161, 1984

65. Bagshawe KD, Lawler SD, Paradinas FJ et al: Gestational trophoblastic tumours following initial diagnosis of partial hydatidiform mole. Lancet 335:1074, 1990

66. Kim DS, Moon H, Kim KT et al: Effects of prophylactic chemotherapy for persistent trophoblastic disease in patients with complete hydatidiform mole. Obstet Gynecol 67:690, 1986

67. Newlands ES, Bagshawe KD, Begent RHJ et al: Results with the EMA/CO (etoposide, methotrexate, actinomycin D, cyclophosphamide, vincristine) regimen in high risk gestational trophoblastic tumours, 1979–1989. Br J Obstet Gynaecol 98:550, 1991

68. Ober WB, Edgcomb JH, Price EB Jr: The pathology of choriocarcinoma. Ann NY Acad Sci 172:299, 1971

69. Sand PK, Lurain JR, Brewer JI: Repeat gestational trophoblastic disease. Obstet Gynecol 63:140, 1984

70. Mutch DG, Soper JT, Babcock CJ et al: Recurrent gestational trophoblastic disease. Cancer 66:978, 1990

71. Wertelecki W, Graham JM, Sergovich FR: The clinical syndrome of triploidy. Obstet Gynecol 47:69, 1976

72. Doshi N, Surti U, Szulman AE: Morphologic anomalies in triploid liveborn fetuses. Hum Pathol 14:716, 1983

73. Surti U, Szulman AE, Wagner K et al: Tetraploid partial hydatidiform moles: two cases with a triple paternal contribution and a 92, XXXY karyotype. Hum Genet 72:15, 1986

74. Vejerslev LO, Sunde L, Hansen BF et al: Hydatidiform mole and fetus with normal karyotype: support of a separate entity. Obstet Gynecol 77:868, 1991

75. Teng NNH, Ballon SC: Partial hydatidiform mole with diploid karyotype: report of 3 cases. Am J Obstet Gynecol 150:961, 1984

76. Crooij MJ, van der Harten JJ, Puyenbroek JI et al: A partial hydatidiform mole, dispersed throughout the placenta, coexisting with a normal living fetus. Br J Obstet Gynecol 92:104, 1985

77. Pool R, Lebethe SJ, Lancaster EJ: Partial hydatidiform mole with a coexistent live full-term fetus: a case report. S Afr Med J 75:186, 1989

78. Davis JR, Kerrigan DP, Way DL et al: Par-

tial hydatidiform moles: deoxyribonucleic acid content and course. Am J Obstet Gynecol 157:969, 1987

79. Lage JM: Placentomegaly with massive hydrops of placental stem villi, diploid DNA content, and fetal omphaloceles: possible association with Beckwith-Wiedemann syndrome. Hum Pathol 22:591, 1991

80. Feinberg RF, Lockwood CJ, Salafia C et al: Sonographic diagnosis of a pregnancy with diffuse hydatidiform mole and coexistent 46,XX fetus: a case report. Obstet Gynecol 72:485, 1988

81. Rice LW, Berkowitz RS, Lage JM et al: Persistent gestational trophoblastic tumor after partial hydatidiform mole. Gynecol Oncol 36:358, 1990

82. Lawler SD, Fisher RA, Pickthall VJ et al: Genetic studies on hydatidiform moles. I. The origin of partial moles. Cancer Genet Cytogenet 5:309, 1982

83. Lage JM, Berkowitz RS, Rice LW ct al: Flow cytometric analysis of DNA content in partial hydatidiform moles with persistent gestational trophoblastic tumor. Obstet Gynecol 77:111, 1991

84. Gardner HAR, Lage JM: Choriocarcinoma following partial hydatidiform mole: a case report. Hum Pathol 23:468, 1992

85. Szulman AE, Philippe E, Boue JG, Boue A: Human triploidy: association with partial hydatidiform moles and nonmolar conceptuses. Hum Pathol 12:1016, 1981

86. Elston CW: The histopathology of trophoblastic tumours, suppl. 29. J Clin Pathol 10:111, 1976

87. Park WW, Lees JC: Choriocarcinoma: a general review with analysis of 516 cases. Arch Pathol 49:73, 205, 1950

88. Brewer JI, Mazur MT: Gestational choriocarcinoma. Its origin in the placenta during seemingly normal pregnancy. Am J Surg Pathol 5:267, 1981

89. Driscoll SG: Choriocarcinoma: an "incidental finding" within a term placenta. Obstet Gynecol 21:96, 1963

90. MacRae DJ: Chorionepithelioma occurring during pregnancy. J Obstet Gynaecol Br Commonw 58:373, 1951

91. Ollendorff DA, Goldberg JM, Abu-Jawdeh GM, Lurain JR: Markedly elevated maternal serum alpha-fetoprotein associated with a normal fetus and choriocarcinoma of the placenta. Obstet Gynecol 76:494, 1990

92. Brewer JI, Gerbie AB: Early development of choriocarcinoma. Am J Obstet Gynecol 94:692, 1966

93. Lage JM, Roberts DR: Choriocarcinoma in a term placenta. Pathologic diagnosis of tumor in an asymptomatic patient with metastatic disease. Int J Obstet Gynecol (in press)

94. Olive DL, Lurain JR, Brewer JI: Choriocarcinoma associated with term gestation. Am J Obstet Gynecol 148:711, 1984

95. Park WW: Choriocarcinoma: A Study of Its Pathology. Heinemann, London; WA Davis, Philadelphia.

96. Brinton LA, Bracken MB, Connelly RR: Choriocarcinoma incidence in the United States. Am J Epidemiol 123:1094, 1986

97. Bracken MB, Brinton LA, Hayashi K: Epidemiology of hydatidiform mole and choriocarcinoma. Epidemiol Rev 6:52, 1984

98. Grimes DA: Epidemiology of gestational trophoblastic disease. Am J Obstet Gynecol 150:309, 1984

99. Elston CW: Trophoblastic tumors of the placenta. p. 368. In Fox H (ed): Pathology of the Placenta. WB Saunders, Philadelphia, 1978

100. Marquez-Monter H, De La Vega GA, Ridaura C et al: Gestational choriocarcinoma in the general hospital of Mexico. Cancer 22:91, 1968

101. Brewer JI, Torok EE, Kahan BD et al: Gestational trophoblastic disease: origin of choriocarcinoma, invasive mole and choriocarcinoma associated with hydatidiform mole, and some immunologic aspects. Adv Cancer Res 27:89, 1978

102. Hallam LA, McLaren KM, El-Jabbour JN et al: Intraplacental choriocarcinoma: a case report. Placenta 11:247, 1990

103. Fox H, Laurini RN: Intraplacental choriocarcinoma: a report of two cases. J Clin Pathol 41:1085, 1988

104. Buckley JD, Henderson BE, Morrow CP et al: Case-control study of gestational choriocarcinoma. Cancer Res 48:1004, 1988

105. Chaganti RS, Koduru PR, Chakraborty R, Jones WB: Genetic origin of a trophoblas-

tic choriocarcinoma. Cancer Res 50:6330, 1990

106. Osada H, Kawata M, Yamada M et al: Genetic identification of pregnancies responsible for choriocarcinomas after multiple pregnancies by restriction fragment length polymorphism analysis. Am J Obstet Gynecol 165:682, 1991

107. Fisher RA, Lawler SD, Povey S, Bagshawe KD: Genetically homozygous choriocarcinoma following pregnancy with hydatidiform mole. Br J Cancer 58:788, 1988

108. Bagshawe DK: Risk and prognostic factors in trophoblastic neoplasia. Cancer 38:1373, 1976

109. Bagshawe DK, Rawlins GJ, Pike MC et al: ABO blood groups in trophoblastic neoplasia. Lancet 1:553, 1971

110. Dawood MY, Teoh ES, Ratnam SG: ABO blood group in patients with malignant trophoblastic disease. Gynecol Obstet Invest 20:23, 1985

111. Fischer HE, Lichtiger B, Cox I: Expression of RhO(D) antigen in choriocarcinoma of the uterus in an RhO(D)-negative patient: report of a case. Hum Pathol 16:1165, 1985

112. Davis JR, Surwit EA, Garay JP et al: Sex assignment in gestational trophoblastic neoplasia. Am J Obstet Gynecol 148:722, 1984

113. Berkowitz RS, Goldstein DP, Bernstein MR: Choriocarcinoma following term gestation. Gynecol Oncol 17:52, 1984

114. Fox MW, Harms RW, Davis DH: Selected neurologic complications of pregnancy. Mayo Clin Proc 65:1595, 1990

115. Hertig AT: Choriocarcinoma. p. 289. In Human Trophoblast. Charles C Thomas, Springfield, IL, 1968

116. Avril MF, Mathieu A, Kalifa C, Caillou C: Infantile choriocarcinoma with cutaneous tumors. J Am Acad Dermatol 14:918, 1986

117. Mazur MT, Kurman RJ: Choriocarcinoma and placental site trophoblastic tumor. p. 45. In Szulman AE, Buchsbaum HJ (eds): Gestational Trophoblastic Disease. Springer-Verlag, New York, 1987

118. Soper JT, Mutch DG, Chin N et al: Renal metastases of gestational trophoblastic disease: a report of eight cases. Obstet Gynecol 72:796, 1988

119. Baquero A, Foote J, Kottle S et al: Inadvertent transplantation of choriocarcinoma into four recipients. Transplant Proc 20:98, 1988

120. Mazur MT, Lurain JR, Brewer JI: Fatal gestational choriocarcinoma. Clinicopathologic study of patients treated at a trophoblastic disease center. Cancer 50:1833, 1982

121. Silva E, Tornos C, Lage J et al: Multiple nodules of intermediate trophoblast, an unusual complication of hydatidiform moles, abstracted. Lab Invest 66:68A, 1992

122. Mazur MT: Metastatic gestational choriocarcinoma. Unusual pathologic variant following therapy. Cancer 63:1370, 1989

123. Nishikawa Y, Kaseki S, Tomoda Y et al: Histopathologic classification of uterine choriocarcinoma. Cancer 55:1044, 1985

124. Lurain JR, Sand PK, Brewer JI: Choriocarcinoma associated with ectopic pregnancy. Obstet Gynecol 68:286, 1986

125. Elston CW, Bagshawe KD: The diagnosis of trophoblastic tumours from uterine curettings. J Clin Pathol 25:111, 1972

126. Parazzini F, LaVecchia C, Pampallona S et al: Reproductive patterns and the risk of gestational trophoblastic disease. Am J Obstet Gynecol 152:866, 1985

127. Jauniaux E, Zucker M, Meuris S et al: Chorangiocarcinoma: an unusual tumour of the placenta. The missing link? Placenta 9:607, 1988

128. Young RH, Kurman RJ, Scully RE: Proliferations and tumors of intermediate trophoblast of the placental site. Semin Diagn Pathol 5:223, 1988

129. Young RH, Kurman RJ, Scully RE: Placental site nodules and plaques. A clinicopathologic analysis of 20 cases. Am J Surg Pathol 14:1001, 1990

130. Scully RE, Young RH: Trophoblastic pseudotumor. A reappraisal. Am J Surg Pathol 5:75, 1981

131. Yeh I-T, Kurman RJ, O'Connor DM: Intermediate trophoblast: further immunocytochemical characterization. Mod Pathol 3:282, 1990

132. Heyderman E, Gibbons AR, Rosen SW: Immunoperoxidase localization of human placental lactogen: a marker for the placental origin of the giant cells in "syncytial

endometritis" of pregnancy. J Clin Pathol 34:303, 1981

133. Ewing J: Chorioma. Surg Gynecol Obstet 10:366, 1910

134. Collins RJ, Hgan HYS, Wong LC: Placental site trophoblastic tumor: with features between an exaggerated placental site reaction and a placental site trophoblastic tumor. Int J Gynecol Pathol 9:170, 1990

135. Carinelli SG, Vendolan, Zanotti F, Benzi G: Placental site nodules. A report of 17 cases. Pathol Res Pract 185:30, 1989

136. Marchand F: Uber die sogenannten "decualen" Geschwulste im Anschloss an normale Geburt, Abort Blasenmole und Extrauterin Schwangerschaft. Monatsschr Geburtshilfe Gynaekol 1:419, 53, 1895

137. Park WW: Possible functions of nonvillous trophoblast. Eur J Obstet Gynecol Reprod Biol 5:1, 35, 1975

138. Kurman RJ, Scully RE, Norris HJ: Trophoblastic pseudotumor of the uterus. An exaggerated form of "syncytial endometritis" simulating a malignant tumor. Cancer 38:1214, 1976

139. McLellan R, Buscema J, Currie JL, Woodruff JD: Placental site trophoblastic tumor in a postmenopausal woman. Am J Clin Pathol 95:670, 1991

140. Young RH, Scully RE: Placental-site trophoblastic tumor. Current status. Clin Obstet Gynecol 27:248, 1984

141. Finkler NJ, Berkowitz RS, Driscoll SG et al: Clinical experience with placental site trophoblastic tumors at the New England Trophoblastic Disease Center. Obstet Gynecol 71:854, 1988

142. Lathrop JC, Lauchlan S, Nayak R, Ambler M: Clinical characteristics of placental site trophoblastic tumor (PSTT). Gynecol Oncol 31:32, 1988

143. Eckstein RP, Paradinas FJ, Bagshawe KD: Placental site trophoblastic tumour (trophoblastic pseudotumour): a study of four cases requiring hysterectomy including one fatal case. Histopathology 6:211, 1982

144. Nagelberg SB, Rosen SW: Clinical and laboratory investigation of a virilized woman with placental-site trophoblastic tumor. Obstet Gynecol 65:527, 1985

145. Nagamani M, Kaspar HG, Van Dinh T et al: Hyperthecosis of the ovaries in a woman with a placental trophoblastic tumor. Obstet Gynecol 76:931, 1990

146. Brewer CA, Adelson MD, Elder RC: Erythrocytosis associated with a placental-site trophoblastic tumor. Obstet Gynecol 79:846, 1992

147. Dessau R, Rustin GJS, Dent RJ et al: Surgery and chemotherapy in the management of placental site tumor. Gynecol Oncol 39:56, 1990

148. Young RH, Scully RE, McCluskey RT: A distinctive glomerular lesion complicating placental site trophoblastic tumor. Report of two cases. Hum Pathol 16:35, 1985

149. Yamamoto Y, Otsuka H, Numoto S et al: Placental-site trophoblastic tumor of the uterus. Clinicopathological and immunohistochemical observations of a case. Acta Pathol Jpn 37:1979, 1987

150. Abdul-Hafeez M, Akhtar M, Baaqeel HS, Kidess EA: Placental site trophoblastic tumor: Report of a case with review of literature. Ann Saudi Med 7:340, 1987

151. Kurman RJ, Young RH, Main CA et al: Immunohistochemical localization of placental lactogen and chorionic gonadotropin in the normal placenta and trophoblastic tumors with emphasis on intermediate trophoblast and the placental-site trophoblastic tumor. Int J Gynecol Pathol 3:101, 1984

152. Blackwell JB, Papadimitriou JM: Trophoblastic pseudotumor of the uterus. Case report and ultrastructure. Cancer 43:1734, 1979

153. Gloor E, Hurlimann J: Trophoblastic pseudotumor of the uterus: clinicopathological report with immunohistochemical and ultrastructural studies. Am J Surg Pathol 5:5, 1981

154. Twiggs LB, Okagaki T, Phillips GL et al: Trophoblastic pseudotumor. Evidence of malignant disease potential. Gynecol Oncol 12:238, 1981

155. Berger G, Verbaere J, Feroldi J: Placental site trophoblastic tumor of the uterus: an ultrastructural and immunohistochemical study. Ultrastruct Pathol 6:319, 1984

156. Hopkins M, Nunez C, Murphy JR, Wentz WB: Malignant placental site trophoblastic tumor. Obstet Gynecol 66:95S, 1985

157. Duncan D, Mazur MT: Trophoblastic tumors. Ultrastructural comparison of choriocarcinoma and placental site tumor, abstracted. Lab Invest 56:20A, 1987

158. Genton CY, Bronz L, Möhr E, Spycher MA: Placental site trophoblastic tumor. Ein fallbericht mit immunohistochemischen and ultrastrukturellen untersuchungen. Pathologe 10:359, 1989

159. Kashimura M, Kashimura Y, Oikawa K et al: Placental site trophoblastic tumor: Immunohistochemical and nuclear DNA study. Gynecol Oncol 38:262, 1990

160. Alvero R, Remmenga S, O'Connor D et al: Metastatic placental site trophoblastic tumor. Gynecol Oncol 37:445, 1990

161. Larsen LG, Theilade K, Skibsted L, Jacobsen GK: Malignant placental site trophoblastic tumor. A case report and a review of the literature, Suppl. APMIS 23:138, 1991

162. Van Bogaert L-J, Staguet J-P: Chorionepitheliosis: a rare benign trophoblastic disease. Acta Obstet Gynecol Scand 56:69, 1977

163. Nickels J, Risberg B, Melander S: Trophoblastic pseudotumor of the uterus. A case report. Acta Pathol Microbiol Scand A 86:14, 1978

164. Rosenshein NB, Wijnen H, Woodruff JD: Clinical importance of the diagnosis of trophoblastic pseudotumors. Am J Obstet Gynecol 136:635, 1980

165. Wetzel WJ: Trophoblastic pseudotumor—an illustrative case. Diagn Gynecol Obstet 2:147, 1980

166. Beukes CA, Middlecote BD, Duyvene Dewit LJ, Lyell HL: Placental-site trophoblastic tumor (trophoblastic pseudotumor). S Afr Med J 66:540, 1984

167. Samlowski W, Abbott TM, Kepas DE, Eyre HJ: Placental-site trophoblastic tumor (trophoblastic pseudotumor)—case report demonstrating failure of chemotherapy, surgery and radiotherapy to control metastatic disease. Gynecol Oncol 21:111, 1985

168. Heintz APM, Schaberg A, Engelsman E, van Hall EV: Placental-site trophoblastic tumor: diagnosis, treatment, and biological behavior. Int J Gynecol Pathol 4:75, 1985

169. Eckstein RP, Russell P, Friedlander ML et al: Metastasizing placental site trophoblastic tumor: a case study. Hum Pathol 16:632, 1985

170. Gloor E, Dialdas J, Hurlimann J et al: Placental site trophoblastic tumor (trophoblastic pseudotumor) of the uterus with metastases and fatal outcome. Clinical and autopsy observations of a case. Am J Surg Pathol 7:483, 1983

171. Orrell JM, Sanders DSA: A particularly aggressive placental site trophoblastic tumour. Histopathology 18:559, 1991

Index

Page numbers followed by f *indicate figures; those followed by* t *indicate tables.*